I0056594

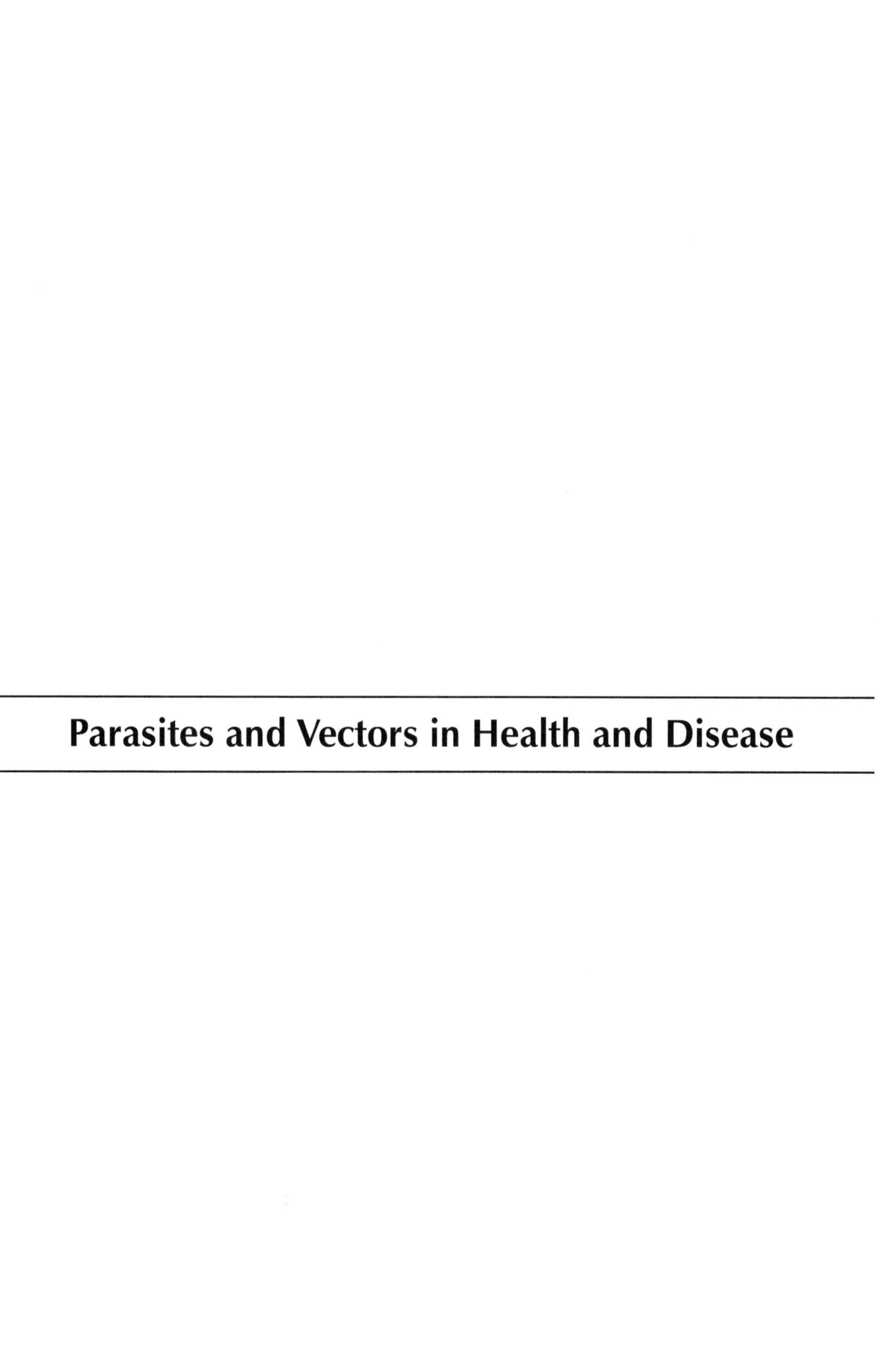

Parasites and Vectors in Health and Disease

Parasites and Vectors in Health and Disease

Editor: Madelyn Goodman

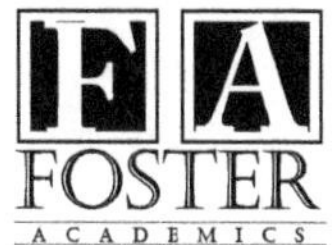

www.fosteracademics.com

www.fosteracademics.com

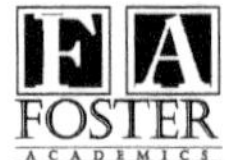

Cataloging-in-Publication Data

Parasites and vectors in health and disease / edited by Madelyn Goodman.
p. cm.
Includes bibliographical references and index.
ISBN 978-1-63242-855-4
1. Communicable diseases--Transmission. 2. Carrier state (Communicable diseases). 3. Parasites.
4. Vector-pathogen relationships. 5. Animals as carriers of disease. 6. Insects as carriers of disease.
I. Goodman, Madelyn.
RC112 .P37 2019
616.9--dc23

Foster Academics,
118-35 Queens Blvd., Suite 400,
Forest Hills, NY 11375, USA

ISBN 978-1-63242-855-4 (Hardback)

Contents

Preface

This book has been an outcome of determined endeavour from a group of educationists in the field. The primary objective was to involve a broad spectrum of professionals from diverse cultural background involved in the field for developing new researches. The book not only targets students but also scholars pursuing higher research for further enhancement of the theoretical and practical applications of the subject.

The agents that carry and transmit infectious pathogens to other living organisms are called vectors. Such agents are usually intermediate parasites or microbes. Parasite refers to the organism which either lives in or on some other organism, benefitting itself by causing harm to that organism. Some common parasites are hookworms, protozoans, mosquitoes, lice, honey fungus, broomrapes, mistletoe and dodder. As they interact with other species, they are well placed to act as vectors of pathogens, which cause diseases. Dengue fever, plague, Lyme disease and West Nile fever are some examples of vector-borne zoonotic diseases. This book is compiled in such a manner, that it will provide in-depth knowledge about the role of parasites and vectors in health and diseases. It presents researches and studies performed by experts across the globe. The book is appropriate for students seeking detailed information in this area as well as for experts.

It was an honour to edit such a profound book and also a challenging task to compile and examine all the relevant data for accuracy and originality. I wish to acknowledge the efforts of the contributors for submitting such brilliant and diverse chapters in the field and for endlessly working for the completion of the book. Last, but not the least; I thank my family for being a constant source of support in all my research endeavours.

Editor

1

Implications of insecticide resistance for malaria vector control with long-lasting insecticidal nets: trends in pyrethroid resistance during a WHO-coordinated multi-country prospective study

Implications of Insecticide Resistance Consortium

Abstract

Background: Increasing pyrethroid resistance has been an undesirable correlate of the rapid increase in coverage of insecticide-treated nets (ITNs) since 2000. Whilst monitoring of resistance levels has increased markedly over this period, longitudinal monitoring is still lacking, meaning the temporal and spatial dynamics of phenotypic resistance in the context of increasing ITN coverage are unclear.

Methods: As part of a large WHO-co-ordinated epidemiological study investigating the impact of resistance on malaria infection, longitudinal monitoring of phenotypic resistance to pyrethroids was undertaken in 290 clusters across Benin, Cameroon, India, Kenya and Sudan. Mortality in response to pyrethroids in the major anopheline vectors in each location was recorded during consecutive years using standard WHO test procedures. Trends in mosquito mortality were examined using generalised linear mixed-effect models.

Results: Insecticide resistance (using the WHO definition of mortality < 90%) was detected in clusters in all countries across the study period. The highest mosquito mortality (lowest resistance frequency) was consistently reported from India, in an area where ITNs had only recently been introduced. Substantial temporal and spatial variation was evident in mortality measures in all countries. Overall, a trend of decreasing mosquito mortality (increasing resistance frequency) was recorded (Odds Ratio per year: 0.79 per year (95% CI: 0.79–0.81, $P < 0.001$). There was also evidence that higher net usage was associated with lower mosquito mortality in some countries.

Discussion: Pyrethroid resistance increased over the study duration in four out of five countries. Insecticide-based vector control may be compromised as a result of ever higher resistance frequencies.

Keywords: Malaria, Vector control, Insecticide resistance, Trends, Bednets, Bioassay

Background

Vector control using indoor residual spraying (IRS) and insecticide-treated nets (ITNs) are core strategies for malaria control and elimination. The huge scale-up of these interventions in the last 20 years has been associated with major reductions in disease burden [1]. Between 2000 and 2015, it is estimated that over 1 billion ITNs were distributed in malaria endemic countries. The proportion of people in sub-Saharan Africa sleeping under a net increased from 30 to 54% between 2010 and 2016, whilst in 2016 an estimated 2.9% of the at-risk population was covered by IRS globally [1]. The increased coverage of vector control is estimated to have been a major contributor to the documented 62% decline in malaria mortality between 2000–2015 [2, 3]. However, between 2015 and 2016, data suggest that malaria mortality have remained the same in the WHO regions of Southeast Asia, the Western Pacific and Africa,

* Correspondence: Jackie.Cook@lshtm.ac.uk
MRC Tropical Epidemiology Group, Department of Infectious Disease Epidemiology, London School of Hygiene and Tropical Medicine, Keppel Street, London WC1E 7HT, UK

and possibly increased in the Eastern Mediterranean and the Americas [1]. There are therefore justified concerns about the emergence and spread of insecticide resistance and the impact this may have on the continued effectiveness of insecticide-based interventions [1, 4].

Resistance has now been detected in malaria vectors to the four classes of public health insecticides used in malaria vector control (pyrethroids, organochlorines, organophosphates and carbamates) [5], and up to October 2016 had been reported in 71 malaria-endemic countries [6]. Until recently, pyrethroids have been the only class used for long-lasting insecticidal nets (LLINs) and accounted for a large proportion of the insecticide used for IRS. This heavy reliance on a single insecticide class prompted the World Health Organization (WHO) to issue a Global Plan for Insecticide Resistance Management (GPIRM) [5] which was subsequently expanded as part of the Global Vector Control Response [7]. The aim of these initiatives is to sustain the advances made in the fight against vector-borne disease through rational use of vector control tools, including insecticide deployment to slow the development of resistance. Country-level implementation of recommended activities and monitoring has been poor due to a combination of limited availability and costs of insecticides with new modes of action; human, financial and infrastructural capacity shortfalls; and insufficient data to determine epidemiological impact of insecticide resistance [8]. To address this latter point the WHO, with funding from the Bill and Melinda Gates Foundation, initiated a multi-country prospective study to assess the impact of insecticide resistance on the effectiveness of LLINs and IRS. The main objectives of the study were: (i) to determine the impact of insecticide resistance in malaria vectors on the protective effectiveness of LLINs and IRS, and hence on malaria disease burden; and (ii) to assess trends in the insecticide resistance status and underlying mechanisms in the main malaria vector species from the study areas in response to different interventions.

The study was conducted in five countries, Benin, Cameroon, India, Kenya and Sudan, with data collection conducted from 2010–2016. Details of the overall study design are given in Kleinschmidt et al. [9]. Overall epidemiological outcomes, presented in Kleinschmidt et al. [10], showed that nets provided protection against malaria irrespective of resistance frequency, indicating that populations in malaria endemic areas should continue to use LLINs to reduce their risk of infection. A number of country-specific analyses from this and other studies corroborate this finding [11–15]. In addition, several studies have published country-specific entomological data relating to the second objective [16–18], with ranges of resistance to pyrethroids reported. In this paper, we describe temporal and spatial trends in insecticide resistance of the main malaria vector species from across the five study countries.

Methods

Study design

The overall study design is described in detail in Kleinschmidt et al. [9]. The five countries included in the study were selected to represent areas of varying transmission intensity where resistance had previously been detected in malaria vectors (Table 1). In 279 study clusters (villages or groups of villages) across 16 areas in the five countries pyrethroid susceptibility in malaria vectors, and malaria infection and disease in children were measured simultaneously over several years. We aimed to assess whether higher levels of resistance are associated with loss of effectiveness of LLINs, and to characterise temporal and spatial trends in insecticide resistance. The numbers of clusters chosen per country are shown in Table 1 and were based on sample size calculations determined by the epidemiological outcomes [9]. Clusters were defined as villages or groups of hamlets with no less than 500 houses and were at least 2 km apart to avoid spill over in outcomes between clusters.

Vector control

LLIN mass distributions were carried out routinely in each site to provide universal coverage for each household (one net per two persons). Nets were distributed in Benin in 2011 (Olyset Net®, Sumitomo Chemical, Tokyo, Japan; 1 g/m^2 permethrin) and 2014 (PermaNet® 2.0, Vestergaard, Lausanne, Switzerland; 55 mg/m^2 deltamethrin), in Cameroon in 2011 and 2015 (PermaNet® 2.0), in India in 2014 (PermaNet® 2.0), in Kenya in 2010 and 2013 (PermaNet® 2.0), and in Sudan in 2011 and 2014 (PermaNet® 2.0). Net usage, defined as the proportion of respondents reporting as having slept under an LLIN the previous night, was determined through cross-sectional surveys which took place at least once in each country during the study period [10]. Cross-sectional household surveys, which consisted of sampling children from random households occurred in 2012 (Kenya, Sudan), 2013 (Cameroon, Sudan), 2014 (Sudan), 2015 (Benin, India) and 2016 (India) [10]. We used net usage as a proxy for the level of local mosquito exposure to pyrethroids. In Sudan half of the clusters were randomised to receive two rounds of IRS with bendiocarb (Ficam®80% WP, Bayer, Leverkusen, Germany; 200 mg active ingredient/m^2). An exception was the Galabat region where clusters received IRS with deltamethrin (25 mg of a.i./m^2; Chema Industries, Alexandria, Egypt) before changing to bendiocarb in subsequent years [15].

Measuring resistance

Phenotypic susceptibility to the pyrethroid deltamethrin, in the main local vector(s), was measured annually in each cluster using WHO adult susceptibility tests and recorded as percent mortality [19]. In Benin, Cameroon, Kenya and Sudan larvae were collected from breeding

Table 1 Details of study sampling and sites including vector control coverage and insecticide resistance prevalence at baseline

	Study sampling sites				
	Benin	Cameroon	India	Kenya	Sudan
Malaria transmission intensity	High	High	Low	High	Low
Study locations	Districts of Ifangni, Sakété, Pobé and Kétou (Departement de Plateau)	Districts of Garoua, Pitoa and Mayo Oulo (North region)	Subdistrict of Keshkal (Kondagaon, Chhattisgarh)	Districts of Teso, Rachuonyo, Nyando and Bondo (western Kenya)	El Hoosh and Hag Abdalla (Gezira State); Galabat (Gedarif State; New Halfa (Kassala State)
Number of clusters sampled	32	38	80	61	79
Entomological sampling points (years)	2011–2015	2012–2015	2013–2016	2011–2015	2011–2014
Main malaria vectors	*Anopheles gambiae* (*s.s.*)[a], *Anopheles coluzzii*[a]	*An. arabiensis*[a], *An. gambiae* (*s.s.*)[a], *An. funestus*	*An. culicfacies*[a]	*An. gambiae* (*s.s.*)[a], *An. arabiensis*[a], *An. funestus*	*An. arabiensis*[a]
Vector control interventions	High coverage of ITNs (primarily PermaNet 2.0) in all clusters	High coverage of ITNs (PermaNet 2.0) in all clusters	High coverage of ITNs (PermaNet 2.0) in all clusters	High coverage of ITNs (PermaNet 2.0 and Olyset Net) in all clusters. Rachuonyo and Nyando received IRS with deltamethrin and lambda-cyhalothrin in 2012, but no IRS was carried out subsequently	High coverage of ITNs (PermaNet 2.0) in all study clusters. In each study area half of clusters randomly allocated to receive additional IRS with bendiocarb
Baseline insecticide resistance information (cluster-specific range)	Kdr frequency by cluster ranged from 44 to 93% (2011) WHO Bioassay mortality to deltamethrin ranged between 20–100% (2011)	Kdr frequency by cluster ranged from 9 to 65% (2011) WHO Bioassay mortality to deltamethrin ranged between 43–100% (2012)	WHO Bioassay mortality to deltamethrin ranged between 86–100%	WHO Bioassay mortality to deltamethrin ranged between 1–100% (2011)	Kdr frequency by cluster ranged from 8.3 to 70.8% (2010); WHO Bioassay mortality to deltamethrin in sentinel clusters ranged between 47–100% (2011)

[a]Mortality results presented for these species in the analyses

sites within each cluster annually and reared to adulthood in insectaries. In India, where larval sites were difficult to locate, resting females were caught [19]. Adult female mosquitoes [of unknown age (India); 2–5 days-old (all other countries)] were exposed for 60 minutes to deltamethrin using WHO impregnated papers at standard concentrations (0.05% deltamethrin). Mosquitoes were kept at temperatures between 23 and 27 °C, with humidity, where measured, between 75–85%. Mortality was measured 24 h post-exposure. In all tests, observed mortality in control mosquitoes was less than 5% therefore Abbott's correction was not applied.

Statistical analysis

Mosquito mortality data were analysed at the level of the individual mosquito, with post-exposure status (dead/alive after 24 h) modelled as the response variable in logistic regression. Explanatory variables of interest were year, years since last LLIN distribution, and cluster- and year-specific LLIN use as measured in cross-sectional household surveys. Susceptibility test data were excluded from the analysis if fewer than 40 mosquitoes were tested. A mortality estimate was calculated per cluster for each time point, with data for each country analysed separately and in an all-country model. Association between cluster mortality estimates was assessed between years using binomial generalised linear models. Separate generalised mixed-effect models were used to assess trends in mortality over time, effect of time since LLIN mass distribution and effect of bednet use, with the cluster specified as the random effect to account for within cluster correlation of responses. Year was modelled as a linear term to investigate trends over time. Where appropriate, a regional identifier was included as a fixed effect to allow for spatial differences in resistance within countries. Where data were available, insectary temperature and humidity during resistance testing were included in country-level models (Cameroon, India, Sudan).

Cluster-level net usage, as a categorical variable (low, < 40%; medium, 40–80%; and high, > 80%), was explored as an explanatory variable in the years where these data were available from concurrent cross-sectional surveys.

As bednet usage was only available for some years, a time variable was not included in these models. To investigate whether the impact of bednet distributions waned over time, models using time since bednet distribution (in years) as the key explanatory variable (as opposed to calendar time) were also examined.

Data from all 5 countries were combined to investigate whether there was evidence for an overall temporal trend in phenotypic resistance, with country added as a fixed effect. As the only data available from 2016 were from India, the all-country analysis was undertaken with and without India.

Results are presented in terms of changes in mortality of mosquitoes by year [Odds Ratios (OR) per year] or with increasing cluster-level category of net usage, with a reduction in mortality indicative of increasing resistance frequency.

Results

Estimates of mortality

More than 90,000 mosquitoes were tested in 911 separate tests across 5 countries and over 6 years. The median number of mosquitoes exposed per cluster per year was 100 [interquartile range (IQR) 84–104]. Median mortality across all tests was 81% (IQR: 63–94%). Insecticide resistance, classified according to the WHO criteria of < 90% mortality, was detected in all tested species, in all five countries and in 87% (n = 793) of tests performed. In only 7% of tests performed (n = 63, from 57 clusters) was 100% mortality observed. There were noticeable differences in the proportions of clusters defined as susceptible across countries. For example, in India, ≥ 98% mortality was observed in 28% (n = 66) of tests compared to only 1% of tests (n = 2) in Sudan. In Benin, Cameroon, Kenya and Sudan, > 50% mortality was recorded in at least 14% of tests recorded; no tests in India had less than 50% mortality.

Temporal and spatial variation

Cluster-specific mosquito mortality showed limited and inconsistent evidence of year-to-year correlation in all countries (Fig. 1). The strongest association was seen between data points from 2014 and 2015 (Kendall's tau coefficient: 0.42, P < 0.001), although this pattern differed by country, with no correlation seen between those years in Benin or India (Sudan ceased data collection in 2014) (Kendall's tau coefficient 0.07, P = 0.677, and 0.02, P = 0.886, respectively). The strongest correlation between years was seen in Cameroon, with Kendall's tau coefficient > 0.3 for all year pairs (P < 0.02), whilst for the other countries correlation was only present in some pairwise comparisons.

Trends in mortality over time

The trends in mortality over the study period differed by country (Table 2, Fig. 2). A decrease in mortality was detected in Benin, Cameroon, Kenya and Sudan. A slight increase in mortality was detected in India [aOR: 1.03 (95% CI: 0.98–1.1), P = 0.08]. The most substantial yearly decrease was detected in Sudan [aOR: 0.67 (95% CI: 0.64–0.70), P < 0.001]. With data from all countries combined, a 21% decrease per year in odds of mortality was detected [aOR 0.79 (95% CI: 0.79–0.81), P < 0.001]. This was not substantially altered with the exclusion of India [aOR 0.77 (95% CI: 0.76–0.79), P < 0.001].

Effect of bednet distributions and bednet use

Bednet distributions occurred in all sites during the study period. Associations between bednet usage and cluster specific mosquito mortality was investigated for each year that epidemiological cross-sectional data were available. Mean net use was above 65% in all countries, with Kenya reporting the highest value (94.2%). Benin, India and Kenya had no clusters with less than 40% net usage. Net usage appeared to have differential impact on mosquito mortality in each country with no association found in Benin and Kenya (P = 0.225 and P = 0.241, respectively); higher mortality found in areas with higher net usage in Cameroon (aOR 1.6 and 1.4 for net usage between 40–80% and above 80% respectively, compared to clusters with net use under 40%, P < 0.001) and strong negative associations found in India and Sudan (Table 3).

Time since bednet distribution was also investigated to establish whether changes associated with bednet distributions waned over time. Differential trends were evident with Benin, India and Sudan demonstrating an increase in odds of mortality (decreasing resistance frequency) for each year post-distribution (P < 0.001 for each) whereas mosquito mortality in Cameroon (aOR: 0.95, P = 0.016) and Kenya (aOR: 0.59; P < 0.001) decreased (increased resistance frequency) with each year post-LLIN distribution (Table 4).

Discussion

Insecticides have been a key component in the public health and agriculture toolbox for over a century, resulting in the inevitable emergence of resistance in mosquito vectors. This study brings together a very large collection of data from a range of transmission settings to investigate the trends in pyrethroid resistance. Whilst year to year variation was substantial, and poor inter-year correlation prevented cluster specific predictions of resistance, a decrease in mosquito mortality was detected in four out of the five countries over the 5-year period of the study suggesting that resistance to pyrethroids has been gradually increasing in these settings.

WHO encourages regular monitoring of resistance frequencies to all insecticides used in country. Consequently, the level of reporting has increased dramatically in recent years with over 30,000 data points now entered

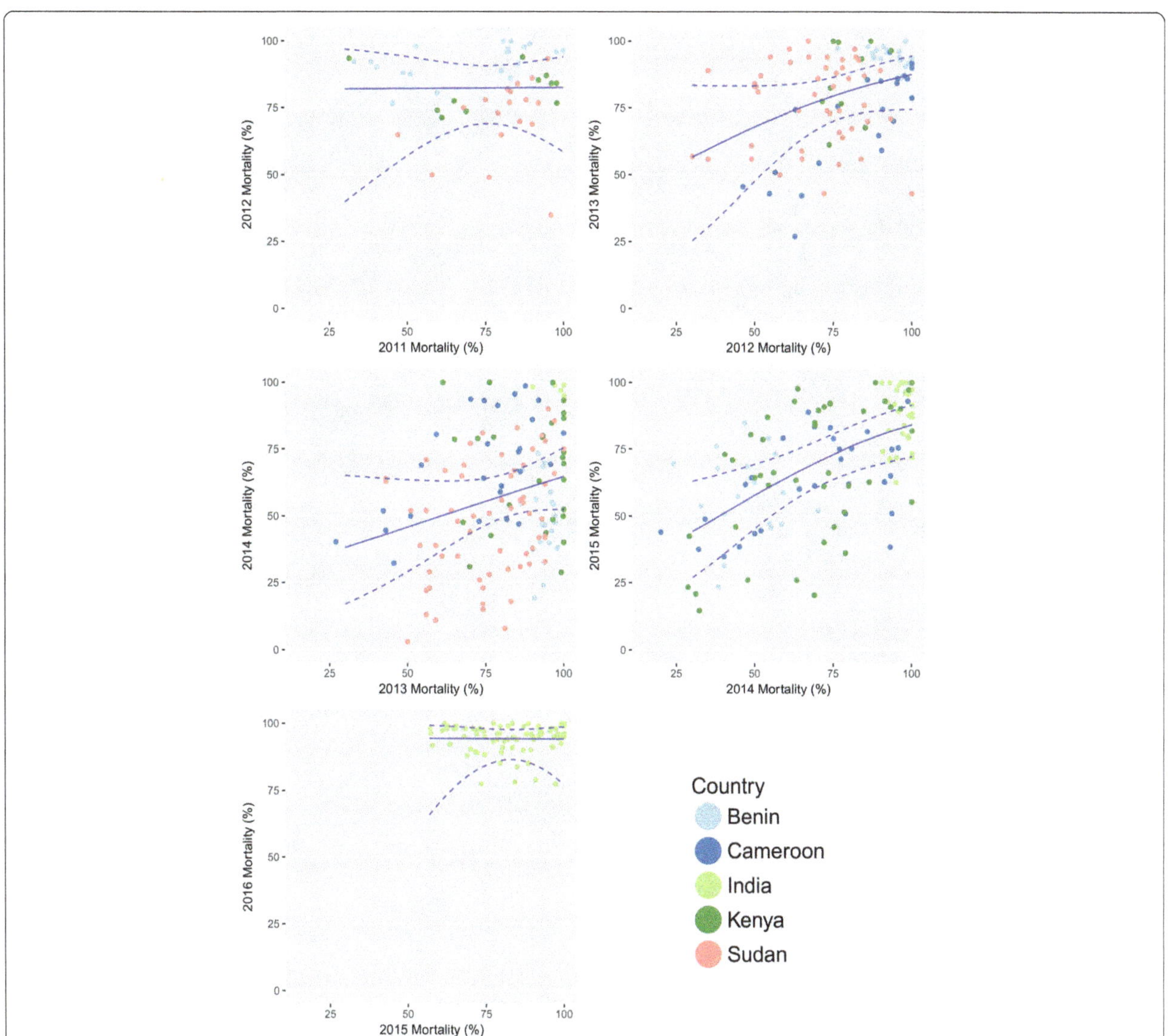

Fig. 1 Association in cluster mortality between years. Scatter diagrams show results for clusters with mortality estimates in consecutive years for each year of the study. The predicted mortality result from binomial generalised linear models is overlaid on each graph with 95% confidence intervals

Table 2 Impact of time on mosquito mortality. Results from generalised linear mixed-effect models examining the impact on mosquito mortality over time (year)

Country	Odds ratio for change in mortality per year (95% CI)	*P*-value
All five countries combined[a]	0.79 (0.79–0.81)	<0.001
Four countries combined (without India)[a]	0.77 (0.76–0.79)	<0.001
Benin[b]	0.74 (0.72–0.76)	<0.001
Cameroon[c]	0.74 (0.69–0.78)	<0.001
India[c]	1.03 (0.98–1.10)	0.08
Kenya[b]	0.88 (0.86–0.90)	<0.001
Sudan[c]	0.67 (0.64–0.70)	<0.001

[a]Adjusted for country
[b]Adjusted for district
[c]Adjusted for district, temperature and humidity
Results are presented in terms of change in odds of mortality of mosquitoes in WHO bioassays by year. Odds ratios are adjusted for locality and temperature and humidity where indicated. The data are shown for each country, as well as all countries combined (with country included as a covariate). Cluster was included as a random effect in all models

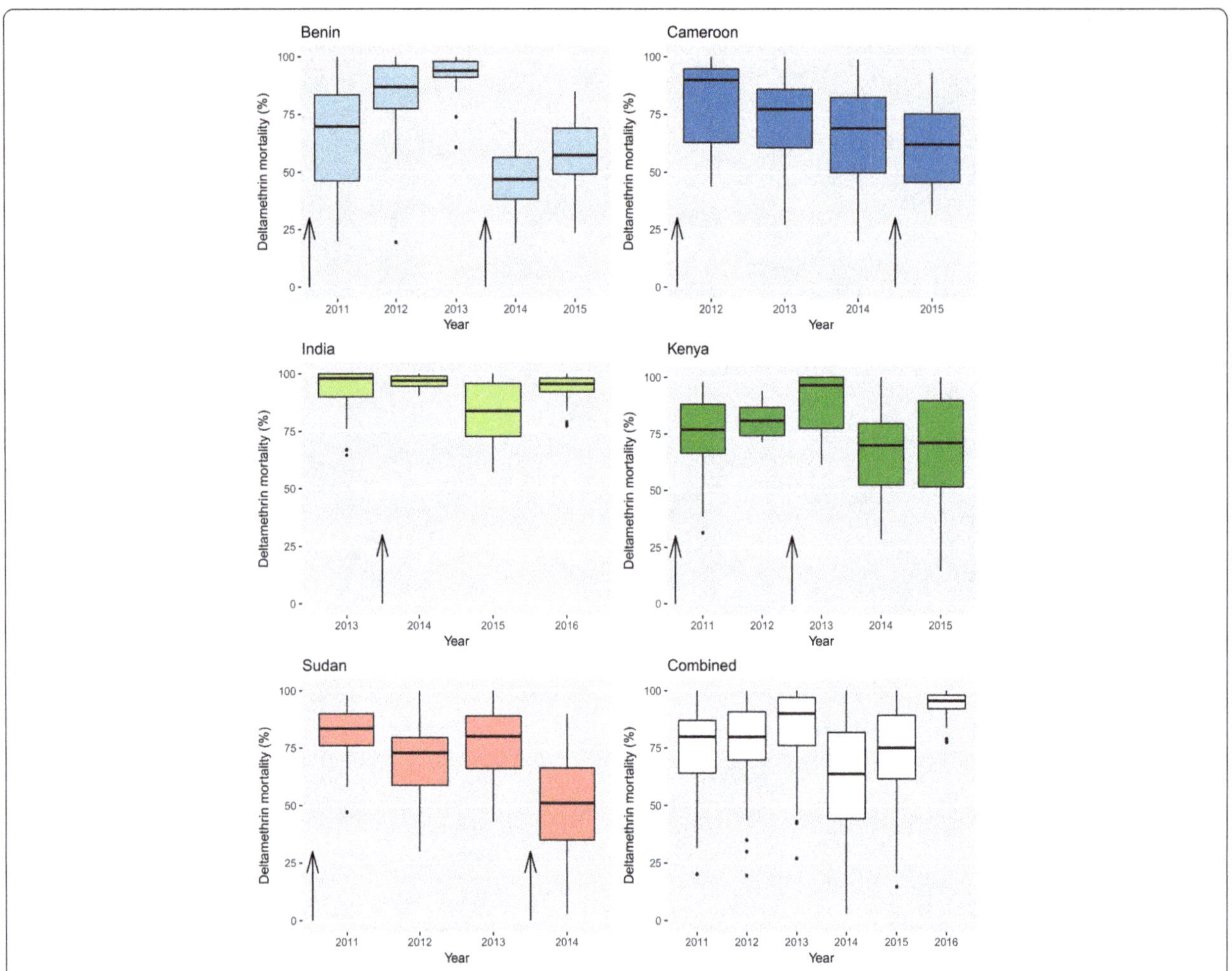

Fig. 2 Box-and-whisker plots showing the range of cluster-level mortality by year and country. Arrows indicate the timing of bednet distributions within country

Table 3 Impact of cluster-level bednet usage on mosquito mortality. Results from generalised mixed-effect models examining the impact of cluster-level bednet usage on mosquito mortality

		All countries combined[a]	Benin[b]	Cameroon[c]	India[c]	Kenya[b]	Sudan[c]
	No. of clusters included (year)	59 (2012); 87 (2013); 143 (2014); 99 (2015); 80 (2016)	19 (2015)	22 (2013); 26 (2014)	80 (2015); 80 (2016)	13(2012); 41 (2014)	46 (2012); 65 (2013); 76 (2014)
	Mean net usage (range) (%)		74.9 (52.5–100)	67.8 (7.0–100)	89.9 (60.9–100)	94.2 (73.7–100)	78.6 (0–100)
Effect of cluster-level net usage on mosquito mortality, OR (95% CI)	< 40%	1 (reference)	–	1 (reference)	–	–	1 (reference)
	40–80%	1.03 (0.89–1.19)	1 (reference)	1.61 (1.21–2.14)	1 (reference)	1 (reference)	0.69 (0.58–0.83)
	> 80%	0.65 (0.57–0.74)	1.59 (0.75–3.37)	1.40 (1.08–1.82)	0.36 (0.29–0.44)	2.38 (0.56–10.1)	0.45 (0.38–0.53)
	P-value	<0.001	0.225	<0.001	<0.001	0.241	<0.001

[a]Adjusted for country
[a]Adjusted for district
[c]Adjusted for district, temperature and humidity
Results are presented in terms of change in mortality of mosquitoes for increasing bednet usage category (< 40%; between 40–80%; and above 80%). Bednet usage was calculated for years where cross-sectional survey data was available. Odds ratios are adjusted for locality and temperature and humidity where indicated. The results are shown for each country, as well as all countries combined (with country included as a covariate). Cluster was included as a random effect in all models

Table 4 Impact of time since bednet distribution (years) on mosquito mortality. Results from generalised mixed-effect models examining the impact time since bednet distribution on mosquito mortality

Country	Odds ratio for change in mortality per year (95% CI)	*P*-value
All countries combined[a]	1.34 (1.31–1.37)	<0.001
Benin[b]	3.20 (3.02–3.39)	<0.001
Cameroon[c]	0.95 (0.90–0.99)	0.016
India[c]	1.62 (1.52–1.73)	<0.001
Kenya[b]	0.59 (0.56–0.62)	<0.001
Sudan[c]	1.60 (1.53–1.67)	<0.001

[a]Adjusted for country
[b]Adjusted for district
[c]Adjusted for district, temperature and humidity
Results are presented in terms of change in mortality of mosquitoes for each year since a mass bednet distribution took place in-country. Odds ratios are adjusted for locality and temperature and humidity where indicated. The results are shown for each country, as well as all countries combined (with country included as a covariate). Cluster was included as a random effect in all models

into global databases such as the WHO Malaria Threats Map [20] and IR-mapper (www.irmapper.com) [21]. The picture that emerges from these summary data [6, 22, 23], as with the present study, is that resistance to pyrethroids is increasing in frequency and geographic extent. However, these global databases often aggregate data with substantially differential sampling effort across years and regions [6] which may obscure the substantial stochasticity in mortality estimates.

It is assumed that the increase in resistance to pyrethroids over the past decade is due in part to the higher coverage of insecticide-based interventions, such as LLINs. However, studies have shown conflicting results with some reports of increasing resistance following bednet distributions [24–27], and other reports of no increases despite sustained insecticidal campaigns [28–30]. Although ascertaining the effect of bednet coverage was not a primary goal of this study, it was possible to investigate the impact of net use through cross-sectional surveys that were conducted concurrently to resistance measurements. Trends were not uniform across countries, perhaps in part reflecting the differing biology of the vector species. *Anopheles arabiensis* (a major vector in Kenya, Cameroon and Sudan study locations) and *An. culicifacies* (primary vector in India study locations) commonly show high rates of zoophily. Obtaining blood meals from sources other than humans means LLINs would potentially have less impact on selective pressure for resistance. However, overall, higher net usage was associated with increasing resistance in mosquitoes. This trend was most evident in Sudan where the widest range of net usage was reported whereas in other settings reported net usage was more uniform, thereby reducing the likelihood of detecting a trend.

We did not discern a consistent trend in mosquito mortality with increasing time post-net distribution. In Benin, India and Sudan, mortality increased every year post-distribution, suggesting that the initial increased coverage of nets may have been a short-term driver for resistance and that as the insecticide on the nets reduced over time, the selection pressure reduced, in turn reducing the proportion of resistant mosquitoes. However, in Cameroon and Kenya, the opposite effect was observed, with mortality decreasing with every year from the date of the distribution. Data from the *An. gambiae* 1000 genome project has revealed that there appear to be numerous instances of localised adaptation to insecticide pressure [31]. The difference we observed in response to LLIN distribution may reflect in part this innate difference of vector populations to respond to insecticide pressure and caution against making generalised predictions.

Moreover, whilst bednet distributions will have increased selection pressure in the study settings, it is also possible that the insecticide resistance could be linked to ongoing agricultural practices [32–34]. In several African countries, including northern Cameroon, the use of pyrethroids for cotton farming has been implicated as a catalyst for the increase in recorded resistance in *An. gambiae* populations [34–36]. Differences in the use of pyrethroids for agricultural purposes in the study settings could further impact the relationship between time of net distribution and insecticide resistance.

Previous studies have also shown resistance to be highly focal [16, 37–39], with large variations over small geographical distances. This is exemplified by the range of mortality measures within each country and highlights the need for multiple sentinel monitoring sites per country and reinforces that extrapolating resistance data from few, widely-dispersed sentinel sites to larger areas is untenable. Spatial heterogeneity in insecticide resistance poses challenges for integrated resistance management and suggests that locally tailored vector control and resistance management programmes are required.

There was considerable temporal heterogeneity with high between year variation at cluster level. This phenomenon has also been reported elsewhere [40–43]. There are several reasons why levels of resistance in a mosquito population may fluctuate over time, for instance, resistance can recede if proper resistance management practices are implemented or if resistance drivers reduce and resistance associated genetic variants are deleterious in the absence of selection pressure [5, 44]. It is possible that in our study settings varying exposure to pyrethroids resulted in fluctuating frequency of resistance in the mosquito population with evidence from some areas suggesting that bednet usage resulted in higher resistance frequencies.

As well as genuine fluctuations in the frequency of resistance, it is possible that the different susceptibility recorded is, in part, an artefact of the method of testing. Longitudinal monitoring is easily influenced by any changes in protocol for measuring mortality and the timings of the tests. Some studies have demonstrated fluctuations in mosquito mortality over a transmission season [45] and whilst all efforts were taken to ensure that tests occurred at the same time each year, differences between seasons may have had an impact. In addition, humidity and temperature are known to have an impact on mortality testing [46]; whilst these were controlled for where data were available, it is possible that differing conditions influenced mortality results.

There is mounting evidence that tests recording mosquito mortality after 24 h may not be the best way to record changes in population resistance, particularly when the level of resistance is high [47]. A number of alternative options are now available for monitoring the presence of resistance, including molecular assays, time/dose response assays and increasing the time post-exposure at which mortality is calculated, all of which are likely to be more sensitive to resistance trends [48–51], but these methods are also more resource intensive. Although as noted by Churcher et al. [4] the strong association between bioassay data and mortality measured in experimental hut trials still supports the use of bioassays as a quantitative test of the impact of resistance on LLIN efficacy. In this multi-country study, to ensure comparability between sites, the test was performed using one insecticide dose and one exposure time, using wild-caught mosquitoes reared in the laboratory. These settings may not reflect adequately the conditions wild mosquitoes experience, such as variations in temperature, food availability and pre-existing pesticide exposure [51]. In addition, the doses used in the resistance tests are not necessarily reflective of the doses mosquitoes would experience in the wild, which can be influenced by age or retreatment of ITN or regularity and coverage of IRS. The dose used for detecting resistance can have a particularly strong effect depending on the prevalence and penetrance of the resistant mechanisms present in the mosquito population. Recording mortality at 24 h may also miss some of the nuances involved with the evolution of resistance which may result in delayed mortality [51]. In addition, mosquito age has been shown to have a big impact on susceptibility, with older mosquitoes showing higher mortality rates compared to their younger counterparts [52]. If insecticides remain effective against mosquitoes old enough to transmit malaria, this may explain why some studies are observing minimal impact on epidemiological outcomes [10–12, 14].

Conclusions

This study demonstrated increasing frequency of resistance to pyrethroids in malaria vectors from 4 out of 5 study countries. Although the increase does not appear linear, if the current trend continues, it is likely to result in a reduction of the effectiveness of pyrethroid-based interventions such as ITN and IRS. There was evidence in some countries of increased selection pressure for pyrethroid resistance in clusters where net use was higher. There are a number of strategies presented within GPIRM to mitigate the increase of insecticide resistance in malaria vectors such as rotations, combinations, mosaics and mixtures [5]. In the short term, two trials have demonstrated improved efficacy of dual-active [53] and pyrethroid-PBO treated LLINs [54], suggesting that we are likely to be able to prolong the useful active life of pyrethroid-based interventions. However, the lack of vector control tools with different modes of actions and their increased costs, means that many endemic countries will continue to struggle to develop and implement insecticide resistance management plans. Whilst new products are currently being trialled [55–57], and some have recently come to market, the fine-scale monitoring of resistance phenotypes and mechanisms will be key to mitigating the impacts of insecticide resistance through informed selection of vector control tools.

Acknowledgements

The Implications of Insecticide Resistance Consortium is a multi-country collaboration. Study country Principal Investigators are denoted by an asterisk.
Writing and analysis team: Jackie Cook[1], Sean Tomlinson[2], *Immo Kleinschmidt[1,3] and *Martin James Donnelly[2].
Benin country team: *Martin Akogbeto[4], Alioun Adechoubou[5], Achile Massougbodji[6], Mariam Okê-Sopoh[5], Vincent Corbel[7], Sylvie Cornelie[7]and Aurore Ogouyemi-Hounto[6].
Cameroon study team: *Josiane Etang[8,9,10], Herman Parfait Awono-Ambene[8], Jude Bigoga[11], Stanislas Elysée Mandeng[8,12], Boris Njeambosay[11], Raymond Tabue[11], Celestin Kouambeng[13] and Etienne Fondjo[13].
India study team: *Kamaraju Raghavendra[14], Rajendra M Bhatt[14], Mehul Kumar Chourasia[14], Dipak K. Swain[14], Sreehari Uragayala14 and Neena Valecha[14].
Kenya study team: *Charles Mbogo[15], Nabie Bayoh[16], Teresa Kinyari[17], Kiambo Njagi[18], Lawrence Muthami[19], Luna Kamau[20], Evan Mathenge[21] and Eric Ochomo[16].
Sudan study team: *Hmooda Toto Kafy[22, 23], Bashir Adam Ismail[24], Elfatih M Malik[25], Khalid Elmardi[22], Jihad Eltaher Sulieman[26] and Mujahid Abdin[22].
Study support: Krishanthi Subramaniam[2], Brent Thomas[2], Philippa West[1] and John Bradley[1].
WHO co-ordination team: Tessa Bellamy Knox[27], Abraham Peter Mnzava[27], Jonathan Lines[28], Michael Macdonald[27]and Zinga José Nkuni[27]
[1]MRC Tropical Epidemiology Group, Department of Infectious Disease Epidemiology, London School of Hygiene and Tropical Medicine, Keppel Street, London, WC1E 7HT, UK. [2]Department of Vector Biology, Liverpool School of Tropical Medicine, Pembroke Place, Liverpool, L3 5QA, UK. [3]School of Public Health, University of the Witwatersrand, Johannesburg, South Africa. [4]Centre de Recherche Entomologique de Cotonou. Cotonou, Benin. [5]Programme National de Lutte conte le Paludisme (PNLP), Ministère de la Santé, Benin. [6]Faculté des Sciences de la Santé, Université d'Abomey Calavi, Cotonou, Benin. [7]Maladies Infectieuses et Vecteurs, Ecologie, Génétique, Evolution et Contrôle (MIVEGEC), Institut de Recherche pour le Développement (IRD), CNRS, University of Montpellier, Montpellier, France. [8]Organisation de Coordination pour la lutte contre les Endemies en Afrique

Centrale (OCEAC), Yaounde, Cameroon. [9]Faculty of Medicine and Pharmaceutical Sciences, University of Douala, PO Box 2701, Douala, Cameroon. [10] Institute for Insect Biotechnology, Justus Liebig University Gießen, Winchesterstr. 2, 35394 Gießen, Germany. [11]National Reference Unit (NRU) for Vector Control, The Biotechnology Center, University of Yaounde I, PO Box 3851, Messa, Yaounde, Cameroon. [12]Laboratory of General Biology, University of Yaounde I, P.O. Box 812, Yaounde, Cameroon. [13]National Malaria Control Program, Ministry of Public Health, PO, Box 14386, Yaounde, Cameroon. [14]National Institute of Malaria Research, Department of Health Research, (GoI), Sector 8, Dwarka, New Delhi 110 077, India. [15]KEMRI Centre for Geographic Medicine Research Coast, PO Box 230 – 80108, Kilifi, Kenya. [16]KEMRI/CDC Research and Public Health Collaboration, PO Box 1578, Kisumu 40100, Kenya. [17]University of Nairobi, School of Medicine, College of Health Sciences, Department of Medical Physiology, Nairobi, Kenya. [18]Ministry of Health, Malaria Control Unit, PO Box 1992–00202, Nairobi, Kenya. [19]KEMRI Centre for Public Health Research, Nairobi, Kenya. [20]KEMRI - Centre for Biotechnology and Research Development, Nairobi, Kenya. [21]KEMRI - Eastern and Southern Africa Centre of International Parasite Control, Nairobi, Kenya. [22]Integrated Vector Management Department, Federal Ministry of Health, PO Box 303, Khartoum, Sudan. [23]School of Biological Sciences, Universiti Sains Malaysia, 11800 USM Pulau Penang, Malaysia. [24]Khartoum Malaria Free Initiative, Khartoum, Sudan. [25]Faculty of Medicine, University of Khartoum, Khartoum, Sudan. [26]Sennar Malaria Research and Training Centre, Sennar, Sudan. [27]Global Malaria Programme, World Health Organization, Avenue Appia 20, 1211 Geneva, Switzerland. [28]Department of Disease Control, London School of Hygiene and Tropical Medicine, Keppel Street, London, WC1E 7HT, UK.

Funding
This study was funded by Bill & Melinda Gates Foundation, UK Medical Research Council, and UK Department for International Development.

Authors' contributions
All authors contributed substantially either to the study design, fieldwork and data collection, analyses or drafting the manuscript. All authors read and approved the final manuscript.

Competing interests
The authors declare that they have no competing interests.

References

1. WHO. World Malaria Report 2017. Geneva: World Health Organisation; 2017.
2. WHO. World Malaria Report 2016. Geneva: World Health Organisation; 2016.
3. Bhatt S, Weiss DJ, Cameron E, Bisanzio D, Mappin B, Dalrymple U, et al. The effect of malaria control on *Plasmodium falciparum* in Africa between 2000 and 2015. Nature. 2015;526:207–11.
4. Churcher TS, Lissenden N, Griffin JT, Worrall E, Ranson H. The impact of pyrethroid resistance on the efficacy and effectiveness of bednets for malaria control in Africa. Elife. 2016;5.
5. WHO. Global plan for insecticide resistance management in malaria vectors. Geneva: World Health Organisation; 2012.
6. Coleman M, Hemingway J, Gleave KA, Wiebe A, Gething PW, Moyes CL. Developing global maps of insecticide resistance risk to improve vector control. Malar J. 2017;16:86.
7. WHO. Global Vector Control Response: 2017–2030. Geneva: World Health Organization; 2017.
8. Mnzava AP, Knox TB, Temu EA, Trett A, Fornadel C, Hemingway J, et al. Implementation of the global plan for insecticide resistance management in malaria vectors: progress, challenges and the way forward. Malar J. 2015;14:173.
9. Kleinschmidt I, Mnzava AP, Kafy HT, Mbogo C, Bashir AI, Bigoga J, et al. Design of a study to determine the impact of insecticide resistance on malaria vector control: a multi-country investigation. Malar J. 2015;14:282.
10. Kleinschmidt I, Bradley J, Knox TB, Mnzava AP, Kafy HT, Mbogo C, et al. Implications of insecticide resistance for malaria vector control with long-lasting insecticidal nets: a WHO-coordinated, prospective, international, observational cohort study. Lancet Infect Dis. 2018;18:640–9.
11. Ochomo E, Chahilu M, Cook J, Kinyari T, Bayoh NM, West P, et al. Insecticide-treated nets and protection against insecticide-resistant malaria vectors in western Kenya. Emerg Infect Dis. 2017;23:758–64.
12. Bradley J, Ogouyemi-Hounto A, Cornelie S, Fassinou J, de Tove YSS, Adeothy AA, et al. Insecticide-treated nets provide protection against malaria to children in an area of insecticide resistance in southern Benin. Malar J. 2017;16:225.
13. Chourasia MK, Kamaraju R, Kleinschmidt I, Bhatt RM, Swain DK, Knox TB, et al. Impact of long-lasting insecticidal nets on prevalence of subclinical malaria among children in the presence of pyrethroid resistance in *Anopheles culicifacies* in central India. Int J Infect Dis. 2017;57:123–9.
14. Lindblade KA, Mwandama D, Mzilahowa T, Steinhardt L, Gimnig J, Shah M, et al. A cohort study of the effectiveness of insecticide-treated bed nets to prevent malaria in an area of moderate pyrethroid resistance, Malawi. Malar J. 2015;14:31.
15. Kafy HT, Ismail BA, Mnzava AP, Lines J, Abdin MSE, Eltaher JS, et al. Impact of insecticide resistance in *Anopheles arabiensis* on malaria incidence and prevalence in Sudan and the costs of mitigation. Proc Natl Acad Sci USA. 2017;114:E11267–75.
16. Ochomo E, Bayoh NM, Kamau L, Atieli F, Vulule J, Ouma C, et al. Pyrethroid susceptibility of malaria vectors in four districts of western Kenya. Parasit Vectors. 2014;7:310.
17. Tabue RN, Awono-Ambene P, Etang J, Atangana J, AN C, Toto JC, et al. Role of *Anopheles* (*Cellia*) *rufipes* (Gough, 1910) and other local anophelines in human malaria transmission in the northern savannah of Cameroon: a cross-sectional survey. Parasit Vectors. 2017;10:22.
18. Ismail BA, Kafy HT, Sulieman JE, Subramaniam K, Thomas B, Mnzava A, et al. Temporal and spatial trends in insecticide resistance in *Anopheles arabiensis* in Sudan: outcomes from an evaluation of implications of insecticide resistance for malaria vector control. Parasit Vectors. 2018;11:122.
19. WHO. Global Malaria Programme. Test procedures for insecticide resistance monitoring in malaria vector mosquitoes. 2nd ed. Geneva: World Health Organization; 2016.
20. Malaria Threats Map: World Health Organisation. www.who.int/malaria/maps/threats/. Accessed 1 Feb 2018
21. Knox TB, Juma EO, Ochomo EO, Pates Jamet H, Ndungo L, Chege P, et al. An online tool for mapping insecticide resistance in major *Anopheles* vectors of human malaria parasites and review of resistance status for the Afrotropical region. Parasit Vectors. 2014;7:76.
22. Ranson H, Lissenden N. Insecticide resistance in African *Anopheles* mosquitoes: a worsening situation that needs urgent action to maintain malaria control. Trends Parasitol. 2016;32:187–96.
23. Dialynas E, Topalis P, Vontas J, Louis C. MIRO and IRbase: IT tools for the epidemiological monitoring of insecticide resistance in mosquito disease vectors. PLoS Negl Trop Dis. 2009;3:e465.
24. Stump AD, Atieli FK, Vulule JM, Besansky NJ. Dynamics of the pyrethroid knockdown resistance allele in western Kenyan populations of *Anopheles gambiae* in response to insecticide-treated bed net trials. Am J Trop Med Hyg. 2004;70:591–6.
25. Reimer LJ, Tripet F, Slotman M, Spielman A, Fondjo E, Lanzaro GC. An unusual distribution of the kdr gene among populations of *Anopheles gambiae* on the island of Bioko, Equatorial Guinea. Insect Mol Biol. 2005;14:683–8.
26. Czeher C, Labbo R, Arzika I, Duchemin JB. Evidence of increasing Leu-Phe knockdown resistance mutation in *Anopheles gambiae* from Niger following a nationwide long-lasting insecticide-treated nets implementation. Malar J. 2008;7:189.
27. Protopopoff N, Verhaeghen K, Van Bortel W, Roelants P, Marcotty T, Baza D, et al. A significant increase in kdr in *Anopheles gambiae* is associated with an intensive vector control intervention in Burundi highlands. Tropical Med Int Health. 2008;13:1479–87.
28. Kulkarni MA, Malima R, Mosha FW, Msangi S, Mrema E, Kabula B, et al. Efficacy of pyrethroid-treated nets against malaria vectors and nuisance-biting mosquitoes in Tanzania in areas with long-term insecticide-treated net use. Tropical Med Int Health. 2007;12:1061–73.
29. Vulule JM, Beach RF, Atieli FK, Mount DL, Roberts JM, Mwangi RW. Long-term use of permethrin-impregnated nets does not increase *Anopheles gambiae* permethrin tolerance. Med Vet Entomol. 1996;10:71–9.
30. Koimbu G, Czeher C, Katusele M, Sakur M, Kilepak L, Tandrapah A, et al. Status of insecticide resistance in Papua New Guinea: an update from

nation-wide monitoring of *Anopheles* mosquitoes. Am J Trop Med Hyg. 2018;98:162–5.

31. *Anopheles gambiae* 1000 Genomes Consortium. Genetic diversity of the African malaria vector *Anopheles gambiae*. Nature 2017;552:96–100.
32. Hemingway J, Jayawardena KG, Herath PR. Pesticide resistance mechanisms produced by field selection pressures on *Anopheles nigerrimus* and *A. culicifacies* in Sri Lanka. Bull World Health Organ. 1986;64:753–8.
33. Abuelmaali SA, Elaagip AH, Basheer MA, Frah EA, Ahmed FT, Elhaj HF, et al. Impacts of agricultural practices on insecticide resistance in the malaria vector *Anopheles arabiensis* in Khartoum State, Sudan. PLoS One. 2013;8: e80549.
34. Chouaibou M, Etang J, Brevault T, Nwane P, Hinzoumbe CK, Mimpfoundi R, et al. Dynamics of insecticide resistance in the malaria vector *Anopheles gambiae* (*s.l.*) from an area of extensive cotton cultivation in northern Cameroon. Trop Med Int Health. 2008;13:476–86.
35. Diabate A, Baldet T, Chandre F, Akoobeto M, Guiguemde TR, Darriet F, et al. The role of agricultural use of insecticides in resistance to pyrethroids in *Anopheles gambiae* (*s.l.*) in Burkina Faso. Am J Trop Med Hyg. 2002;67:617–22.
36. N'Guessan R, Corbel V, Akogbeto M, Rowland M. Reduced efficacy of insecticide-treated nets and indoor residual spraying for malaria control in pyrethroid resistance area, Benin. Emerg Infect Dis. 2007;13:199–206.
37. Kabula B, Tungu P, Matowo J, Kitau J, Mweya C, Emidi B, et al. Susceptibility status of malaria vectors to insecticides commonly used for malaria control in Tanzania. Trop Med Int Health. 2012;17:742–50.
38. Cisse MB, Keita C, Dicko A, Dengela D, Coleman J, Lucas B, et al. Characterizing the insecticide resistance of *Anopheles gambiae* in Mali. Malar J. 2015;14:327.
39. Matowo NS, Munhenga G, Tanner M, Coetzee M, Feringa WF, Ngowo HS, et al. Fine-scale spatial and temporal heterogeneities in insecticide resistance profiles of the malaria vector, *Anopheles arabiensis* in rural south-eastern Tanzania. Wellcome Open Res. 2017;2:96.
40. Foster GM, Coleman M, Thomsen E, Ranson H, Yangalbe-Kalnone E, Moundai T, et al. Spatial and temporal trends in insecticide resistance among malaria vectors in Chad highlight the importance of continual monitoring. PLoS One. 2016;11:e0155746.
41. Badolo A, Traore A, Jones CM, Sanou A, Flood L, Guelbeogo WM, et al. Three years of insecticide resistance monitoring in *Anopheles gambiae* in Burkina Faso: resistance on the rise? Malar J. 2012;11:232.
42. Djegbe I, Boussari O, Sidick A, Martin T, Ranson H, Chandre F, et al. Dynamics of insecticide resistance in malaria vectors in Benin: first evidence of the presence of L1014S kdr mutation in *Anopheles gambiae* from West Africa. Malar J. 2011;10:261.
43. Yahouedo GA, Cornelie S, Djegbe I, Ahlonsou J, Aboubakar S, Soares C, et al. Dynamics of pyrethroid resistance in malaria vectors in southern Benin following a large scale implementation of vector control interventions. Parasit Vectors. 2016;9:385.
44. Raghavendra K, Verma V, Srivastava HC, Gunasekaran K, Sreehari U, Dash AP. Persistence of DDT, malathion & deltamethrin resistance in *Anopheles culicifacies* after their sequential withdrawal from indoor residual spraying in Surat district, India. Indian J Med Res. 2010;132:260–4.
45. Mbepera S, Nkwengulila G, Peter R, Mausa EA, Mahande AM, Coetzee M, et al. The influence of age on insecticide susceptibility of *Anopheles arabiensis* during dry and rainy seasons in rice irrigation schemes of northern Tanzania. Malar J. 2017;16:364.
46. Glunt KD, Paaijmans KP, Read AF, Thomas MB. Environmental temperatures significantly change the impact of insecticides measured using WHOPES protocols. Malar J. 2014;13:350.
47. Bagi J, Grisales N, Corkill R, Morgan JC, N'Fale S, Brogdon WG, et al. When a discriminating dose assay is not enough: measuring the intensity of insecticide resistance in malaria vectors. Malar J. 2015;14:210.
48. Muller P, Chouaibou M, Pignatelli P, Etang J, Walker ED, Donnelly MJ, et al. Pyrethroid tolerance is associated with elevated expression of antioxidants and agricultural practice in *Anopheles arabiensis* sampled from an area of cotton fields in northern Cameroon. Mol Ecol. 2008;17:1145–55.
49. Mawejje HD, Wilding CS, Rippon EJ, Hughes A, Weetman D, Donnelly MJ. Insecticide resistance monitoring of field-collected *Anopheles gambiae* (*s.l.*) populations from Jinja, eastern Uganda, identifies high levels of pyrethroid resistance. Med Vet Entomol. 2013;27:276–83.
50. Toe KH, Jones CM, N'Fale S, Ismail HM, Dabire RK, Ranson H. Increased pyrethroid resistance in malaria vectors and decreased bed net effectiveness, Burkina Faso. Emerg Infect Dis. 2014;20:1691–6.
51. Viana M, Hughes A, Matthiopoulos J, Ranson H, Ferguson HM. Delayed mortality effects cut the malaria transmission potential of insecticide-resistant mosquitoes. Proc Natl Acad Sci USA. 2016;113:8975–80.
52. Jones CM, Sanou A, Guelbeogo WM, Sagnon N, Johnson PC, Ranson H. Aging partially restores the efficacy of malaria vector control in insecticide-resistant populations of *Anopheles gambiae s.l.* from Burkina Faso. Malar J. 2012;11:24.
53. Tiono AB, Ouedraogo A, Ouattara D, Bougouma EC, Coulibaly S, Diarra A, et al. Efficacy of Olyset Duo, a bednet containing pyriproxyfen and permethrin, *versus* a permethrin-only net against clinical malaria in an area with highly pyrethroid-resistant vectors in rural Burkina Faso: a cluster-randomised controlled trial. Lancet. 2018. https://doi.org/10.1016/S0140-6736(18)31711-2 .
54. Protopopoff N, Mosha JF, Lukole E, Charlwood JD, Wright A, Mwalimu CD, et al. Effectiveness of a long-lasting piperonyl butoxide-treated insecticidal net and indoor residual spray interventions, separately and together, against malaria transmitted by pyrethroid-resistant mosquitoes: a cluster, randomised controlled, two-by-two factorial design trial. Lancet. 2018;391: 1577–88.
55. N'Guessan R, Odjo A, Ngufor C, Malone D, Rowland M. A Chlorfenapyr Mixture Net Interceptor(R) G2 shows high efficacy and wash durability against resistant mosquitoes in West Africa. PLoS One. 2016;11:e0165925.
56. Sternberg ED, Ng'habi KR, Lyimo IN, Kessy ST, Farenhorst M, Thomas MB, et al. Eave tubes for malaria control in Africa: initial development and semi-field evaluations in Tanzania. Malar J. 2016;15:447.
57. Qualls WA, Muller GC, Traore SF, Traore MM, Arheart KL, Doumbia S, et al. Indoor use of attractive toxic sugar bait (ATSB) to effectively control malaria vectors in Mali, West Africa. Malar J. 2015;14:301.

2

Improvement of mosquito identification by MALDI-TOF MS biotyping using protein signatures from two body parts

Anubis Vega-Rúa[1*], Nonito Pagès[2,3], Albin Fontaine[4,5], Christopher Nuccio[6], Lyza Hery[1], Daniella Goindin[1], Joel Gustave[7] and Lionel Almeras[4,5]

Abstract

Background: Matrix-assisted laser desorption/ionization time-of-flight mass spectrometry technology (MALDI-TOF MS) is an innovative tool that has been shown to be effective for the identification of numerous arthropod groups including mosquitoes. A critical step in the implementation of MALDI-TOF MS identification is the creation of spectra databases (DB) for the species of interest. Mosquito legs were the body part most frequently used to create identification DB. However, legs are one of the most fragile mosquito compartments, which can put identification at risk. Here, we assessed whether mosquito thoraxes could also be used as a relevant body part for mosquito species identification using a MALDI-TOF MS biotyping strategy; we propose a double DB query strategy to reinforce identification success.

Methods: Thoraxes and legs from 91 mosquito specimens belonging to seven mosquito species collected in six localities from Guadeloupe, and two laboratory strains, *Aedes aegypti* BORA and *Aedes albopictus* Marseille, were dissected and analyzed by MALDI-TOF MS. Molecular identification using *cox*1 gene sequencing was also conducted on representative specimens to confirm their identification.

Results: MS profiles obtained with both thoraxes and legs were highly compartment-specific, species-specific and species-reproducible, allowing high identification scores (log-score values, LSVs) when queried against the in-house MS reference spectra DB (thorax LSVs range: 2.260–2.783, leg LSVs range: 2.132–2.753).

Conclusions: Both thoraxes and legs could be used for a double DB query in order to reinforce the success and accuracy of MALDI-TOF MS identification.

Keywords: Mosquitoes, Culicidae, Identification, Guadeloupe, MALDI-TOF MS, Innovative strategy

Background

Despite centuries of control efforts, the past three decades have witnessed a dramatic spread of many mosquito-borne diseases worldwide. Today, they constitute a major public health problem accounting for more than 1.5 million deaths per year [1, 2]. This burden irrefutably demonstrates the need for appropriate mosquito surveillance programmes where specimens are accurately identified at the species level. Mosquito species are primarily identified using morphological traits and dichotomous keys. This identification approach is limited by the damage to the specimens, morphological interspecies similarities, availability of an appropriate identification key and entomological skills [3]. In cases with such limitations, PCR-based methods have proved their efficacy as they can be used with damaged specimens and allow discrimination of morphologically undistinguishable mosquito species and closely related species groups (i.e. *Culex pipiens* form *pipiens*, *Culex pipiens* form *molestus* and hybrids) [3, 4]. However, molecular approaches are expensive and time-consuming, limiting large-scale implementation in the frame of entomological surveillance [5]. In addition, molecular identification requires information on gene target sequences that are frequently unavailable in the corresponding databases. In this context, the use of an alternative cheap and rapid tool, allowing for large scale and high-quality monitoring of

* Correspondence: anubis.vega-rua@pasteur.fr
[1]Laboratory of Vector Control Research, Environment and Health Unit, Institut Pasteur de la Guadeloupe, 97183 Les Abymes, Guadeloupe, France
Full list of author information is available at the end of the article

culicid populations, is required to revolutionize entomological surveillance.

Matrix-assisted laser desorption/ionization time-of-flight mass spectrometry technology (MALDI-TOF MS) has recently emerged as an innovative tool that has been shown to be effective for rapid and low-cost identification of numerous arthropod groups, including mosquitoes (Culicidae) [6, 7], phlebotomine flies (Psychodidae) [8–10], tsetse flies (Glossinidae) [11], biting midges (Ceratopogonidae) [12], fleas (Siphonaptera) [13] and hard ticks (Ixodidae) [14, 15]. In addition, the sensitivity and specificity of MALDI-TOF MS biotyping allow a correct identification of immature arthropod stages [16, 17] and closely related species, which would otherwise be indistinguishable using morphological and/or molecular approaches (i.e. cryptic *Anopheles gambiae* species) [18].

The efforts conducted over the past five years have yielded improvements to protocols and standardization of methods for this kind of protein-based identification [19, 20]. These guidelines should facilitate the comparison and exchange of MS spectra between teams all over the world. For the mosquito identification at adult stages, legs were repeatedly chosen for the creation of MS reference spectra databases and specimens identification [6, 7, 21]. However, mosquito legs are breakable and the loss of one or several legs occurs frequently during mosquito sampling, transportation or storage. If only three or fewer legs are available for a single specimen, the identification by MALDI-TOF MS could be compromised [22]. In such cases, the selection of another adult mosquito body part for MALDI-TOF MS analysis could solve species identification when failure occurred with mosquito legs.

The abdomen is generally excluded for MS specimen identification due to the high heterogeneity of MS profiles generated by this body part. Indeed, according to the gravid or feeding status (unfed, recently fed or blood meal under digestion) of arthropods, abdomen MS profiles could be drastically different among specimens from the same species [12, 18, 23]. Moreover, MS profiles from freshly engorged mosquitoes can differ according to the source of the recently ingested blood meal [23, 24]; consequently, the mosquito abdomen cannot be considered as a suitable body part for species identification using MALDI-TOF. Because the mosquito head is frequently used to evaluate vector competence (i.e. efficient dissemination of pathogens beyond the midgut barrier) [25–27], the only remaining body part which is not prone to degradation during collection, transportation or storing and that could be used for species identification is the thorax.

The aim of the present study was to assess whether thoraxes from adult mosquitoes can produce species-specific protein signatures that can be used for mosquito species identification, as previously reported for legs (species reproducibility and species specificity of MS spectra). The creation of an MS spectra reference database containing a double entry for queried paired-MS spectra from each specimen is likely to improve user confidence in this method. This may result in popularization of this innovative strategy for entomological studies.

Results

Morphological identification and molecular confirmation

Among mosquitoes trapped in 6 distinct sites from Guadeloupe (Fig. 1), eight specimens were selected per species and collection site. These mosquitoes were morphologically identified as seven distinct mosquito species (Table 1). Two *Aedes* species, *Ae. aegypti* and *Ae. albopictus*, reared in laboratory were also added as controls. A total of 91 mosquito specimens were included in the present study.

Two out of eight morphologically identified specimens per species and collection site (25%) were submitted to *cox*1 gene sequencing to confirm their identification. The absence of *cox*1 sequences for *Cx. atratus* and *Deinocerites magnus* on GenBank resulted in unreliable identification (similarity with top match < 97%); *cox*1 sequences obtained for *Cx. atratus* and *D. magnus* were deposited in the GenBank database as new sequences with accession numbers MH376749/MH376750 and MH376751/MH376752, respectively. The query of the remaining *cox*1 sequences in the GenBank database, using the BLAST function, allowed us to obtain reliable mosquito species identification for 10 out of 14 samples, with sequence coverage and identity ranges of 87–92% and 99–100%, respectively (Table 1). The four specimens morphologically identified as *Cx. quinquefasciatus* did not reach the identity sequence threshold of 97% for reliable classification. The first two top-ranking hits of species identification were *Cx. p. pipiens* and *Cx. quinquefasciatus*, both obtaining 96% of *cox*1 sequence similarity. These specimens were therefore classified as *Culex* genus.

In the Barcode of Life Data Systems (BOLD) database, *cox*1 sequences from the seven mosquito species were available (Table 1). The query of the *cox*1 sequences from specimens of six mosquito species corroborated morphological identification, notably for *D. magnus* (similarity > 99.4%) and *Cx. quinquefasciatus* specimens (similarity > 98.9%), and confirmed the four other species identified using the sequences in the GenBank DB. The *cox*1 sequences of specimens morphologically identified as *Cx. atratus* failed to match any species in the BOLD system. The high similarity (> 99% on 649 bp) of *cox*1 sequences from specimens morphologically identified as *Cx. atratus*

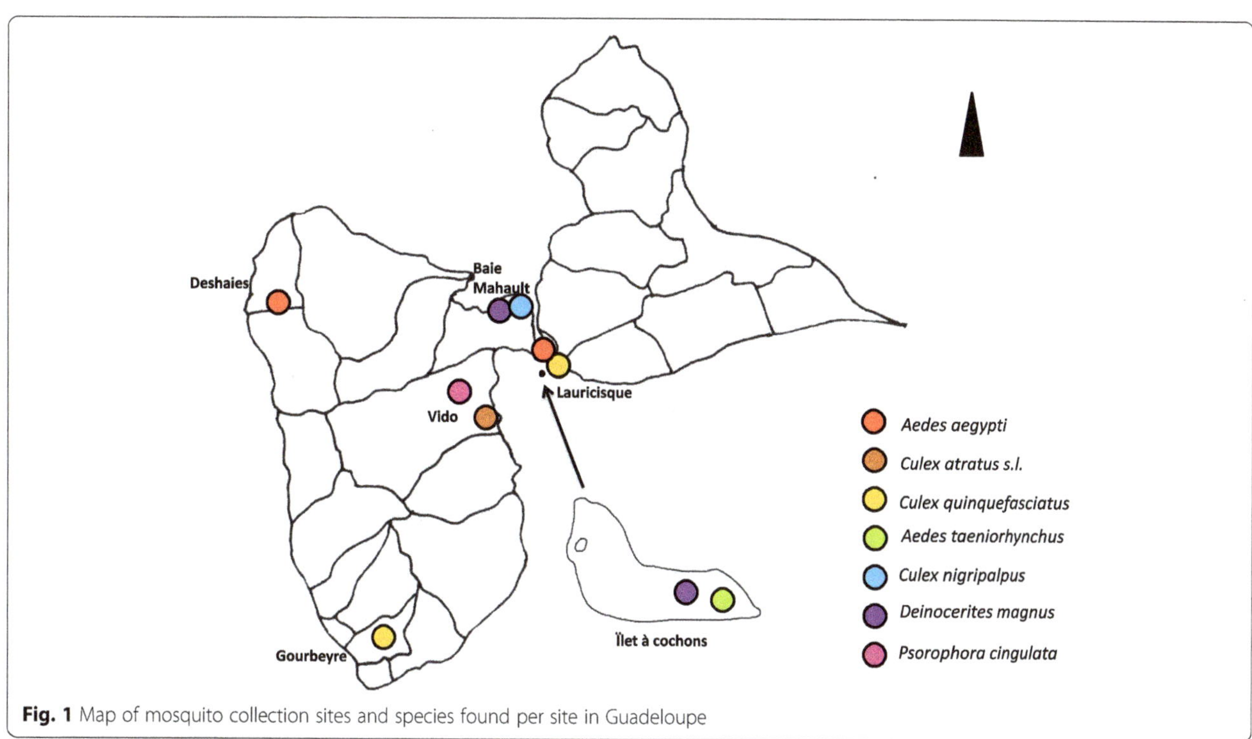

Fig. 1 Map of mosquito collection sites and species found per site in Guadeloupe

supported that these mosquito specimens were conspecific. The alignment of *cox*1 sequences of *Cx. atratus* collected in Guadeloupe with those from BOLD revealed a low similarity rate (< 89% on 649 bp). The description of several members in the *Cx. atratus* complex could explain *cox*1 sequence heterogeneity [28]. Based on the lack of specific molecular sequences distinguishing species from *Cx. atratus* complex and the absence of diagnostic morphological character states for female mosquitoes, we classified these specimens as *Cx. atratus* (*s.l.*).

Reproducible and specific MS spectra from both mosquito body parts

Legs and thoraxes from each of the 91 mosquitoes were dissected prior to MS analysis. Unfortunately, legs from 3 specimens (1 *Cx. atratus* and 2 *Cx. quinquefasciatus*) were missing, probably broken during transport and/or storing, and one thorax from *Psorophora cingulata* was lost during the dissection step. Finally, legs and thoraxes from 88 and 90 specimens, respectively, were submitted to MALDI-TOF MS analysis. The comparison of MS

Table 1 Overview of mosquito origins and subgroup identification by *cox*1 molecular typing

Morphological identification	Locality	No. of specimens included (sequenced)	Species identified *via* GenBank (accession number)	*cox*1 sequence coverage (%)/ similarity (%)	Species identified *via* BOLD	*cox*1 sequence similarity (%)
Ae. aegypti	Deshaies, Lauricisque	16 (4)	*Ae. aegypti* (AY432106.1)	92/100	*Ae. aegypti*	100
Cx. quinquefasciatus	Gourbeyre, Lauricisque	15[b] (4)	No reliable ID	–	*Cx. quinquefasciatus*	98.9
Cx. nigripalpus	Baie Mahault	8 (2)	*Cx. nigripalpus* (KM592992.1)	87/99	*Cx. nigripalpus*	99.7
Cx. atratus (*s.l.*)	Vido	8 (2)	No reliable ID[a]	–	No reliable ID	–
D. magnus	Baie Mahault, Ilet à cochons	16 (4)	No reliable ID[a]	–	*D. magnus*	99.4
Ae. taeniorhynchus	Ilet à cochons	8 (2)	*Ae. taeniorhynchus* (JX259676.1)	88/99	*Ae. taeniorhynchus*	99.0
P. cingulata	Vido	8 (2)	*P. cingulata* (KM592989.1)	88/99	*P. cingulata*	99.1
Ae. aegypti (Bora)	Laboratory reared	8 (–)	–		–	
Ae. albopictus (MRS)	Laboratory reared	4 (–)	–	–	–	

[a]Mosquito species for which *cox1* sequences were not available in the database (30th March 2018)
[b]Specimens identified morphologically as *Cx. quinquefasciatus* at Lauricisque ($n = 7$) and Gourbeyre ($n = 8$)
Abbreviations: No reliable ID, similarity with top match < 97%; BOLD, Barcode of Life Data Systems; *cox*1, cytochrome *c* oxidase subunit 1; MRS, Marseille strain

spectra from legs (Fig. 2a) and thoraxes (Fig. 2b) between mosquito species revealed protein profiles of high intensity (> 2000 a.u.) and were visually reproducible for specimens of the same species according to body part.

To assess the reproducibility and specificity of the MS spectra from legs and thoraxes per species according to body parts, a cluster analysis was performed. Two specimens per species and site plus both *Aedes* laboratory-reared species were used for building MSP dendrograms. The clustering of leg (Fig. 3a) and thorax (Fig. 3b) MS spectra according to mosquito species confirmed the reproducibility and specificity of the protein profiles. The clustering of specimens of the same species, independent of the trapping location site or origin (field or laboratory reared), in each body part, confirmed the high species-specificity of MS spectra. Furthermore, a total of 54 and 56 species-specific mass peaks were found with ClinProTools software between these mosquito species for legs and thoraxes, respectively (Additional file 1: Table S1 and Additional file 2: Table S2). MS spectra generated from legs, thoraxes and a mix of legs and thoraxes from the laboratory reared mosquito species *Ae. albopictus* were also compared (Additional file 3: Figure S1a, b). Interestingly, MS spectra from mixed compartments (i.e. legs and thorax) were similar to thorax counterparts. The more abundant *Ae. albopictus* MS peak obtained with legs (m/z = 8191.5) was nearly undetectable in the MS profiles from mixed legs and thoraxes (Additional file 3: Figure S1c, d).

It is interesting to note that MSP dendrogram generated with mosquito paired body parts were not superimposable between legs and thoraxes (Fig. 3). All specimens of the genus *Culex* were grouped in the same part of the MSP dendrogram for thoraxes, whereas for the leg MSP dendrogram, *Cx. atratus* specimens were isolated from other mosquitoes of the genus. Moreover, *Ae. taeniorhynchus*, a species from the genus *Aedes*, was

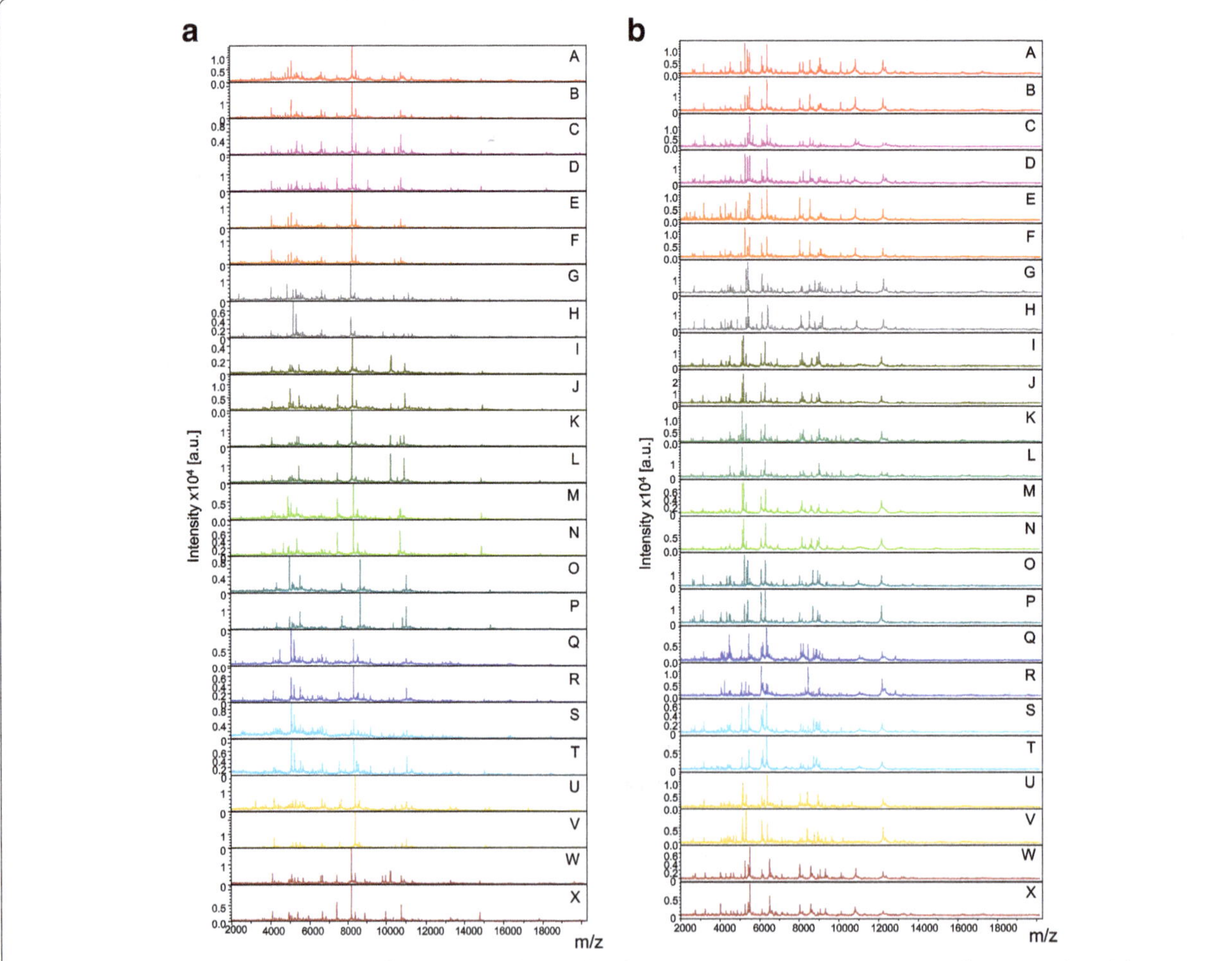

Fig. 2 Comparison of MALDI-TOF MS spectra for legs (**a**) and thoraxes (**b**) of mosquitoes. Representative MS spectra of *Ae. aegypti* (Bora) laboratory-reared (A, B) or collected at Deshaies (C, D) and Lauricisque (E, F), *Ae. taeniorhynchus* collected at Ilet à cochons (G, H), *Cx. quinquefaciatus* collected at Gourbeyre (I, J) and Lauricisque (K, L), *Cx. nigripalpus* collected at Baie Mahault (M, N), *Cx. atratus (s.l.)* collected at Vido (O, P), *D. magnus* collected at Ilet à cochons (Q, R) and Baie Mahault (S, T), *P. cingulata* collected at Vido (U, V) and *Ae. albopictus* (Marseille strain) laboratory-reared (W, X). *Abbreviations*: a.u., arbitrary units; m/z, mass to charge ratio

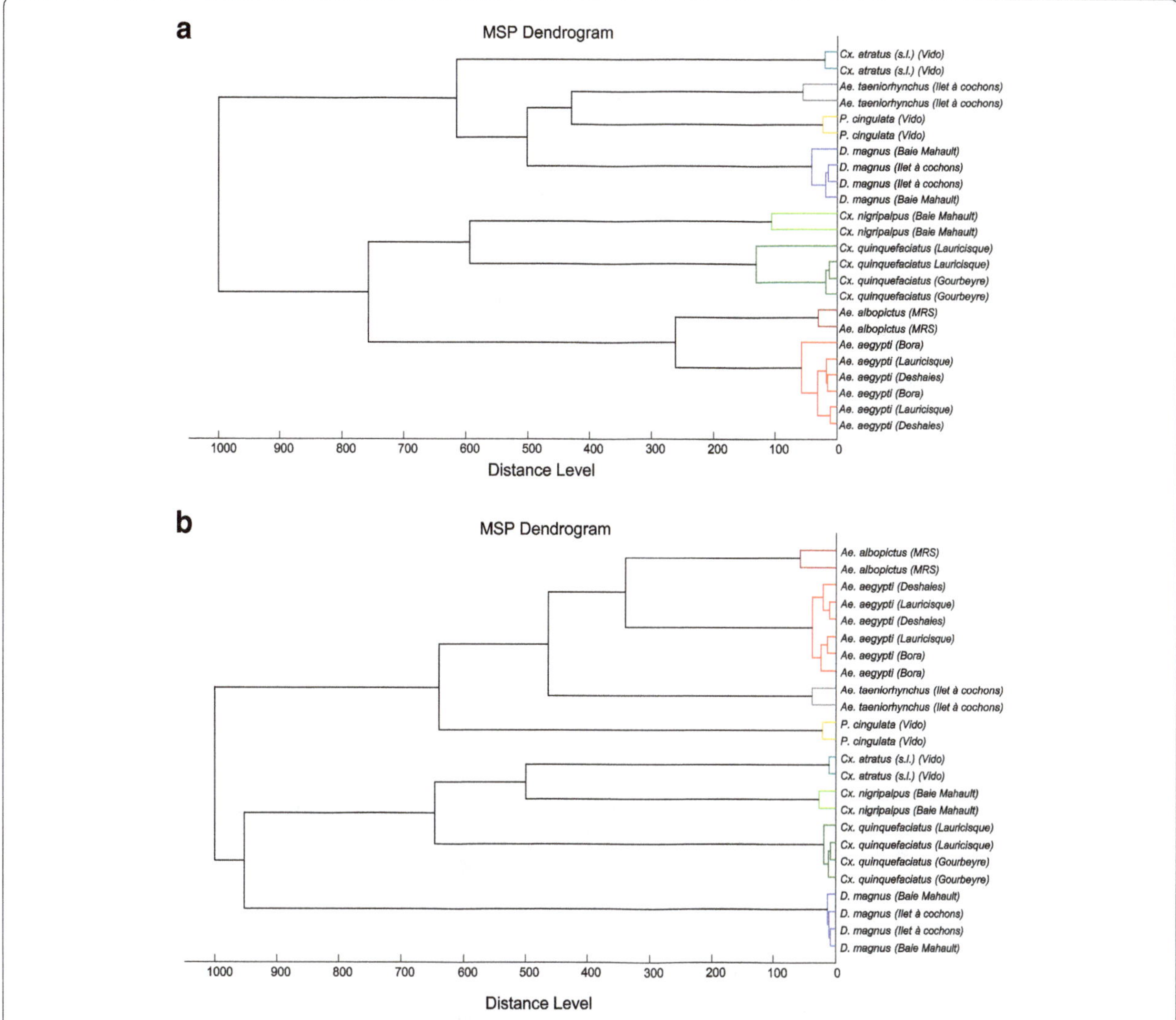

Fig. 3 MSP dendrogram of MALDI-TOF MS spectra for legs (**a**) and thoraxes (**b**) of mosquitoes. Two specimens per collection site were used to construct the dendrogram. The dendrogram was created using Biotyper v3.0 software and distance units correspond to the relative similarity of MS spectra. Mosquito sampling locations are given within parentheses. *Abbreviation*: MRS, Marseille

found at close proximity to other members of this genus solely in the MSP dendrogram from thoraxes.

MS spectra reproducibility from legs and thoraxes were confirmed by CCI matrix highlighting a good correlation between spectra for specimens of the same species whatever their origin (catching location, field-caught or laboratory-reared). Moreover, the low CCI obtained for the comparisons of MS spectra between species using leg (mean ± SD: 0.14 ± 0.08; Fig. 4a) and thorax (0.17 ± 0.16; Fig. 4b) MS spectra supported the species-specificity of the protein profiles.

Interestingly, paired comparisons of legs and thoraxes MS profiles for each species showed clearly distinct protein patterns (Fig. 2). To visualize specificity of the MS spectra according to body part per species, principal components analyses (PCAs) were performed (Additional file 4: Figure S2). PCAs revealed a clear separation of the points corresponding to MS spectra from the legs and thoraxes, confirming a specificity of MS profiles between these two compartments for the seven species tested.

MS reference spectra database creation and validation step

MS spectra for legs and thoraxes from the 24 specimens used for MSP cluster analysis, including at least 2 specimens per species and location site, identified morphologically and molecularly, were used as reference MS spectra for the database (DB) creation. The remaining 64 and 66 MS spectra from legs and thoraxes, respectively, were queried against this DB. Log-score values (LSVs) from legs ranged between 2.132–2.753 and from thoraxes ranged between 2.260–2.783. MS spectra were

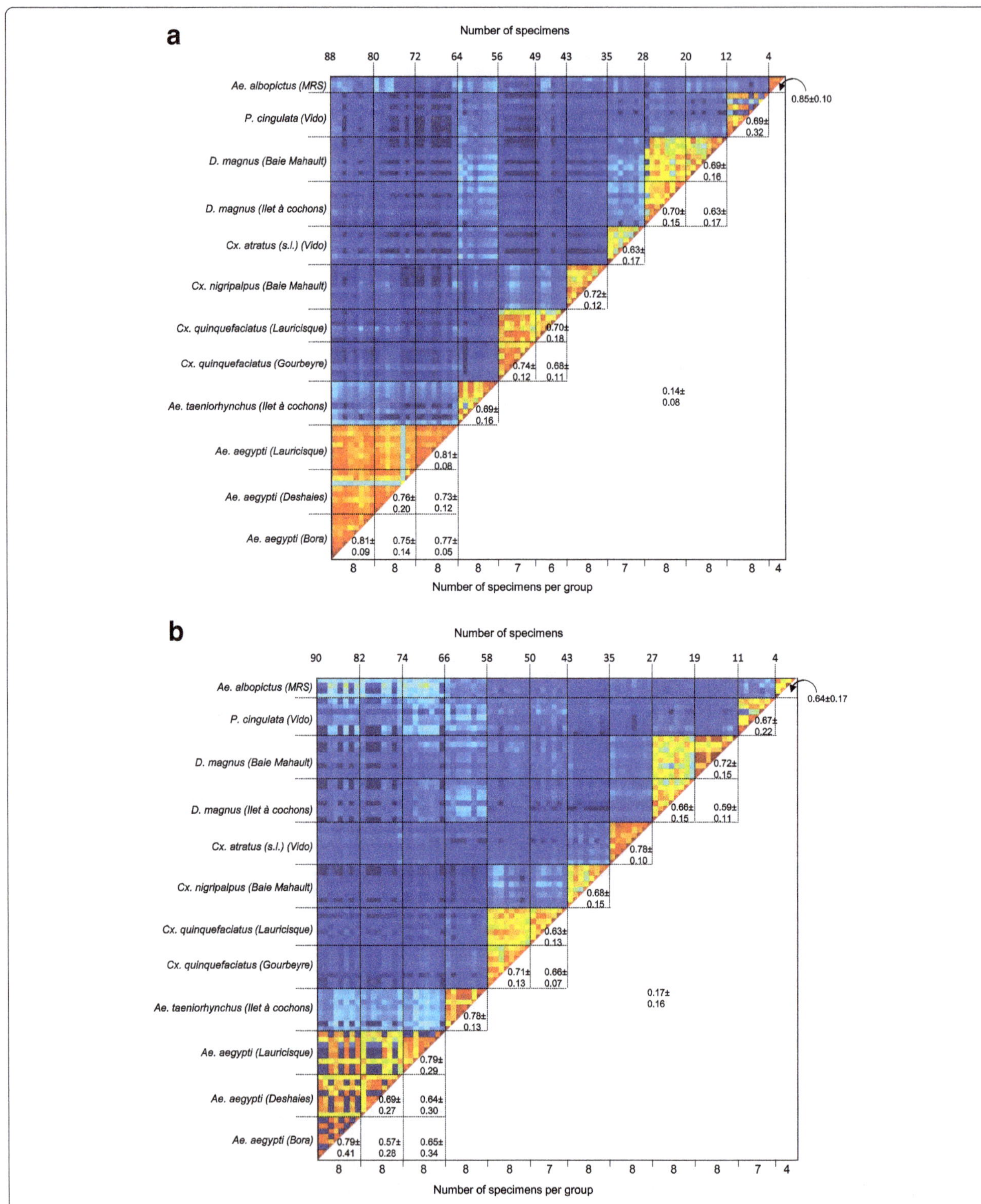

Fig. 4 Assessment of the reproducibility of MS spectra for legs (**a**) and thoraxes (**b**) according to mosquito species using the composite correlation index (CCI). MS spectra from four to eight specimens per collection site were analysed using the CCI tool. Levels of MS spectra reproducibility are indicated in red and blue showing relatedness and incongruence between spectra, respectively. CCI matrix was calculated using MALDI-Biotyper v3.0 software with default settings (mass range 3.0–12.0 kDa; resolution 4; 8 intervals; auto-correction off). The values correspond to the mean coefficient correlation and respective standard deviations obtained for paired condition comparisons. CCI are expressed as the mean ± standard deviation. Mosquito sampling locations are given within parentheses. *Abbreviation*: MRS, Marseille

higher than the threshold value (LSVs > 1.8) for reliable identification [6, 20] for all the samples tested (Fig. 5). For paired samples, concordant species identification (100%) was obtained using MS spectra from legs and thoraxes which were in agreement with morphological classification. The four specimens for which only one body part (legs or thoraxes) was submitted to MS, also provided concordant results with entomological identification.

To verify that reliable identification was achieved for the reference MS spectra whatever the collection site of specimens, a comparison of LSVs resulting from a DB query containing MS spectra from two specimens per species and location site or two specimens per species from a single location site, was done. As expected, a decrease of LSVs was observed when only specimens from one site were included in the DB, compared to all sites (Additional file 5: Figure S3). Nevertheless, identification scores remained sufficiently high (LSVs > 1.8) to unambiguously classify all specimens, using either mosquito legs or thoraxes. Interestingly, reliable identification could be made when unique MS spectra from legs or thoraxes of laboratory-reared *Ae. aegypti* (Bora) were included in the DB (Additional file 5: Figure S3a, b). These results underline that these two body parts can be used for identification, independent of specimen origin, within mosquitoes from the same species.

Discussion

The present study constitutes a representative example of the requirement for an innovative method for arthropod identification. Although morphological analysis remains the "gold standard" for mosquito identification [22], this time-consuming method is reliant on entomologist skills and mosquito integrity which are drawbacks for its widespread use. In regions such as the Caribbean, morphological identification is even more complex due to a generalized lack of recent culicid fauna inventories (most of them were conducted in the 1960s and 1970s) [29, 30] and updated identification keys. Effectively, the absence of morphological dichotomous keys adapted to local fauna impedes the correct morphological diagnosis of closely-related species such as members belonging to a species complex. Moreover, for these closely-related species (i.e. *Culex* spp.), dissection steps (i.e. male genitalia) are often required for a reliable identification at species level, due to the absence of discriminative external morphological characters [31]. Well-trained personnel possessing expertise is, therefore, critical for successful morphological identification. In the present study, initial morphological observation failed to confidently categorize female specimens from the *Cx. atratus* complex, which were then classified as *Cx. atratus* (*s.l.*). In the USA, the distinction of *Cx. atratus* (*s.s.*) from *Cx. atratus* B is based on the inspection of the cibarial armature, a small structure located at the base of the pharyngeal pump, requiring mosquito head dissection [28]. Two types of cibarial armatures were described for each member of *Cx. atratus* complex, increasing the risk of misidentification [28]. In addition, species composition of the *Cx. atratus* complex in the Neartic region (e.g. the USA) is different to that of the Neotropical region (e.g. the Caribbean). Therefore, it was uncertain at the time the study was implemented to discern whether different cibarial armature states could be confidently associated with a particular species of the Neotropical *Cx. atratus* complex, as other local species from the complex were unavailable.

To circumvent the limitations of morphological identification, molecular strategies based on DNA-barcoding using *cox*1 gene sequencing are generally applied [32, 33]. However, this expensive and time-consuming approach was inefficient in the identification of all specimens collected in Guadeloupe in the frame of the present study. Here, the query of the *cox*1 sequences against the

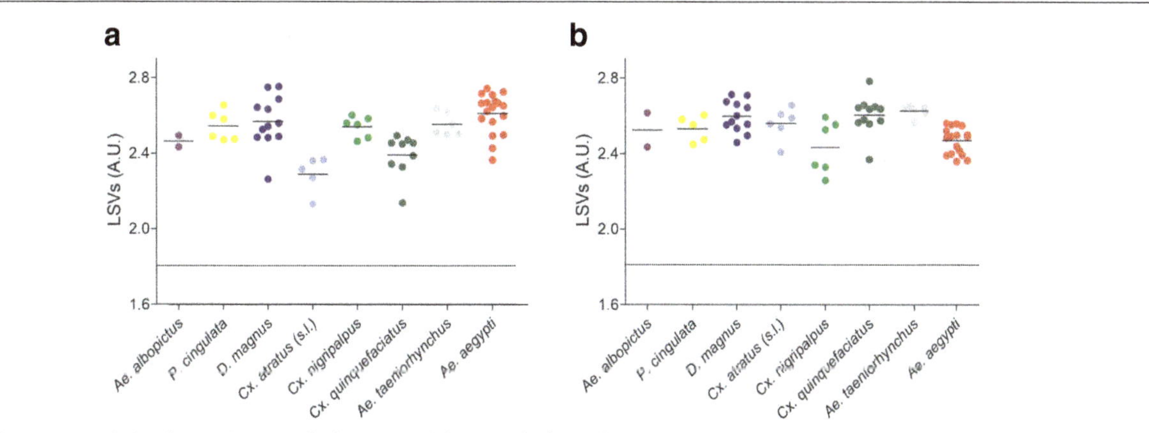

Fig. 5 Comparison of LSVs from MS spectra for legs (**a**) and thoraxes (**b**) from all mosquito species studied. Dashed lines represent the threshold value for relevant identification (LSVs > 1.8). *Abbreviation*: LSV, log-score value

GenBank DB did not successfully identify *Cx. quinquefasciatus* specimens, despite the presence of counterpart *cox*1 sequences. The low percentage of *cox*1 sequences similarity (about 96%) between *Cx. quinquefasciatus* field-collected specimens from Guadeloupe and counterpart species on GenBank allowed identification solely to the genus level (*Culex* sp.). Conversely, the same *cox*1 sequences queried against the BOLD DB confirmed that these specimens belonged to *Cx. quinquefasciatus* with a relevant similarity rate (98.9%). These results underlined that identification success could be dependent of the genomic DB used. The inability to identify certain species was attribute to the absence of the concerned *cox*1 sequences in the DB [i.e. *Cx. atratus* (*s.l.*)] and to the representativeness of *cox*1 gene diversity within a given species (i.e. *Cx. quinquefasciatus*). Indeed, genetic variations in the *cox*1 gene have been reported between specimens from the same mosquito species (i.e. *Cx. bidens*, *Cx. interfor*) collected in different provinces of Argentina, allowing the identification of different haplotypes [31]. Even if this genetic diversity is lower when compared to that of other genes (i.e. the *nad*4 gene), it can influence the molecular identity rate obtained after DB query as observed here.

MS spectra variations between specimens from the same species with a different geographical origin was also observed. This phenomenon was reported for mosquitoes at the adult [6, 18] and larval stages [16], as well as for other arthropod groups such as tsetse flies [11]. MS profile variations according to mosquito origin were also observed in the present study. It was highlighted by the decrease of LSVs depending on the geographical location of the specimens included in the reference MS DB. Nevertheless, these intraspecific variations of MS spectra were moderate and did not negatively affect the correctness and reliability of counterpart specimen identification. Moreover, the exact identification of field-caught *Ae. aegypti* by inclusion in the reference MS DB of MS spectra from laboratory-reared *Ae. aegypti* (Bora) specimens underlined the robustness of this approach.

For *Cx. atratus* (*s.l.*) and *D. magnus*, *cox*1 sequences were not available in the GenBank DB, which resulted in failure to confirm the morphological identification. The lack of complete *cox*1 sequences in a public genomic DB frequently occurs, requiring the sequencing of other reference genes (i.e. ribosomal), or of several *cox*1 gene fragments [31], when possible, to achieve identification. Conversely, the same *cox*1 sequences queried against the BOLD DB allowed the identification of six out of seven species, confirming the morphological identification, including *D. magnus* specimens. Only specimens morphologically identified as *Cx. atratus* (*s.l.*) failed to be validated with *cox*1 sequence similarity lower than 97% following a query in BOLD. Nevertheless, as observed for *Cx. quinquefasciatus* in the GenBank DB, *Cx. atratus* (*s.l.*) *cox*1 sequences were available in the BOLD DB. However, it was not indicated to which member of the *Cx. atratus* complex corresponded the available *cox*1 sequences, i.e. *Cx. atratus* (*s.s.*) or *Cx. atratus* B [28]. The low *cox*1 sequence similarity (< 89%) between *Cx. atratus* (*s.l.*) specimens from Guadeloupe and those available in the BOLD DB could suggest that the former belong to a different species of the *Cx. atratus* complex. The absence of another gene sequence target allowing to distinguish members of the *Cx. atratus* complex in the GenBank DB or the BOLD DB, did not allow us to definitively identify the specimens collected in Guadeloupe. However, the high homology of the *cox*1 sequences between specimens allowed us to consider them conspecific but as *Cx. atratus* (*s.l.*). The reproducibility of MS spectra, for each compartment, from specimens identified as *Cx. atratus* (*s.l.*), in addition to the elevated CCI obtained for both legs and thoraxes, were supplementary arguments to claim that these specimens could be considered as same species. The high efficiency of MALDI-TOF MS biotyping to distinct cryptic species has been repeatedly reported, notably distinguishing *An. gambiae* (*s.s.*) from *An. coluzzi*, corresponding to *An. gambiae M* and *S* molecular forms, respectively [18, 20, 34]. In the future, this proteomic approach could be evaluated to differentiate members from the *Cx. atratus* complex.

A critical step in the implementation of MALDI-TOF MS identification is the creation of MS reference spectra DB for the species of interest. The majority of the existing adult mosquito identification MS DB have been created using mosquito legs [6]. However, legs are one of the most fragile mosquito compartments and they are easily lost during specimen handling and/or storage, which compromises their identification. In the present study, three specimens had all the legs missing, which required identification based on thorax MS spectra to corroborate morphological classification. Moreover, for several other specimens, one or more legs were missing which could have prejudiced their identification. The use of another mosquito compartment to create MS reference DB as a complement of MS spectra obtained from mosquito legs could be an alternative to counteract this technical problem and reinforce the quality of the identification (Additional file 6: Figure S4). The present study demonstrated that mosquito thoraxes could also be used as a suitable and relevant body part for mosquito species identification using MALDI-TOF MS biotyping strategy.

The comparison of MS profiles obtained with legs, thoraxes and a mix of legs and thoraxes from *Ae. albopictus* specimens revealed similar MS profiles between mixed compartments and thorax counterparts. In MS profiling, mainly abundant ionizable proteins are detectable. As proteins from legs were proportionally less abundant than those from the thorax, their protein quantities were insufficient to drastically change thorax MS profiles. Nevertheless, under the hypothesis that thorax MS profiles would be changed by the addition of legs for other species, it is probable that intensity of MS peaks corresponding to legs in the mixture could be variable according to the number of legs included. In such conditions, the reference MS spectra database from mixed legs and thoraxes would not be suitable to identify specimens which had lost several or all legs. Conversely, when legs were submitted alone, the MS profile was unchanged whatever the number of legs and only a decrease of the MS profile intensity was observed according to the number of legs used. For specimens with one or two legs remaining, the low ratio intensity of MS peaks/background can hinder peak detection, compromising their identification. The MS submission of a second compartment, such as the thorax, could then reveal specimen identity, especially for specimens which have lost several legs or for closely-related species.

This new strategy consisting of submitting two body compartments per specimen to MALDI-TOF MS analysis, thereby producing distinct but species-specific MS spectra, should improve identification confidence. Moreover, the distinct topologies of the MSP dendrograms for each body part from paired specimens, pointed out that the proximity of MS spectra between mosquito species were different for legs and thoraxes. These MS pattern properties reinforce the species identification accuracy and reduce the risk of misidentification. The MS spectra specificity according to body part used, was also reported in others arthropods such as ticks [35] and it has been recommended to submit legs and half-idiosome from the same tick specimen to MS for MS reference DB creation or to strengthen specimen identification [35].

In addition to the standardization of sample preparation protocols [19, 20, 36], the creation of a standardized MS reference spectra DB for mosquito identification composed of paired legs and thoraxes MS spectra for each species becomes compulsory. The double MS spectra query strategy remains compatible with the use of remaining body parts of the specimen to obtain additional information. For instance, the remaining abdomen could still be used to detect the blood meal source in the case of an engorged mosquito female [23], while the head can be used for pathogen detection [36], both by a MALDI-TOF biotyping approach.

Conclusions

The present study points out MALDI-TOF biotyping strategy as an innovative and alternative tool for mosquito identification that could lead to a dramatic positive impact in the mosquito surveillance field worldwide. The double MS spectra DB query should reinforce identification quality and, in the case of missing legs, identification remains possible by the use of the thorax. To achieve this, the development of an international comprehensive and accessible mosquito spectra database is essential.

Methods

Mosquitoes

Adult female mosquitoes, collected in the field or laboratory-reared, were used for this study. Field collection of mosquitoes was undertaken in 6 distinct sites from the Caribbean Island of Guadeloupe using BG sentinel traps (Fig. 1). Collected specimens were stored at -20 °C from a few months to one year. Mosquito species were determined by morphological identification under a binocular loupe at a magnification of 56× (Leica M80, Leica, Nanterre, France) using morphological descriptions [37–39]. In each collection site, 8 specimens per species were selected for MS analysis. *Aedes aegypti* (Bora strain) and *Ae. albopictus* (Marseille strain, MRS) mosquitoes were raised in the laboratory using standard methods as previously described [40, 41]. Only imago non-engorged female mosquitoes were included in the study. The mosquitoes were sedated and stored at -20 °C until future analysis.

Mosquito dissection

Legs and thoraxes from mosquitoes were processed as previously described [36]. Briefly, specimens were individually dissected with a sterile surgical blade under a binocular loupe. For each specimen, legs and thorax (without wings) were removed and transferred separately in 1.5 ml Eppendorf tubes for MALDI-TOF MS analysis. The remaining body parts (abdomens and heads) were used for molecular analyses. A nomenclature was established to pair body parts from the same specimen. In addition, paired legs and thorax (without wings) from five *Ae. albopictus* specimens were mixed prior to MALDI-TOF MS analysis.

Molecular identification of mosquitoes

DNA was individually extracted from the head and abdomen of 2 mosquito specimens per species selected for MS reference database creation (n = 24) using the QIAamp DNA tissue extraction kit (Qiagen, Hilden, Germany) according to the manufacturer's instructions. Molecular identification of mosquito at the species level was performed by sequencing the PCR product of a fragment of the cytochrome *c* oxidase 1 gene (*cox*1) using the primers LCO1490 (forward) (5'-GGT CAA CAA ATC ATA AAG ATA TTG G-3') and HC02198 (reverse) (5'-TAA ACT TCA GGG TGA CCA AAA AAT CA-3') as previously described [42, 43]. The sequences were assembled and analyzed using the ChromasPro software version 1.7.7 (Technelysium Pty. Ltd., Tewantin, Australia). All sequences were compared with sequences in the GenBank database using BLAST (http://blast.ncbi.nlm.nih.gov/Blast.cgi) and the Barcode of Life Data Systems (BOLD; http://www.barcodinglife.org; [44]) to assign unknown *cox*1 sequences to mosquito species.

Sample homogenization and MALDI-TOF MS analysis

Each compartment dissected was individually homogenized 3 × 1 min at 30 Hz using TissueLyser (Qiagen) and glass powder (Sigma-Aldrich, Lyon, France) in a homogenization buffer composed of a mix (50/50) of 70% (v/v) formic acid (Sigma-Aldrich, Lyon, France) and 50% (v/v) acetonitrile (Fluka, Buchs, Switzerland) for protein extraction according to the standardized automated setting described by Nebbak et al. [20]. Respectively, 30 μl and 50 μl of the homogenization buffer were used for legs and thoraxes. For samples containing a mix of legs and thorax from the same individual, 60 μl of the homogenization buffer were used. After sample homogenization, a quick spin centrifugation at 200× *g* for 1 min was then performed and 1 μl of the supernatant of each sample was loaded on the MALDI-TOF steel target plate in quadruplicate (Bruker Daltonics, Wissembourg, France). After air-drying, 1 μl of matrix solution composed of saturated α-cyano-4-hydroxycinnamic acid (Sigma-Aldrich, Lyon, France), 50% (v/v) acetonitrile, 2.5% (v/v) trifluoroacetic acid (Sigma-Aldrich, Dorset, UK) and HPLC-grade water was added. To control matrix quality (i.e. absence of MS peaks due to matrix buffer impurities) and MALDI-TOF apparatus performance, matrix solution was loaded in duplicate onto each MALDI-TOF plate alone and with a bacterial test standard (Bruker Bacterial Test Standard, ref: #8255343). Moreover, legs or thoraxes from two *Ae. albopictus* specimens reared at the laboratory and stored at -20 °C were included on each plate and were used as homogenization positive controls.

MALDI-TOF MS parameters

Protein mass profiles were obtained using a Microflex LT MALDI-TOF Mass Spectrometer (Bruker Daltonics, Bremen, Germany), with detection in the linear positive-ion mode at a laser frequency of 50 Hz within a mass range of 2–20 kDa. The setting parameters of the MALDI-TOF MS apparatus were identical to those previously used [19]. The spectrum profiles obtained were visualized with Flex analysis v.3.3 software and exported to ClinProTools version v.2.2 and MALDI-Biotyper v.3.0 (Bruker Daltonics, Germany) for data processing (smoothing, baseline subtraction, peak picking) and evaluation with cluster analysis.

MS spectra analysis

MS spectra profiles were first controlled visually with flexAnalysis v.3.3 software (Bruker Daltonics, Bremen, Germany). MS spectra were then exported to ClinProTools v.2.2 and MALDI-Biotyper v.3.0. (Bruker Daltonics, Bremen, Germany) for data processing (smoothing, baseline subtraction, peak picking). MS spectra reproducibility was assessed by the comparison of the average spectral profiles (main spectrum profile, MSP) obtained from the four spots for each specimen according to body part with MALDI-Biotyper v.3.0 software (Bruker Daltonics, Bremen, Germany). MS spectra reproducibility and specificity taking into account mosquito body part were demonstrated using clustering analyses and the composite correlation index (CCI) tool. In addition, ClinProTools software was used to identify discriminatory peaks among the 8 mosquito species for each body-part. Cluster analyses (MS dendrogram) were performed based on comparison of the MSP given by MALDI-Biotyper v.3.0. software and clustered according to protein mass profile (i.e. their mass signals and intensities). The CCI tool from MALDI-Biotyper v.3.0 software was also used to assess the spectral variations within and between each sample group, according to the body part, as previously described [20, 45]. Higher correlation values (expressed as the mean ± standard deviation, SD) reflecting higher reproducibility for the MS spectra, were used to estimate MS spectra distance between species for each body part. To visualize MS spectra distribution from mosquitoes according to body part, principal components analysis (PCA) from ClinProTools v.2.2 software was performed for each species.

Database creation and blind tests

The reference MS spectra were created using spectra from legs and thoraxes of two specimens per species collected in each site or reared at the laboratory using MALDI-Biotyper software v.3.0. (Bruker Daltonics, Bremen, Germany) [10]. MS spectra were created with an unbiased algorithm using information on the peak position, intensity and frequency. Raw MS spectra from legs and thoraxes of mosquitoes included in the MS reference database used in the present study are provided for free use (Additional file 7). MS spectra from mosquito legs and thoraxes were tested against the in-house MS reference spectra DB. The reliability of species identification was estimated using the log-score values (LSVs) obtained from the MALDI Biotyper software v.3.0, which ranged from 0 to 3. According to previous studies [6, 20], LSVs greater than 1.8 were considered reliable for species identification. Data were analyzed by using GraphPad Prism software v.5.01 (GraphPad, San Diego, CA, USA).

Additional files

Additional file 1: Table S1. Mass peak list distinguishing mosquito species using legs as biological material, based on the Genetic Algorithm model analysis of ClinProTools. The list includes unique species-specific mass peaks. *Abbreviations*: Da, Daltons; m/z, mass to charge ratio. (DOCX 16 kb)

Additional file 2: Table S2. Mass peak list distinguishing mosquito species using thoraxes as biologic material, based on the Genetic Algorithm model analysis of ClinProTools. The list includes unique species-specific mass peaks. *Abbreviations*: Da, Daltons; m/z, mass to charge ratio. (DOCX 17 kb)

Additional file 3: Figure S1. Resulting MS spectra for legs (red), thoraxes (green) and mix of legs and thoraxes (blue) from *Ae. albopictus* specimens. Five specimens per condition, loaded in quadruplicate, were tested. **a** Overlay of the mean MS profile per condition. **b** Gel view of the MS profiles per condition. An enlargement of the m/z window including the more intense MS peak from *Ae. albopictus* legs is presented as a MS spectra overlay (**c**), and gel view (**d**). (TIF 23971 kb)

Additional file 4: Figure S2. Principal components analysis (PCA) from MS spectra for mosquito legs and thoraxes. PCA 3-dimensional (PCA1-PCA3) image from MS spectra of legs (red dots) and thoraxes (green dots) from *Ae. aegypti* (**a**), *Cx. quinquefasciatus* (**b**), *Ae. taeniorynchus* (**c**), *P. cingulata* (**d**), *Cx. atratus* (*s.l.*) (**e**), *Cx. nigripalpus* (**f**) and *D. magnus* (**g**). (TIF 44631 kb)

Additional file 5: Figure S3. Geographical reproducibility of the MS spectra from legs (**a**, **c**, **e**) and thoraxes (**b**, **d**, **f**) included in the DB per mosquito species. LSVs obtained for *Ae. aegypti* (**a**, **b**), *Cx. quinquefasciatus* (**c**, **d**) and *D. magnus* (**e**, **f**), according to origins of the MS spectra from specimens of the same species included in the DB are shown. The dashed line represents the threshold value for relevant identification (LSVs > 1.8). *Abbreviation*: LSV, log-score value. (TIF 35156 kb)

Additional file 6: Figure S4. Experimental design for mosquito identification using two distinct compartments by MALDI-TOF MS. The advantages of the creation of a MS reference database (DB) including mosquito legs and thoraxes are indicated. (PDF 95 kb)

Additional file 7: Raw MS spectra from legs and thoraxes of mosquitoes included in the MS reference database. MS spectra were obtained using a Microflex LT MALDI-TOF Mass Spectrometer (Bruker Daltonics). (7Z 4576 kb)

Abbreviations
CCI: Composite correlation index; LSV: Log-score value; MALDI-TOF MS: Matrix-assisted laser desorption/ionization time-of-flight mass spectrometry; PCR: Polymerase chain reaction

Acknowledgments
We thank Christelle Delannay and the vector control staff of the Regional Health Agency of Guadeloupe for their assistance during certain sampling campaigns. We thank Ken Giraud-Girard and Loïc Jacquet-Cretides for mosquito field collections and Angéline Kernalléguen for her advice on MALDI-TOF MS adjustment and calibration.

Funding
This work has been supported by the Vector Control Service of Health Regional Agency of Guadeloupe and by a FEDER grant, financed by the European Union and Guadeloupe Region (Programme Opérationnel FEDER-Guadeloupe-Conseil Régional 2014–2020, grant number 2015-FED-192) and by the Délégation Générale pour l'Armement (DGA, MoSIS project, grant number PDH-2-NRBC-2-B-2113).

Authors' contributions
AVR and LA designed and performed the research, analyzed the data and wrote the paper. NP participated in sampling campaigns, morphological identification of specimens and manuscript review. AF participated in specimen molecular identification and data analysis. CN provided technical support for MALDI-TOF MS acquisitions. DG, LH, CR and JG participated in mosquito collection, rearing and identifications. All authors read and approved the final manuscript.

Competing interests
The authors declare that they have no competing interests.

Author details
[1]Laboratory of Vector Control Research, Environment and Health Unit, Institut Pasteur de la Guadeloupe, 97183 Les Abymes, Guadeloupe, France. [2]CIRAD, UMR ASTRE, F-97170 Petit Bourg, Guadeloupe, France. [3]ASTRE, CIRAD, INRA, University of Montpellier, Montpellier, France. [4]Unité de Parasitologie et Entomologie, Département des Maladies Infectieuses, Institut de Recherche Biomédicale des Armées, Marseille, France. [5]Aix Marseille Université, IRD, AP-HM, SSA, UMR Vecteurs - Infections Tropicales et Méditerranéennes (VITROME), IHU - Méditerranée Infection, 19–21 bd Jean Moulin, 13385 Marseille, cedex 5, France. [6]Aix Marseille Université, INSERM, SSA, IRBA, MCT, 13005 Marseille, France. [7]Vector Control Service of Guadeloupe, Regional Health Agency, Airport Zone South Raizet, 97139 Les Abymes, Guadeloupe, France.

References
1. WHO. Global Health Day: about vector borne diseases. 2014. http://www.who.int/campaigns/world-health-day/2014/vector-borne-diseases/en/. Accessed 21 May 2018.
2. UNICEF/WHO. Reversing the incidence of malaria 2000–2015. WHO Global Malaria Program. Geneva: World Health Organization. p. 2015. http://apps.who.int/iris/bitstream/10665/184521/1/9789241509442_eng.pdf?ua=1. Accessed 21 May 2018
3. Kent RJ, Deus S, Williams M, Savage HM. Development of a multiplexed polymerase chain reaction-restriction fragment length polymorphism (PCR-RFLP) assay to identify common members of the subgenera *Culex* (*Culex*) and *Culex* (*Phenacomyia*) in Guatemala. Am J Trop Med Hyg. 2010;83:285–91.
4. Amraoui F, Tijane M, Sarih M, Failloux A-B. Molecular evidence of *Culex pipiens* form *molestus* and hybrids *pipiens/molestus* in Morocco, North Africa. Parasit Vectors. 2012;5:83.
5. Freiwald A, Sauer S. Phylogenetic classification and identification of bacteria by mass spectrometry. Nat Protoc. 2009;4:732–42.
6. Yssouf A, Parola P, Lindström A, Lilja T, L'Ambert G, Bondesson U, et al. Identification of European mosquito species by MALDI-TOF MS. Parasitol Res. 2014;113:2375–8.
7. Raharimalala FN, Andrianinarivomanana TM, Rakotondrasoa A, Collard JM, Boyer S. Usefulness and accuracy of MALDI-TOF mass spectrometry as a supplementary tool to identify mosquito vector species and to invest in development of international database. Med Vet Entomol. 2017. https://doi.org/10.1111/mve.12230.
8. Dvorak V, Halada P, Hlavackova K, Dokianakis E, Antoniou M, Volf P. Identification of phlebotomine sand flies (Diptera: Psychodidae) by matrix-assisted laser desorption/ionization time of flight mass spectrometry. Parasit Vectors. 2014;7:21.
9. Mathis A, Depaquit J, Dvořák V, Tuten H, Bañuls A-L, Halada P, et al. Identification of phlebotomine sand flies using one MALDI-TOF MS reference database and two mass spectrometer systems. Parasit Vectors. 2015;8:266.
10. Lafri I, Almeras L, Bitam I, Caputo A, Yssouf A, Forestier CL, et al. Identification of Algerian field-caught phlebotomine sand fly vectors by MALDI-TOF MS. PLoS Negl Trop Dis. 2016;10:e0004351.
11. Hoppenheit A, Murugaiyan J, Bauer B, Steuber S, Clausen PH, Roesler U. Identification of tsetse (*Glossina* spp.) using matrix-assisted laser desorption/ionisation time of flight mass spectrometry. PLoS Negl Trop Dis. 2013;7:e2305.
12. Kaufmann C, Schaffner F, Ziegler D, Pflüger V, Mathis A. Identification of field-caught *Culicoides* biting midges using matrix-assisted laser desorption/ionization time of flight mass spectrometry. Parasitology. 2012;139:248–58.
13. Yssouf A, Socolovschi C, Leulmi H, Kernif T, Bitam I, Audoly G, et al. Identification of flea species using MALDI-TOF/MS. Comp. Immunol Microbiol Infect Dis. 2014;37:153–7.
14. Karger A, Kampen H, Bettin B, Dautel H, Ziller M, Hoffmann B, et al. Species determination and characterization of developmental stages of ticks by whole-animal matrix-assisted laser desorption/ionization mass spectrometry. Ticks Tick Borne Dis. 2012;3:78–89.

15. Kumsa B, Laroche M, Almeras L, Mediannikov O, Raoult D, Parola P. Morphological, molecular and MALDI-TOF mass spectrometry identification of ixodid tick species collected in Oromia, Ethiopia. Parasitol Res. 2016;115:4199–210.
16. Dieme C, Yssouf A, Vega-Rúa A, Berenger J-M, Failloux A-B, Raoult D, et al. Accurate identification of Culicidae at aquatic developmental stages by MALDI-TOF MS profiling. Parasit Vectors. 2014;7:544.
17. Suter T, Flacio E, Fariña BF, Engeler L, Tonolla M, Müller P. First report of the invasive mosquito species *Aedes koreicus* in the Swiss-Italian border region. Parasit Vectors. 2015;8:402.
18. Müller P, Pflüger V, Wittwer M, Ziegler D, Chandre F, Simard F, et al. Identification of cryptic *Anopheles* mosquito species by molecular protein profiling. PLoS One. 2013;8:e57486.
19. Nebbak A, El Hamzaoui B, Berenger JM, Bitam I, Raoult D, Almeras L, et al. Comparative analysis of storage conditions and homogenization methods for tick and flea species for identification by MALDI-TOF MS. Med Vet Entomol. 2017;31:438–48.
20. Nebbak A, Willcox AC, Bitam I, Raoult D, Parola P, Almeras L. Standardization of sample homogenization for mosquito identification using an innovative proteomic tool based on protein profiling. Proteomics. 2016;16:3148–60.
21. Yssouf A, Socolovschi C, Flaudrops C, Ndiath MO, Sougoufara S, Dehecq JS, et al. Matrix-assisted laser desorption ionization - time of flight mass spectrometry: an emerging tool for the rapid identification of mosquito vectors. PLoS One. 2013;8:e72380.
22. Yssouf A, Almeras L, Raoult D, Parola P. Emerging tools for identification of arthropod vectors. Future Microbiol. 2016;11:549–66.
23. Niare S, Berenger J-M, Dieme C, Doumbo O, Raoult D, Parola P, et al. Identification of blood meal sources in the main African malaria mosquito vector by MALDI-TOF MS. Malar J. 2016;15:87.
24. Niare S, Tandina F, Davoust B, Doumbo O, Raoult D, Parola P, et al. Accurate identification of *Anopheles gambiae* Giles trophic preferences by MALDI-TOF MS. Infect Genet Evol. 2017;63:410–9.
25. Fansiri T, Fontaine A, Diancourt L, Caro V, Thaisomboonsuk B, Richardson JH, et al. Genetic mapping of specific interactions between *Aedes aegypti* mosquitoes and dengue viruses. PLoS Genet. 2013;9:e1003621.
26. Vega-Rua A, Zouache K, Girod R, Failloux AB, Lourenco-de-Oliveira R. High level of vector competence of *Aedes aegypti* and *Aedes albopictus* from ten American countries as a crucial factor in the spread of chikungunya virus. J Virol. 2014;88:6294–306.
27. Chouin-Carneiro T, Vega-Rua A, Vazeille M, Yebakima A, Girod R, Goindin D, et al. Differential susceptibilities of *Aedes aegypti* and *Aedes albopictus* from the Americas to Zika virus. PLoS Negl Trop Dis. 2016;10:e0005453.
28. Williams MR, Savage HM. Identification of *Culex* (*Melanoconion*) species of the United States using female cibarial armature (Diptera: Culicidae). J Med Entomol. 2009;46:745–52.
29. Belkin JN, Heinemann SJ. Collection records of the project "Mosquitoes of Middle America." 3. Bahama Is. (BAH), Cayman Is. (CAY), Cuba (CUB), Haiti (HAC, HAR, HAT) and Lesser Antilles (LAR). Mosq Syst. 1975;7:367–93.
30. Belkin JN, Heinemann SJ. Collection records of the project "Mosquitoes of Middle America." 4. Leeward Islands: Anguilla (ANG), Antigua (ANT), Barbuda (BAB), Montserrat (MNT), Nevis (NVS), St. Kitts (KIT). Mosq Syst. 1976;8:123–62.
31. Laurito M, Ayala AM, Almirón WR, Gardenal CN. Molecular identification of two *Culex* (*Culex*) species of the neotropical region (Diptera: Culicidae). PLoS One. 2017;12:e0173052.
32. Versteirt V, Nagy ZT, Roelants P, Denis L, Breman FC, Damiens D, et al. Identification of Belgian mosquito species (Diptera: Culicidae) by DNA barcoding. Mol Ecol Resour. 2015;15:449–57.
33. Batovska J, Blacket MJ, Brown K, Lynch SE. Molecular identification of mosquitoes (Diptera: Culicidae) in southeastern Australia. Ecol Evol. 2016;6:3001–11.
34. Sawadago S, Costantini C, Pennetier C, Diabate A, Gibson G, Dabire R. Differences in timing of mating swarms in sympatric populations of *Anopheles coluzzii* and *Anopheles gambiae s.s.* (formerly *An. gambiae* M and S molecular forms) in Burkina Faso, West Africa. Parasit Vectors. 2013;6:275.
35. Boyer PH, Boulanger N, Nebbak A, Collin E, Jaulhac B, Almeras L. Assessment of MALDI-TOF MS biotyping for *Borrelia burgdorferi s.l.* detection in *Ixodes ricinus*. PLoS One. 2017;12:e0185430.
36. Tahir D, Almeras L, Varloud M, Raoult D, Davoust B, Parola P. Assessment of MALDI-TOF mass spectrometry for filariae detection in *Aedes aegypti* mosquitoes. PLoS Negl Trop Dis. 2017;11:e0006093.
37. Theobald F. A monograph of the Culicidae, or mosquitoes. London: British Museum (Natural History); 1901.
38. Clark-Gil S, Darsie R. The mosquitoes of Guatemala. Their identification, distribution and bionomics, with keys to adult females and larvae. Mosq. Syst. 1983;15:151–284.
39. Darsie RF. The occurrence of *Psorophora cingulata* and *Uranotaenia apicalis* in Guatemala (Diptera: Culicidae). Mosq Syst. 1983;15:28–32.
40. Goindin D, Delannay C, Gelasse A, Ramdini C, Gaude T, Faucon F, et al. Levels of insecticide resistance to deltamethrin, malathion, and temephos, and associated mechanisms in *Aedes aegypti* mosquitoes from the Guadeloupe and Saint Martin islands (French West Indies). Infect Dis Poverty. 2017;6:38.
41. Tahir D, Davoust B, Almeras L, Berenger JM, Varloud M, Parola P. Anti-feeding and insecticidal efficacy of a topical administration of dinotefuran–pyriproxyfen–permethrin spot-on (Vectra® 3D) on mice against *Stegomyia albopicta* (= *Aedes albopictus*). Med Vet Entomol. 2017;31:351–7.
42. Nebbak A, Koumare S, Willcox AC, Berenger JM, Raoult D, Almeras L, et al. Field application of MALDI-TOF MS on mosquito larvae identification. Parasitology. 2017;145:677–87.
43. Folmer O, Black M, Hoeh W, Lutz R, Vrijenhoek R. DNA primers for amplification of mitochondrial cytochrome c oxidase subunit I from diverse metazoan invertebrates. Mol Mar Biol Biotechnol. 1994;3:294–9.
44. Ratnasingham S, Hebert PDN. bold: The Barcode of Life Data System (http://www.barcodinglife.org). Mol Ecol Notes. 2007;7:355–64.
45. Diarra AZ, Almeras L, Laroche M, Berenger JM, Koné AK, Bocoum Z, et al. Molecular and MALDI-TOF identification of ticks and tick-associated bacteria in Mali. PLoS Negl Trop Dis. 2017;11:e0005762.

3

Diverse target gene modifications in *Plasmodium falciparum* using Bxb1 integrase and an intronic *attB*

Praveen Balabaskaran-Nina[1,2] and Sanjay A. Desai[1*]

Abstract

Genetic manipulation of the human malaria parasite *Plasmodium falciparum* is needed to explore pathogen biology and evaluate antimalarial targets. It is, however, aggravated by a low transfection efficiency, a paucity of selectable markers and a biased A/T-rich genome. While various enabling technologies have been introduced over the past two decades, facile and broad-range modification of essential genes remains challenging. We recently devised a new application of the Bxb1 integrase strategy to meet this need through an intronic *attB* sequence within the gene of interest. Although this *attB* is silent and without effect on intron splicing or protein translation and function, it allows efficient gene modification with minimal risk of unwanted changes at other genomic sites. We describe the range of applications for this new method as well as specific cases where it is preferred over CRISPR-Cas9 and other technologies. The advantages and limitations of various strategies for endogenous gene editing are also discussed.

Keywords: Malaria, DNA transfection, Intron, Bxb1 integrase, Gene editing

Background

Despite advances from combination therapies and public health measures such as bednets, more than 400,000 people still die of malaria annually. Since *Plasmodium falciparum*, a virulent human malaria parasite, acquires resistance to most antimalarial drugs quickly, new drug targets and a better understanding of resistance mechanisms are needed to sustain advances in global health. These goals depend on transfection studies in cultured *P. falciparum* parasites [1–3]. Because transfection efficiencies are low, selectable markers are required; the available markers have facilitated functional analyses [4], but their relatively small number adds to the difficulties faced in molecular and biochemical studies of this pathogen.

Gene manipulation in this system requires single or double crossover homologous recombination into the haploid genome as the parasite lacks the enzymes to carryout non-homologous end joining. Historically, these experiments relied on infrequent, coincidental genome breaks at or near the target site, often necessitating many months of continuous cultivation and drug-cycling to obtain detectable levels of integration [5]. Further aggravating this process, the circular plasmids required for stable retention in transfected parasites tend to concatemerize under drug selection, reducing the likelihood of integration and complicating interpretation of some phenotypes [6, 7].

Subsequent implementation of *piggyBac* transposase and mycobacteriophage Bxb1 integrase facilitated stable integration of transgenes and reporters [8, 9], but these approaches have not been used to edit specific genes of interest. The advent of sequence-specific nucleases then opened the door to directed gene editing in *P. falciparum*, with zinc finger nucleases (ZFN) and clustered regulatory interspaced short palindromic repeats (CRISPRs) successfully used to study parasite biology [10–15]. Gene editing with ZFN is expensive and requires a new enzyme design for each target locus. As with many other organisms, CRISPR-Cas9 is quickly becoming the preferred strategy because of simplicity and cost, but several important

* Correspondence: sdesai@niaid.nih.gov
[1]The Laboratory of Malaria and Vector Research, National Institute of Allergy and Infectious Diseases, National Institutes of Health, Rockville, MD 20852, USA
Full list of author information is available at the end of the article

concerns prevent the full spectrum of molecular modifications. Among these, off-target effects due to Cas9-mediated cleavage at unwanted genomic sites and the dependence on specific recognition motifs (known as protospacer adjacent motifs or PAMs) are considered the most problematic in many organisms [16].

To address these concerns and to add another option for DNA transfection in *P. falciparum*, we recently implemented a novel application of the Bxb1 integrase transposition technology to permit targeted gene replacements [17]. Our approach achieves rapid site-specific integration, allows the full spectrum of native gene modifications, and has a distinct set of advantages when compared to other methods including CRISPR-Cas9. Our strategy is based on the introduction of a silent *attB* element into an intron of the target gene; we found that this 40 bp insertion is well-tolerated as it does not adversely affect either intron splicing or subsequent translation and function of the encoded protein. Once integrated, this *attB* element permits rapid recombination with an *attP* site on subsequent transfection plasmids to replace the downstream sequence with desired modifications. Although our strategy requires an additional transfection to first introduce the *attB* site, it then enables an unlimited array of distal modifications including site-directed mutations, insertions, deletions, epitope tagging, and conditional knockdown through the introduction of ddFKBP or EcDHFR-based destabilization domains, the TetR aptamer module, or the *glmS* riboswitch [18–21]. After describing our procedures, we summarize the advantages and limitations of this approach when compared to currently available methods.

Mechanism of *attB-attP* recombination and conventional application in *P. falciparum*

Bxb1 integrase is a mycobacteriophage serine integrase that catalyses recombination between an *attP* sequence in the phage and an *attB* sequence in the *Mycobacterium smegmatis groEL1* gene with minimal fully effective sequences of 48 and 38 bp, respectively. This recombination enables phage integration into the bacterial genome [22–24]. Recombination begins when Bxb1 dimers bind to each of these sites with high affinity (K_d estimated at 70 nM); these dimers then interact with each other to form a synaptic tetramer, a process known as synapsis [25]. All four DNA strands are then cleaved within a central 8 bp core conserved between *attB* and *attP* (Fig. 1a); cleavage occurs asymmetrically at a non-palindromic 5'-GT dinucleotide to ensure faithful exchange of phage *attP* and bacterial *attB* sequences and prevent incorrect joining of half-sites [24]. A conserved serine in Bxb1 forms a

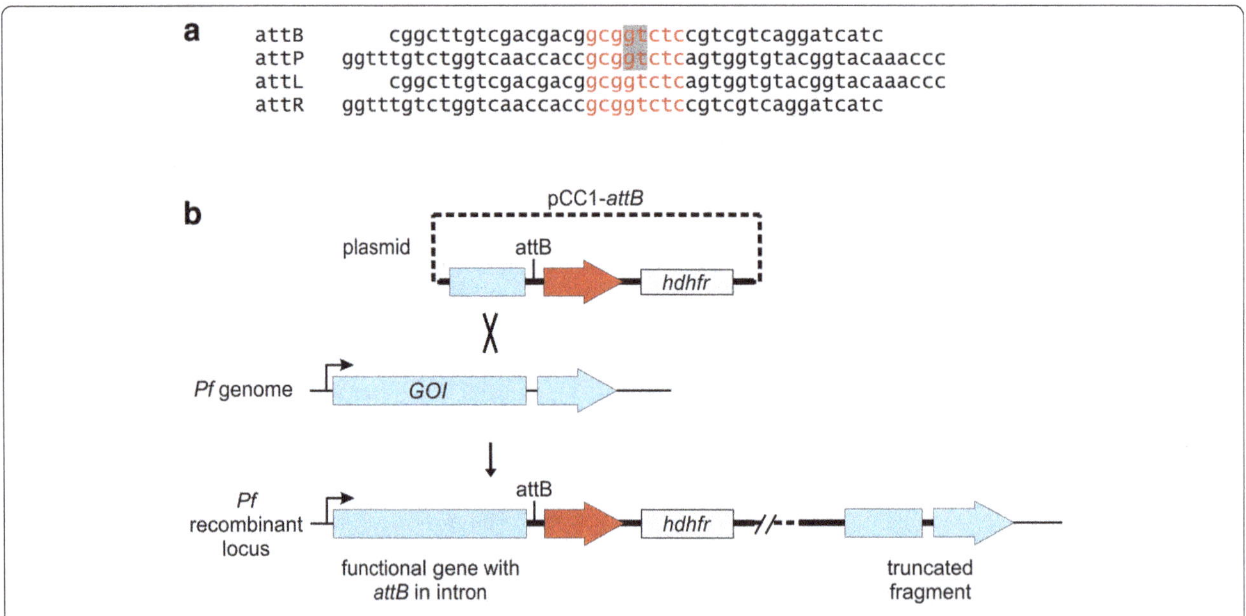

Fig. 1 Introduction of silent *attB* element to enable gene editing. **a** Sequences of *attB* and *attP* used in *P. falciparum* transfections. Integrase-mediated recombination yields *attL* and *attR* elements as shown. The conserved 8 bp core sequence is shown in red; a non-palindromic 5'-GT dinucleotide (grey highlight) prevents self-ligation after cleavage by Bxb1 integrase and promotes efficient strand exchange. **b** Strategy for introducing *attB* into the intron of a gene of interest (GOI). The *pCC1-attB* plasmid carries an upstream sequence (light blue) to facilitate homologous recombination into the parasite genome, an intron with an inserted *attB*, and a recodonized version of the remainder of the gene (red). The *hdhfr* cassette permits selection of successfully transfected parasites. Recombination of the plasmid into the parasite genome yields the required *attB*-carrying parasite without affecting target gene transcription or associated phenotypes

covalent bond with the cleaved DNA, allowing rotation and re-ligation of the two double-stranded DNA polymers. The resulting sites, termed *attL* and *attR*, differ from one another and do not match the original *attB* and *attP* elements as they carry swapped flanking sequences. This reaction is generally considered irreversible, but auxiliary proteins known as the recombination directionality factors (RDFs) can facilitate the reverse reaction and excision of the phage from the host genome [26]. Structural studies have revealed extensive contacts between the recombinase domain, an unusual zinc ribbon domain, and *att* sequences that confer specificity for *attB-attP* recombination and prevent the reverse *attL-attR* recombination reaction [27]. Kinetic and mutagenesis experiments have led to a model of highly coordinated formation of a synaptic complex between a tetrameric recombinase complex and two *att* sites, controlled cleavage and rotation, hybridization and religation [28–31]. When compared to tyrosine integrases, serine integrases do not require DNA super coiling, divalent cations or bacterial host factors for integrase activity, making their use in heterologous systems more attractive.

Nkrumah et al. [9] demonstrated this system's utility in malaria parasites by showing efficient recombination of an *attP*-containing plasmid with an engineered *attB* in the parasite genome; Bxb1 integrase was expressed from a co-transfected helper plasmid. The *attB* sequence, otherwise not present in *P. falciparum*, was introduced into the nonessential *cg6* gene; several such *cg6-attB* lines have been generated in distinct genetic backgrounds [32]. These studies reported a rapid appearance of recombinants with a near-homogeneous population of integrant parasites within 2–4 weeks of the second transfection [9]. Nevertheless, several concerns have limited the utility of this technology. Most importantly, in cases where the desired transgene on the *attP* plasmid is a modified version of a parasite gene, the endogenous copy is not affected by transfection and is expected to remain functional, yielding a merodiploid whose phenotype may be more difficult to study. Expression levels for the transgene may also confound interpretation: genomic site effects due to expression from a heterologous *cg6* locus or concatemerization of the *attP* plasmid prior to integration may lead to unanticipated transcript levels. Another concern is that the phenotype under study may be affected by disruption of the *cg6* gene. Production of lines that carry *attB* at nonessential loci other than *cg6* could address some of these concerns, but this has not been undertaken to our knowledge.

While Cre recombinase, a distinct phage recombinase from the tyrosine integrase family [33], has been used in various parasites [34–36], use of Bxb1 integrase has not been described for Apicomplexan parasites other than *Plasmodium* spp.

Integrase strategy for native gene manipulation in *Plasmodium falciparum*

To address these limitations and enable rapid and essentially unlimited manipulation of an endogenous parasite gene, we devised and used a modified version of this Bxb1 integrase strategy [17]. Our approach entails introducing *attB* into an intron of the gene of interest (Fig. 1b); we found that this relatively short element did not adversely affect mRNA splicing, transcription or translation of *clag3*, an intensively studied gene linked to malaria parasite nutrient uptake [37–39]. As changes to the intronic sequence are silent, the encoded protein should be faithfully translated without mutation or changes in associated phenotypes. Consistent with this prediction, our studies with the *clag3* target revealed expression of a full-length unmodified protein, unchanged trafficking of the encoded protein to the host membrane, and preserved channel-mediated solute uptake and pharmacology [17]. As knockdown or modification of the *clag3* gene product is associated with a significant fitness cost [40, 41], these findings suggest that most essential genes will tolerate addition of an intronic *attB* sequence.

We envision that this approach will be broadly applicable to study of *P. falciparum* genes. Approximately half of this parasite's genes have one or more introns with a small average size, 179 bp [42], simplifying addition of *attB* and *attP* sequences. This cloning step can be performed either through DNA synthesis or through hybridization of complementary oligonucleotides in cases where the introns are small. Consistent with previous additions of short sequences to this parasite's introns [43], these small silent insertions are generally well-tolerated in *P. falciparum*. Although we have not examined the effect of position within the intron systematically, we suggest a central placement within the intron and preferably at least 60 nucleotides upstream of the 3' end of the intron as splicing branch points have been observed up to 57 nucleotides from the 3' intron-exon boundary [42]. For genes that lack introns, insertion of a heterologous intron carrying the *attB* sequence into the open reading frame (ORF) offers excellent prospects for introduction of a silent *attB* without requiring modifying the encoded protein's sequence; our *clag3 attB* intron has been validated and should work in most cases based on studies confirming faithful recognition and splicing of heterologous introns [43].

We originally introduced the *attB*-loaded intron into *clag3 via* single crossover recombination, but this may be simplified by CRISPR-Cas9 transfection with a donor plasmid that contains homology arms of 200–300 bp on either side of the intron; if CRISPR-Cas9 is used, it is critical to select the single guide RNA (sgRNA) and cleavage site carefully with proximity to the intron and on-target efficiency score the most critical factors in *P. falciparum* transfections [44]. After parasites grow out in this first transfection, it is important to use limiting dilution cloning to obtain a clonal population carrying the *attB* sequence. Although some workers have argued that limiting dilution cloning is not required because subpopulations without this integration event will be removed by cloning after the second transfection, we caution against this because genome-level modifications at non-target sites may grow preferentially in the second transfection, aggravating attempts to identify the desired final clone.

After the silent *attB* site has been successfully introduced, the full range of target gene modifications can be generated with a second transfection with two plasmids (Fig. 2a, pLN-*attP* and pINT). The pLN-*attP* plasmid carries the *attP* element followed by the distal intronic sequence with a 3' splice site for faithful splicing after integration. Any sequence following this *attP*-intron will be inserted into the genome upon *attB-attP* recombination as facilitated by the Bxb1 integrase expressed from the pINT helper plasmid.

The use of a silent *attB* in a target gene's intron distinguishes our approach from previous use of this technology in malaria research and has two important consequences. It disrupts the target gene by inserting the entire pLN-*attP* plasmid in the gene after the modified intron. It also achieves a promoter-trap because the sequence inserted distal to the intron upon recombination will be spliced in frame behind the native promoter and gene sequence upstream of the intron. Thus, the outcome in most cases is an effective gene replacement.

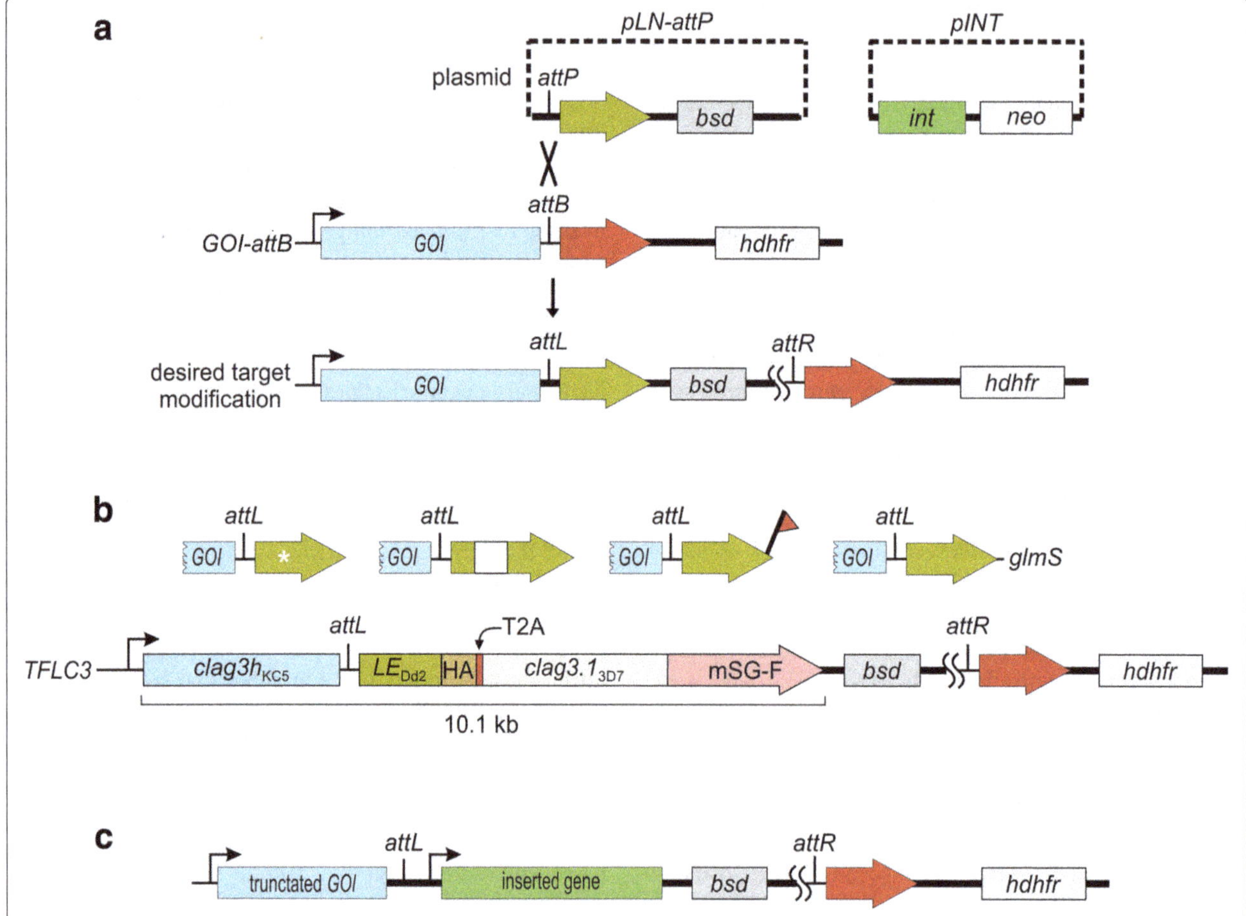

Fig. 2 A broad range of gene modifications using the intronic *attB*. **a** Strategy for Bxb1 integrase-mediated recombination to produce diverse changes to a target gene. The *pLN-attP* plasmid carries the *attP* element, the downstream intronic sequence and desired downstream modifications. *bsd*, *neo* and *hdhfr* are selectable markers; *int* represents Bxb1 integrase gene as expressed from the *pINT* helper plasmid. Transfection of the *GOI-attB* parasite replaces the downstream ORF (red arrow) with a desired modification (yellow arrow) of the gene of interest (*GOI*). Recombination between *attB* and *attP* elements yields *attL* and *attR* sites. **b** Example modifications. Top row shows a site-directed mutation, an insertion, an epitope tag, and the *glmS* riboswitch in the 3' untranslated region (left to right, respectively). Second row shows production of the *TFLC3* parasite expressing two full-length CLAG3 proteins (Dd2 and 3D7 isoforms) with distinct epitope tags (HA and mSG-F) under a single *clag3* promoter; the two proteins are separated during translation through insertion of a viral skip peptide (T2A, [52]). **c** Gene replacement approach showing insertion of a full-length gene with promoter and terminator sequences after the silent *attB*. This approach simultaneously disrupts the *GOI* and integrates a cloned gene downstream of the target site

In one application, this distal sequence could be the remainder of the gene with desired modifications. These modifications may include site-directed mutations, internal insertions or deletions (indels), domain swaps, addition of C-terminal epitope tags on the encoded protein, modified codon usage, and/or altered transcriptional regulatory elements (e.g. removal of distal introns or addition of the *glmS* riboswitch into the 3' untranslated region). To demonstrate the range of possible modifications, we reported the production of a merodiploid parasite that expresses two CLAG3 proteins with distinct functional properties and separate epitope tags using this approach; although these *clag3* genes are large (5.3 kb each) and we desired distinct epitope tags on two proteins expressed under a single promoter, our strategy and use of the *clag3-attB* line permitted facile introduction with a single plasmid (Fig. 2b, *TFLC3*; [17]).

In another application, the promoter trap enabled by the silent *attB*-intron is disregarded, and the pLN-*attP* plasmid may carry an entire gene cassette with required 5' and 3' untranslated regions (Fig. 2c). This may be particularly useful for examining whether other genes (e.g. paralogs) can adequately replace essential activities of the target gene carrying the *attB*-intron. For such applications, an important caveat is that the sequence upstream of the intron will typically still be transcribed and translated, yielding a truncated protein. For large genes such as *clag3*, the effect of the residual upstream protein may be significant, yielding either preserved activity or a dominant-negative effect due to protein-protein interactions with the truncated protein. This theoretical concern may be largely avoided by introducing the *attB* into an intron near the start of the target gene. If such an intron is not available, a heterologous *attB*-containing intron may be inserted at any desired position as described above.

Comparison to other methods available for targeted gene modifications

While there are several methods for expression of transgenes in *P. falciparum* [45], there are only a few options for directed modification of a target gene of interest. Table 1 summarizes these options along with the required components, advantages and limitations of each method. Although CRISPR-Cas9 is the most straightforward to implement and allows rapid gene editing suitable for most applications [11, 12, 44], use of Bxb1 integrase with an engineered intronic *attB* site may be preferred for large insertions and has several other advantages.

Our use of an intronic *attB* site resembles the recent description of *loxP* insertion into introns for conditional editing of a target gene [43], but there are important differences that confer greater versatility to *attB-attP* technology. Both use a target gene intron to introduce short DNA elements that enable enzyme-mediated DNA recombination. The DiCre-*loxP* system sites uses two halves of Cre recombinase linked to distinct rapamycin binding proteins; addition of rapamycin stimulates dimerization of the two halves, allowing conditional Cre activity and recombination at two properly oriented *loxP* sites. This system permits conditional knockout or modification such as addition of an epitope tag or site-directed mutation [43]. The main strength of this system relative to our *attB*-intron system is that it allows conditional modifications dependent on small molecule addition. At the same time, a key limitation is that facilitated recombination between the two *loxP* sites is reversible, in contrast to irreversible recombination between *attB* and *attP* sites [26]. This reversibility prevents use of a single initial transfectant with a *loxP*-intron for multiple distinct modifications: a plasmid carrying a *loxP* with desired distal modifications, analogous to our pLN-*attP* plasmid (Fig. 2a), would likely undergo cycles of integration and excision due to the reversibility of *loxP* recombination. This results in an inefficient integration reaction; although various strategies have been devised to overcome this inefficiency [46], these have not been implemented in malaria research to our knowledge. Thus, multiple distinct modifications cannot be performed with a single engineered *loxP* parasite: each desired modification requires a *de novo* transfection to introduce the *loxP*-intron cassette into the parasite genome.

As increasingly acknowledged by workers, CRISPR-Cas9 technology will be the method of choice for most gene modifications in *P. falciparum*. This system largely bypasses the need for introduction of DNA motifs such as *attB* or *attP*; it requires expression of Cas9, an RNA-guided endonuclease, and a small single-stranded RNA molecule known as the single guide RNA or sgRNA to achieve site-specific modification of the genome [47]. The sgRNA binds Cas9 and identifies the cleavage site through Watson-Crick base pairing over a 20 bp recognition sequence; gene editing results from blunt-end cleavage within the recognition sequence. Although a protospacer adjacent domain (PAM) must be present immediately after the chosen recognition sequence, there are nearly 663,000 canonical PAM sites in the *P. falciparum* genome [44]; thus, almost any genomic site can be targeted. Nevertheless, we considered two important cases where CRISPR-Cas9 may not be the ideal method for target gene modifications. One problematic situation arises when a gene of interest is a member of a multigene family. If the site to be modified in the target gene is conserved amongst paralogs that should not be edited, it may be difficult to find an sgRNA that does not cleave one or more of these paralogs; such "off-target" cleavage sites may be predicted and avoided with a newly devised paralog specificity score [44]. If multiple modifications of a target gene are envisioned, use of the CRISPR system may still require

Table 1 Strategies for target gene modification in *P. falciparum*

Method	Mechanism	Required elements	Advantages	Key limitations
Single or double crossover (with or without SLI)	Homologous recombination between a targeting sequence on transfection plasmid and the gene of interest	1 or 2 large homology arms on the plasmid	(i) Does not require expression of heterologous nucleases or enzymes; (ii) The foundation of allelic replacement strategies in malaria research	(i) Depends on coincidental genome breaks near the target; (ii) Cannot prevent gradual loss of the desired modification due to plasmid loop-out (avoided by SLI); (iii) Requires months, usually with rounds of drug cycling to select for genomic integration (reduced with SLI)
Zinc-finger nuclease (ZFN)	Engineered ZFN produces a double-stranded break, which is repaired by homologous recombination with plasmid	(i) Custom engineered ZFN for each target site; (ii) 2 homology arms for HDR, typically on a separate plasmid	(i) Rapid gene editing; (ii) No sequence-specific restrictions such as PAM; (iii) Longer track-record of use than CRISPR-Cas9, including clinical trials in humans	(i) Expensive; (ii) Requires custom ZFN production for each target site; (iii) Off-target nuclease activity may be comparable to CRISPR-Cas9
CRISPR-Cas9	sgRNA directs Cas9 nuclease to produce a double-stranded break, which is repaired by homologous recombination with plasmid	(i) Cas9 nuclease; (ii) sgRNA expressed under a U6 promoter or by heterologous T7 polymerase; (iii) 2 homology arms for HDR, typically on a separate plasmid	(i) Rapid gene editing (ii) Easy to implement in most labs	(i) Cleavage limited to sites adjacent to PAM sequence; (ii) Requires careful consideration of on-target efficiency score for optimal design; (iii) Off-target cleavage
Bxb1 integrase and intronic *attB*	*attB* introduced into target gene intron (or via an engineered synthetic intron) undergoes specific recombination with *attP* element on transfection plasmid, facilitated by Bxb1 integrase	(i) Intronic *attB*; (ii) Bxb1 integrase; (iii) Desired gene modification is placed distal to *attP* on plasmid	(i) Rapid gene editing; (ii) Allows diverse modifications on a gene of interest; (iii) Does not depend on HDR, so avoids cloning of AT-rich homology arms; (iv) Little or no risk of off-target recombination; (v) Permits larger target site insertions than CRISPR-Cas9	(i) Requires production of cloned parasite with intronic *attB* for each gene of interest; (ii) Location of intronic *attB* within the target gene must be carefully selected to enable desired gene modifications

greater effort and cost because confident production of each modification will require screening of limiting dilution clones to identify parasites with the desired target gene modification and no unwanted edits to paralogs. The *attB*-intron strategy reduces labor and expense because the identification of a clone without unwanted *attB* introduction into paralogs need only be done once: subsequent transfections with *attP*-containing plasmids will then be highly specific for the desired target gene, confidently avoiding paralogs.

Even for genes not within multigene families, off-target effects remain a concern with CRISPR-Cas9 editing because the Cas9 nuclease can recognize and cleave at sites carrying one or more mismatches relative to the selected 20 bp recognition sequence. This limitation has led to the development of predictive off-target scoring algorithms and Cas9 mutants with ongoing improvements in specificity [16, 48]. The targeted genome break produced by Cas9 nuclease may also lead to chromosome repair by production of large deletions or more complex rearrangements [49], although these have not been reported to date in malaria research. Promiscuous recombination and target site rearrangements have not been reported with the Bxb1 integrase, presumably because of the highly coordinated *attB-attP* recombination process [50].

Another important case where the *attB*-intron strategy will be preferred over technologies such as CRISPR-Cas9 and selection-linked integration (SLI, [51]) is exemplified by the production of a parasite carrying two *clag3* genes under the native promoter (*TLFC3* parasite in Fig. 2b). SLI selects specifically for homologous recombination at the target site by using a promoter trap to drive expression of the selectable marker gene. Because both CRISPR-Cas9 and SLI depend on homologous recombination, both would require fully re-codonized versions of the two *clag3* genes to produce *TFLC3* to avoid internal recombination events that bypass introduction of desired tags on the two *clag3* alleles ("HA" and "mSG-F" in Fig. 2b *TFLC3* ribbon). This re-codonization would require custom synthesis of a 6.3 kb DNA, which is both prohibitively expensive and time-consuming for most research labs.

Conclusions

DNA transfection technologies represent an important tool for basic and translational malaria research. We remain limited by a low transfection efficiency, relatively slow parasite replication, a paucity of selection markers, and other difficulties specific to this important pathogen. Ongoing improvements in the methods available for generating parasite lines with desired genome modifications make this is an exciting time for malaria research. While CRISPR-Cas9 is currently the method-of-choice for most gene editing experiments, other strategies such as our *attB*-intron method should be considered, especially for labs that have committed to specific genes and require a broad collection of gene modifications for biochemical and/or structural studies.

Abbreviations

Bsd: Blasticidin S deaminase selectable marker; Cas9: CRISPR associated protein 9; *Clag3*: Cytoadherence linked asexual gene 3; CRISPR: Clustered regularly interspaced short palindromic repeats; GOI: Gene of interest; *hdhfr*: Human dihydrofolate reductase selectable marker; HDR: Homology directed repair; indels: Internal insertions or deletions; *neo*: Neomycin selectable marker; ORF: Open reading frame; PAM: Protospacer adjacent motif; sgRNA: Single guide RNA; SLI: Selection linked integration; *TFLC3*: Tandem full-length *clag3* parasite; ZFN: Zinc finger nuclease

Funding

This work was supported by the Intramural Research Program of National Institutes of Health (NIH), National Institute of Allergy and Infectious Diseases (NIAID), USA.

Authors' contributions

PBN drafted the first version of the manuscript. Both authors edited, read and approved the final manuscript.

Competing interests

The authors declare that they have no competing interests.

Author details

[1]The Laboratory of Malaria and Vector Research, National Institute of Allergy and Infectious Diseases, National Institutes of Health, Rockville, MD 20852, USA. [2]Present Address: Department of Epidemiology and Public Health, Central University of Tamil Nadu, Thiruvarur, India.

References

1. Waterkeyn JG, Crabb BS, Cowman AF. Transfection of the human malaria parasite *Plasmodium falciparum*. Int J Parasitol. 1999;29:945–55.
2. Gardiner DL, Skinner-Adams TS, Spielmann T, Trenholme KR. Malaria transfection and transfection vectors. Trends Parasitol. 2003;19:381–3.
3. Balu B, Adams JH. Advancements in transfection technologies for *Plasmodium*. Int J Parasitol. 2007;37:1–10.
4. Mamoun CB, Gluzman IY, Goyard S, Beverley SM, Goldberg DE. A set of independent selectable markers for transfection of the human malaria parasite *Plasmodium falciparum*. Proc Natl Acad Sci USA. 1999;96:8716–20.
5. Crabb BS, Rug M, Gilberger TW, Thompson JK, Triglia T, Maier AG, et al. Transfection of the human malaria parasite *Plasmodium falciparum*. Methods Mol Biol. 2004;270:263–76.
6. Kadekoppala M, Cheresh P, Catron D, Ji D, Deitsch K, Wellems TE, et al. Rapid recombination among transfected plasmids, chimeric episome formation and trans gene expression in *Plasmodium falciparum*. Mol Biochem Parasitol. 2001;112:211–8.
7. O'Donnell RA, Preiser PR, Williamson DH, Moore PW, Cowman AF, Crabb BS. An alteration in concatameric structure is associated with efficient segregation of plasmids in transfected *Plasmodium falciparum* parasites. Nucleic Acids Res. 2001;29:716–24.
8. Balu B, Adams JH. Functional genomics of *Plasmodium falciparum* through transposon-mediated mutagenesis. Cell Microbiol. 2006;8:1529–36.

9. Nkrumah LJ, Muhle RA, Moura PA, Ghosh P, Hatfull GF, Jacobs WR Jr, Fidock DA. Efficient site-specific integration in *Plasmodium falciparum* chromosomes mediated by mycobacteriophage Bxb1 integrase. Nat Methods. 2006;3:615–21.
10. Straimer J, Lee MC, Lee AH, Zeitler B, Williams AE, Pearl JR, et al. Site-specific genome editing in *Plasmodium falciparum* using engineered zinc-finger nucleases. Nat Methods. 2012;9:993–8.
11. Ghorbal M, Gorman M, Macpherson CR, Martins RM, Scherf A, Lopez-Rubio JJ. Genome editing in the human malaria parasite *Plasmodium falciparum* using the CRISPR-Cas9 system. Nat Biotechnol. 2014;32:819–21.
12. Wagner JC, Platt RJ, Goldfless SJ, Zhang F, Niles JC. Efficient CRISPR-Cas9-mediated genome editing in *Plasmodium falciparum*. Nat Methods. 2014;11:915–8.
13. Veiga MI, Dhingra SK, Henrich PP, Straimer J, Gnadig N, Uhlemann AC, et al. Globally prevalent PfMDR1 mutations modulate *Plasmodium falciparum* susceptibility to artemisinin-based combination therapies. Nat Commun. 2016;7:11553.
14. Ito D, Schureck MA, Desai SA. An essential dual-function complex mediates erythrocyte invasion and channel-mediated nutrient uptake in malaria parasites. Elife. 2017;6:e23485.
15. Bansal A, Molina-Cruz A, Brzostowski J, Mu J, Miller LH. *Plasmodium falciparum* calcium-dependent protein kinase 2 is critical for male gametocyte exflagellation but not essential for asexual proliferation. MBio. 2017;8:e01656–17.
16. Doench JG, Fusi N, Sullender M, Hegde M, Vaimberg EW, Donovan KF, et al. Optimized sgRNA design to maximize activity and minimize off-target effects of CRISPR-Cas9. Nat Biotechnol. 2016;34:184–91.
17. Gupta A, Balabaskaran-Nina P, Nguitragool W, Saggu GS, Schureck MA, Desai SA. CLAG3 self-associates in malaria parasites and quantitatively determines nutrient uptake channels at the host membrane. mBio. 2018;9: e02293–17.
18. Armstrong CM, Goldberg DE. An FKBP destabilization domain modulates protein levels in *Plasmodium falciparum*. Nat Methods. 2007;4:1007–9.
19. Muralidharan V, Oksman A, Iwamoto M, Wandless TJ, Goldberg DE. Asparagine repeat function in a *Plasmodium falciparum* protein assessed via a regulatable fluorescent affinity tag. Proc Natl Acad Sci USA. 2011; 108:4411–6.
20. Ganesan SM, Falla A, Goldfless SJ, Nasamu AS, Niles JC. Synthetic RNA-protein modules integrated with native translation mechanisms to control gene expression in malaria parasites. Nat Commun. 2016;7:10727.
21. Prommana P, Uthaipibull C, Wongsombat C, Kamchonwongpaisan S, Yuthavong Y, Knuepfer E, et al. Inducible knockdown of *Plasmodium* gene expression using the *glmS* ribozyme. PLoS One. 2013;8:e73783.
22. Kim AI, Ghosh P, Aaron MA, Bibb LA, Jain S, Hatfull GF. Mycobacteriophage Bxb1 integrates into the *Mycobacterium smegmatis* groEL1 gene. Mol Microbiol. 2003;50:463–73.
23. Groth AC, Calos MP. Phage integrases: biology and applications. J Mol Biol. 2004;335:667–78.
24. Ghosh P, Bibb LA, Hatfull GF. Two-step site selection for serine-integrase-mediated excision: DNA-directed integrase conformation and central dinucleotide proofreading. Proc Natl Acad Sci USA. 2008;105:3238–43.
25. Rutherford K, Van Duyne GD. The ins and outs of serine integrase site-specific recombination. Curr Opin Struct Biol. 2014;24:125–31.
26. Ghosh P, Wasil LR, Hatfull GF. Control of phage Bxb1 excision by a novel recombination directionality factor. PLoS Biol. 2006;4:e186.
27. Rutherford K, Yuan P, Perry K, Sharp R, Van Duyne GD. Attachment site recognition and regulation of directionality by the serine integrases. Nucleic Acids Res. 2013;41:8341–56.
28. Keenholtz RA, Grindley ND, Hatfull GF, Marko JF. Crossover-site sequence and DNA torsional stress control strand interchanges by the Bxb1 site-specific serine recombinase. Nucleic Acids Res. 2016;44:8921–32.
29. Olorunniji FJ, McPherson AL, Rosser SJ, Smith MCM, Colloms SD, Stark WM. Control of serine integrase recombination directionality by fusion with the directionality factor. Nucleic Acids Res. 2017;45:8635–45.
30. Rowley PA, Smith MC, Younger E, Smith MC. A motif in the C-terminal domain of phiC31 integrase controls the directionality of recombination. Nucleic Acids Res. 2008;36:3879–91.
31. Farruggio AP, Calos MP. Serine integrase chimeras with activity in *E. coli* and HeLa cells. Biol Open. 2014;3:895–903.
32. Ke H, Morrisey JM, Ganesan SM, Painter HJ, Mather MW, Vaidya AB. Variation among *Plasmodium falciparum* strains in their reliance on mitochondrial electron transport chain function. Eukaryot Cell. 2011;10:1053–61.
33. Fogg PC, Colloms S, Rosser S, Stark M, Smith MC. New applications for phage integrases. J Mol Biol. 2014;426:2703–16.
34. Brecht S, Erdhart H, Soete M, Soldati D. Genome engineering of *Toxoplasma gondii* using the site-specific recombinase Cre. Gene. 1999;234:239–47.
35. Santos RERS, Silva GLA, Santos EV, Duncan SM, Mottram JC, Damasceno JD, et al. A DiCre recombinase-based system for inducible expression in *Leishmania major*. Mol Biochem Parasitol. 2017;216:45–8.
36. Wampfler PB, Faso C, Hehl AB. The Cre/*loxP* system in *Giardia lamblia*: genetic manipulations in a binucleate tetraploid protozoan. Int J Parasitol. 2014;44:497–506.
37. Nguitragool W, Bokhari AA, Pillai AD, Rayavara K, Sharma P, Turpin B, et al. Malaria parasite *clag3* genes determine channel-mediated nutrient uptake by infected red blood cells. Cell. 2011;145:665–77.
38. Rovira-Graells N, Crowley VM, Bancells C, Mira-Martinez S, Ribas de PL, Cortes A. Deciphering the principles that govern mutually exclusive expression of *Plasmodium falciparum clag3* genes. Nucleic Acids Res. 2015; 43:8243–57.
39. Nguitragool W, Rayavara K, Desai SA. Proteolysis at a specific extracellular residue implicates integral membrane CLAG3 in malaria parasite nutrient channels. PLoS One. 2014;9:e93759.
40. Sharma P, Wollenberg K, Sellers M, Zainabadi K, Galinsky K, Moss E, et al. An epigenetic antimalarial resistance mechanism involving parasite genes linked to nutrient uptake. J Biol Chem. 2013;288:19429–40.
41. Sharma P, Rayavara K, Ito D, Basore K, Desai SA. A CLAG3 mutation in an amphipathic transmembrane domain alters malaria parasite nutrient channels and confers leupeptin resistance. Infect Immun. 2015;83:2566–74.
42. Zhang X, Tolzmann CA, Melcher M, Haas BJ, Gardner MJ, Smith JD, et al. Branch point identification and sequence requirements for intron splicing in *Plasmodium falciparum*. Eukaryot Cell. 2011;10:1422–8.
43. Jones ML, Das S, Belda H, Collins CR, Blackman MJ, Treeck M. A versatile strategy for rapid conditional genome engineering using *loxP* sites in a small synthetic intron in *Plasmodium falciparum*. Sci Rep. 2016;6:21800.
44. Ribeiro JM, Garriga M, Potchen N, Crater AK, Gupta A, Ito D, et al. Guide RNA selection for CRISPR-Cas9 transfections in *Plasmodium falciparum*. Int J Parasitol. 2018. https://doi.org/10.1016/j.ijpara.2018.03.009.
45. de Koning-Ward TF, Gilson PR, Crabb BS. Advances in molecular genetic systems in malaria. Nat Rev Microbiol. 2015;13:373–87.
46. Araki K, Araki M, Yamamura K. Site-directed integration of the *cre* gene mediated by Cre recombinase using a combination of mutant *lox* sites. Nucleic Acids Res. 2002;30:e103.
47. Wright AV, Nunez JK, Doudna JA. Biology and applications of CRISPR systems: harnessing nature's toolbox for genome engineering. Cell. 2016; 164:29–44.
48. Chen JS, Dagdas YS, Kleinstiver BP, Welch MM, Sousa AA, Harrington LB, et al. Enhanced proofreading governs CRISPR-Cas9 targeting accuracy. Nature. 2017;550:407–10.
49. Kosicki M, Tomberg K, Bradley A. Repair of double-strand breaks induced by CRISPR-Cas9 leads to large deletions and complex rearrangements. Nat Biotechnol. 2018;36:765–71.
50. Singh S, Ghosh P, Hatfull GF. Attachment site selection and identity in Bxb1 serine integrase-mediated site-specific recombination. PLoS Genet. 2013;9: e1003490.
51. Birnbaum J, Flemming S, Reichard N, Soares AB, Mesen-Ramirez P, Jonscher E, et al. A genetic system to study *Plasmodium falciparum* protein function. Nat Methods. 2017;14:450–6.
52. Kim JH, Lee SR, Li LH, Park HJ, Park JH, Lee KY, et al. High cleavage efficiency of a 2A peptide derived from porcine teschovirus-1 in human cell lines, zebrafish and mice. PLoS One. 2011;6:e18556.

4

Influence of ecological factors on the presence of a triatomine species associated with the arboreal habitat of a host of *Trypanosoma cruzi*

Sofía Ocaña-Mayorga[1], Simón E. Lobos[1,2], Verónica Crespo-Pérez[3], Anita G. Villacís[1], C. Miguel Pinto[1,4] and Mario J. Grijalva[1,5*]

Abstract

Background: The white-naped squirrel, *Simosciurus nebouxii* (previously known as *Sciurus stramineus*), has recently been identified as an important natural host for *Trypanosoma cruzi* in Ecuador. The nests of this species have been reported as having high infestation rates with the triatomine vector *Rhodnius ecuadoriensis*. The present study aims to determine the levels of nest infestation with *R. ecuadoriensis*, the ecological variables that are influencing the nest site selection, and the relationship between *R. ecuadoriensis* infestation and trypanosome infection.

Results: The study was carried out in transects in forest patches near two rural communities in southern Ecuador. We recorded ecological information of the trees that harbored squirrel nests and the trees within a 10 m radius. Manual examinations of each nest determined infestation with triatomines. We recorded 498 trees ($n = 52$ with nests and $n = 446$ without nests). *Rhodnius ecuadoriensis* was present in 59.5% of the nests and 60% presented infestation with nymphs (colonization). Moreover, we detected *T. cruzi* in 46% of the triatomines analyzed.

Conclusions: We observed that tree height influences nest site selection, which is consistent with previous observations of squirrel species. Factors such as the diameter at breast height and the interaction between tree height and tree species were not sufficient to explain squirrel nest presence or absence. However, the nest occupancy and tree richness around the nest were significant predictors of the abundance of triatomines. Nevertheless, the variables of colonization and infection were not significant, and the data observed could be expected because of chance alone (under the null hypothesis). This study ratifies the hypothesis that the ecological features of the forest patches around rural communities in southern Ecuador favor the presence of nesting areas for *S. nebouxii* and an increase of the chances of having triatomines that maintain *T. cruzi* populations circulating in areas near human dwellings. Additionally, these results highlight the importance of including ecological studies to understand the dynamics of *T. cruzi* transmission due to the existence of similar ecological and land use features along the distribution of the dry forest of southern Ecuador and northern Peru, which implies similar challenges for Chagas disease control.

Keywords: Vector-borne disease, Chagas disease, *Rhodnius ecuadoriensis*, *Sciurus stramineus*, *Simosciurus nebouxii*, Nest site preferences, Ecuador

* Correspondence: grijalva@ohio.edu
[1]Centro de Investigación para la Salud en América Latina (CISeAL), Escuela de Ciencias Biológicas, Facultad de Ciencias Exactas y Naturales, Pontificia Universidad Católica del Ecuador, Calle San Pedro y Pamba Hacienda, 170530 Nayón, Ecuador
[5]Infectious and Tropical Disease Institute, Department of Biomedical Sciences, Heritage College of Osteopathic Medicine, Ohio University, Athens, OH 45701, USA
Full list of author information is available at the end of the article

Background

Vector-borne diseases involve complex interactions among multiple sets of host, vector and pathogen species. Chagas disease is representative of such complex interactions. This disease is caused by the parasite *Trypanosoma cruzi* and is transmitted by the feces of triatomine bugs. In natural conditions, the parasite populations are maintained through systemic infections of mammalian hosts through a mechanic infection by skin contaminated with infected feces of triatomine bugs or by oral transmission due to the ingestion of infected vectors [1].

As in other host-parasite interactions, *T. cruzi* infections in vertebrate and invertebrate hosts occur in three overlapping and interchangeable cycles: domestic, peridomestic and sylvatic [2]. Although, these cycles have some particular characteristics, e.g. species more adapted to life inside the houses), the discrimination of these habitats is somewhat arbitrary, particularly with the peridomestic and sylvatic area boundaries. In general, the domestic cycle occurs when infected triatomines infest the human dwellings, e.g. bedrooms, kitchens, while the peridomestic cycle occurs when they infest man-built structures surrounding a house, e.g. chicken coops, piles of material. The sylvatic cycle occurs in vertebrate nests and burrows (used by birds and small mammals) in areas separate from what is defined as a human dwelling but where human activities can take place (e.g. crop fields, forest patches) [3, 4].

In southern Ecuador, the presence of parasites of the genus *Trypanosoma* (*T. cruzi* and *T. rangeli*) has been reported circulating in triatomine vectors and mammalian hosts [3–7]. The most abundant triatomine species in this region is *Rhodnius ecuadoriensis*, which is involved in all three transmission cycles (domestic, peridomestic and sylvatic) [4]. In the sylvatic cycle, an interesting association with the nests of the white-naped squirrel *Simosciurus nebouxii*, previously lumped with the Guayaquil squirrel *Sciurus stramineus* [8], has been reported [3, 9]. These squirrels, *S. nebouxii* and *S. stramineus*, have been identified as hosts for *T. cruzi* in coastal and southern Ecuador [3, 9–12]. They are considered important hosts because they inhabit areas surrounding human dwellings and their nests are suitable habitats for triatomines [13]. Additional evidence of a close relationship between *R. ecuadoriensis* and these squirrels was revealed by a spatial analysis that found that changes in land use and dispersal patterns of the squirrels influence triatomine abundance and *T. cruzi* persistence [12]. Therefore, the study of ecological dynamics of vector-host-pathogen interactions can provide novel insights into the mechanisms of emergence, maintenance and spread of diseases [14]. However, the interactions among invertebrate and vertebrate hosts and their influence on Chagas disease transmission have not yet been thoroughly evaluated. Notably, the understanding of ecological preferences, e.g. nesting habitat selection, of the squirrels is essential to assess vector and parasite dynamics, especially in areas where the increasing presence of human settlements near sylvatic environments challenges the effectiveness of Chagas disease control strategies.

The objectives of this study were to determine (i) the level of nest infestation of the squirrel *S. nebouxii* with the vector *R. ecuadoriensis*; (ii) the ecological variables that influence squirrel nest site selection; and (iii) the relationships between ecological variables and the abundance, colonization, and trypanosome infection of *R. ecuadoriensis* associated with squirrels.

Results

Along the three transects of this study, a total of 498 trees were sampled. Of these, 52 trees presented one or more squirrel nests. Thirty species of trees [≥ 0.1 m of diameter at breast height (DBH)] were identified. *Vachellia macracantha* (*Fabaceae*, common name: faique) was the most abundant tree (38%), followed by 21% of *Pisonia aculeata* (*Nyctaginaceae*, common name: pego-pego) and 12% of *Morus celtidifolia* (*Moraceae*, common name: palo blanco). Fifteen percent of the sampled trees could not be identified (Additional file 1: Table S1).

Entomological indices, population structure and natural trypanosome infection rates of triatomines

We examined 42 squirrel nests. Of these, 25 (60%) were infested with triatomines. We collected 298 individuals of *R. ecuadoriensis* from all infested nests. Overall triatomine density was 7.1 bugs per searched nest; crowding was 11.9 bugs per infested nest; and the overall colonization index was 60% (Table 1). Population structure analyses showed that nymphs III, IV and NV were more abundant than NI, NII and adults (females and males) (Table 1).

We analyzed the infection with trypanosomes in a subset (145 individuals) of the collected triatomines. High infection rates were detected with *T. cruzi* (46%) and *T. rangeli* (59%), including mixed infection with both parasites (Table 1). Parasite infection was reported at all developmental stages.

Predictors of nesting-habitat preferences of the white-naped squirrel

We analyzed nesting-habitat preferences only for trees that had no missing values for any independent variable, totaling 310 trees, of which 44 harbored squirrel nests (Additional file 1: Table S1). Multi-model inference analysis revealed that the most parsimonious model for explaining squirrel nest presence/absence was one that included only tree height as an explanatory variable (AIC = 190.82) (Table 2). A model including tree height, diameter at breast height and the interaction between tree height and plant species also had good explanatory power, although with a slightly higher AIC

Table 1 Entomological indices and natural trypanosome infection rates of triatomines collected on squirrel's nests in two rural communities in southern Ecuador

Community	Squirrel nests			Triatomines															
				Nymphs					Adults			Entomological indices				*Trypanosoma* infection (%)			
	N	Infested	With nymphs	I	II	III	IV	V	F	M	Total	In (%)	D	CW	C (%)	Total	TC	TR	Mx
Bellamaría	26	15	9	14	19	39	44	70	34	28	248	57.7	9.5	16.5	60	117	23.9	43.6	19.7
Bellamaría Chico	6	5	3	5	10	0	0	0	1	1	17	83.3	2.8	3.4	60	10	60.0	40.0	0.0
Chaquizcha	10	5	3	1	12	12	3	0	0	5	33	50.0	3.3	6.6	60	18	50.0	38.9	5.6
Total	42	25	15	20	41	51	47	70	35	34	298	59.5	7.1	11.9	60	145	29.7	42.8	16.6

Abbreviations: *F* female, *M* male, *In* infestation index, *D* density, *CW* crowding, *C* colonization, *TC T. cruzi*, *TR*, *T. rangeli*, *Mx* mixed infection *T. cruzi* + *T. rangeli*

(191.07) than just using tree height alone (Table 2). Finally, the model-averaged importance of term analysis revealed that tree height had the highest relative importance, followed by the diameter at breast height, and the interaction between the two variables, although only the former had importance higher than 80% (Fig. 1a).

Predictors of nests-habitat features on triatomine abundance, colonization and their infection with trypanosome species

To analyze the predictors of triatomine abundance, we included only trees with nests that had no missing data ($n = 31$) (Additional file 2: Table S2). Model inference analyses revealed that the most parsimonious model was one that included only nest occupancy, tree height, and tree richness around the nest (Table 3). Also, according to the model-averaged importance of term analysis, nest occupancy and tree richness around the nest were both equally important and had very high support. Tree height also had high support, although lower than the other two variables (Fig. 1b).

The analysis of the predictors of triatomine colonization and their infection with trypanosome species was calculated for trees with the presence of both nest and triatomines ($n = 20$) (Additional file 2: Table S2). The analyses found that no model explains the response better than a null model and that none of the explanatory variables has a significant effect on the response.

Table 2 Results of the multi-model inference analysis of nest presence/absence, for the tree models with the lowest AIC

Model	AIC	Δ AIC[a]	LRT[b]	*P*-value
TH	190.82	73.68	66.30	0.60
TH + DBH + SPP:TH	191.07	73.43	16.54	1
TH + DBH + SPP:DBH	191.53	72.97	17.01	1

Abbreviations: *TH* tree height, *DBH* diameter at breast height, *SPP* tree species
[a]Δ AIC is the difference between the Akaike Information Criterion (AIC) for the complete model and the reduced model
[b]Likelihood ratio test (LRT) and associated *P*-value test the hypothesis that the reduced model provides no worse fit than the complete model

Discussion

The high triatomine infestation rates and densities of vectors found in this study confirm the white-naped squirrel (*S. nebouxii*) as an important natural food source for triatomines in the southern Andean region of Ecuador [3, 9]. Despite the extensive distribution of the vector *R. ecuadoriensis*, its presence in different habitats and its close association with other arboreal vertebrates, e.g. birds, rodents) [3], reaches its highest abundance in squirrel (*S. nebouxii*) nests [3, 9, 10, 12]. Also, other squirrel species of the genus *Sciurus* and the vector extensively overlap in both range and habitat, across the equatorial Pacific region of western Ecuador and northwestern Peru between 0–2000 masl [8, 15].

Our results reveal that ecological features of squirrel nests, such as tree height and tree richness in the surrounding forest, could favor the presence of triatomines. Although *R. ecuadoriensis* may not be specialized to *S. nebouxii*, ecological and environmental conditions might favor an overlap in geographical distribution of the two species [13, 16, 17], and thus, their interaction. Nevertheless, the high infestation rates could suggest that *S. nebouxii* favors *R. ecuadoriensis* population persistence in relation to other sympatric vertebrate hosts, where conditions are suitable. Furthermore, phenotypic variability in *R. ecuadoriensis* [17] could be a critical factor in the optimal exploitation of all available resources (i.e. host species) for successful vector colonization and multiplication [18].

Infestation of squirrel nest with triatomines

We detected a high infection rate (60%) and found only one species (*R. ecuadoriensis*) of the four species of triatomine reported for southern Ecuador. This finding is in accordance with other reports of *R. ecuadoriensis* (instars and adults) in sylvatic environments associated with squirrel nests. However, the infestation rate is higher than previously reported: 14% [9] and 12% [3].

In this study, triatomine population structure, with the presence of all nymphal stages and adults, revealed long-term colonization of triatomines. Considering that temperature influences the duration of triatomine life-cycle [19] and that *R. ecuadoriensis* requires around

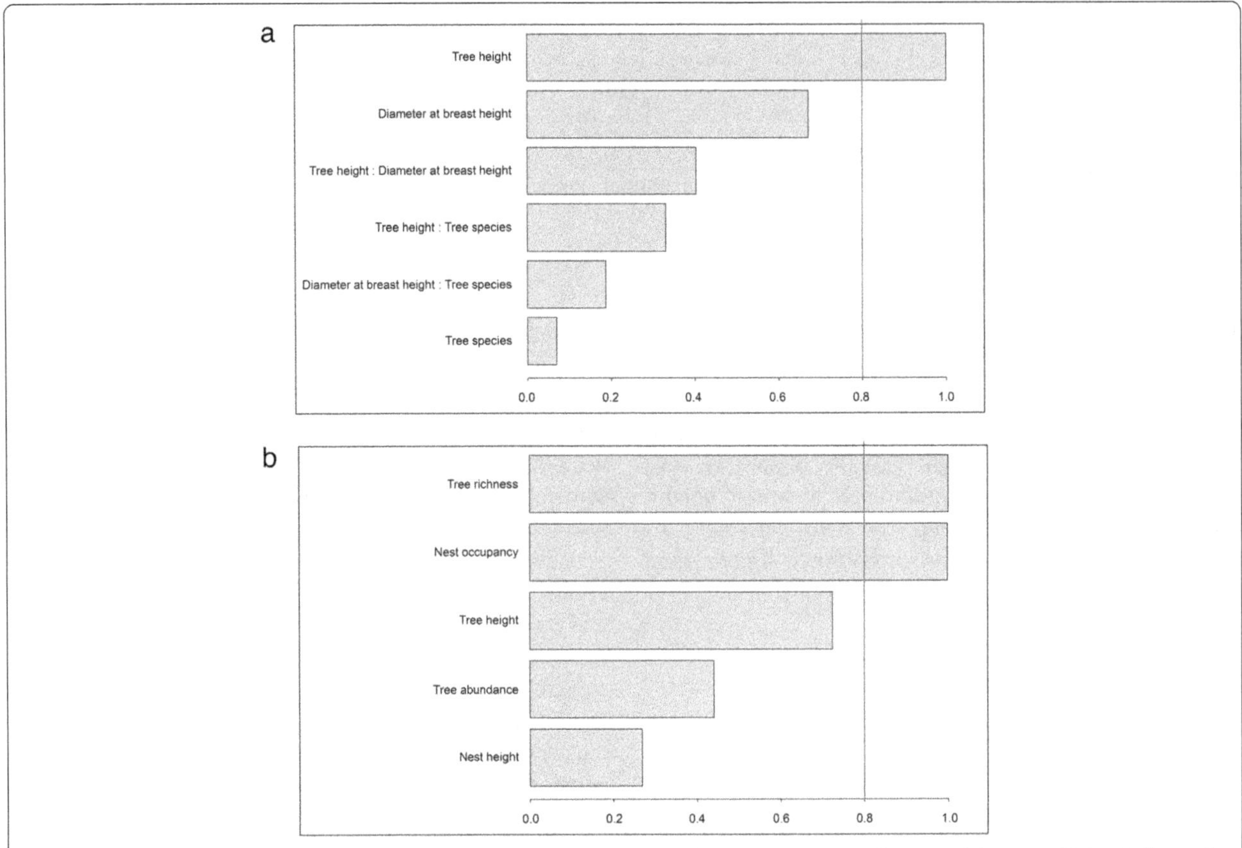

Fig. 1 Multi-model inference analysis. Model-average importance of term results for nesting-habitat preferences of the squirrel (**a**) and effects of nests-habitat features on triatomine abundance (**b**)

six months to reach the adult stage [20], the presence of nymphs could thus indicate stable conditions for triatomines in squirrel nests. The effectiveness of triatomines at colonizing nests of a particular host species could be primarily related to adult oviposition rate, offspring performance [21] and availability of at least one blood meal to molt [20]. Survival under those conditions and within a seasonal environment, with a mortality risk during nymphal development, could be significantly maximized by biotic (e.g. protection against predation, intra- and interspecific competition) and abiotic (e.g. adequate temperature and humidity conditions) features of squirrel nest.

Table 3 Results of the multi-model inference analysis on triatomine abundance, for the tree models with the lowest AIC_c

Model	AIC_c	Δ AIC_c[a]	LRT[b]	*P*-value
NO + TH + TR	609.33	2.81	3.15	0.21
NO + TH + TA + TR	610.08	2.06	1.05	0.31
NO + NH + TH + TR	611.21	0.93	2.18	0.14

Abbreviations: *NO* nest occupancy, *TH* tree height, *TR* tree richness, *TA* tree abundance, *NH* nest height

[a]Δ AIC_c is the difference between the corrected Akaike Information Criterion (AIC_c) for the complete model and the reduced model

[b]Likelihood ratio test (LRT), and associated *P*-value test the hypothesis that the reduced model provides no worse fit than the complete model

Trypanosome infection of triatomines

We detected *T. cruzi* and *T. rangeli* in 89% of the analyzed triatomines, of which more than half were nymphs (57%). The higher trypanosome prevalence in nymphs, along with nymph limited dispersal capacity [22, 23], suggests that they acquired the parasites from infected squirrels and/or the opportunistic rodents that use the abandoned nests. The effective parasite transmission could be related to the primary infection route through contact with triatomine feces (i.e. stercorarian transmission). However, the most effective pathway of infection for wildlife in sylvatic cycles is predation on infected bugs, as it happens in other natural hosts (e.g. raccoons, opossums) [24]. Nevertheless, mammalian host immunity should be further explored in order to understand the influence of trypanosome parasitemia and the degree of tolerance to repeated triatomine exposure.

Selection of nesting sites by squirrels

Some species of tree squirrels, including the white-naped squirrel, build nests on trees. Nests are important resources, and they are used for sleeping, resting, and provide protection against weather conditions and predators, and serve as places to raise offspring [25, 26]. *Simosciurus nebouxii* nests are loosely constructed of woven sticks of about 30 cm in diameter [13]. Nesting site selection depends on many factors (i.e. position, biome composition, the height of the tree) and can be a limiting factor for squirrel distribution [27]. Our results demonstrated that tree height (TH) is an important variable for nesting site selection of *S. nebouxii,* together with the diameter at breast height (DBH), although to a lesser extent. These findings are in accordance with other studies of tree squirrels (i.e. Albert's squirrel, Virginia northern flying squirrel) that reported TH and DBH as important variables for nesting site selection [27, 28].

In this analysis, tree species did not explain the absence or presence of squirrel nests. Only 30 species of trees (≥ 0.1 m of DBH) were identified. Of these, 22 species are higher than 800 cm up to almost 30 meters. Despite the diversity of tree species, only two species (*Vachellia macracantha* and *Pisonia aculeata*) accounted for 57% of trees and harbored the 48% of squirrels' nests. The selection of a nesting site could explain this result is more related to the availability of trees than to a specific preference for tree species. In other squirrel species (e.g. Albert's squirrel), tree size and access routes appear to be more important to the selection of nest sites than tree species [28].

Features of nesting habitat in relation to triatomine abundance and trypanosome presence

Wild and synanthropic rodents are important for *T. cruzi* transmission in several regions; however, their role varies with time and place [29]. Biotic factors (i.e. nutritional status, age, stress conditions, abundance) are important in host-vector-parasite interaction [30] and the particular association of squirrel-triatomines-*T. cruzi* has been previously reported [3, 10, 12, 31, 32]. Nevertheless, little information is available about the ecological characteristics of this association.

Multi-model inference analysis revealed that tree height, nest occupancy and tree richness influence the presence of triatomines in squirrel nests. The importance of tree height has been demonstrated in previous studies that reported higher triatomine abundance in squirrel nests located five meters above ground level and close to human dwellings [3, 10]. At the same time, nest occupancy is an important factor due to the availability of blood, which is essential for triatomine development [20, 33]. In sylvatic environments as well as in environments near human dwellings, squirrels are not the only available host. Other arboreal rodents could, eventually, use the abandoned squirrel nest and serve as blood sources for triatomines. Within this context, the importance of tree richness might have an impact on vertebrate host diversity and the dynamics on rodents, which implies opportunistic behavior of other rodent species to use the squirrel nests and serve as an alternative blood source for triatomines.

Despite the role of other rodent species, it has been demonstrated that squirrels have a very important impact on triatomine abundance and distribution. Previous studies in sylvatic environment reported a triatomine infestation rate > 14% in squirrel nests, and much lower infestation rates in other habitats, such as bird and mouse/rat nests [3, 9]. Additionally, it has been shown that triatomines are associated with squirrels all year round and closely related to human activities such as cultivation of maize. Therefore, land use constitutes an important factor in the dispersal patterns of sylvatic triatomines, particularly of *R. ecuadoriensis*, which is temporally and spatially more closely related to squirrel dynamics than those of other available hosts [12]. Moreover, land use impact might also be reflected in the presence of a pathogen within the host species, depending on the specific biology of the host-parasite relationship [34, 35]. Also, as important as the association of this squirrel species with triatomine abundance, it would be important to unveil the side effects of the use of abandoned nest by opportunistic rodents because of the generation of new habitats.

Conclusions

The interaction between hosts (vertebrate and invertebrate) and parasites represents a complex scenario. This study revealed that particular ecological characteristics of the white-naped squirrel (*S. nebouxii)* have local implications for the maintenance of triatomines and trypanosomes and thus, constitute a risk factor to consider when there are near human settlements. Indeed, these results might be considered when assessing transmission risk of *T. cruzi* in areas with similar ecological and land use features along the distribution of the dry forest in southern Ecuador and northern Peru, which might face similar challenges when triatomine control strategies are applied. This study corroborates *S. nebouxii* as the main factor for the maintenance of *T. cruzi* circulating in areas near human dwellings. Moreover, squirrel presence favors the preservation of triatomine populations, especially *R. ecuadoriensis*, that may, eventually, colonize human dwellings. Further studies on the ecology of vertebrate hosts are essential for understanding the dynamics of *T. cruzi* transmission, especially in areas where classic control strategies have shown limited effectiveness. Therefore, long-term Chagas disease control strategies must consider the ecological characteristics of the surrounding areas because those represent a source of triatomines that can invade human dwellings. In this regard, house improvement activities in order to generate physical barriers for the entrance of triatomines, the detection of possible sources of triatomines in forest patches around the houses, together with the involvement of the community in prevention activities and surveillance are key for a sustainable strategy to control Chagas disease transmission.

Methods

Study area

We carried out data collection during June and July of 2012 and 2013. The study area includes three forest fragments, in two rural communities of Loja Province, located on the slopes of the southwestern Ecuadorian Andes: Bellamaria (4°11'27.6"S, 79°37'15.599"W; 1150 meters above sea level, masl) and Chaquizhca (4°13'30"S, 79°35'52.799"W; 1162 masl) (Fig. 2). These communities were selected based on previous reports of high infection rates with trypanosomatids of sylvatic *Rhodnius ecuadoriensis* populations, associated with *Simosciurus nebouxii* nests [3, 9], and also due to ease of access and permission by owners.

Within the study area, households are scattered amongst a mosaic of small forest fragments surrounded by crop plantations (maize, kidney beans, yucca, coffee and peanuts), pastures, and dirt roads [3]. The study area is part of the neotropical, seasonal, dry forest and has vegetation of both the Central Andes Coast and Central Inter-Andean Valleys floristic groups [36]. Its native vegetation is dominated by *Cedrela fissilis* (*Meliaceae*; Spanish name: cedro), *Vachellia macracantha* (*Fabaceae*; Spanish name: faique) and *Pisonia aculeata* (*Nyctaginaceae*; Spanish name: pego-pego).

Data collection

We followed a transect approximately one-kilometer-long in each forest fragment included in the study (two transects in Bellamaria and one in Chaquizhca) (Fig. 2). Along each transect, all the trees that harbored squirrels' nests were georeferenced and assigned a field code. For all those trees, we collected the following variables: tree species (SPP) (samples were collected for taxonomic identification at the QCA herbarium at PUCE), tree height (TH, which was measured with a clinometer model PM-5/1520, Suunto, Vantaa, Finland), tree diameter at breast height (DBH, measured at 1.30 m above the ground with a measuring tape), height of the nest on the tree (NH) and nest occupancy (NO), defined as the presence of a squirrel in the nest at the time of inspection or conclusive evidence

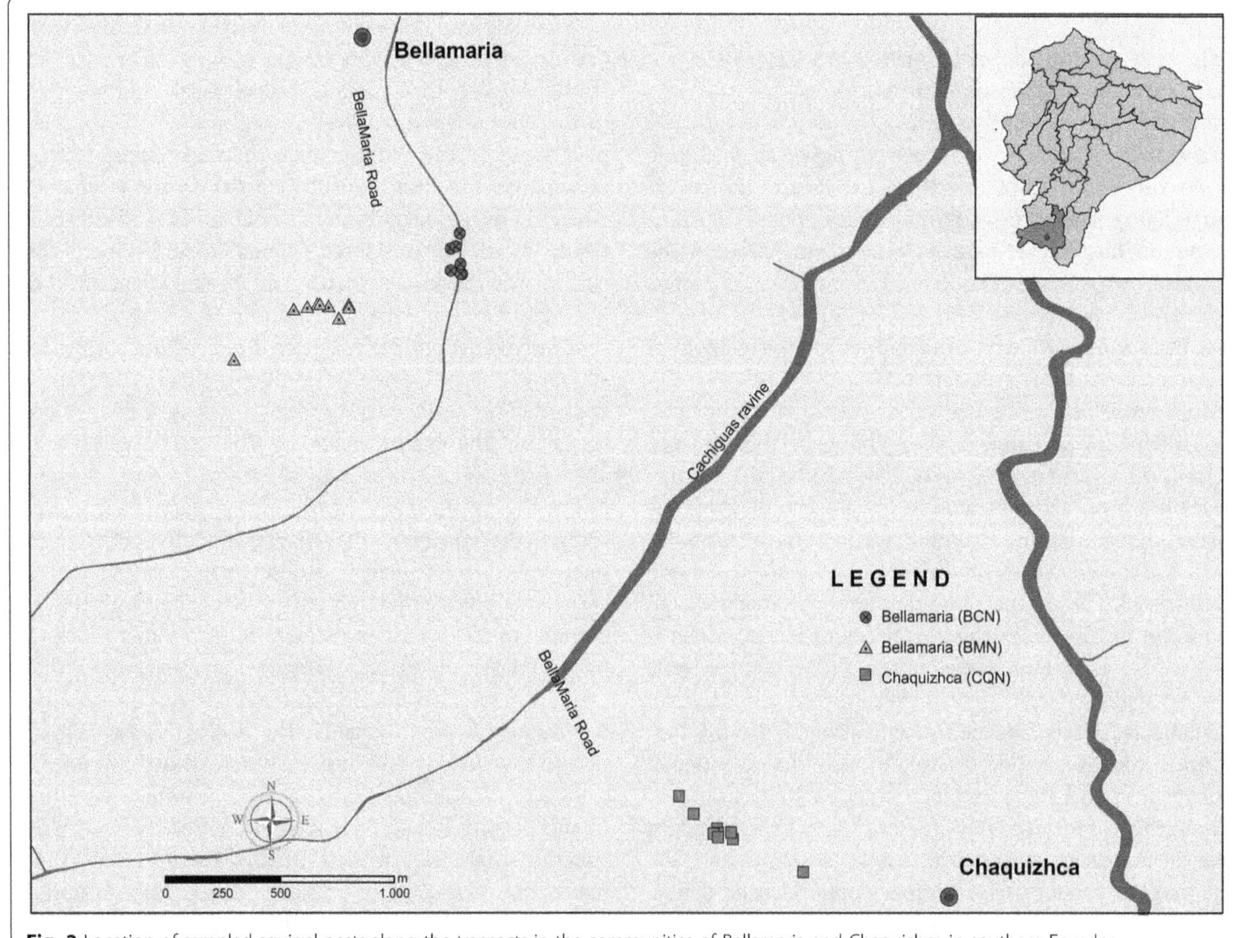

Fig. 2 Location of sampled squirrel nests along the transects in the communities of Bellamaria and Chaquizhca in southern Ecuador

of current occupancy (e.g. urine odor, presence of fur). Additionally, information about SPP, TH, DBH, tree species richness (TR) and abundance (TA) was recorded within a 10 m radius around the focal tree (note that we only included trees ≥ 0.1 m of DBH).

Triatomine searches

We conducted triatomine searches on the nests that could be taken from tree branches. A search effort of 10 min/person/nest was performed following all safety standards as previously described [10]. A nest was considered positive when at least one live triatomine of any developmental stage was found. The triatomines were placed in labeled plastic containers and transported to the insectary at the Center for Research on Health for Latin America at Pontifical Catholic University of Ecuador (CISeAL, PUCE) for species identification and stage classification (NI-NV for nymphal stages or male/female for adults).

Entomological indices

We estimated entomological indices with four standard calculations, according to the WHO recommendations [37] (i) infestation rate (IIn): number of infested nests/number of searched nests × 100; (ii) density (D): number of captured triatomines/number of searched nests; (iii) crowding (CW): number of captured triatomines/number of infested nests; and colonization index (C): nests with presence of nymphs/number of infested nests × 100.

Natural infection of triatomines with trypanosomes

Intestinal contents from captured triatomines were isolated for detection of trypanosomes. Detection was carried through PCR amplification of the conserved domain of minicircle of kinetoplast DNA (kDNA), as described in [6, 38]. The differential detection of *T. cruzi* and *T. rangeli* was based on the size of the PCR products. A band of 330 bp was expected for *T. cruzi*, whereas a band of 760 bp together with bands of 300–450 bp defined *T. rangeli*. Infection rates for *T. cruzi* and *T. rangeli* were calculated by dividing the number of positive samples by the total number of analyzed samples.

Nesting habitat preferences of the white-naped squirrel *S. nebouxii*

We used a multi-model inference approach to test the effect of TH, DBH and SPP on the presence or absence of squirrel nests (NEST). We fitted binomial, generalized linear models (GLM, containing all possible subsets of the explanatory variables and all the possible interactions between them) with a logit link function, using the *glmulti* package of R [39]. The most parsimonious model was identified using the Akaike Information Criterion (AIC). Also, we used likelihood ratio tests (with the *lrtest* function of the *lmtest* package of R) to analyze the difference between the null model (with only an intercept, NEST ~ 1) and the fitted models in order to determine if the fitted models predicted the response significantly better than by chance. Finally, the *glmulti* package also allowed us to determine the relative importance of the various independent variables, by summing the weights/probabilities of the models in which each variable appeared. These values can be regarded as the overall support for each variable across all models [40]. The dataset used for this analysis is detailed in Additional file 1: Table S1.

Effects of nest-habitat features on triatomine abundance, colonization and their infection with trypanosome species

We followed a similar approach (multi-model inference) to understand which variables explain triatomine abundance (ABUND), colonization (COL, presence/absence of nymphs) and infection by trypanosome species (INF). We fitted GLMs to test the effect of tree height (TH), nest height (NH), nest occupancy (NO), tree richness (TR) and tree abundance (TA) on each response variable. In the case of triatomine abundance, we fitted Poisson log-linear models. For the other two response variables, we fitted binomial models with a logit link function. We did not include interactions for these analyses because the number of possible models became too large and the resulting models were too complex and difficult to interpret. The more parsimonious model was identified using the corrected Akaike Information Criterion (AIC_c), which is recommended for small sample sizes (see [41]). Also, we used likelihood ratio tests to analyze the difference between null models and the fitted models. Finally, as for nest presence/absence, we determined the relative importance of the various model variables (see above). The dataset used for this analysis is detailed in Additional file 2: Table S2.

Abbreviations

ABUND: Triatomine abundance; AIC: Akaike Information Criterion; C: Colonization index; COL: Presence/absence of nymphs; CW: Crowding; D: Density; DBH: Tree diameter at breast height; GLM: Generalized Linear Model; IIn: Infestation rate; INF: Infection with trypanosomes; kDNA: Kinetoplast DNA; masl: Meters above sea level; NEST: Presence or absence of squirrel nest; NH: Height of nest on the tree; NO: Nest occupancy; SPP: Tree species; TA: Tree abundance; TH: Tree height; TR: Tree species richness

Acknowledgements

Special thanks to the inhabitants of the visited communities, especially to Dionisio Jiménez who collaborated during the fieldwork and to the personnel of the National Chagas Control Program-National Vector Borne-Disease Control Service, Ecuadorian Ministry of Health who collaborated in the collection of the triatomines. Technical assistance was provided by César Yumiseva, Nelly Muñoz, Santiago Alemán, Dino Sánchez, Anabel Padilla from the Center for Research on Health in Latin America (CISeAL), Álvaro Pérez from the QCA Herbarium at PUCE and Alejandra Lovato.

Funding

Financial support was received from the Pontifical Catholic University of Ecuador (I13048, J13049), the Global Infectious Diseases Training Grant-Fogarty International Center-National Institutes of Health (D43TW008261), the Divisions of Microbiology and Infectious Diseases, National Institute of Allergy and Infectious Diseases, National Institutes of Health (DMID, NIAID, NIH) (AI077896-01) and PEW Latin American Fellows Program in the Biomedical Sciences (ID:00026195). The funders had no role in study design, data collection and analysis, decision to publish, or preparation of the manuscript.

Authors' contributions

SBO participated in the conception and design of the study, the analysis of the parasite of the triatomines collected, the analysis and interpretation of data and the writing of the paper. SEL participated in the conception and design of the study, the collection of field specimens in 2012 and 2013, the analysis and interpretation of data and the writing of the paper. VCP participated in the analysis and interpretation of data and the writing of the paper. AGV participated in data collection, identification of the collected specimens in 2012 and 2013, the analysis and interpretation of data and the writing of the paper. CMP participated in the analysis and interpretation of data and the writing of the paper. MJG participated in the design of the study, the collection of field specimens in 2012 and 2013, and the revision of the manuscript. All authors read and approved the final manuscript.

Competing interests

The authors declare that they have no competing interests.

Author details

[1]Centro de Investigación para la Salud en América Latina (CISeAL), Escuela de Ciencias Biológicas, Facultad de Ciencias Exactas y Naturales, Pontificia Universidad Católica del Ecuador, Calle San Pedro y Pamba Hacienda, 170530 Nayón, Ecuador. [2]Museo de Zoología, Escuela de Ciencias Biológicas, Facultad de Ciencias Exactas y Naturales, Pontificia Universidad Católica del Ecuador, Av. 12 de octubre 1076 y Roca, 170525 Quito, Ecuador. [3]Laboratorio de Entomología, Escuela de Ciencias Biológicas, Facultad de Ciencias Exactas y Naturales, Pontificia Universidad Católica del Ecuador, Av. 12 de octubre 1076 y Roca, 170525 Quito, Ecuador. [4]Instituto de Ciencias Biológicas, Escuela Politécnica Nacional, Ladrón de Guevara E11-254, 170517 Quito, Ecuador. [5]Infectious and Tropical Disease Institute, Department of Biomedical Sciences, Heritage College of Osteopathic Medicine, Ohio University, Athens, OH 45701, USA.

References

1. Klotz SA, Dorn PL, Mosbacher M, Schmidt JO. Kissing bugs in the United States: risk for vector-borne disease in humans. Environ Health Insights. 2014;8(Suppl. 2):49–59.
2. Coura JR. Chagas disease: control, elimination and eradication. Is it possible? Mem Inst Oswaldo Cruz. 2013;108:962–7.
3. Grijalva MJ, Suarez-Davalos V, Villacis AG, Ocana-Mayorga S, Dangles O. Ecological factors related to the widespread distribution of sylvatic *Rhodnius ecuadoriensis* populations in southern Ecuador. Parasit Vectors. 2012;5:17.
4. Grijalva MJ, Villacis AG, Ocana-Mayorga S, Yumiseva CA, Moncayo AL, Baus EG. Comprehensive survey of domiciliary triatomine species capable of transmitting chagas disease in Southern Ecuador. PLoS Negl Trop Dis. 2015; 9:e0004142.
5. Pinto CM, Ocana-Mayorga S, Lascano MS, Grijalva MJ. Infection by trypanosomes in marsupials and rodents associated with human dwellings in Ecuador. J Parasitol. 2006;92:1251–5.
6. Ocana-Mayorga S, Aguirre-Villacis F, Pinto CM, Vallejo GA, Grijalva MJ. Prevalence, genetic characterization, and 18S small subunit ribosomal RNA diversity of *Trypanosoma rangeli* in triatomine and mammal hosts in endemic areas for Chagas disease in Ecuador. Vector Borne Zoonotic Dis. 2015;15:732–42.
7. Pinto CM, Ocana-Mayorga S, Tapia EE, Lobos SE, Zurita AP, Aguirre-Villacis F, et al. Bats, trypanosomes, and triatomines in Ecuador: new insights into the diversity, transmission, and origins of *Trypanosoma cruzi* and Chagas disease. PLoS One. 2015;10:e0139999.
8. de Vivo M, Carmignotto AP, Family Sciuridae G. Fisher, 1817. In: Patton JL, Pardiñas UFJ, D'Elía G, editors. Mammals of South America, vol. 2. Chicago: The University of Chicago Press; 2015. p. 43–7.
9. Grijalva MJ, Villacis AG. Presence of *Rhodnius ecuadoriensis* in sylvatic habitats in the southern highlands (Loja Province) of Ecuador. J Med Entomol. 2009;46:708–11.
10. Suarez-Davalos V, Dangles O, Villacis AG, Grijalva MJ. Microdistribution of sylvatic triatomine populations in central-coastal Ecuador. J Med Entomol. 2010;47:80–8.
11. Grijalva MJ, Villacis AG, Ocana-Mayorga S, Yumiseva CA, Baus EG. Limitations of selective deltamethrin application for triatomine control in central coastal Ecuador. Parasit Vectors. 2011;4:20.
12. Grijalva MJ, Teran D, Dangles O. Dynamics of sylvatic Chagas disease vectors in coastal Ecuador is driven by changes in land cover. PLoS Negl Trop Dis. 2014;8:e2960.
13. Merrick MJ, Koprowski JL, Gwinn RN. *Sciurus stramineus* (Rodentia: Sciuridae). Mamm Species. 2012;44:44–50.
14. Plowright RK, Sokolow SH, Gorman ME, Daszak P, Foley JE. Causal inference in disease ecology: investigating ecological drivers of disease emergence. Front Ecol Environ. 2008;6:420–9.
15. Cuba CA, Abad-Franch F, Roldan Rodriguez J, Vargas Vasquez F, Pollack Velasquez L, Miles MA. The triatomines of northern Peru, with emphasis on the ecology and infection by trypanosomes of *Rhodnius ecuadoriensis* (Triatominae). Mem Inst Oswaldo Cruz. 2002;97:175–83.
16. Agosta SJ. On ecological fitting, plant-insect associations, herbivore host shifts, and host plant selection. Oikos. 2006;114:556–65.
17. Villacis AG, Grijalva MJ, Catala SS. Phenotypic variability of *Rhodnius ecuadoriensis* populations at the Ecuadorian central and southern Andean region. J Med Entomol. 2010;47:1034–43.
18. Agosta SJ, Klemens JA. Ecological fitting by phenotypically flexible genotypes: implications for species associations, community assembly and evolution. Ecol Lett. 2008;11:1123–34.
19. da Silva IG, da Silva HH. The influence of temperature on the biology of Triatominae. IX. *Rhodnius nasutus* Stal, 1859 (Hemiptera, Reduviidae). Mem Inst Oswaldo Cruz. 1989;84:377–82.
20. Villacis AG, Arcos-Teran L, Grijalva MJ. Life-cycle, feeding and defecation patterns of *Rhodnius ecuadoriensis* (Lent & Leon 1958) (Hemiptera: Reduviidae: Triatominae) under laboratory conditions. Mem Inst Oswaldo Cruz. 2008;103:690–5.
21. Guidobaldi F, Guerenstein PG. Oviposition in the blood-sucking insect *Rhodnius prolixus* is modulated by host odors. Parasit Vectors. 2015;8:265.
22. Lent H, Wygodzinsky P. Revision of the Triatominae (Hemiptera, Reduviidae), and their significance as vectors of Chagas' disease. Bull Am Mus Nat Hist. 1979;163:123–520.
23. Abrahan LB, Gorla DE, Catala SS. Dispersal of *Triatoma infestans* and other Triatominae species in the arid Chaco of Argentina: flying, walking or passive carriage? The importance of walking females. Mem Inst Oswaldo Cruz. 2011;106:232–9.
24. Roellig DM, Ellis AE, Yabsley MJ. Oral transmission of *Trypanosoma cruzi* with opposing evidence for the theory of carnivory. J Parasitol. 2009;95:360–4.
25. Tittensor AM. Red squirrel drey. Notes Mamm Soc. 1970;21:528–33.
26. Steele M, Koprowski JC. North American Tree Squirrels. Washington: Smithsonian Institution Press; 2001.
27. Menzel JM, Ford WM, Edwards JW, Menzel MA. Nest tree use by endangered Virginia northern flying squirrel in the Central Appalachian Mountains. Amer Midl Nat. 2004;151:355–68.
28. Edelman AJ, Koprowski JL. Selection of drey sites by Albert's squirrel in an introduced population. J Mammal. 2005;86:1220–6.

29. Bezerra CM, Cavalcanti LP, Souza Rde C, Barbosa SE, Xavier SC, Jansen AM, et al. Domestic, peridomestic and wild hosts in the transmission of *Trypanosoma cruzi* in the Caatinga area colonised by *Triatoma brasiliensis*. Mem Inst Oswaldo Cruz. 2014;109:887–98.
30. Noireau F, Diosque P, Jansen AM. *Trypanosoma cruzi*: adaptation to its vectors and its hosts. Vet Res. 2009;40:26.
31. Navin TR, Roberto RR, Juranek DD, Limpakarnjanarat K, Mortenson EW, Clover JR, et al. Human and sylvatic *Trypanosoma cruzi* infection in California. Am J Public Health. 1985;75:366–9.
32. Lainson R, Brigido Mdo C, Silveira FT. Blood and intestinal parasites of squirrels (Rodentia: Sciuridae) in Amazonian Brazil. Mem Inst Oswaldo Cruz. 2004;99:577–9.
33. Nattero J, Rodriguez CS, Crocco L. Effects of blood meal source on food resource use and reproduction in *Triatoma patagonica* Del Ponte (Hemiptera, Reduviidae). J Vector Ecol. 2013;38:127–33.
34. Patz JA, Daszak P, Tabor GM, Aguirre AA, Pearl M, Epstein J, et al. Unhealthy landscapes: policy recommendations on land use change and infectious disease emergence. Environ Health Perspect. 2004;112:1092–8.
35. Roque AL, Xavier SC, da Rocha MG, Duarte AC, D'Andrea PS, Jansen AM. *Trypanosoma cruzi* transmission cycle among wild and domestic mammals in three areas of orally transmitted Chagas disease outbreaks. Am J Trop Med Hyg. 2008;79:742–9.
36. Banda-R K, Delgado-Salinas A, Dexter KG, Linares-Palomino R, Oliveira A, Prado D, et al. Plant diversity patterns in Neotropical dry forests and their conservation implications. Science. 2016;353:1383–7.
37. WHO. Control of Chagas disease. World Health Organ Tech Rep Ser. 2002; 905:1–109.
38. Virreira M, Alonso-Vega C, Solano M, Jijena J, Brutus L, Bustamante Z, et al. Congenital Chagas disease in Bolivia is not associated with DNA polymorphism of *Trypanosoma cruzi*. Am J Trop Med Hyg. 2006;75:871–9.
39. R Development Core Team. R: A language and environment for statistical computing. Vienna: R Foundation for Statistical Computing; 2016. https://www.r-project.org/.
40. Calcagno V: Glmulti: Model Selection and Multimodel Inference Made Easy. 1.0.7 edn2013: R package. https://cran.r-project.org/web/packages/glmulti/glmulti.pdf.
41. Venables WN, Ripley BD. Modern Applied Statistics with S. New York: Springer-Verlag; 2002.

5

Mitochondrial genomes of two diplectanids (Platyhelminthes: Monogenea) expose paraphyly of the order Dactylogyridea and extensive tRNA gene rearrangements

Dong Zhang[1,2], Wen X. Li[1], Hong Zou[1], Shan G. Wu[1], Ming Li[1], Ivan Jakovlić[3], Jin Zhang[3], Rong Chen[3] and Gui T. Wang[1*]

Abstract

Background: Recent mitochondrial phylogenomics studies have reported a sister-group relationship of the orders Capsalidea and Dactylogyridea, which is inconsistent with previous morphology- and molecular-based phylogenies. As Dactylogyridea mitochondrial genomes (mitogenomes) are currently represented by only one family, to improve the phylogenetic resolution, we sequenced and characterized two dactylogyridean parasites, *Lamellodiscus spari* and *Lepidotrema longipenis*, belonging to a non-represented family Diplectanidae.

Results: The *L. longipenis* mitogenome (15,433 bp) contains the standard 36 flatworm mitochondrial genes (*atp*8 is absent), whereas we failed to detect *trnS*1, *trnC* and *trnG* in *L. spari* (14,614 bp). Both mitogenomes exhibit unique gene orders (among the Monogenea), with a number of tRNA rearrangements. Both long non-coding regions contain a number of different (partially overlapping) repeat sequences. Intriguingly, these include putative tRNA pseudogenes in a tandem array (17 *trnV* pseudogenes in *L. longipenis*, 13 *trnY* pseudogenes in *L. spari*). Combined nucleotide diversity, non-synonymous/synonymous substitutions ratio and average sequence identity analyses consistently showed that *nad*2, *nad*5 and *nad*4 were the most variable PCGs, whereas *cox*1, *cox*2 and *cytb* were the most conserved. Phylogenomic analysis showed that the newly sequenced species of the family Diplectanidae formed a sister-group with the Dactylogyridae + Capsalidae clade. Thus Dactylogyridea (represented by the Diplectanidae and Dactylogyridae) was rendered paraphyletic (with high statistical support) by the nested Capsalidea (represented by the Capsalidae) clade.

Conclusions: Our results show that *nad*2, *nad*5 and *nad*4 (fast-evolving) would be better candidates than *cox*1 (slow-evolving) for species identification and population genetics studies in the Diplectanidae. The unique gene order pattern further suggests discontinuous evolution of mitogenomic gene order arrangement in the Class Monogenea. This first report of paraphyly of the Dactylogyridea highlights the need to generate more molecular data for monogenean parasites, in order to be able to clarify their relationships using large datasets, as single-gene markers appear to provide a phylogenetic resolution which is too low for the task.

Keywords: Phylogenomics, Gene rearrangement, Molecular markers, Gene loss, Pseudo tRNA gene tandem array

* Correspondence: gtwang@ihb.ac.cn
[1]Key Laboratory of Aquaculture Disease Control, Ministry of Agriculture, and State Key Laboratory of Freshwater Ecology and Biotechnology, Institute of Hydrobiology, Chinese Academy of Sciences, Wuhan 430072, People's Republic of China
Full list of author information is available at the end of the article

Background

Monogeneans of the family Diplectanidae (Dactylogyridea: Dactylogyrinea) are parasites found on the gills of (mostly) marine perciform fishes [1]. The family comprises approximately 250 species and is mainly studied for the adverse health effects these parasites cause to the hosts; the fixation of their opisthaptors on the gills causes haemorrhages and a white mucoid exudate, which often leads to secondary fungal, bacterial and/or viral infections [2, 3]. An example is *Diplectanum aequans* (Wagener, 1857), which can cause high mortality of juvenile European sea bass in the Mediterranean aquaculture [2].

Traditionally used phylogenetic markers, morphology and single-genes, are often not suitable for resolving evolutionary history with high confidence; morphological traits can be homoplastic, which often causes taxonomic and phylogenetic artifacts [4–6] and, due to the small amount of information (phylogenetic signal) they carry, single-gene molecular markers may have limited resolving power [7]. This is reflected in the unresolved phylogeny of Monogenean parasites [8–11]. Specifically, studies based on spermatozoal ultrastructural characters [12, 13], the *18S rRNA* gene [9–11], and a combination of three unlinked nuclear genes [5], supported a phylogenetically closer relationship between monogenean orders Capsalidea and Gyrodactylidea than (either of the two) to the Dactylogyridea. However, 66 homologous series of morphological characters resolved the Gyrodactylidea and Dactylogyridea as sister groups [14]. Therefore, molecular markers carrying more powerful phylogenetic signals are needed to resolve their phylogenetic relationships with high resolution. Mitogenome is a good candidate marker, with an approximately ten times larger nucleotide alignment length than commonly used single-gene molecular markers (ITS, *18S* and *28S rRNA*). Although their applicability for studies of the Neodermata is still hampered by their relative scarcity, they are increasingly used in population genetics [15], phylogenetics [16, 17] and diagnostics [7, 18] of parasitic flatworms, despite this limitation. Intriguingly, recent researches [4, 19, 20] relying on the mitochondrial (mt) phylogenomics approach consistently resolved the Dactylogyridea and Capsalidea as sister-groups, thereby further complicating phylogenetic hypotheses for the three aforementioned orders.

As the resolution power of mitochondrial genomics is still limited by the very low number of sequenced monogenean mitogenomes available, where many taxonomic categories remain poorly represented or unrepresented (only one dactylogyridean family represented), we sequenced and characterized two complete mitochondrial genomes belonging to a non-represented dactylogyridean family, the Diplectanidae: *Lamellodiscus spari* (Zhukov, 1970) and *Lepidotrema longipenis* (Yamaguti, 1934), collected from the gills of two marine fish species. Their availability shall enable us to employ mitochondrial phylogenomics to investigate relationships of these three orders with improved resolution.

Methods

Specimen collection and identification

According to the records in Zhang et al. [21], we searched for diplectanid parasites by exploring fish markets in several coastal cities in the southern China. *Lepidotrema longipenis* was obtained from *Terapon jarbua* (Forsskål, 1775) (Perciformes: Terapontidae) bought at a local market in Zhanjiang city, Guangdong Province (21° 15'5"-21°15'16"N, 110°23'46"-110°24'12"E), on the 18th June 2016. *Lamellodiscus spari* was obtained from the black sea bream *Acanthopagrus schlegelii* (Bleeker, 1854) (Perciformes: Sparidae) caught by fishermen in Daya Bay, Guangdong Province (22°42'58"-22°42'56"N, 114° 32'16"-114°32'25"E) on the 10th July 2017. Discriminative morphological characteristics for the Diplectanidae are their opisthaptor equipped by three transversal bars connected to two pairs of central hooks, 14 marginal hooks and accessory adhesive organ (lamellodisc or squamodisc) that can be present or absent [22, 23]. Parasites were further morphologically identified to the genus level as described in Domingues & Boeger [23], and to the species level under a light microscope according to the traits described in Ogawa & Egusa [24] for *L. spari*, and the traits described in Zhang et al. [21] for *L. longipenis*. Additionally, to confirm the taxonomic identity, the *28S rRNA* gene was amplified using universal primers [25] (Additional file 1: Dataset S1); both species share a very high identity of 99.6% with corresponding conspecific homologs available in GenBank: 744/747 identical bp for *L. longipenis* (EF100563), and (837/840) for *L. spari* (DQ054823). All sampled and identified parasites were first washed in 0.6% saline and then stored in 100% ethanol at 4 °C.

DNA extraction, amplification and sequencing

Due to the small size of these parasites, we used two kinds of genomic DNA to ensure a sufficient amount for amplification and sequencing, both extracted using a TIANamp MicroDNA Kit (Tiangen Biotech, Beijing, China): mixture DNA (20 parasite specimens) and individual DNA (a single parasite specimen). Mixture DNA was first used to amplify the whole mitogenome. First, we selected 14 monogenean mitogenomes from GenBank, aligned them using ClustalX [26], and designed degenerate primer pairs (Additional file 1: Dataset S1) matching the generally conserved regions of mitochondrial genes (*16S*, *12S*, *cox*1, *cox*2, *nad*1, *nad*4 and *cytb*). On the basis of these obtained fragments, specific primers were then designed using

Primer Premier 5 [27], and the remaining mitogenome was amplified and sequenced in several PCR steps (Additional file 1: Dataset S1). Both mitogenomes were amplified exactly following the procedures previously described [4, 17, 19, 28]; detailed PCR conditions are provided in Additional file 1: Dataset S1. PCR products were sequenced bi-directionally using both degenerate and specific primers mentioned above on an ABI 3730 automatic sequencer (Sangon, Shanghai, China) using the Sanger method. During the sequencing we paid close attention to chromatograms, carefully examining them for double peaks, or any other sign of the existence of two different sequences. A BLAST [29] check was used to confirm that all amplicons are the actual target sequences. To address the possibility of intraspecific sequence variation present in the mixture DNA, we then used individual DNA and long-range PCR to verify the obtained sequences (primers used are listed in Additional file 1: Dataset S1). If we found two different sequences, we used the DNA extracted from a single individual to infer the mitogenomic sequence, thereby ensuring that each sequence belongs to a single specimen.

Sequence annotation and analyses

Both mitogenomes were assembled and annotated following a previously described procedure [4, 17, 19, 28] using DNAstar v.7.1 software [30], MITOS [31], ARWEN [32] and DOGMA [33] web tools, so detailed methodology is provided in Additional file 1: Dataset S1. Codon usage and relative synonymous codon usage (RSCU) for 12 protein-encoding genes (PCGs) of the two studied diplectanids, two dactylogyrids (*Dactylogyrus lamellatus* Achmerov, 1952 and *Tetrancistrum nebulosi* Young, 1967) and three capsalids (*Neobenedenia melleni* MacCallum, 1927, *Benedenia seriolae* Yamaguti, 1934 and *B. hoshinai* Ogawa, 1984) were computed and sorted using MitoTool [34] (an in-house GUI-based software), and finally the RSCU figure drawn using the ggplot2 [35] plugin. Non-synonymous (dN) / synonymous (dS) mutation rate ratios among the 12 PCGs of the two studied diplectanid mitogenomes were calculated with DnaSP v.5 [36]. The same software was also employed to conduct the sliding window analysis: a sliding window of 200 bp and a step size of 20 bp were implemented to estimate the nucleotide divergence Pi between the mitogenomes of *L. longipenis* and *L. spari*. Tandem Repeats Finder [37] was employed to find tandem repeats in the long non-coding regions (LNCR), and their secondary structures were predicted by Mfold software [38]. Rearrangement events in the mitogenomes and pairwise comparisons of gene orders of all 20 available monogeneans were calculated with the CREx program [39] using the common intervals measurement. Due to limitations of the CREx algorithm, and to facilitate comparative analyses of gene orders, we provisionally added the gene block *trnS1-trnC-trnG* to the gene order sequence of *L. spari*, corresponding to the position where these genes were found in *L. longipenis* (between *nad*5 and *cox*3). Genetic distances (identity) among mitogenomic sequences were calculated with the "DistanceCalculator" function in Biopython using the "identity" model.

Phylogenetic analyses

Phylogenetic analyses were conducted using the two newly sequenced diplectanid mitogenomes and all 18 monogenean mitogenomes available in GenBank (5th May 2018). Two species of the order Tricladida, *Crenobia alpina* (Dana, 1766) (KP208776) and *Obama* sp. (NC_026978), were used as outgroups, thus making a total of 22 mitogenomes (Additional file 2: Table S1). Two datasets were used for phylogenetic analysis: amino acid alignment of 12 protein-coding genes (PCGAA) and codon-based alignment of nucleotide sequences of 12 protein-coding genes + secondary structure alignment of 22 tRNAs and 2 rRNAs (PCGRT). As data processing was conducted as previously described [4, 17, 19, 28, 40], using MitoTool, MAFFT [41] and Gblocks [42]; details are given in Additional file 1: Dataset S1. The heterogeneity of sequence divergence within data sets was analyzed using AliGROOVE [43], wherein indels in nucleotide dataset were treated as ambiguity, and a BLOSUM62 matrix was used for amino acids. Best partitioning scheme and evolutionary models were selected using PartitionFinder2 [44], with greedy algorithm and AICc criterion. Phylogenetic analyses were conducted using two different algorithms: maximum likelihood (ML) and Bayesian inference (BI). Based on the Akaike information criterion implemented in ProtTest [45], MTART+I+G+F was chosen as the optimal evolutionary model for the downstream phylogenetic analyses. Under this optimal model and partition model, ML analysis was conducted in RAxML [46] using a ML+rapid bootstrap (BS) algorithm with 1000 replicates. Bayesian inference analyses with the empirical MTART model were conducted using PhyloBayes (PB) MPI 1.5a [47]. For each analysis, two MCMC chains were run after the removal of invariable sites from the alignment, and the analysis was stopped when the conditions considered to indicate a good run (according to the PhyloBayes manual) were reached: maxdiff < 0.1 and minimum effective size > 300. Phylograms and gene orders were visualized and annotated by iTOL [48] with the help of several dataset files generated by MitoTool, as described in our recent papers [4, 17].

Results and discussion

Genome organization and base composition

The full circular mitochondrial genome of *L. longipenis* (GenBank: MH328203), at 15,433 bp, is the longest among the monopisthocotylids characterized so far (Additional file 2: Table S1). The mitogenome of *L. spari* is 14,614 bp in size (GenBank: MH328204). The *L. longipenis* mitogenome contains the standard [49] 36 flatworm mitochondrial genes, including 12 protein-encoding genes (PCGs; *atp*8 is absent), 22 tRNA genes, and two rRNA genes, whereas *trnS*1, *trnC* and *trnG* genes are missing in *L. spari* (Table 1 and Fig. 1). The architecture, gene contents and similarity of orthologous sequences for the two studied mitogenomes are summarized in Table 1. Average sequence similarity of PCGs between the two studied mitogenomes ranged from 55.58 (*nad*5) to 79.45% (*cox*1) (Table 1). In comparison to PCGs, average sequence similarity values between the rRNAs of the two species were higher: 75.43% for *rrnL* and 70.87% for *rrnS*.

Protein-coding genes and codon usage

Eleven out of 12 PCGs of the two studied mitogenomes used ATG or GTG as the initial codons. However, it proved difficult to determine the initial codon of the *nad*2 gene in both species. On the basis of results reported for other related species, as a working hypothesis we proposed TTG and ATT as the initial codon of *nad*2 for *L. longipenis* and *L. spari*, respectively. Similarly, ATT was proposed as the start codon for *nad*2 in *B. hoshinai* (Ogawa, 1984) and *Aglaiogyrodactylus forficulatus* (Kritsky, Vianna & Boeger, 2007) [20, 50], and TTG as the start codon for *cox*2 in *Paragyrodactylus variegatus* (You, King, Ye & Cone, 2014) [51] (also see Additional file 3: Table S2). Canonical stop codons for the genetic code 9 (echinoderm and flatworm mitochondrion), TAA and TAG, were found in all 12 PCGs (Table 1 and Additional file 3: Table S2). Codon usage, RSCU, and codon family (corresponding to the amino acids) proportions were investigated among the seven available capsalids (three species) and dactylogyrids (four species) (Additional file 4: Figure S1). The third codon position exhibited the highest A+T bias (Table 2). Amino acids encoded by adenosine and thymine-rich codon families (such as Phe, Leu2 and Ile) were strongly preferred, whereas amino acids encoded by guanine and cytosine-rich codon families (such as Arg, Pro and Ala) appear to be selected against (Additional file 4: Figure S1).

Loss of *trnS*1, *trnC* and *trnG* from the *L. spari* mitogenome

Both ARWEN and MITOS algorithms failed to detect *trnS*1, *trnC* and *trnG* in the *L. spari* mitogenome. We made several attempts to corroborate that this is not an artifact. First, we carefully checked (*via* alignments with monogenean *trnS*1, *trnC* and *trnG* homologs) all intergenic sequences (including the LNCR). As these missing tRNA genes are located between *nad*5 and LNCR in *L. longipenis* (Table 1, Fig. 2), and as *trnC* is located between two rRNA genes in many other monogeneans (Fig. 2), we focused specifically on these two fragments. None of these sequences showed appreciable similarity with the queried homologs. Secondly, we re-sequenced the fragment between *nad*5 and *cox*3 using both mixture DNA and individual DNA, and checked the chromatograms carefully [52]. We did not find any evidence for sequence variability. Thirdly, referring to *L. longipenis* and other closely related monogeneans, as well as cestodes and trematodes in most of which *trnG* is located between *nad*5 and *cox*3 (Fig. 2, Additional file 5: Figure S2), we designed two primer pairs (Additional file 1: Dataset S1) to assess whether *trnG* is located between these two genes (or in their vicinity) in *L. spari*: (i) one forward primer (LS-GlyF) matching the most conserved region of *trnG* and two reverse primers (LSR1-6 and LSR1-8) matching the conserved regions of *cox*3 to amplify the fragment between *trnG* and *cox*3; and (ii) two forward primers (LSF17-0 and LSF17) matching *nad*5 and one reverse primer (LS-GlyR) matching *trnG* to amplify the fragment between *nad*5 and *trnG*. None of these primer pairs could generate a PCR product, which indicates that *trnG* is either not in the vicinity of these two genes in *L. spari*, or that its sequence is highly divergent, or that it is completely missing from the mitogenome. On the basis of these tests and high quality of chromatograms of the fragment between *nad*5 and *cox*3 [52], we suspect that all three tRNAs (*trnS*1-*trnC*-*trnG*) might be missing from the mitogenome of *L. spari*. These results would have to be corroborated either by resequencing of this mitogenome, or by sequencing of other closely related species. Loss of tRNA genes was also reported in many other metazoan taxa [53–57]. Given that the amino acid usage frequency of serine (AGN), glycine and cysteine is analogous between *L. spari* and other monogeneans (Additional file 4: Figure S1), there are at least three possible explanations for the missing tRNAs: (i) they are imported from the nucleus, as is common in mitochondria [58]; (ii) they are encoded in the mitogenome, but undergo extensive post-transcriptional RNA editing [54], so they could not be identified from their coding sequences; and (iii) they are encoded on a separate minicircle of mtDNA.

Non-coding regions

A putative control region, or long non-coding region (LNCR), was found between *nad*5 and *cox*3 genes in both mitogenomes (disregarding the three missing tRNAs; Table 1 and Fig. 1). The LNCR of *L. longipenis* (1993 bp) was the longest among the monogeneans characterized so far [4, 7, 16, 19, 20, 50, 51, 59–67]. The A+T content of both LNCRs (*L. longipenis* = 93.8%, *L. spari* = 92.5%) was much higher than in other parts of the mitogenomes (Table 2). Both LNCRs contained a highly repetitive region (HRR): the HRR of *L. longipenis* was composed of 18 tandem repeats (TRs), where repeat

Table 1 Comparison of the annotated mitochondrial genomes of *Lamellodiscus spari* and *Lepidotrema longipenis*

Gene	Position		Size	Intergenic nucleotides	Codon		Strand	Identity
	From	To			Start	Stop		
Lepidotrema longipenis/Lamellodiscus spari								
cox1	1/1	1548/1557	1548/1557		GTG/GTG	TAA/TAG	H/H	79.45
trnT	1553/1581	1609/1641	57/61	4/23			H/H	61.9
rrnL	1610/1642	2582/2593	973/952				H/H	73.19
rrnS	2609/2599	3328/3335	720/737	26/5			H/H	69.43
cox2	3361/3336	3936/3917	576/582	32/-	ATG/ATG	TAG/TAA	H/H	70.79
trnL1	3970/3920	4039/3985	70/66	33/2			H/H	56.58
trnS2	4040/3985	4104/4050	65/66	-/-1			H/H	70.15
trnE	4105/4051	4171/4118	67/68				H/H	77.14
nad6	4175/4119	4624/4577	450/459	3/-	ATG/GTG	TAA/TAA	H/H	62.75
trnL2	4628/4584	4697/4648	70/65	3/6			H/H	64.29
trnY	4700/4662	4767/4727	68/66	2/13			H/H	72.86
trnR	4769/4725	4836/4789	68/65	1/-3			H/H	72.06
nad5	4840/4790	6366/6193	1527/1404	3/-	ATG/GTG	TAA/TAA	H/H	55.58
trnS1	6368/-	6427/-	60/-	1/-			H/-	–
trnC	6431/-	6496/-	66/-	3/-			H/-	–
trnG	6503/-	6567/-	65/-	6/-			H/-	–
LNCR	6568/6194	8560/7966	1993/1773				H/H	60.71
cox3	8561/7967	9214/8617	654/651		ATG/ATG	TAA/TAA	H/H	71.41
trnH	9218/8619	9285/8682	68/64	3/1			H/H	76.47
cytb	9286/8683	10,374/9771	1089/1089		ATG/ATG	TAG/TAG	H/H	74.93
nad4L	10,422/9764	10,670/10,018	249/255	47/-8	ATG/ATG	TAG/TAG	H/H	65.89
nad4	10,640/9991	11,857/11,166	1218/1176	-31/-28	ATG/ATG	TAA/TAG	H/H	59.5
trnQ	11,874/11,313	11,935/11,375	62/63	16/75			H/H	85.71
trnF	11,936/11,173	12,003/11,237	68/65	-/6			H/H	77.94
trnM	12,000/11,389	12,063/11,453	64/65	-4/13			H/H	67.69
atp6	12,064/11,454	12,579/11,966	516/513		ATG/ATG	TAA/TAG	H/H	69.56
nad2	12,629/11,962	13,525/12,810	897/849	49/-5	TTG/ATT	TAA/TAA	H/H	56.16
trnA	13,559/12,817	13,624/12,878	66/62	33/6			H/H	68.18
trnD	13,633/12,880	13,697/12,941	65/62	8/1			H/H	83.08
trnV	13,698/12,944	13,763/13,010	66/67	-/2			H/H	86.76
nad1	13,764/13,012	14,660/13,905	897/894	-/1	GTG/ATG	TAG/TAA	H/H	69.56
trnN	14,661/13,909	14,726/13,971	66/63	-/3			H/H	74.63
trnI	14,759/14,056	14,827/14,123	69/68	32/11			H/H	77.14
trnP	14,854/13,978	14,920/14,044	67/67	26/6			H/H	79.41
trnK	14,923/14,130	14,986/14,197	64/68	2/6			H/H	69.12
nad3	15,018/14,200	15,386/14,550	369/351	31/2	ATG/ATG	TAG/TAG	H/H	63.44
trnW	15,367/14,549	15,433/14,614	67/66	-20/-2			H/H	66.18

Abbreviation: LNCR, large non-coding region

units 2–18 were identical (91 bp) and unit 1 was 1 bp longer with a nucleotide insertion at the 16th position; the HRR of *L. spari* contained 20 TRs with the consensus size of 87 bp, but sizes and sequences of the repeat units were variable, exhibiting nucleotide mutations, deletions and insertions. This is the second report of TRs with high repeat numbers and large size in the subclass Monopisthocotylea; the first report was also in a

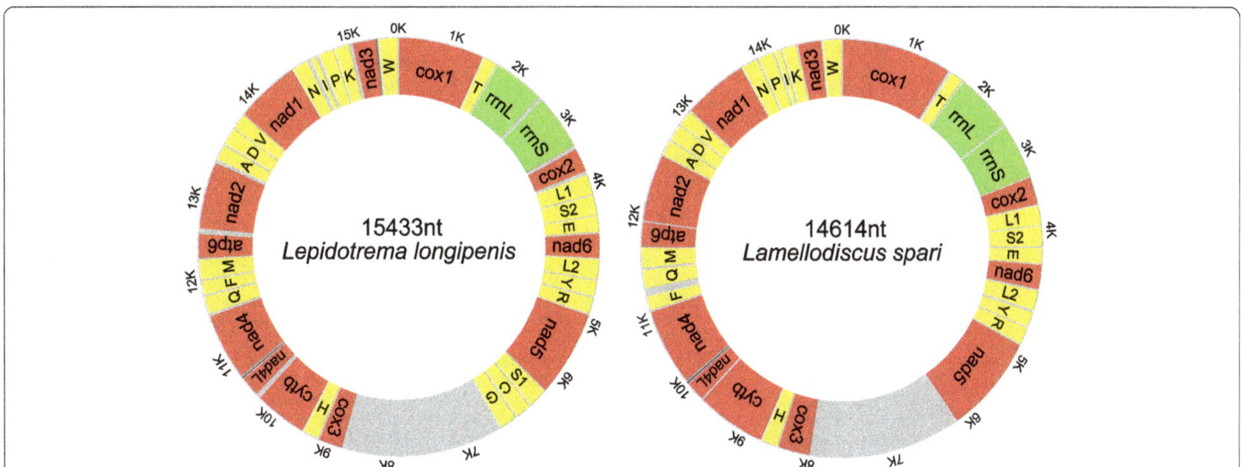

Fig. 1 Visual representation of the circular mitochondrial genomes of *Lepidotrema longipenis* and *Lamellodiscus spari*. *Key*: Red, protein-coding genes; yellow, tRNAs; green, rRNAs; grey, non-coding regions

Table 2 Nucleotide composition and skewness comparison of different elements of the mitochondrial genomes of *Lamellodiscus spari* and *Lepidotrema longipenis*

Regions	Size (bp)	T(U)	C	A	G	AT (%)	GC (%)	GT (%)	AT skew	GC skew
Lepidotrema longipenis/Lamellodiscus spari										
PCGs	9990/9780	47.3/47.7	7.9/8.5	28.5/26.7	16.3/17.1	75.8/74.4	24.2/25.6	63.6/64.8	-0.248/-0.281	0.347/0.336
1st codon position	3330/3260	41.2/40.3	8.2/9.0	30.4/29.5	20.2/21.3	71.6/69.8	28.4/30.3	61.4/61.6	-0.151/-0.154	0.425/0.407
2nd codon position	3330/3260	48.9/49.1	12.2/12.7	21.1/20.0	17.9/18.2	70.0/69.1	30.1/30.9	66.8/67.3	-0.398/-0.420	0.189/0.176
3rd codon position	3330/3260	51.7/53.7	3.4/3.8	34.0/30.7	10.8/11.8	85.7/84.4	14.2/15.6	62.5/65.5	-0.207/-0.273	0.523/0.516
atp6	516/513	49.0/51.9	8.7/9.2	25.0/23.6	17.2/15.4	74.0/75.5	25.9/24.6	66.2/67.3	-0.325/-0.375	0.328/0.254
cox1	1548/1557	44.4/45.6	10.2/10.6	26.0/25.3	19.4/18.5	70.4/70.9	29.6/29.1	63.8/64.1	-0.261/-0.286	0.310/0.272
cox2	576/582	42.0/43.5	9.7/8.9	29.3/26.1	18.9/21.5	71.3/69.6	28.6/30.4	60.9/65.0	-0.178/-0.249	0.321/0.412
cox3	654/651	52.1/50.4	6.0/7.2	26.6/25.3	15.3/17.1	78.7/75.7	21.3/24.3	67.4/67.5	-0.324/-0.331	0.439/0.405
cytb	1089/1089	45.7/46.2	9.6/11.1	27.4/24.9	17.4/17.8	73.1/71.1	27.0/28.9	63.1/64.0	-0.251/-0.300	0.290/0.232
nad1	897/894	46.9/47.9	6.4/7.8	28.2/26.1	18.5/18.2	75.1/74.0	24.9/26.0	65.4/66.1	-0.249/-0.295	0.489/0.399
nad2	897/849	51.3/50.8	7.4/6.9	30.2/28.5	11.1/13.8	81.5/79.3	18.5/20.7	62.4/64.6	-0.259/-0.281	0.205/0.330
nad3	369/351	48.5/45.9	4.6/5.1	31.2/33.0	15.7/16.0	79.7/78.9	20.3/21.1	64.2/61.9	-0.218/-0.162	0.547/0.514
nad4	1218/1176	48.1/48.7	8.9/8.6	28.7/26.7	14.4/16.0	76.8/75.4	23.3/24.6	62.5/64.7	-0.253/-0.292	0.237/0.301
nad4L	249/255	50.2/47.8	4.8/7.5	31.3/25.9	13.7/18.8	81.5/73.7	18.5/26.3	63.9/66.6	-0.232/-0.298	0.478/0.433
nad5	1527/1404	46.6/47.3	6.4/7.5	31.6/28.8	15.5/16.3	78.2/76.1	21.9/23.8	62.1/63.6	-0.192/-0.242	0.413/0.367
nad6	450/459	48.9/49.0	6.9/5.4	27.8/29.8	16.4/15.7	76.7/78.8	23.3/21.1	65.3/64.7	-0.275/-0.243	0.410/0.485
rrnL	973/952	41.7/40.1	8.6/9.5	34.0/34.3	15.6/16.1	75.7/74.4	24.2/25.6	57.3/56.2	-0.102/-0.078	0.288/0.259
rrnS	720/737	39.7/38.8	9.6/10.2	35.3/33.9	15.4/17.1	75.0/72.7	25.0/27.3	55.1/55.9	-0.059/-0.067	0.233/0.254
LNCR	1993/1773	46.3/40.3	2.6/2.8	47.5/52.2	3.6/4.7	93.8/92.5	6.2/7.5	49.9/45.0	0.013/0.128	0.161/0.263
tRNAs	1448/1237	40.2/40.4	7.9/8.4	37.0/34.2	14.9/17.0	77.2/74.6	22.8/25.4	55.1/57.4	-0.041/-0.083	0.309/0.338
rRNAs	1693/1689	40.9/39.6	9.0/9.8	34.6/34.2	15.5/16.5	75.5/73.8	24.5/26.3	56.4/56.1	-0.084/-0.073	0.264/0.257
Full genome	15,433/14,614	45.8/45.3	7.3/7.9	32.6/31.5	14.3/15.4	78.4/76.8	21.6/23.3	60.1/60.7	-0.169/-0.180	0.326/0.323

Abbreviation: LNCR, large non-coding region

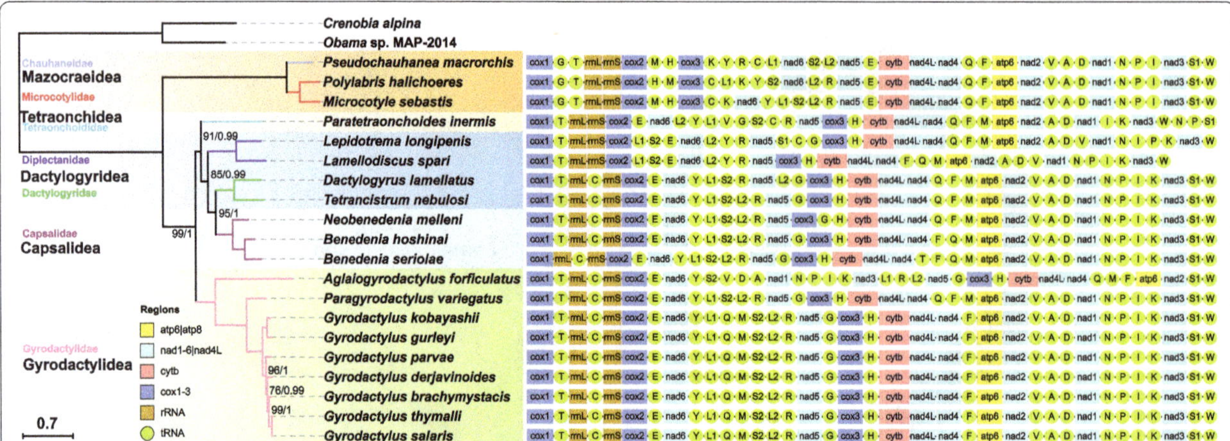

Fig. 2 Phylogeny and mitogenomic architecture of the class Monogenea. The phylogram was constructed using MTART model on the basis of concatenated amino acid sequences of 20 monogenean mitogenomes. *Crenobia alpina* and *Obama* sp. are outgroups. The scale-bar corresponds to the estimated number of substitutions per site. Statistical support values are shown above the nodes, except for nodes with maximum support. Monogenean families are shown in different colors. Gene order is displayed to the right of the tree

dactylogyridean species, *D. lamellatus* [19]. These findings consistently reject the hypothesis that monopisthocotylids possess fewer and smaller (in size) TRs in the LNCR than polyopisthocotylids [61]. As in other monogeneans [19, 64] and cestodes [68, 69], both consensus repeat patterns of the HRRs in *L. longipenis* and *L. spari* are capable of forming stem-loop structures (Additional file 6: Figure S3). Since the presence of tandem repeats forming stable secondary structure is often associated with replication origin in mitochondria [64, 70, 71], it appears likely that these repeat regions are embedded within the control region.

Aside from these TRs, the LNCR of *L. longipenis* also harbored 17 identical *trnV* pseudogenes, whereas the LNCR of *L. spari* contained 13 *trnY* pseudogenes (identified using ARWEN and DOGMA algorithms), all of which were located on the minus strand. These pseudogenes and HRR repeat patterns were two separate features, although the pseudogenes partially overlapped with the repeat patterns of HRR. Among the 13 *trnY* pseudogenes, six were 80 bases-long, and seven were 82

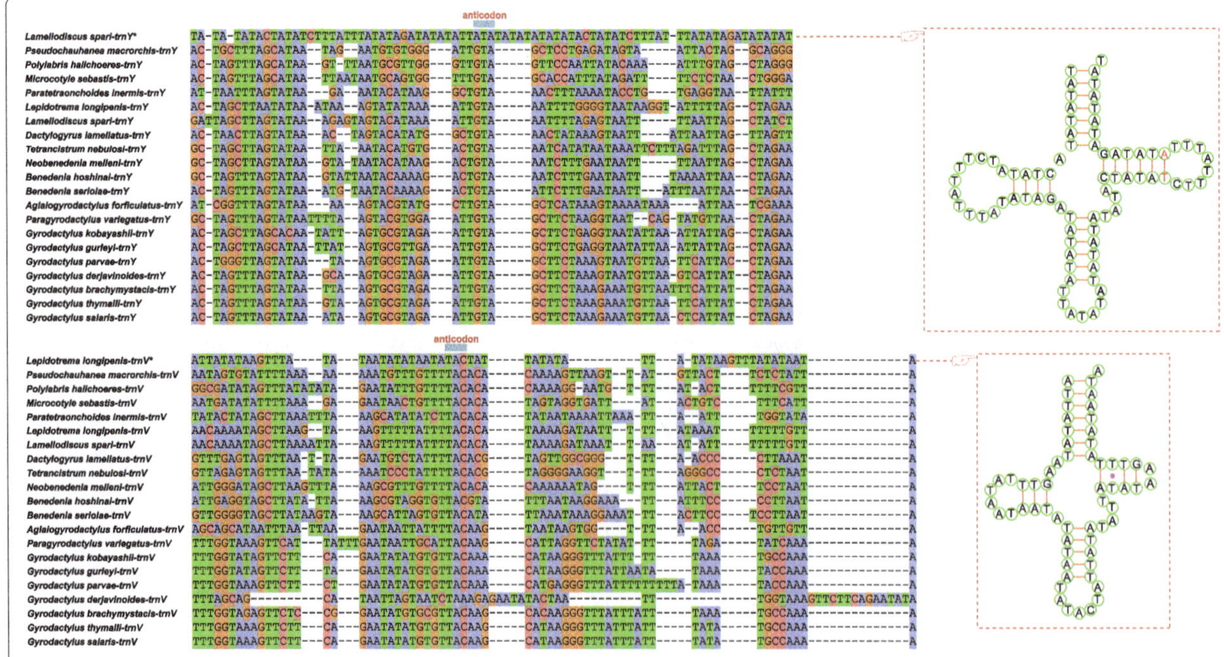

Fig. 3 Alignment of *trnV* and *trnY* pseudogenes with the corresponding functional monogenean tRNA homologs. Cloverleaf structures of the two pseudogenes are shown on the right of alignment. Two red bases in *trnY* indicate nucleotide insertions in the TΨC stem

bases-long, with two bases inserted in the TΨC stem. *trnV* pseudogene had a standard TAC anticodon, whereas *trnY* contained modified standard anticodon (ATA). The cloverleaf structures of the two pseudogenes and the alignment with the corresponding functional monogenean tRNA homologs is shown in Fig. 3. Average sequence similarity values of the alignment for *trnV* and *trnY* were 40.78 ± 3.87% and 39.91 ± 4.13%, respectively. As the amino acid usage frequencies of valine and tyrosine for *L. longipenis* and *L. spari* were analogous with other monogeneans (Additional file 4: Figure S1), we hypothesise that the presence of these pseudogenes is non-adaptive, and that they may not be functional. A tRNA pseudogene was also found in the LNCR of *Paratetraonchoides inermis* (Bychowsky, Gussev & Nagibina, 1965) [4], but such a large accumulation of tRNA pseudogenes in tandem arrays is much more common in plastid genomes [72] and prokaryotes [73] than in mitochondrial genomes of metazoans. It might be of interest to sequence mitogenomes of other closely related species to infer whether they also harbor this feature, and study its evolutionary history and mutational rate.

Nucleotide diversity and evolutionary rate analysis

The sliding window analysis was conducted using concatenated alignments of 12 PCGs, two rRNAs and 19 coalescent tRNAs of the two diplectanids (*trnS*1, *trnC* and *trnG* were removed due to their absence from *L. spari*). The plot of sequence variation ratio exhibited highly variable nucleotide diversity between the two diplectanids, with Pi values for the 200 bp windows ranging from 0.201 to 0.411 (Fig. 4a). *cox*1 (0.201), tRNAs (0.215), *rrnS* (0.221), *rrnL* (0.224) and *cytb* (0.251) exhibited a comparatively low sequence variability, whereas *nad*2 (0.411), *nad*5 (0.392), *nad*4 (0.381) and *nad*6 (0.354) had a comparatively high sequence variability. This was corroborated by the non-synonymous/synonymous (dN/dS) ratio (omega) analysis, which showed that *cox*1 (0.163), *cytb* (0.167), *nad*4L (0.213) and *cox*2 (0.229) are evolving comparatively slowly, whereas *nad*2

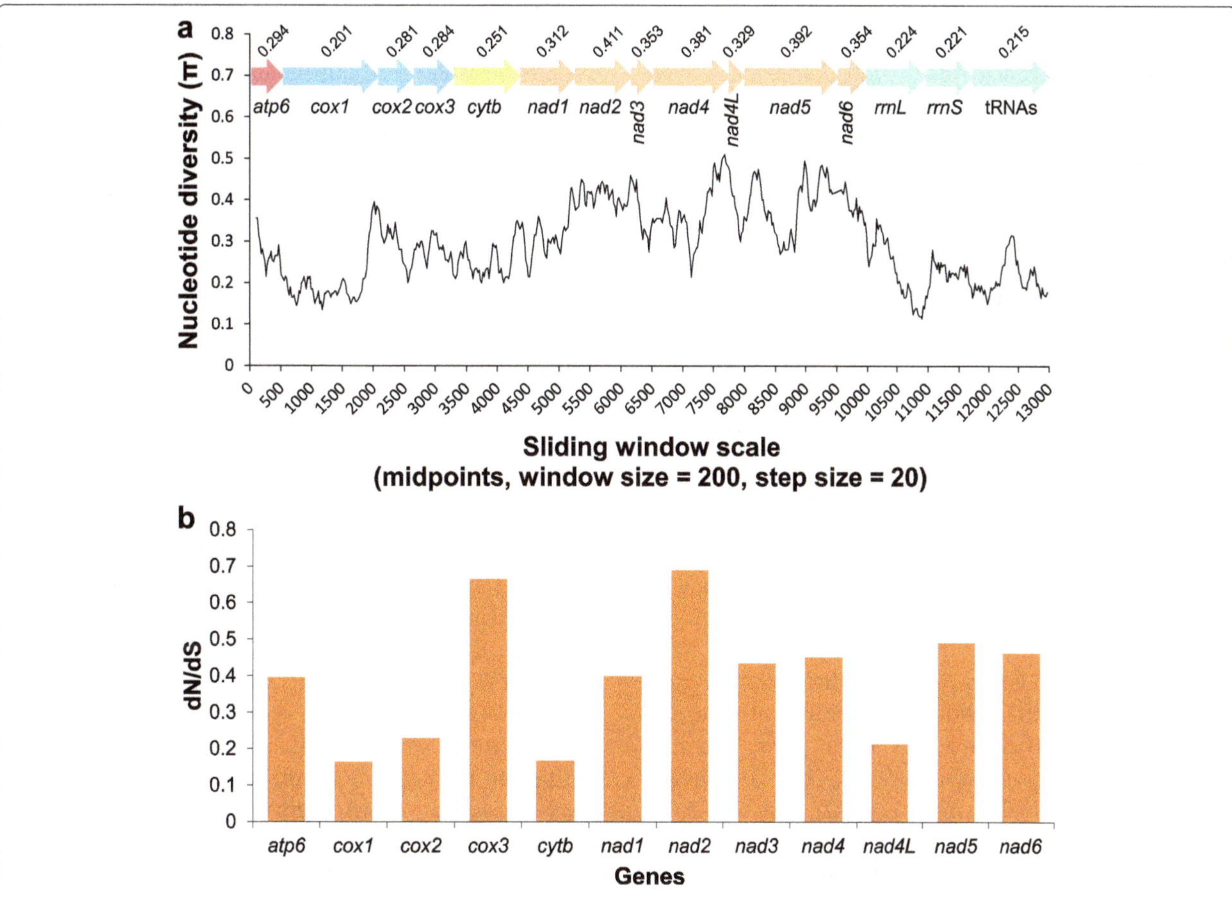

Fig. 4 Sliding window and selection pressure analyses of the mitogenomes of *Lepidotrema longipenis* and *Lamellodiscus spari*. **a** Sliding window analysis was conducted on concatenated alignments of 12 PCGs, 2 rRNAs and 19 coalescent tRNAs (missing tRNAs, *trnS*1, *trnC* and *trnG*, were removed). The black line represents the value of nucleotide diversity (window size = 200 bp, step size = 20 bp, with the value inserted at its midpoint). Gene names, boundaries/direction (colored arrows) and average nucleotide diversity values are indicated above the graph. **b** Ratios of non-synonymous (dN) to synonymous (dS) substitution rates calculated for protein-coding genes

(0.69), *nad*5 (0.49), *nad*6 (0.462) and *nad*4 (0.451) are evolving comparatively fast (Fig. 4b). Therefore, these analyses consistently indicate that *cox*1, which is often used as a universal barcode for species identification [74], as well as population genetics in monogeneans [75–78], is the slowest evolving and least variable gene. As rapidly evolving genes are more suitable for analyzing relationships among closely related species [79], we propose that the fast-evolving *nad*2, *nad*5, *nad*6 and *nad*4 would be better molecular markers than *cox*1 for diplectanids.

Phylogeny

Regardless of the dataset and model used, all analyses produced phylograms with concordant branch topologies (Fig. 2 and Additional file 7: Figure S4 and S5). As the AliGROOVE analysis indicated that the PCGAA dataset exhibits lower heterogeneity than PCGRT (Additional file 7: Figure S6), we displayed only the results of PCGAA in Fig. 2. As expected, the two diplectanids, *L. longipenis* and *L. spari*, constituted a monophyletic group with maximum support. In accordance with previous results based on mitochondrial phylogenomics [4, 19, 20], the two dactylogyrids (*D. lamellatus* and *T. nebulosi*; Dactylogyridea: Dactylogyridae) formed a sister-group with the three capsalids (*N. melleni*, *B. hoshinai* and *B. seriolae*; Capsalidea: Capsalidae). The two newly-sequenced diplectanids (Diplectanidae) formed a sister-group with this (Dactylogyridae + Capsalidae) clade. As the family Diplectanidae was classified into the order Dactylogyridea in the classifications proposed by Bychowsky [80], Lebedev [81] and Boeger & Kritsky [82], this topology rendered Dactylogyridea paraphyletic by the nested Capsalidea clade. In these taxonomic systems, the Dactylogyridae and Diplectanidae were assigned to the same order Dactylogyridea (or suborder Dactylogyrinea within the order Dactylogyridea in Bychowsky [80]), whereas the Capsalidae was classified into the order Capsalidea (or suborder Monopisthocotylinea within the order Dactylogyridea in Bychowsky [80]). A number of subsequent morphology- and molecular data-based studies further supported the closer phylogenetic relationship between the Dactylogyridae and Diplectanidae than either of the two with Capsalidae: chaetotaxy and ciliated cells of the oncomiracidium [83], spermatozoon ultrastructure [12, 13], comprehensive morphological characters [14, 82], *28S* rRNA [8] and *18S* rRNA [9–11]. Regarding the phylogenetic position of the Capsalidae, it was either resolved as phylogenetically closely related to the Gyrodactylidea (families Gyrodactylidae and/or Udonellidae) based on the evidence of spermatozoon ultrastructure [12, 13], *28S* rRNA gene [8], *18S* rRNA gene [9–11], and a combination of three unlinked nuclear genes (*28S* rRNA, *Histone 3* and *Elongation Factor 1α*) [5], or was resolved as basal to the Gyrodactylidea and Dactylogyridea on the basis of comprehensive morphological characters [14, 82]. However, as argued before, morphological traits are liable to cause taxonomic and phylogenetic artifacts in (parasitic) microscopic animals [4–6] and single gene-based molecular markers may not provide sufficient resolution power to infer the relationships among these species with high precision [7, 84]. These discrepancies could also be a result of discrepant evolutionary rates between mitochondrial and nuclear sequences, which can produce differing evolutionary signals [85, 86]. Although our phylogenetic analysis was based on relatively limited mitogenomic data (four species belonging to two families for Dactylogyridea, and three species/one family for Capsalidea), the paraphyly of the Dactylogyridea with reasonably high support values (BS = 85, PB = 0.99) suggests that their relationships should be further explored using a larger number of monogenean mitogenomes and large nuclear datasets.

Gene order

The order of tRNA genes of the two studied diplectanids exhibits notable rearrangements in comparison to all other sequenced monogenean mitogenomes (Fig. 2, Additional file 8: Table S4). Disregarding the three missing tRNAs, the gene order of the two diplectanids was very similar, with only two transposition events: position interchanges of *trnF* and *trnQ*, and *trnP* and *trnI* (Fig. 2 and Additional file 8: Table S4). This unique gene order pattern of the two diplectanids is further manifested by low pairwise similarity values in comparison with those observed among other monogeneans: the highest, between *L. spari* and *B. hoshinai*, is only 354 over 1254 (Additional file 8: Table S4). The transformational pathway from *L. spari* to the most similar gene arrangement, belonging to *B. hoshinai*, required one transposition, one TDRL (tandem-duplication-random-loss) and two coupled transposition events (Additional file 9: Figure S7). The transformational pathway from *L. longipenis* to the most similar gene arrangement found in *T. nebulosi* and *P. variegatus* (similarity value: 322 over 1254; gene orders of *T. nebulosi* and *P. variegatus* were identical) required two transpositions, one TDRL and two coupled transposition events (Additional file 9: Figure S7). In addition to the patterns summarized in our recent paper [4], we assigned pattern 1c to the gene order of the two diplectanids, which seems to be synapomorphic to the family Diplectanidae (Additional file 5: Figure S2).

Conserved gene arrangement is considered to be a typical feature of mitochondrial genomes [87–89], but our results suggest that extensive gene order rearrangements are not rare events in the class Monogenea. As five out of six proposed main patterns are found in the

Monogenea (1a, 1b, 3, 4 and the new pattern 1c; Additional file 5: Figure S2), this further confirms the hypothesis [4] that gene order in monogeneans is evolving at a relatively rapid rate. However, evidence is emerging that the evolution of mitogenomic gene order arrangements is discontinuous in monogeneans, as some taxonomic categories appear to be particularly prone to mitogenomic rearrangements (diplectanids, tetraonchids and *A. forficulatus*), whereas others exhibit relatively conserved gene orders. Of course, our conclusions should be interpreted within the context of the limited number of monogenean mitogenomes currently available. Discontinuity in mitogenomic architecture evolution was also found in nematodes [28], snails [90], insects [91] and vertebrates [92]. Although gene order is sometimes used as a tool for inferring phylogenetic relationships [93, 94], this discontinuity in gene order rearrangements in monogeneans might produce misleading evolutionary signals, such as disproportionately long branches, which in turn might cause long branch attraction artifacts. Thus, gene order may only be used for phylogenetic analyses in this group of animals with this limitation in mind. The provisional addition of three missing tRNAs certainly affected the similarity values and transformational pathways between *L. spari* and other monogeneans, but it would not affect the assignment of a new gene order pattern to diplectanids, nor our conclusion that diplectanids are prone to mitogenomic rearrangements.

Conclusions

The present study reports four findings worthy of emphasis. First, on the basis of nucleotide diversity, dN/dS and average sequence identity, we propose that *nad*2, *nad*5 and *nad*4 genes are better-suited as molecular markers for species identification and population genetics studies of diplectanids than the commonly used *cox*1. Secondly, the long non-coding region of both mitogenomes contains two interesting features: (i) a highly repetitive region, which is often associated with replication origin in mitochondria; and (ii) tRNA pseudogenes in tandem arrays, which is common in plastid genomes and prokaryotes, but rare in metazoan mitogenomes. Thirdly, phylogenetic analysis showed that the two new diplectanids (Dactylogyridea) formed a sister group with a clade comprised of two other dactylogyrids (Dactylogyridea) and three capsalids (Capsalidea). Thus, Dactylogyridea was rendered paraphyletic by the nested Capsalidea clade. Fourthly, due to the extensive tRNA gene rearrangements in the two diplectanids, we assigned them a new gene order pattern, and concluded that the evolution of mitogenomic gene order arrangements is discontinuous in monogeneans. However, our confidence in the unorthodox phylogeny produced here, and understanding of genomic architecture evolution, is curbed by the scarcity of available mitogenomes (only four dactylogyrideans and 20 monogeneans), so we encourage researchers to accumulate more samples and molecular data (especially large molecular data) for monogenean parasites in order to infer their evolutionary history with confidence.

Abbreviations

ORF: open reading frame; RSCU: relative synonymous codon usage; PCGs: protein-encoding genes; ML: maximum likelihood; BI: Bayesian inference; dN: non-synonymous mutation rate; dS: synonymous mutation rate; LNCR: long non-coding regions; BS: bootstrap; PB: PhyloBayes; HRR: highly repetitive region; TRs: tandem repeats; TDRL: tandem-duplication-random-loss

Acknowledgements

The authors would like to thank MSc Run Q. Wang for their assistance in sampling the monogeneans. We would also like to thank the editor and the two anonymous reviewers for the time they invested in reviewing our manuscript.

Funding

This work was funded by the National Natural Science Foundation of China (31872604, 31572658), the Earmarked Fund for China Agriculture Research System (CARS-45-15) and the Major Scientific and Technological Innovation Project of Hubei Province (2015ABA045).

Authors' contributions

GTW, WXL and DZ designed the study. DZ, HZ, JZ and RC conducted the experiments. DZ conducted the data analysis. DZ, WXL and IJ wrote the paper. All authors revised the manuscript critically for important intellectual content, read and approved the final manuscript.

Competing interests

The authors declare that they have no competing interests.

Author details

[1]Key Laboratory of Aquaculture Disease Control, Ministry of Agriculture, and State Key Laboratory of Freshwater Ecology and Biotechnology, Institute of Hydrobiology, Chinese Academy of Sciences, Wuhan 430072, People's Republic of China. [2]University of Chinese Academy of Sciences, Beijing, People's Republic of China. [3]Bio-Transduction Lab, Biolake, Wuhan 430075, People's Republic of China.

References

1. Oliver G. Les Diplectanidae Bychowsky, 1957 (Monogenea, Monopisthocotylea, Dactylogyridea). Systématique. Biologie. Ontogénie. Écologie. Essai de phylogénèse. Thesis. France: Université des Sciences et Techniques du Languedoc; 1987.
2. Dezfuli BS, Giari L, Simoni E, Menegatti R, Shinn AP, Manera M. Gill histopathology of cultured European sea bass, *Dicentrarchus labrax* (L.), infected with *Diplectanum aequans* (Wagener, 1857) Diesing 1958 (Diplectanidae: Monogenea). Parasitol Res. 2007;100:707–13.
3. Cone DK. Monogenea (Phylum Platyhelminthes). In: Woo PTK, editor. Fish Diseases and Disorders: Protozoan and Metazoan Infections. Wallingford: CAB International; 1995. p. 289–327.
4. Zhang D, Zou H, Wu SG, Li M, Jakovlić I, Zhang J, et al. Sequencing of the complete mitochondrial genome of a fish-parasitic flatworm *Paratetraonchoides inermis* (Platyhelminthes: Monogenea): tRNA gene arrangement reshuffling and implications for phylogeny. Parasit Vectors. 2017;10:462.
5. Perkins EM, Donnellan SC, Bertozzi T, Chisholm LA, Whittington ID. Looks can deceive: molecular phylogeny of a family of flatworm ectoparasites (Monogenea: Capsalidae) does not reflect current morphological classification. Mol Phylogenet Evol. 2009;52:705–14.
6. Poulin R, Morand S. The diversity of parasites. Q Rev Biol. 2000;75:277–93.
7. Huyse T, Buchmann K, Littlewood DT. The mitochondrial genome of *Gyrodactylus derjavinoides* (Platyhelminthes: Monogenea) - a mitogenomic approach for *Gyrodactylus* species and strain identification. Gene. 2008;417:27–34.
8. Mollaret I, Jamieson BG, Justine J-L. Phylogeny of the Monopisthocotylea and Polyopisthocotylea (Platyhelminthes) inferred from 28S rDNA sequences. Int J Parasitol. 2000;30:171–85.
9. Olson P, Littlewood D. Phylogenetics of the Monogenea - evidence from a medley of molecules. Int J Parasitol. 2002;32:233–44.
10. Simkova A, Plaisance L, Matejusova I, Morand S, Verneau O. Phylogenetic relationships of the Dactylogyridae Bychowsky, 1933 (Monogenea: Dactylogyridea): the need for the systematic revision of the Ancyrocephalinae Bychowsky, 1937. Syst Parasitol. 2003;54:1–11.
11. Plaisance L, Littlewood DTJ, Olson PD, Morand S. Molecular phylogeny of gill monogeneans (Platyhelminthes, Monogenea, Dactylogyridae) and colonization of Indo-West Pacific butterflyfish hosts (Perciformes, Chaetodontidae). Zool Scr. 2005;34:425–36.
12. Justine J-L. Cladistic study in the Monogenea (Platyhelminthes), based upon a parsimony analysis of spermiogenetic and spermatozoal ultrastructural characters. Int J Parasitol. 1991;21:821–38.
13. Justine J-L, Lambert A, Mattei X. Spermatozoon ultrastructure and phylogenetic relationships in the monogeneans (Platyhelminthes). Int J Parasitol. 1985;15:601–8.
14. Boeger WA, Kritsky DC. Phylogenetic relationships of the Monogenoidea. In: Littlewood DTJ, Bray RA, editors. Interrelationships of the Platyhelminthes. London: Taylor & Francis; 2001. p. 92–102.
15. Yin M, Zheng HX, Su J, Feng Z, McManus DP, Zhou XN, et al. Co-dispersal of the blood fluke *Schistosoma japonicum* and *Homo sapiens* in the Neolithic Age. Sci Rep. 2015;5:18058.
16. Perkins EM, Donnellan SC, Bertozzi T, Whittington ID. Closing the mitochondrial circle on paraphyly of the Monogenea (Platyhelminthes) infers evolution in the diet of parasitic flatworms. Int J Parasitol. 2010;40: 1237–45.
17. Li WX, Zhang D, Boyce K, Xi BW, Zou H, Wu SG, et al. The complete mitochondrial DNA of three monozoic tapeworms in the Caryophyllidea: a mitogenomic perspective on the phylogeny of eucestodes. Parasit Vectors. 2017;10:314.
18. Jia W-Z, Yan H-B, Guo A-J, Zhu X-Q, Wang Y-C, Shi W-G, et al. Complete mitochondrial genomes of *Taenia multiceps*, *T. hydatigena* and *T. pisiformis*: additional molecular markers for a tapeworm genus of human and animal health significance. BMC Genomics. 2010;11:447.
19. Zhang D, Zou H, Wu SG, Li M, Jakovlic I, Zhang J, et al. Sequencing, characterization and phylogenomics of the complete mitochondrial genome of *Dactylogyrus lamellatus* (Monogenea: Dactylogyridae). J Helminthol. 2018;92:455–66.
20. Bachmann L, Fromm B, de Azambuja LP, Boeger WA. The mitochondrial genome of the egg-laying flatworm *Aglaiogyrodactylus forficulatus* (Platyhelminthes: Monogenoidea). Parasit Vectors. 2016;9:285.
21. Zhang JY, Yang TB, Liu L. Monogeneans of Chinese Marine Fishes. Beijing: Agriculture Press; 2001.
22. Sánchez-García N, Padrós F, Raga JA, Montero FE. Comparative study of the three attachment mechanisms of diplectanid monogeneans. Aquaculture. 2011;318:290–9.
23. Domingues MV, Boeger WA. Phylogeny and revision of Diplectanidae Monticelli, 1903 (Platyhelminthes: Monogenoidea). Zootaxa. 2008;1698:1–40.
24. Ogawa K, Egusa S. Three species of *Lamellodiscus* (Monogenea: diplectanidae) from the gills of the Japanese black sea bream, *Acanthopagrus schlegeli* (Bleeker). Bull Jap Soc Sci Fish. 1978;44:607–12.
25. Wu XY, Li AX, Zhu XQ, Xie MQ. Description of *Pseudorhabdosynochus seabassi* sp. n. (Monogenea: Diplectanidae) from *Lates calcarifer* and revision of the phylogenetic position of *Diplectanum grouperi* (Monogenea: Diplectanidae) based on rDNA sequence data. Folia Parasitol. 2005;52:231.
26. Thompson JD, Gibson TJ, Higgins DG. Multiple sequence alignment using ClustalW and ClustalX. Curr Protoc Bioinformatics. 2002;Chapter 2:Unit 2.3.
27. Lalitha S. Primer Premier 5. Biot Soft Int Rep. 2000;1:270–2.
28. Zou H, Jakovlic I, Chen R, Zhang D, Zhang J, Li WX, et al. The complete mitochondrial genome of parasitic nematode *Camallanus cotti*: extreme discontinuity in the rate of mitogenomic architecture evolution within the Chromadorea class. BMC Genomics. 2017;18:840.
29. Altschul SF, Gish W, Miller W, Myers EW, Lipman DJ. Basic local alignment search tool. J Mol Biol. 1990;215:403–10.
30. Burland TG. DNASTAR's Lasergene sequence analysis software. Methods Mol Biol. 2000;132:71–91.
31. Bernt M, Donath A, Juhling F, Externbrink F, Florentz C, Fritzsch G, et al. MITOS: improved *de novo* metazoan mitochondrial genome annotation. Mol Phylogenet Evol. 2013;69:313–9.
32. Laslett D, Canback BARWEN. a program to detect tRNA genes in metazoan mitochondrial nucleotide sequences. Bioinformatics. 2008;24:172–5.
33. Wyman SK, Jansen RK, Boore JL. Automatic annotation of organellar genomes with DOGMA. Bioinformatics. 2004;20:3252–5.
34. Zhang D. MitoTool software. 2016. https://github.com/dongzhang0725/MitoTool. Accessed 22 July 2018.
35. Hadley W. ggplot2: Elegant graphics for data analysis. New York: Springer; 2009.
36. Librado P, Rozas J. DnaSP v5: a software for comprehensive analysis of DNA polymorphism data. Bioinformatics. 2009;25:1451–2.
37. Benson G. Tandem repeats finder: a program to analyze DNA sequences. Nucleic Acids Res. 1999;27:573.
38. Zuker M. Mfold web server for nucleic acid folding and hybridization prediction. Nucleic Acids Res. 2003;31:3406–15.
39. Bernt M, Merkle D, Ramsch K, Fritzsch G, Perseke M, Bernhard D, et al. CREx: inferring genomic rearrangements based on common intervals. Bioinformatics. 2007;23:2957–8.
40. Liu F-F, Li Y-P, Jakovlic I, Yuan X-Q. Tandem duplication of two tRNA genes in the mitochondrial genome of *Tagiades vajuna* (Lepidoptera: Hesperiidae). Eur J Entomol. 2017;114:407–15.
41. Katoh K. Standley DM. MAFFT multiple sequence alignment software version 7: improvements in performance and usability. Mol Biol Evol. 2013; 30:772–80.
42. Talavera G, Castresana J. Improvement of phylogenies after removing divergent and ambiguously aligned blocks from protein sequence alignments. Syst Biol. 2007;56:564–77.
43. Kück P, Meid SA, Groß C, Wägele JW, Misof B. AliGROOVE - visualization of heterogeneous sequence divergence within multiple sequence alignments and detection of inflated branch support. BMC Bioinformatics. 2014;15:294.
44. Lanfear R, Frandsen PB, Wright AM, Senfeld T, Calcott B. PartitionFinder 2: new methods for selecting partitioned models of evolution for molecular and morphological phylogenetic analyses. Mol Biol Evol. 2017;34:772–3.
45. Abascal F, Zardoya R, Posada D. ProtTest: selection of best-fit models of protein evolution. Bioinformatics. 2005;21:2104–5.
46. Stamatakis A. RAxML version 8: a tool for phylogenetic analysis and post-analysis of large phylogenies. Bioinformatics. 2014;30:1312–3.
47. Lartillot N, Rodrigue N, Stubbs D, Richer J. PhyloBayes MPI: phylogenetic reconstruction with infinite mixtures of profiles in a parallel environment. Syst Biol. 2013;62:611–5.
48. Letunic I, Bork P. Interactive tree of life (iTOL) v3: an online tool for the display and annotation of phylogenetic and other trees. Nucleic Acids Res. 2016;44:W242–5.
49. Wey-Fabrizius AR, Podsiadlowski L, Herlyn H, Hankeln T. Platyzoan mitochondrial genomes. Mol Phylogenet Evol. 2013;69:365–75.
50. Kang S, Kim J, Lee J, Kim S, Min GS, Park JK. The complete mitochondrial

genome of an ectoparasitic monopisthocotylean fluke *Benedenia hoshinai* (Monogenea: Platyhelminthes). Mitochondrial DNA. 2012;23:176–8.

51. Ye F, King SD, Cone DK, You P. The mitochondrial genome of *Paragyrodactylus variegatus* (Platyhelminthes: Monogenea): differences in major non-coding region and gene order compared to *Gyrodactylus*. Parasit Vectors. 2014;7:377.
52. Zhang D. The chromatograms of the fragments between *nad5* and *cox3*. 2018. https://figshare.com/articles/The_chromatograms_of_the_fragments_between_nad5_and_cox3/6363965. Accessed 26 May 2018.
53. Doublet V, Ubrig E, Alioua A, Bouchon D, Marcade I, Marechal-Drouard L. Large gene overlaps and tRNA processing in the compact mitochondrial genome of the crustacean *Armadillidium vulgare*. RNA Biol. 2015;12:1159–68.
54. Kilpert F, Podsiadlowski L. The complete mitochondrial genome of the common sea slater, *Ligia oceanica* (Crustacea, Isopoda) bears a novel gene order and unusual control region features. BMC Genomics. 2006;7:241.
55. Kumazawa Y, Miura S, Yamada C, Hashiguchi Y. Gene rearrangements in gekkonid mitochondrial genomes with shuffling, lossand reassignment of tRNA genes. BMC Genomics. 2014;15:930.
56. Wu X, Xu X, Yu Z, Kong X. Comparative mitogenomic analyses of three scallops (Bivalvia: Pectinidae) reveal high level variation of genomic organization and a diversity of transfer RNA gene sets. BMC Res Notes. 2009;2:69.
57. Domes K, Maraun M, Scheu S, Cameron SL. The complete mitochondrial genome of the sexual oribatid mite *Steganacarus magnus*: genome rearrangements and loss of tRNAs. BMC Genomics. 2008;9:532.
58. Huot JL, Enkler L, Megel C, Karim L, Laporte D, Becker HD, et al. Idiosyncrasies in decoding mitochondrial genomes. Biochimie. 2014;100:95–106.
59. Huyse T, Plaisance L, Webster BL, Mo TA, Bakke TA, Bachmann L, et al. The mitochondrial genome of *Gyrodactylus salaris* (Platyhelminthes: Monogenea), a pathogen of Atlantic salmon (*Salmo salar*). Parasitology. 2007;134:739–47.
60. Plaisance L, Huyse T, Littlewood DT, Bakke TA, Bachmann L. The complete mitochondrial DNA sequence of the monogenean *Gyrodactylus thymalli* (Platyhelminthes: Monogenea), a parasite of grayling (*Thymallus thymallus*). Mol Biochem Parasitol. 2007;154:190–4.
61. Zhang J, Wu X, Xie M, Li A. The complete mitochondrial genome of *Pseudochauhanea macrorchis* (Monogenea: Chauhaneidae) revealed a highly repetitive region and a gene rearrangement hot spot in Polyopisthocotylea. Mol Biol Rep. 2012;39:8115–25.
62. Zhang J, Wu X, Xie M, Xu X, Li A. The mitochondrial genome of *Polylabris halichoeres* (Monogenea: Microcotylidae). Mitochondrial DNA. 2011;22:3–5.
63. Zhang J, Wu X, Li Y, Zhao M, Xie M, Li A. The complete mitochondrial genome of *Neobenedenia melleni* (Platyhelminthes: Monogenea): mitochondrial gene content, arrangement and composition compared with two *Benedenia* species. Mol Biol Rep. 2014;41:6583–9.
64. Park JK, Kim KH, Kang S, Kim W, Eom KS, Littlewood DT. A common origin of complex life cycles in parasitic flatworms: evidence from the complete mitochondrial genome of *Microcotyle sebastis* (Monogenea: Platyhelminthes). BMC Evol Biol. 2007;7:11.
65. Zhang D, Zou H, Zhou S, Wu SG, Li WX, Wang GT. The complete mitochondrial genome of *Gyrodactylus kobayashii* (Platyhelminthes: Monogenea). Mitochondrial DNA Part B. 2016;1:146–7.
66. Zhang J, Wu X, Li Y, Xie M, Li A. The complete mitochondrial genome of *Tetrancistrum nebulosi* (Monogenea: Ancyrocephalidae). Mitochondrial DNA Part B. 2016;27:22–3.
67. Zou H, Zhang D, Li W, Zhou S, Wu S, Wang G. The complete mitochondrial genome of *Gyrodactylus gurleyi* (Platyhelminthes: Monogenea). Mitochondrial DNA Part B. 2016;1:383–5.
68. Kim K, Jeon H, Kang S, Sultana T, Kim GJ, Eom KS, et al. Characterization of the complete mitochondrial genome of *Diphyllobothrium nihonkaiense* (Diphyllobothriidae: Cestoda), and development of molecular markers for differentiating fish tapeworms. Mol Cells. 2007;23:379.
69. von Nickisch-Rosenegk M, Brown WM, Boore JL. Complete sequence of the mitochondrial genome of the tapeworm *Hymenolepis diminuta*: gene arrangements indicate that platyhelminths are eutrochozoans. Mol Biol Evol. 2001;18:721–30.
70. Le TH, Blair D, McManus DP. Mitochondrial genomes of parasitic flatworms. Trends Parasitol. 2002;18:206–13.
71. Fumagalli L, Taberlet P, Favre L, Hausser J. Origin and evolution of homologous repeated sequences in the mitochondrial DNA control region of shrews. Mol Biol Evol. 1996;13:31–46.
72. Amiryousefi A, Hyvonen J, Poczai P. The chloroplast genome sequence of bittersweet (*Solanum dulcamara*): plastid genome structure evolution in *Solanaceae*. PLoS One. 2018;13:e0196069.
73. Tran TT, Belahbib H, Bonnefoy V. Talla E. A comprehensive tRNA genomic survey unravels the evolutionary history of tRNA arrays in prokaryotes. Genome Biol Evol. 2015;8:282–95.
74. Hebert PD, Cywinska A, Ball SL. Biological identifications through DNA barcodes. Proc Biol Sci. 2003;270:313–21.
75. Hansen H, Bachmann L, Bakke TA. Mitochondrial DNA variation of *Gyrodactylus* spp. (Monogenea, Gyrodactylidae) populations infecting Atlantic salmon, grayling, and rainbow trout in Norway and Sweden. Int J Parasitol. 2003;33:1471–8.
76. Hansen H, Martinsen L, Bakke T, Bachmann L. The incongruence of nuclear and mitochondrial DNA variation supports conspecificity of the monogenean parasites *Gyrodactylus salaris* and *G. thymalli*. Parasitology. 2006;133:639–50.
77. Meinilä M, Kuusela J, Ziętara MS, Lumme J. Initial steps of speciation by geographic isolation and host switch in salmonid pathogen *Gyrodactylus salaris* (Monogenea: Gyrodactylidae). Int J Parasitol. 2004;34:515–26.
78. Blasco-Costa I, Miguez-Lozano R, Sarabeev V, Balbuena JA. Molecular phylogeny of species of *Ligophorus* (Monogenea: Dactylogyridae) and their affinities within the Dactylogyridae. Parasitol Int. 2012;61:619–27.
79. Goldstein DB, Linares AR, Cavalli-Sforza LL, Feldman MW. An evaluation of genetic distances for use with microsatellite loci. Genetics. 1995;139:463–71.
80. Bychowsky BE. Monogenetic Trematodes, their systematics and phylogeny. Moscow-Leningrad, USSR: Academy of Sciences; 1957 (In Russian; English translation by Hargis WJ, Oustinoff PC, 1961. American Institute of Biological Sciences, Washington).
81. Lebedev B. Monogenea in the light of new evidence and their position among platyhelminths. Angew Parasitol. 1988;29:149–67.
82. Boeger WA, Kritsky DC. Phylogeny and a revised classification of the Monogenoidea Bychowsky, 1937 (Platyhelminthes). Syst Parasitol. 1993;26:1–32.
83. Lambert A. Oncomiracidiums et phylogénèse des Monogènes (Plathelminthes), 2ème partie: Structures argyrophiles des oncomiracidiums et phylogénèse des Monogenea. Ann Parasitol Hum Comp. 1980;55:281–326.
84. Delsuc F, Tsagkogeorga G, Lartillot N, Philippe H. Additional molecular support for the new chordate phylogeny. Genesis. 2008;46:592–604.
85. Park S, Ruhlman TA, Weng ML, Hajrah NH, Sabir JSM, Jansen RK. Contrasting patterns of nucleotide substitution rates provide insight into dynamic evolution of plastid and mitochondrial genomes of *Geranium*. Genome Biol Evol. 2017;9:1766–80.
86. Grechko VV. The problems of molecular phylogenetics with the example of squamate reptiles: mitochondrial DNA markers. Mol Biol. 2013;47:55–74.
87. Boore JL. The duplication/random loss model for gene rearrangement exemplified by mitochondrial genomes of deuterostome animals. In: Sankoff D, Nadeau JH, editors. Comparative Genomics. Dordrecht: Kluwer Academic Publishers; 2000. p. 133–47.
88. Black WC 4th, Roehrdanz RL. Mitochondrial gene order is not conserved in arthropods: prostriate and metastriate tick mitochondrial genomes. Mol Biol Evol. 1998;15:1772–85.
89. Li H, Liu H, Shi A, Stys P, Zhou X, Cai W. The complete mitochondrial genome and novel gene arrangement of the unique-headed bug *Stenopirates* sp. (Hemiptera: Enicocephalidae). PLoS One. 2012;7:e29419.
90. Wang JG, Zhang D, Jakovlic I, Wang WM. Sequencing of the complete mitochondrial genomes of eight freshwater snail species exposes pervasive paraphyly within the Viviparidae family (Caenogastropoda). PLoS One. 2017; 12:e0181699.
91. Xiong H, Barker SC, Burger TD, Raoult D, Shao R. Heteroplasmy in the mitochondrial genomes of human lice and ticks revealed by high throughput sequencing. PLoS One. 2013;8:e73329.
92. Mueller RL, Boore JL. Molecular mechanisms of extensive mitochondrial gene rearrangement in plethodontid salamanders. Mol Biol Evol. 2005;22:2104–12.
93. Boore J. The use of genome-level characters for phylogenetic reconstruction. Trends Ecol Evol. 2006;21:439–46.
94. Sultana T, Kim J, Lee S-H, Han H, Kim S, Min G-S, et al. Comparative analysis of complete mitochondrial genome sequences confirms independent origins of plant-parasitic nematodes. BMC Evol Biol. 2013;13:12.

6

A new blood parasite of leaf warblers: molecular characterization, phylogenetic relationships, description and identification of vectors

Carolina Romeiro Fernandes Chagas*, Dovilė Bukauskaitė, Mikas Ilgūnas, Tatjana Iezhova and Gediminas Valkiūnas

Abstract

Background: Blood parasites of the genus *Haemoproteus* Kruse, 1890 are cosmopolitan, might be responsible for mortality in non-adapted birds, and often kill blood-sucking insects. However, this group remains insufficiently investigated in the wild. This is particularly true for the parasites of leaf warblers of the Phylloscopidae Alström, Ericson, Olsson & Sundberg the common small Old World passerine birds whose haemoproteid parasite diversity and vectors remain poorly studied. This study reports a new species of *Haemoproteus* parasitizing leaf warblers, its susceptible vector and peculiar phylogenetic relationships with other haemoproteids.

Methods: Wood warblers (*Phylloscopus sibilatrix* Bechstein) were caught in Lithuania during spring migration, and blood films were examined microscopically. Laboratory reared *Culicoides nubeculosus* Meigen were exposed experimentally by allowing them to take blood meals on one individual harbouring mature gametocytes of the new *Haemoproteus* species (lineage hPHSIB2). To follow sporogonic development, the engorged insects were dissected at intervals. The parasite lineage was distinguished using sequence data, and morphological analysis of blood and sporogonic stages was carried out. Bayesian phylogeny was constructed in order to determine the phylogenetic relationships of the new parasite with other haemoproteids.

Results: *Haemoproteus* (*Parahaemoproteus*) *homopalloris* n. sp. was common in wood warblers sampled after arrival to Europe from their wintering grounds in Africa. The new parasite belongs to a group of avian haemoproteid species with macrogametocytes possessing pale staining cytoplasm. All species of this group clustered together in the phylogenetic analysis, indicating that intensity of the cytoplasm staining is a valuable phylogenetic character. Laboratory-reared biting midges *C. nubeculosus* readily supported sporogony of new infections. Phylogenetic analysis corroborated vector experiments, placing the new parasite in the clade of *Haemoproteus* (*Parahaemoproteus*) parasites transmitted by biting midges.

Conclusions: *Haemoproteus homopalloris* n. sp. is the third haemoproteid, which is described from and is prevalent in wood warblers. Phylogenetic analysis identified a clade containing seven haemoproteids, which are characterised by pale staining of the macrogametocyte cytoplasm and with ookinetes maturing exceptionally rapidly (between 1 to 1.5 h after exposure to air). Both these features may represent valuable phylogenetic characters. Studies targeting mechanisms of sporogonic development of haemoproteids remain uncommon and should be encouraged. *Culicoides nubeculosus* is an excellent experimental vector of the new parasite species.

Keywords: *Haemoproteus*, New species, *Haemoproteus homopalloris* n. sp., Phylogenetic relationships, *Culicoides*, Vectors, Sporogony

* Correspondence: crfchagas@gmail.com
Institute of Ecology, Nature Research Centre, Akademijos 2, 21, LT-09412 Vilnius, Lithuania

Background

Blood parasites of the genus *Haemoproteus* Kruse, 1890 (Haemosporida: Haemoproteidae) are distributed worldwide and are among the most extensively studied blood parasites of birds, particularly in the temperate regions [1]. They are transmitted by biting midges (Ceratopogonidae) and louse flies (Hippoboscidae) [2]. *Haemoproteus* species were considered relatively benign to their avian hosts [3]. However, several recent studies demonstrated the negative influence of these parasites and even mortality due to haemoproteosis not only in non-adaptative birds [4–11], but also in blood-sucking insects [12, 13].

Numerous studies addressed morphological and molecular characterization, distribution and genetic diversity of haemoproteids [14–20]. However, some bird groups remain insufficiently investigated. This is particularly true for leaf warblers of genus *Phylloscopus* Boie belonging to the Phylloscopidae Alström, Ericson, Olsson & Sundberg. The wood warbler, *Phylloscopus sibilatrix* Bechstein, is a common European passerine bird wintering in sub-Saharan Africa [21]. Despite its broad range of occurrence, only two haemoproteid species, *Haemoproteus majoris* Laveran, 1902 [2, 22–24] and *Haemoproteus belopolskyi* Valkiūnas, 1989 [25], have been reported in this bird.

Several research groups successfully used molecular techniques to detect haemoproteids in wild caught insects [26–31]. PCR-based protocols detect the presence of parasite DNA in the insect, but do not provide information on which development stage the parasite is present. In other words, these tools are insufficiently sensitive to conclude if invasive stages (sporozoites) develop in the PCR-positive insect and if insects can act as vectors and transmit the parasites [32]. Observation of infective sporozoites in salivary glands strongly suggests the vectorial capacity of blood-sucking insects. Experimental infections provide the opportunity to follow parasite development and to morphologically characterize each life stage [33, 34].

Studies addressing the sporogonic development and transmission of avian *Haemoproteus* species are few [29, 35–38]. Vector species and complete life-cycle remains unknown for the great majority of *Haemoproteus* parasites and their lineages [1, 38, 39]. *Culicoides* species have been used in experimental studies addressing parasite development [33, 34]. These insects are abundant in mixed forest zone in eastern Europe [37]. Despite of their diminutive size and difficulties to maintain in colonies [40], *Culicoides nubeculosus* Meigen and several other species have been kept in laboratory colonies successfully [41, 42]. *Culicoides nubeculosus* has been used to study the sporogonic development of *Haemoproteus handai* Maqsood, 1943 [43], *Haemoproteus tartakovskyi* Valkiūnas, 1986 [34], *Haemoproteus noctuae* Celli & Sanfelice, 1891 and *Haemoproteus syrnii* Mayer, 1910 [33].

During this study, we discovered a new *Haemoproteus* species that infects wood warblers. This parasite is described using morphology of blood stages and molecular data of partial cytochrome *b* (*cytb*) gene sequence. To access information about sporogonic development, we experimentally infected the biting midge *Culicoides nubeculosus.* The main objectives of this study were (i) to characterize the new *Haemoproteus* species morphologically; (ii) to develop its molecular characterization based on partial *cytb* sequence; (iii) to determine phylogenetically closely related parasite species; and (iv) to follow sporogonic development in experimentally infected vector.

Methods

Collection and examination of bird blood samples

We collected blood samples from 16 adult wood warblers (*Phylloscopus sibilatrix*) at the Ornithological Station in Ventės Ragas, Lithuania (55°20'28.1"N, 21° 11'25.3"E) during May in 2015, 2016 and 2017. The birds were caught with mist nets. Approximately 30 μl of blood was withdrawn from the brachial vein using a sterile syringe needle and capillary tubes. Several drops were used immediately for preparation of blood smears on three glass slides, and the remaining blood was stored in SET buffer (0.05 M tris, 0.15 M NaCl, 0.5 M EDTA, pH 8.0) for molecular diagnostics. Blood smears were air-dried, fixed with absolute methanol, and stained with Giemsa [44]. Preparations of good quality and sufficient parasite intensity with single infection, as determined both by microscopic examination and PCR-based testing, were used for morphological characterization of the new species.

Olympus BX41 microscope equipped with PixeLINK and imaging software Megapixel FireWire Camera Release 3.2 were used to examine the blood films and prepare illustrations. Measurements were taken from the images using the calibrated Motic Images Plus 2.0. The slides were examined for 15–20 min at low magnification (×400), and then at least 100 fields were studied at high magnification (×1000). Parasite identification follows the guidelines of Valkiūnas [2]. All measurements are given in micrometres. Images of positive preparations were collected for measurement. Representative preparations were deposited in the Nature Research Centre, Vilnius, Lithuania (accession number 49021 NS and 49022 NS). The analyses were carried out using the Statistica 7 package. A parahapantotype blood film with gametocytes of closely related haemoproteid *Haemoproteus palloris* Dimitrov, Iezhova, Zehtindjiev, Bobeva, Ilieva, Kirilova, Bedev, Sjohölm & Valkiūnas, 2016 (deposited at Nature Research Centre, Vilnius, accession number 48832 NS) was used for comparisons with the new *Haemoproteus* species.

Parasitemia was estimated as a percentage by actual counting the number of parasites per 1000 red blood cells or per 10,000 red blood cells during light infections (i.e. < 0.1%) [45]. Morphology of gametocytes of the new species was also compared with the type-specimens deposited in Institute of Nature Research Centre, Vilnius, Lithuania, of *Haemoproteus majoris* (accession number 48893 NS, from *Phylloscopus trochilus* Linnaeus) and *Haemoproteus belopolskyi* (accession number 435.85p, from *Hippolais icterina* Vieillot) the only two *Haemoproteus* parasites reported in *P. sibillatrix* so far. Hapantotype material of the new species was also compared with other *Haemoproteus* species with pale staining macrogametocytes: *Haemoproteus pallidus* Valkiūnas & Iezhova, 1991 (accession number 963.89, from *Ficedula hypoleuca* Pallas), *Haemoproteus pallidulus* Križanauskienė, Pérez-Tris, Palinaukas, Hellgren, Bensch & Valkiūnas, 2010 (accession number 5420 NS, from *Sylvia atricapilla* Linnaeus), *Haemoproteus minutus* Valkiūnas & Iezhova, 1992 (accession number 245.85p, from *Turdus merula* Linnaeus), *Haemoproteus concavocentralis* Dimitrov, Zehtindjiev, Bensch, Ilieva, Iezhova & Valkiūnas, 2014 (accession number 48756 NS, from *Coccothraustes coccothraustes* Linnaeus) and *Haemoproteus vacuolatus* Valkiūnas, Iezhova, Loiseau, Chasar, Smith & Sehgal, 2008 (accession number 42415 NS, from *Andropadus latirostris* Strickland).

Sporogonic development experimental design

A naturally infected wood warbler with single infection with the new *Haemoproteus* lineage was used as a donor of gametocytes to expose *Culicoides nubeculosus* biting midges. The presence of a single infection in the donor bird was confirmed by microscopic examination (see above) and PCR-based testing, as described below. Insects were reared in the laboratory according to Boorman et al. [41]. Experimental procedures were according to Bukauskaitė et al. [13]. Briefly, biting midges were kept in card boxes covered with fine mesh bolting silk. For the experiment, a box with unfed insects was gently pressed to the feather-free area on pectoral muscles of infected bird. *Culicoides nubeculosus* took blood meals through the bolting silk, with the great majority of females being fully engorged within 30–40 min. Then, biting midges were transferred to a bigger cage made of bolting silk (12 × 12 × 12 cm), males and non-fed females were removed. Remaining insects were kept in a room with controlled temperature (22° C), relative humidity (75 ± 5%) and light-dark photoperiod of 17:7 h. Insects were supplied with a 10% sugar solution offered in cotton pads.

Dissection of biting midges, preparations of parasites and microscopic examination

Experimentally exposed biting midges were dissected, and preparation of ookinetes, oocysts and sporozoites were made. First, the insects were anesthetized by placing them in a tube covered with cotton-wool pads moistened with 96% ethanol. Biting midges were dissected on intervals in order to follow the development of the parasite in the insect. We examined midgut contents for ookinetes 0.5–12 h post exposure, midgut wall for oocysts 2–5 days post exposure (dpe), and salivary glands for sporozoites 7–8 dpe.

For visualizing ookinetes, midgut was dissected and gently crushed on the slide; the preparations were fixed and stained the same way as blood films. For oocyst observation, temporary preparations were made. Midguts were isolated on a glass slide and a drop of 2% mercurochrome solution was placed on the guts, which was then covered with coverslips. This simplified observation of oocysts. To visualize sporozoites, preparation was made by extracting the salivary glands from biting midges and gently crashing them to prepare small thin smears, which were fixed with absolute methanol and stained with 4% Giemsa solution for 1 h. After each insect dissection, residual parts of their bodies were fixed in 96% ethanol and used for PCR-based analysis to confirm presence of corresponding parasite lineage in vectors. Dissected needles were disinfected in fire to prevent contamination after each dissection.

All vector preparations were examined using Olympus BX43 light microscope equipped with Olympus SZX2-FOF digital camera and imaging software QCapture Pro 6.0, Image Pro Plus (Tokyo, Japan). All preparations were examined as described above for blood smears, and the representative preparations were deposited in the Nature Research Centre, Vilnius, Lithuania (accession numbers 49023 NS and 49024 NS).

DNA extraction, PCR, sequencing and phylogenetic analysis

Blood samples from the donor bird and residual parts of infected biting midges were examined for haemosporidian parasites by PCR amplification. Total DNA was extracted from both materials using a standard ammonium acetate method [46] and quantified by NanoPhotometer® P330 (IMPLEN). A nested PCR protocol was used to amplify a *cytb* gene fragment [47, 48]. The first pair of primers (HaemFNI/HaemNR3) amplifies sequences of *Plasmodium*, *Haemoproteus* and *Leucocytozoon*. The second pair of primers (HaemF/HaemR2) is specific for *Plasmodium* and *Haemoproteus* parasites. We performed PCR amplification in 25 μl total volume including 50 ng of total genomic DNA template (2 μl), 12.5 μl of Phusion High-Fidelity PCR Master Mix (Thermo Fisher Scientific, Vilnius, Lithuania), 8.5 μl nuclease-free water and 1 μl of each primer (10 μM concentration). One positive (infection confirmed by microscopy analysis) and one negative control (ultrapure water) were used. Positive results were visualized by electrophoresing 2 μl of the final PCR product on a 2% agarose gel. Amplicons of proper length (approximately 500 bp) were precipitated and sequenced from both ends using Big

Dye Terminator V3.1 cycle Sequencing Kit and ABI PRISM^{TM} 3100 capillary sequencing robot (Applied Biosystems, Foster City, California). Sequences were edited and aligned using the BioEdit program [49] and deposited in the GenBank database (accession number MH513601). The presence of double peaks in sequence chromatograms was considered a co-infection.

A Bayesian phylogeny of parasite lineages was constructed based on alignment of 45 *cytb* lineages (33 *Haemoproteus* spp. and 11 *Plasmodium* spp.) using MrBayes version 3.2 [50]. One lineage of *Leucocytozoon* sp. (lineage lSISKIN2) was used as the outgroup. All lineages were carefully selected based on studies that provided morphological identification of parasites. We used the General Time Reversible model (GTR) selected by the software jModelTest 2 [51] as the best-fit model under the Bayesian Information Criterion. Gaps and missing data in the alignment were discarded prior to analyses. Two simultaneous runs were conducted with a sample frequency of every 100th generation over 3 million generations. We discarded 25% of the trees as 'burn in' period. The remaining trees were used to construct a majority rule consensus tree. The phylogenies were visualized using Fig Tree 1.4 [52]. The codes of *cytb* lineages are given according to MalAvi database, with a letter 'h' starting codes of *Haemoproteus* spp. lineages and a letter 'p' starting codes of *Plasmodium* spp. lineages. The sequence divergence between different lineages was calculated using Jukes-Cantor model of substitution, with all substitutions weighted equally (uniform rates), implemented in the program MEGA7 [53].

Results

Microscopic and molecular analysis of blood samples

In all, 43.8% of wood warbler tested by PCR and microscopy were infected with *Haemoproteus* parasites. All infections were detected by both methods equally. We reported two different lineages of *Haemoproteus* species in tested birds: hPHSIB1 (*Haemoproteus majoris*) and hPHSIB2 (*Haemoproteus homopalloris* n. sp.). The prevalence of infection with lineage hPHSIB2 was 31%. Two individuals harboured double haemosporidian infection, one with two *Haemoproteus* species, and another one with *Haemoproteus* and *Plasmodium* species. These double infections were detected also by PCR.

Phylogenetic analysis confirmed that morphological characteristics of gametocytes are of phylogenetic value because the lineage hPHSIB2 was readily distinguishable both morphologically (Fig. 1) and in the tree (Fig. 2). The lineage hPHSIB2 clustered with other so-called pale staining haemoproteid species, with a high (100%) posterior probability (Fig. 2, clade B): *Haemoproteus pallidus*, *H. palloris*, *H. minutus*, *H. pallidulus*, *H. vacuolatus* and *Haemoproteus concavocentralis*. It is worth noting that the mean genetic distance among *cytb* lineages within this clade was low (1.5%), but all parasites in this clade have unique morphological characters, based on which they can be distinguished from each other (see Fig. 3 and the Remarks below).

Family Haemoproteidae Doflein, 1916
Genus *Haemoproteus* Kruse, 1890

***Haemoproteus (Parahaemoproteus) homopalloris* n. sp.**

***Type-host*:** *Phylloscopus sibilatrix* Bechstein, 1793 (Passeriformes, Phylloscopidae), wood warbler.
***Type-locality*:** Ornithological Station in Ventės Ragas (55°20'28.1"N, 21°11'25.3"E), Lithuania.
***Type-specimens*:** Hapantotypes (accession numbers 49021 NS and 49022 NS, adult bird *Phylloscopus sibilatrix*; parasitaemia 0.1%, 5.vi.2017, Ornithological Station Ventės Ragas, collected by M. Ilgūnas) were deposited in the Institute of Ecology of Nature Research Centre, Vilnius, Lithuania. Parahapantotype (accession number G466204, other data as for the hapantotype) was deposited in the Queensland Museum, Brisbane, Australia. Co-infection with microfilaria is present in the type-material.
***Site of infection*:** Mature erythrocytes; no other data.
***Prevalence*:** 31% (5 out of 16 examined wood warblers were infected).
***Representative DNA sequence*:** Mitochondrial *cytb* lineage hPHSIB2 (478 bp, GenBank accession number MH513601).
***Vector*:** Sporogony completed and sporozoites developed in experimentally infected biting midges *Culicoides nubeculosus*. This insect is a convenient experimental vector. Natural vectors remain unknown. Representative preparations of sporogonic stages are deposited in the Institute of Ecology of Nature Research Centre, Vilnius, Lithuania, with the accession numbers of 49023 NS and 49024 NS.
***ZooBank registration*:** To comply with the regulations set out in article 8.5 of the amended 2012 version of the *International Code of Zoological Nomenclature* (ICZN) [54], details of the new species have been submitted to ZooBank. The Life Science Identifier (LSID) of the article is urn:lsid:zoobank.org:pub:AC9794B3-D735-4D36-BB6E-5CDF1CF2BA3F. The LSID for the new name *Haemoproteus (Parahaemoproteus) homopalloris* is urn:lsid:zoobank.org:act:5481116F-3F96-40D2-956E-96C710C64F29.
***Etymology*:** The species name refers to the morphological and morphometric similarity of the new species with *Haemoproteus palloris*, a closely related haemoproteid infecting a closely related avian host, the willow warbler *Phylloscopus trochilus*.

Description (Fig. 1a-l, Table 1)

Young gametocytes. Rarely seen in the type-material (Fig. 1a, b). Elongate, with even outline and prominent

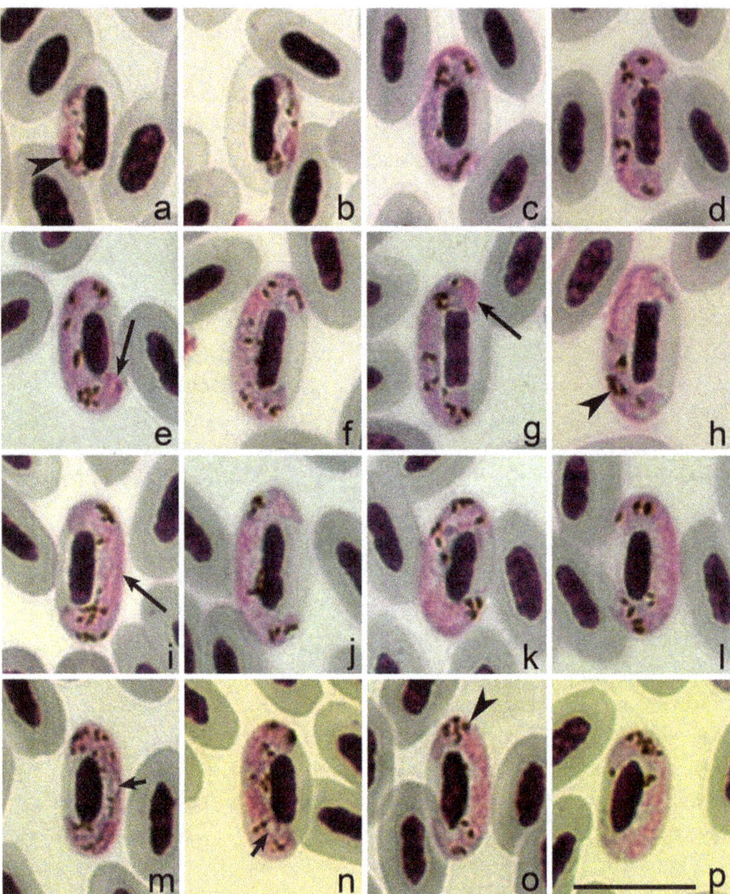

Fig. 1 Gametocytes of two species of haemoproteids described from leaf warbles, Phylloscopidae. *Haemoproteus homopalloris* n. sp. (**a**-**l**) and *Haemoproteus palloris* (**m**-**p**). Young gametocytes (**a**, **b**), macrogametocytes (**c**-**g**, **m**, **n**) and microgametocytes (**h**-**l**, **o**, **p**). Long arrows: gametocyte nuclei; short arrows: vacuole-like spaces in macrogametocytes; arrowheads: pigment granules. Giemsa-stained thin blood films. *Scale-bar*: **a**-**p**, 10 μm

pigment granules. Develop in mature erythrocytes; advanced growing gametocytes closely adhere to erythrocyte nuclei and extend longitudinally along nuclei.

Macrogametocytes. Develop in mature erythrocytes. Cytoplasm staining pale-blue, heterogeneous in appearance, lacking volutin granules. Outline even or slightly wavy (Fig. 1c-g). Vacuoles or vacuole-like spaces absent in the cytoplasm. Gametocytes grow along nuclei of infected erythrocytes, enclose nuclei with their ends, but do not encircle them completely (Fig. 1c-g). Advanced and fully grown macrogametocytes closely appressed both to nuclei and envelop of host cell. Fully grown gametocytes fill erythrocytes up to their poles, not displacing or only slightly displacing nuclei of infected cells laterally. Parasite nucleus relatively small (Table 1), of variable form and position; usually in subterminal position in gametocytes (Fig. 1c, d, f), but also observed in strictly terminal position (Fig. 1e, g) in 12% of macrogametocytes, a characteristic feature of this species development. Nucleolus not seen. Pigment granules roundish or oval, predominantly of medium size (0.5–1.0 μm), usually randomly scattered throughout the cytoplasm. Influence of gametocytes on host cell is non-pronounced (Table 1).

Microgametocytes. General configuration as in macrogametocytes with the usual haemosporidian sexual dimorphic characters, i.e. with large diffuse nuclei and relatively pale staining of the cytoplasm (Fig. 1h-l). Outline often even, but markedly irregular terminal gametocyte edges were also commonly observed (Fig. 1h).

Remarks

So far, *H. homopalloris* has only been recorded in *Phylloscopus sibilatrix*. One sequence with 100% similarity is deposited in GenBank (accession KJ488925), it was also reported in *P. sibilatrix*, in Western Greater Caucasus [55].

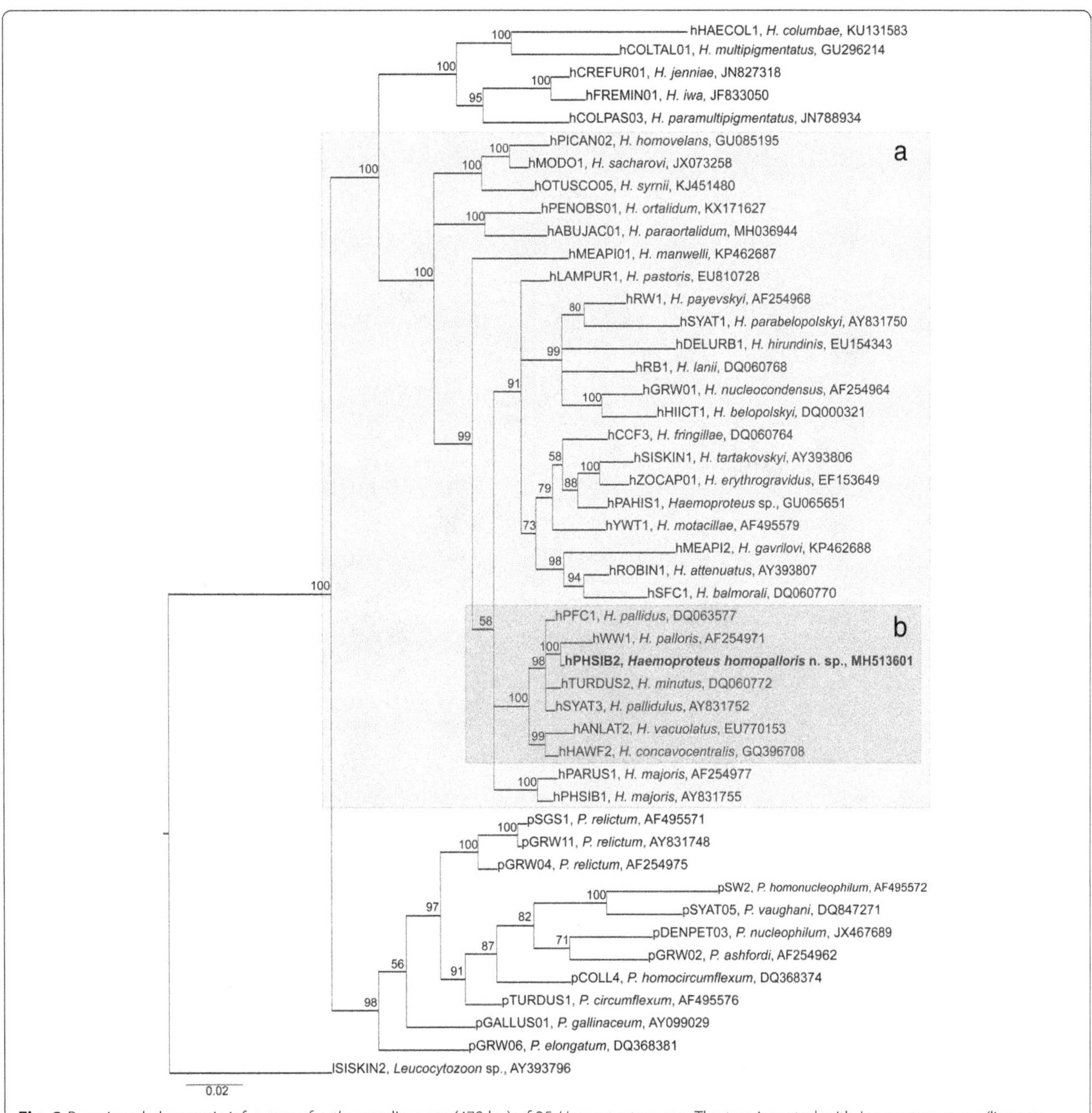

Fig. 2 Bayesian phylogenetic inference of *cytb* gene lineages (479 bp) of 35 *Haemoproteus* spp. The tree is rooted with *Leucocytozoon* sp. (lineage lSISKIN2). Clades A and B indicate species of the subgenus *Parahaemoproteus* (**a**) and haemoproteids with pale-staining cytoplasm of gametocytes (**b**). MalAvi lineage codes are provided, followed by parasite species names and GenBank accession numbers. Nodal support values indicate Bayesian posterior probabilities. New species is given in bold

A characteristic feature of *H. homopalloris* n. sp. is the relatively pale staining of the cytoplasm in macrogametocytes, so that macro- and microgametocytes are relatively poorly distinguishable based on this character (compare Fig. 1f and Fig. 1i or l). Gametocytes with pale staining cytoplasm have been described in several species of *Haemoproteus* [2, 56–58]. These parasites seem to be common in African birds and can be often encountered in migrant European birds wintering in Africa [2, 56–58]. The pale staining cytoplasm is particularly different in cases of co-infections with two species (one with pale-stained and second with dark-stained macrogametocytes) present in same blood films.

Among the haemoproteids of passerine birds, *H. homopalloris* n. sp. is most similar to *Haemoproteus palloris*, lineage hWW1 (Fig. 1m-p). These parasites develop in closely related avian hosts, the wood warbler and the willow warbler *Phylloscopus trochilus*, so should be distinguished. They can be differentiated due to the presence of vacuoles or vacuole-like spaces in the majority (80%) of the

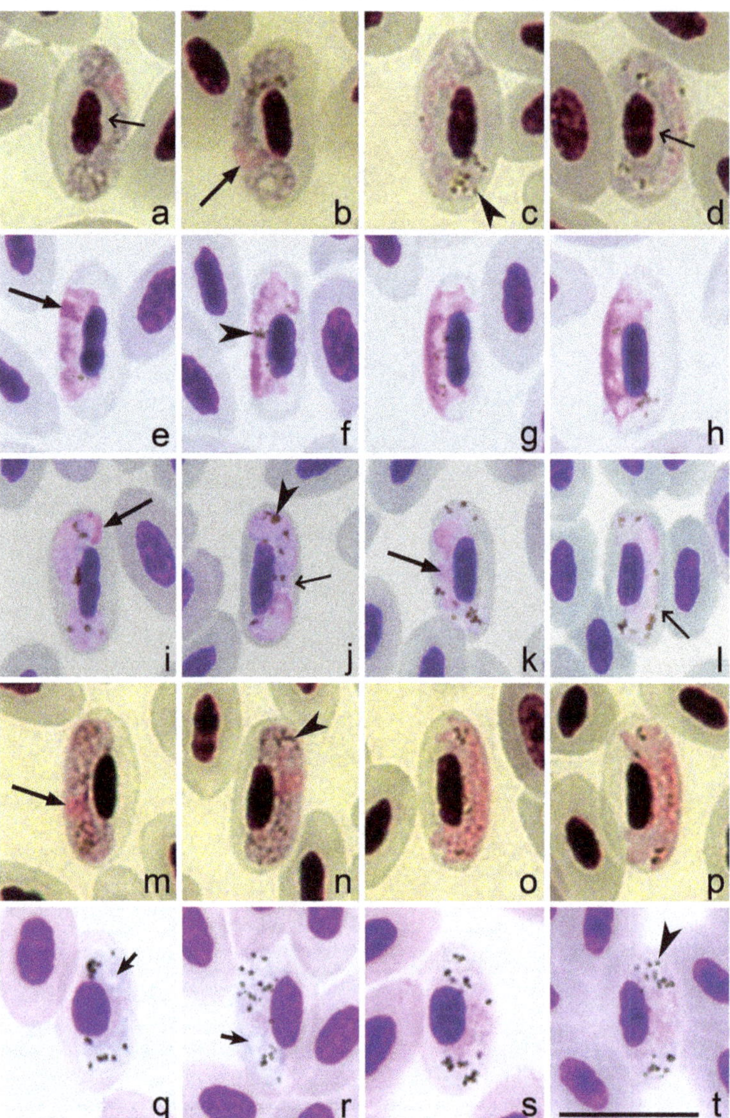

Fig. 3 *Haemoproteus* spp. with pale staining of macrogametocyte cytoplasm. *Haemoproteus concavocentralis* (**a**-**d**), *H. minutus* (**e**-**h**), *H. pallidus* (**i**-**l**), *H. pallidulus* (**m**-**p**) and *H. vacuolatus* (**q**-**t**). Macrogametocytes (**a**, **b**, **e**, **f**, **i**, **j**, **m**, **n**, **q**, **r**), microgametocytes (**c**, **d**, **g**, **h**, **k**, **l**, **o**, **p**, **s**, **t**). Note the following valuable diagnostic features of the parasites: presence of a space between the nucleus of the infected erythrocyte and the growing gametocyte in *H. concavocentralis* (**a**); clearly irregular outline of mature gametocytes, which do not touch the poles of infected erythrocytes in *H. minutus* (**e**-**h**); gametocyte which are closely appressed to the nucleus of erythrocyte but do not touch the envelope of erythrocyte along their entire margin in *H. pallidus* (**j**, **l**); small pigment granules in mature gametocytes of *H. pallidulus* (**m**-**p**); presence of one prominent vacuole in the cytoplasm of each advanced macrogametocyte in *H. vacuolatus* (**q**-**t**). All these features are not characteristics of *H. homopalloris* n. sp. (see Fig. 1). Long simple arrows: gametocyte nuclei; short simple arrows: vacuole-like spaces in macrogametocytes; arrowheads: pigment granules; long simple wide arrows: space present between the parasite and an infected erythrocyte nucleus (**a**, **d**) and space between the parasite and the envelope of infected erythrocyte (**j**, **l**). Giemsa-stained thin blood films. *Scale-bar*: **a**-**t**, 10 μm

advanced macrogametocytes of *H. palloris* (Fig. 1m, n) whereas such structures are absent in gametocytes of *H. homopalloris* n. sp. The second taxonomically distinctive character is the pattern of growth of gametocytes in these two parasites. In *H. palloris* (Fig. 1o), an unfilled space is usually present between the gametocyte and the erythrocyte nucleus [15]. This is not characteristic for *H. homopalloris* n. sp. The presence of nuclei in strictly terminal position in 12% of *H. homopalloris* magrogametocytes is another difference between these two species since this has not been reported in *H. palloris*. Despite of the presence of distinguishing morphological features, gametocytes of *H. palloris* and *H. homopalloris* n. sp. are similar (compare Fig. 1c-l with Fig. 1m-p) and the genetic difference among these two lineages is small (1.1% or 5 bp in 479 bp of the *cytb* gene sequence).

Table 1 Morphometric data (in μm) for host cells, mature gametocytes and sporozoites of *Haemoproteus homopalloris* n. sp., lineage hPHSIB2

Feature	Range (Mean ± SD) (*n* = 21)
Uninfected erythrocyte	
Length	10.9–12.8 (11.6 ± 0.6)
Width	5.6–6.5 (6.1 ± 0.3)
Area	48.7–64.3 (57.2 ± 4.2)
Uninfected erythrocyte nucleus	
Length	5.0–6.6 (5.8 ± 0.4)
Width	1.9–2.5 (2.2 ± 0.1)
Area	9.4–14.4 (11.6 ± 1.5)
Macrogametocyte	
Infected erythrocyte	
Length	11.0–13.0 (12.1 ± 0.4)
Width	5.2–6.6 (6.0 ± 0.3)
Area	53.1–65.6 (60.3 ± 3.8)
Infected erythrocyte nucleus	
Length	5.0–7.2 (6.2 ± 0.5)
Width	1.7–2.5 (2.1 ± 0.2)
Area	9.6–16.6 (11.5 ± 1.5)
Gametocyte	
Length	13.2–17.9 (15.1 ± 1.2)
Width	1.8–2.8 (2.4 ± 0.3)
Area	30.7–39.4 (35.9 ± 2.7)
Gametocyte nucleus	
Length	1.8–3.6 (2.5 ± 0.5)
Width	0.9–2.8 (1.4 ± 0.5)
Area	1.9–5.1 (3.3 ± 0.8)
Pigment granules	12–20 (15 ± 1.8)
NDR	0.6–1.1 (0.8 ± 0.1)
Microgametocytes	
Infected erythrocyte	
Length	11.3–14.0 (12.4 ± 0.6)
Width	5.2–6.6 (6.1 ± 0.4)
Area	53.9-74.3 (62.7 ± 5.0)
Infected erythrocyte nucleus	
Length	5.3–7.2 (6.1 ± 0.5)
Width	1.7–2.5 (2.1 ± 0.2)
Area	10.4–13.8 (11.4 ± 0.9)
Gametocyte	
Length	14.8–18.0 (16.4 ± 0.9)
Width	1.9–2.9 (2.3 ± 0.3)
Area	31.0–43.1 (38.3 ± 2.3)
Gametocyte nucleus [a]	
Length	–
Width	–
Area	–
Pigment granules	9–18 (13 ± 2.6)
NDR	0.6–1.0 (0.8 ± 0.1)
Sporozoites	
Length	6.4–10.0 (7.9 ± 1.1)
Width	1.1–1.9 (1.5 ± 0.2)
Area	6.9–12.0 (9.1 ± 1.5)

[a]Gametocyte nucleus was not well defined and is difficult to measure
Abbreviations: *NDR* nucleus displacement ratio according to Bennett & Campbell (1972), *SD* standard deviation

Haemoproteus majoris (lineage hPHSIB1) has been often reported in wood warblers [22–24]. Phylogenetic analysis showed that *cytb* lineage hPHSIB1 is significantly divergent from the lineage hPHSIB2 of *H. homopalloris* n. sp. (4.5% difference in 17 bp of *cytb* gene fragment) and parasites are morphologically different (compare Fig. 1c-l with Fig. 4a-d). The most distinctive difference between *H. majoris* and *H. homopalloris* is the presence of dumbbell-shaped growing gametocytes in the former ([2], see Fig. 4a), but such gametocytes are absent in *H. homopalloris* n. sp. Additionally, fully grown gametocytes of *H. majoris* markedly displace host cell nuclei laterally (NDR = 0.4 ± 0.1) [2], but this is not a case for *H. homopalloris* n. sp. (NDR = 0.8 ± 0.1) (compare Fig. 1c-l with Fig. 4b-d).

Haemoproteus homopalloris n. sp. (hPHSIB2) can be also readily distinguished from other *Haemoproteus* species with pale staining macrogametocytes. *Haemoproteus concavocentralis* (hHAWF2) has a characteristic space between nucleus of infected erythrocyte and parasite in growing gametocytes [58] (see Fig. 3a-d). *Haemoproteus minutus* (hTURDUS2) possesses a clearly irregular outline, and it does not touch the poles of infected erythrocytes [2, Fig. 3e-h]. *Haemoproteus pallidus* (hPFC1) gametocytes are closely appressed to the nucleus of erythrocyte but usually do not touch the envelope of erythrocyte along their entire margin [2, Fig. 3i-l]. Gametocytes of *Haemoproteus pallidulus* (hSYAT3) possess small pigment granules even in mature gametocytes ([57], Fig. 3m-p). *Haemoproteus vacuolatus* (hANLAT2) possesses one prominent vacuole in the cytoplasm of each advanced macrogametocyte ([56], Fig. 3q, r). None of these features are characters of *H. homopalloris* n. sp.

Sporogony in biting midges

The presence of numerous sporozoites in salivary glands confirms that *H. homopalloris* n. sp. can complete

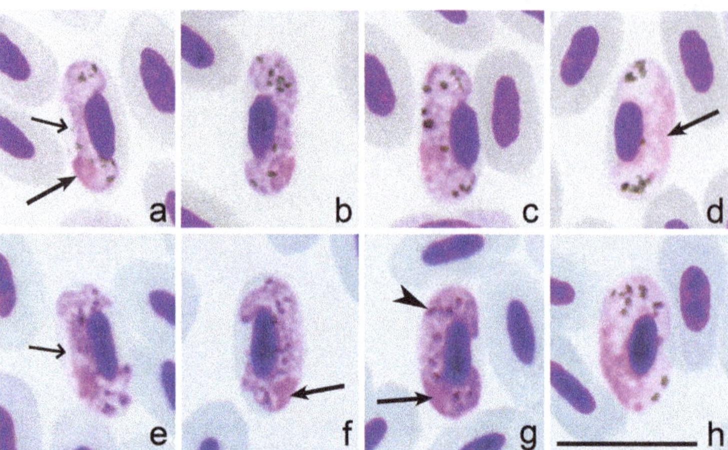

Fig. 4 Gametocytes of two species of haemoproteids, which have been reported in the wood warbler *Phylloscopus sibilatrix*. Macrogametocytes (**a-c**, **e-g**) and microgametocytes (**d**, **h**) of *Haemoproteus majoris* (**a-d**) and *H. belopolskyi* (**e-h**). Note that the intensity of staining of the cytoplasm is different in macro- and microgametocytes. Long arrows: gametocyte nuclei; short arrows: vacuole-like spaces in macrogametocytes; arrowheads: pigment granules. Giemsa-stained thin blood films. *Scale-bar*: **a-h**, 10 μm

sporogony in *C. nubeculosus*. Ookinetes were not reported in preparations, but zygotes were numerous 8 h post-exposure (Fig. 5a). Oocysts were seen in midgut in temporary preparations 4 dpe. Sporozoites were detected in salivary glands preparations 7 dpe (Fig. 5b). The sporozoites possess fusiform bodies with centrally located nuclei and approximately equally pointed ends (Fig. 5b, Table 1). The PCR-based analysis and sequencing confirmed the presence of hPHSIB2 lineage in experimentally infected biting midges at sporozoite stage.

Discussion

Haemoproteus homopalloris n. sp. is the third species of haemoproteid parasite identified in wood warblers. The infection prevalence was high in the studied bird population. It is interesting to note that all birds were caught with stationary mist nets. In other words, the birds flew in the nets themselves, so they were actively moving individuals and looked healthy from this point of view.

The new species clustered with seven *Haemoproteus* species, which all possess the pale staining cytoplasm in macrogametocytes in the phylogenetic analysis based on *cytb* data (compare Figs. 1 and 3 with Fig. 4). This is not characteristic of the great majority of haemosporidian parasites, in which the cytoplasm of macrogametocytes stains more intensively than in microgametocytes (Fig. 4) [59].

The pale staining of the cytoplasm in *H. homopalloris* n. sp. (Fig. 1) and related species (Fig. 3) might be due to the approximately similar density of organelles in the cytoplasm of macrogametocytes in comparison to microgametocytes, resulting in accumulation of similar amount of stain in both types of cells during staining procedures. Additional electron microscope studies are needed to test this hypothesis. Different cellular structure of macro- and microgametocytes can be explained from the point of view of life span of these cells. Numerous cell organelles are needed for a long survival of macrogametocyte cells, which are relatively long-lived cells in comparison to microgametocytes. After fertilization, each macrogametocyte, transforms to zygote and then the same cell develops into ookinete and further, to relatively long living oocyst [2]. Microgametocytes are relatively short-lived cells; they only produce microgametocytes, which develop within several minutes in vectors. This suggests that haemoproteids with pale staining of the macrogametocyte cytoplasm should develop fast during sporogony in comparison to the species with intense staining of the cytoplasm. Available experimental observations support this and show that complete ookinete formation of *H. minutus* and *H. pallidus*, which macrogametocytes are pale-stained (Fig. 1c-l and Fig. 3), occur within 1 to 1.5 h both *in vitro* and *in vivo* at 18 to 20° C [2, 38]. These parasites also have tiny ookinetes (approximately 10 μm in length), which probably facilitates their rapid movement. The biological

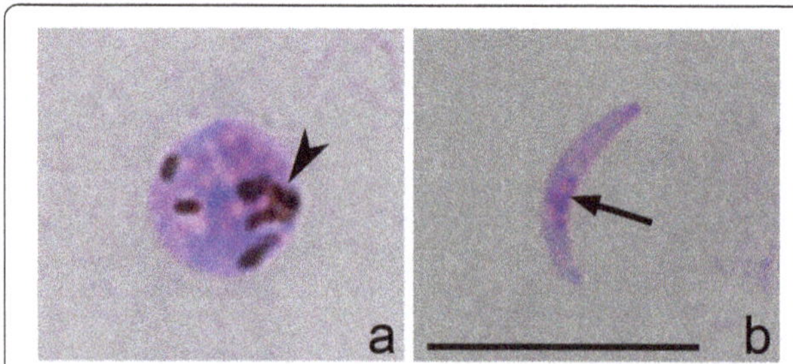

Fig. 5 Sporogonic stages of *Haemoproteus homopalloris* n. sp. in the biting midge *Culicoides nubeculosus*. Zygote (**a**) and sporozoite (**b**). Arrowhead: pigment granules; arrow: sporozoite nucleus. Methanol-fixed and Giemsa-stained thin films. *Scale-bar*: **a**, **b**, 10 μm

meaning of this phenomenon remains unclear. Because pale staining parasites cluster together in the phylogenetic tree (Fig. 2), it is possible that the rapid development of ookinetes might also occur in all other species in this clade. There is no explanation why this pattern is so applicable for the group of pale staining haemoproteid parasites. However, this pattern does not apply for other species like *H. majoris*, *Haemoproteus tartakovskyi* and *H. belopolskyi*, in which macrogametocytes are densely stained with Giemsa (Fig. 4) and mature ookinetes develop relatively slowly (between 6–24 h at the same conditions) [2, 38].

Morphological descriptions of *Haemoproteus homopalloris* n. sp. species was accompanied by DNA sequence information and phylogenetic hypothesis for its relationship with already described parasites. It has been suggested [60] and then confirmed by several other studies [15, 58, 61] that *Haemoproteus* lineages, which differ over 5% in partial *cytb* sequence (479 bp), are likely to be morphologically differentiated and can be distinguished on gametocyte stage. However, it was also shown that some *cytb* lineages of *Haemoproteus* spp. with difference of just two nucleotides (or 0.7%) could be identified based on morphological features of their gametocytes ([56, 62]; this study). This is particularly recognisable in closely related species (Figs. 1 and 3) with pale staining of macrogametocyte cytoplasm [15, 56–58]. The greatest divergence among the seven described species of this group is 3.1%.

The lineage hPHSIB2 of *H. homopalloris* n. sp. clustered with other lineages of the subgenus *Parahaemoproteus* (Fig. 2, clade A) and with other pale staining parasites (Fig. 2, clade B). Interestingly, this group of parasites forms a congruent monophyletic group with low *cytb* genetic divergence (up to 3.1%), but with clearly distinguishable morphological features (Fig. 3). The majority of haemoproteid species with pale staining of macrogametocytes have been reported in European birds wintering in sub-Saharan Africa or resident bird species in this region [2, 15, 56–58]. It might be that they originally evolved in countries with warm climates where they are diverse. Interestingly, *H. homopalloris* n. sp. and *H. minutus* readily complete sporogony in European biting midges at relatively low temperatures (close to 20° C) ([38]; this study), an indication that there are no obstacles to their transmission in the Palaearctic from the point of view of vector availability and temperature needed for sporogony.

It is important to note that one species of haemoproteid with pale staining cytoplasm in macrogametocytes, *H. minutus*, causes mortality of captive parrots in Europe [9, 63]. The mortality is due to heart damage by tissue exo-erythrocytic meronts of this parasite, which abort development before development of parasitemia [11]. *Haemoproteus minutus* is broadly distributed in the Palaearctic region, and several closely related lineages of this pathogen have been identified [63]. It is possible that other closely related to *H. minutus* parasites of clade B (Fig. 2) also might be virulent in non-adapted avian hosts. It is not clear if *H. homopalloris* n. sp. is virulent as the former species; the pathology of this parasite should be investigated in the future.

In this study, two birds were co-infected with different haemosporidian species, and the double infections were detected by both PCR diagnostics and microscopic examination. Various combinations of mixed infections are common in wild naturally infected birds [58, 64–68]. It is important to note that presence of mixed infections often markedly vary among different bird populations. Such infections might predominate and represent more than 80% in some bird species [64]. Mixed infections have been reported to be highly virulent in avian hosts [68, 69]. However, the currently used general primers often underestimate the prevalence of mixed infections [65, 70, 71], and this calls for application of new PCR protocols, which are sensitive to detect mixed infections of *Haemoproteus* and *Plasmodium* parasites [72]. However, all currently available PCR-based protocols remain insensitive to read mixed infections of several haemosporidian species belonging to the same genus or subgenus, suggesting essential need of application of microscopic examination and morphological identification in parasite biodiversity studies in the wild [44].

Four *Haemoproteus* species can complete sporogony in *C. nubeculosus*. These are *Haemoproteus handai*, *Haemoproteus noctuae*, *Haemoproteus syrnii* and *Haemoproteus tartakovskyi* [33, 34, 43]. This study adds *H. homopalloris* n. sp. to this list of haemoproteid species transmitted by this biting midge and reinforces the importance of *C. nubeculosus* in experimental vector research. The pattern of sporogony in *Culicoides impuctatus* seems to be similar in different *Haemoproteus* species under experimental conditions. During sporogonic development of *H. balmorali* Peirce, 1984, *H. belopolskyi*, *H. dolniki* Valkiūnas & Iezhova, 1992, *H. fringillae* Labbé, 1894, *H. lanii* Mello, 1936, *H. minutus*, *H. parabelopolskyi* Valkiūnas, Križanauskienė, Iezhova, Hellgren & Bensch, 2007 and *H. tartakovskyi* ookinetes can be reported between 6 h and 3 dpe and sporozoites between 5 and 7 dpe, indicating asynchronous development ([2, 33, 38]; this study). In *C. nubeculosus* sporogony of *H. homopalloris* n. sp., *H. noctuae*, *H. syrnii* and *H. tartakovskyi* occurs at similar rates: oocysts can be seen 3 dpe until 5 dpe, and sporozoites about 7 dpe ([33, 34]; this study). Interestingly, the sporogony rate of *Haemoproteus* species inhabiting phylogenetically distantly related birds belong to different orders (Passeriformes and Strigiformes) is similar in same species of biting midges ([33, 34]; this study).

The presence of few oocysts in temporary preparations was likely due to the low parasitemia in the donor bird during this study (0.1%). Heavy *Haemoproteus* parasitemia is markedly virulent in blood-sucking insects, and such infections might kill them due to the damage by numerous migrating ookinetes [12]. When performing experimental infections with vectors it is important to use donor birds with light *Haemoproteus* sp. parasitemia (about 0.1%). If parasitemia is high (≥ 1%) in the blood meal, mortality is usually high in biting midges and other blood-sucking insects, resulting in rapid death of experimental groups [13]. Thus, donor birds should be carefully selected for experimental vector research. Interestingly, mainly light parasitemia (< 1%) usually is present in wild-caught birds [16, 19, 58, 73, 74], and such infections are particularly important for transmission. This explains the biological meaning of persistence of haemosporidian parasites in birds at stage of low parasitemia from the viewpoint of parasite transmission.

Conclusions

Haemoproteus homopalloris n. sp. (lineage hPHSIB2) is the third haemoproteid species reported in wood warblers. The new species belongs to the subgenus *Parahaemoproteus* based on the morphology of the sporogonic stages, susceptibility of *Culicoides* biting midges and phylogeny. The phylogenetic analysis identified a well-supported clade containing seven haemoproteids, including the new species, which possess pale staining macrogametocytes and develop exceptionally rapidly at ookinete stage; biological meaning of these characters remains unclear. Studies targeting mechanisms of sporogonic development of haemoproteids and other wildlife haemosporidian parasites remain uncommon and should be encouraged. *Culicoides nubeculosus* is an excellent experimental vector of *H. homopalloris* n. sp. and several other avian haemoproteids. This insect is relatively easy to rear, and it is recommended in laboratory experimental research.

Acknowledgments

We thank V. Jusys and V. Eigirdas (Ventės Ragas Ornithological Station, Lithuania) for support during field work and R. Bernotienė, for assistance in the laboratory. Institute for Animal Health, Pirbright Laboratory for providing *Culicoides nubeculosus* for establishing our colony as part of a grant funded by the Biotechnology and Biological Sciences Research Council (BBS/E/I/00001701), UK.

Funding

This study was funded by the Research Council of Lithuania (nr. DOTSUT-137-09.3.3-LMT-K-712-02-0004) and also supported by the Open Access to research infrastructure of the Nature Research Centre under Lithuanian open access network initiative.

Authors' contributions

Experimental conception and design: GV and CRFC. Biting midge experiments, dissection and laboratory maintenance: DB. Donor bird collection and testing: GV, MI and TI. Morphological analysis: CRFC, GV and TAI. Phylogenetic analysis and its discussion: CRFC and GV. Paper writing: CRFC and GV. All authors read and approved the final manuscript.

Competing interests

The authors declare that they have no competing interests.

References

1. Clark NJ, Clegg SM, Lima MR. A review of global diversity in avian haemosporidians (*Plasmodium* and *Haemoproteus*: Haemosporida): new insights from molecular data. Int J Parasitol. 2014;44:329–38.
2. Valkiūnas G. Avian Malaria Parasites and Other Haemosporidia. Boca Raton: CRC Press; 2005.
3. Bennett GF, Peirce MA, Ashford RW. Avian haematozoa: mortality and pathogenicity. J Nat Hist. 1993;27:993–1001.
4. Marzal A, De Lope F, Navarro C, Møller AP. Malarial parasites decrease reproductive success: an experimental study in a passerine bird. Oecologia. 2005;142:541–5.
5. Dunn JC, Goodman SJ, Benton TG, Hamer KC. Avian blood parasite infection during the non-breeding season: an overlooked issue in declining populations? BMC Ecol. 2013;13:30.
6. Cardona CJ, Ihejirika A, McClellan L. *Haemoproteus lophortyx* infection in bobwhite quail. Avian Dis. 2002;46:249–55.
7. Ferrell ST, Snowden K, Marlar AB, Garner M, Lung NP. Fatal hemoprotozoal infections in multiple avian species in a zoological park. J Zoo Wildl Med. 2007;38:309–16.
8. Donovan TA, Schrenzel M, Tucker TA, Pessier AP, Stalis IH. Hepatic hemorrhage, hemocoelom, and sudden death due to *Haemoproteus* infection in passerine birds: eleven cases. J Vet Diagn Invest. 2008;20:304–13.
9. Olias P, Wegelin M, Zenker W, Freter S, Gruber AD, Klopfleisch R. Avian malaria deaths in parrots, Europe. Emerg Infect Dis. 2011;17:950–2.
10. Cannell BL, Krasnec KV, Campbell K, Jones HI, Miller RD, Stephens N. The pathology and pathogenicity of a novel *Haemoproteus* spp. infection in wild little penguins (*Eudyptula minor*). Vet Parasitol. 2013;205:416.
11. Valkiūnas G, Iezhova TA. Exo-erythrocytic development of avian malaria and related haemosporidian parasites. Malar J. 2017;16:101.
12. Valkiūnas G, Kazlauskienė R, Bernotienė R, Bukauskaitė D, Palinauskas V, Iezhova TA. *Haemoproteus* infections (Haemosporida, Haemoproteidae) kill bird-biting mosquitoes. Parasitol Res. 2014;113:1011–8.
13. Bukauskaitė D, Bernotienė R, Iezhova TA, Valkiūnas G. Mechanisms of mortality in *Culicoides* biting midges due to *Haemoproteus* infection. Parasitology. 2016;143:1748–54.
14. Chagas CR, Guimarães L de O, Monteiro EF, Valkiūnas G, Katayama MV, Santos SV, et al. Hemosporidian parasites of free-living birds in the São Paulo Zoo, Brazil. Parasitol Res. 2016;115:1443–52.
15. Dimitrov D, Iezhova TA, Zehtindjiev P, Bobeva A, Ilieva M, Kirilova M, et al. Molecular characterisation of three avian haemoproteids (Haemosporida, Haemoproteidae), with the description of *Haemoproteus* (*Parahaemoproteus*) *palloris* n. sp. Syst Parasitol. 2016;93:431–49.
16. Matta NE, Pacheco MA, Escalante AA, Valkiūnas G, Ayerbe-Quiñones F, Acevedo-Cendales LD. Description and molecular characterization of *Haemoproteus macrovacuolatus* n. sp. (Haemosporida, Haemoproteidae), a morphologically

unique blood parasite of black-bellied whistling duck (*Dendrocygna autumnalis*) from South America. Parasitol Res. 2014;113:2991–3000.

17. Mantilla JS, González AD, Lotta IA, Moens M, Pacheco MA, Escalante AA, et al. *Haemoproteus erythrogravidus* n. sp. (Haemosporida, Haemoproteidae): description and molecular characterization of a widespread blood parasite of birds in South America. Acta Trop. 2016;159:83–94.
18. Chagas CR, Valkiūnas G, de Oliveira Guimarães L, Monteiro EF, Guida FJ, Simões RF, et al. Diversity and distribution of avian malaria and related haemosporidian parasites in captive birds from a Brazilian megalopolis. Malar J. 2017;16:83.
19. Valkiūnas G, Pendl H, Olias P. New *Haemoproteus* parasite of parrots, with remarks on the virulence of haemoproteids in naive avian hosts. Acta Trop. 2017;176:256–62.
20. Ferreira-Junior FC, Dutra DA, Martins NRS, Valkiūnas G, Braga EM. *Haemoproteus paraortalidum* n. sp. in captive Black-fronted Piping-guans *Aburria jacutinga* (Galliformes, Cracidae): high prevalence in a population reintroduced into the wild. Acta Trop. 2018;188:93–100.
21. BirdLife International. *Phylloscopus sibilatrix*. The IUCN Red List of Threatened Species. 2016; https://doi.org/10.2305/IUCN.UK.2016-3.RLTS.T22715260A87668662.en. Accessed 22 May 2018.
22. Waldenström J, Bensch S, Kiboi S, Hasselquist D, Ottosson U. Cross-species infection of blood parasites between resident and migratory songbirds in Africa. Mol Ecol. 2002;11:1545–54.
23. Hellgren O, Waldenström J, Peréz-Tris J, Szöll E, Si O, Hasselquist D, et al. Detecting shifts of transmission areas in avian blood parasites: a phylogenetic approach. Mol Ecol. 2007;16:1281–90.
24. Bensch S, Hellgren O, Pérez-Tris J. MalAvi: a public database of malaria parasites and related haemosporidians in avian hosts based on mitochondrial cytochrome b lineages. Mol Ecol Resour. 2009;9:1353–8.
25. Shurulinkov P, Golemansky V. Haemoproteids (Haemosporida: Haemoproteidae) of wild birds in Bulgaria. Acta Protozool. 2002;41:359–74.
26. Ishtiaq F, Guillaumot L, Clegg SM, Phillimore AB, Black RA, Owens IPF, et al. Avian haematozoan parasites and their associations with mosquitoes across Southwest Pacific Islands. Mol Ecol. 2008;17:4545–55.
27. Kim KS, Tsuda Y, Sasaki T, Kobayashi M, Hirota Y. Mosquito blood-meal analysis for avian malaria study in wild bird communities: laboratory verification and application to *Culex sasai* (Diptera: Culicidae) collected in Tokyo, Japan. Parasitol Res. 2009;105:1351–7.
28. Njabo KY, Cornel AJ, Bonneaud C, Toffelmier E, Sehgal RN, Valkiūnas G, et al. Nonspecific patterns of vector, host and avian malaria parasite associations in a central African rainforest. Mol Ecol. 2011;20:1049–61.
29. Martínez-de la Puente J, Martínez J, Rivero de Aguilar J, Herrero J, Merino S. On the specificity of avian blood parasites: revealing specific and generalist relationships between haemosporidians and biting midges. Mol Ecol. 2011; 20:3275–87.
30. Ferraguti M, Martinez-de la Puente J, Ruiz S, Soriguer R, Figuerola J. On the study of the transmission network of blood parasites from SW Spain: diversity of avian haemosporidians in the biting midge *Culicoides circumscriptus* and wild birds. Parasit Vectors. 2013;6:208.
31. Bobeva A, Zehtindjiev P, Ilieva M, Dimitrov D, Mathis A, Bensch S. Host preferences of ornithophilic biting midges of the genus *Culicoides* in the eastern Balkans. Med Vet Entomol. 2015;29:290–6.
32. Valkiūnas G, Kazlauskienė R, Bernotienė R, Palinauskas V, Iezhova TA. Abortive long-lasting sporogony of two *Haemoproteus* species (Haemosporida, Haemoproteidae) in the mosquito *Ochlerotatus cantans*, with perspectives on haemosporidian vector research. Parasitol Res. 2013;113:2159–69.
33. Bukauskaitė D, Žiegytė R, Palinauskas V, Iezhova TA, Dimitrov D, Ilgūnas M, et al. Biting midges (*Culicoides*, Diptera) transmit *Haemoproteus* parasites of owls: evidence from sporogony and molecular phylogeny. Parasit Vectors. 2015;8:303.
34. Žiegytė R, Bernotienė R, Palinauskas V, Valkiūnas G. *Haemoproteus tartakovskyi* (Haemoproteidae): complete sporogony in *Culicoides nubeculosus* (Ceratopogonidae), with implications for avian haemoproteid experimental research. Exp Parasitol. 2016;160:17–22.
35. Levin II, Valkiūnas G, Santiago-Alarcon D, Cruz LL, Iezhova TA, O'Brien SL, et al. Hippoboscid-transmitted *Haemoproteus* parasites (Haemosporida) infect Galapagos pelecaniform birds: evidence from molecular and morphological studies, with a description of *Haemoproteus iwa*. Int J Parasitol. 2011;41:1019–27.
36. Santiago-Alarcon D, Palinauskas V, Schaefer HM. Diptera vectors of avian haemosporidian parasites: untangling parasite life cycles and their taxonomy. Biol Rev Camb Philos Soc. 2012;87:928–64.
37. Bobeva A, Zehtindjiev P, Bensch S, Radrova J. A survey of biting midges of the genus *Culicoides* Latreille, 1809 (Diptera: Ceratopogonidae) in NE Bulgaria, with respect to transmission of avian haemosporidians. Acta Parasitol. 2013;58:585–91.
38. Žiegytė R, Palinauskas V, Bernotienė R, Iezhova TA, Valkiūnas G. *Haemoproteus minutus* and *Haemoproteus belopolskyi* (Haemoproteidae): complete sporogony in the biting midge *Culicoides impunctatus* (Ceratopogonidae), with implications on epidemiology of haemoproteosis. Exp Parasitol. 2014;145:74–9.
39. Atkinson CT. *Haemoproteus*. In: Atkinson CT, Thomas NJ, Hunter BC, editors. Parasitic Diseases of Wild Birds. Ames: Wiley-Blackwell; 2008. p. 13–35.
40. Nayduch D, Cohnstaedt LW, Saski C, Lawson D, Kersey P, Fife M, et al. Studying *Culicoides* vectors of BTV in the post-genomic era: resources, bottlenecks to progress and future directions. Virus Res. 2014;182:43–9.
41. Boorman J. The maintenance of laboratory colonies of *Culicoides variipenniss* (Coq.), *C. nubeculosus* (Mg.) and *C. riethi* Kieff. (Diptera, Ceratopogonidae). Bull Entomol Res. 1974;64:371–7.
42. Pages N, Breard E, Urien C, Talavera S, Viarouge C, Lorca-Oro C, et al. *Culicoides* midge bites modulate the host response and impact on bluetongue virus infection in sheep. PLoS One. 2014;9:e83683.
43. Miltgen F, Landau I, Ratanaworabhan N, Yenbutra S. *Parahaemoproteus desseri* n. sp.; Gametogonie et shizogonie chez l'hote naturel: *Psittacula roseate* de Thailande, et sporogonie experimentale chez *Culicoides nubeculosus*. Ann Parasitol Hum Comp. 1981;56:123–30.
44. Valkiūnas G, Iezhova TA, Križanauskienė A, Palinauskas V, Sehgal RNM, Bensch S. A comparative analysis of microscopy and PCR-based detection methods for blood parasites. J Parasitol. 2008;94:1395–401.
45. Godfrey RD, Fedynich AM, Pence DB. Quantification of hematozoa in blood smears. J Wildl Dis. 1987;23:558–65.
46. Richardson DS, Jury FL, Blaakmeer K, Komdeur J, Burke T. Parentage assignment and extra-group paternity in a cooperative breeder: the Seychelles warbler (*Acrocephalus sechellensis*). Mol Ecol. 2001;10:2263–73.
47. Bensch S, Stjernman M, Hasselquist D, Ostman O, Hansson B, Westerdahl H, et al. Host specificity in avian blood parasites: a study of *Plasmodium* and *Haemoproteus* mitochondrial DNA amplified from birds. Proc Biol Sci. 2000; 267:1583–9.
48. Hellgren O, Waldenström J, Bensch S. A new PCR assay for simultaneous studies of *Leucocytozoon*, *Plasmodium* and *Haemoproteus* from avian blood. J Parasitol. 2004;90:797–802.
49. Hall TA. BioEdit: a user-friendly biological sequence alignment editor and analysis program for Windows 95/98/NT. Nucl Acids Symp Ser. 1999;41:95–8.
50. Ronquist F, Heulsenbeck JP. MrBayes 3: Bayesian phylogenetic inference under mixed models. Bioinformatics. 2003;19:1572–4.
51. Nylander JAA. MrModeltest v2. Program distributed by the author. Software available at https://github.com/nylander/MrModeltest2. Accessed 10 Apr 2018.
52. Rambaut A. FigTree: Tree Figure Drawing Tool Version 1.4.0. 2006–2012. Institute of Evolutionary Biology, University of Edinburgh. http://tree.bio.ed.ac.uk/software/figtree/.
53. Kumar S, Stecher G, Tamura K. MEGA7: Molecular Evolutionary Genetics Analysis Version 7.0 for Bigger Datasets. Mol Biol Evol. 2016;33:1870–4.
54. ICZN. International Commission on Zoological Nomenclature: Amendment of articles 8, 9, 10, 21 and 78 of the International Code of Zoological Nomenclature to expand and refine methods of publication. Bull Zool Nomencl. 2012;69:161–9.
55. Drovetski SV, Aghayan SA, Mata VA, Lopes RJ, Mode NA, Harvey JA, et al. Does the niche breadth or trade-off hypothesis explain the abundance-occupancy relationship in avian haemosporidia? Mol Ecol. 2014;23:3322–9.
56. Valkiūnas G, Iezhova TA, Loiseau C, Chasar A, Smith TB, Sehgal RNM. New species of haemosporidian parasites (Haemosporida) from African rainforest birds, with remarks on their classification. Parasitol Res. 2008;103:1213–28.
57. Križanauskienė A, Pérez-Tris J, Palinauskas V, Hellgren O, Bensch S, Valkiūnas G. Molecular phylogenetic and morphological analysis of haemosporidian parasites (Haemosporida) in a naturally infected European songbird, the blackcap *Sylvia atricapilla*, with description of *Haemoproteus pallidulus* sp. nov. Parasitology. 2010;137:217–27.
58. Dimitrov D, Zehtindjiev P, Bensch S, Ilieva M, Iezhova TA, Valkiūnas G. Two new species of *Haemoproteus* Kruse, 1890 (Haemosporida, Haemoproteidae) from European birds, with emphasis on DNA barcoding for detection of haemosporidians in wildlife. Syst Parasitol. 2014;87:135–51.
59. Valkiūnas G, Iezhova TA. Keys to the avian malaria parasites. Malar J. 2018;17:212.

60. Hellgren O, Krizanauskiene A, Valkiūnas G, Bensch S. Diversity and phylogeny of mitochondrial cytochrome B lineages from six morphospecies of avian *Haemoproteus* (Haemosporida: Haemoproteidae). J Parasitol. 2007;93:889–96.
61. Valkiūnas G, Križanauskienė A, Iezhova TA, Hellgren O, Bensch S. Molecular phylogenetic analysis of circumnuclear hemoproteids (Haemosporida: Haemoproteidae) of sylvid birds, with a description of *Haemoproteus parabelopolskyi* sp. nov. J Parasitol. 2007;93:680–7.
62. Levin II, Valkiūnas G, Iezhova TA, O'Brien SL, Parker PG. Novel *Haemoproteus* species (Haemosporida: Haemoproteidae) from the swallow-tailed gull (Laridae), with remarks on the host range of hippoboscid-transmitted avian hemoproteids. J Parasitol. 2012;98:847–54.
63. Palinauskas V, Iezhova TA, Križanauskienė A, Markovets MY, Bensch S, Valkiūnas G. Molecular characterization and distribution of *Haemoproteus minutus* (Haemosporida, Haemoproteidae): a pathogenic avian parasite. Parasitol Int. 2013;62:358–63.
64. Valkiūnas G, Iezhova TA, Shapoval AP. High prevalence of blood parasites in hawfinch *Coccothraustes coccothraustes*. J Nat Hist. 2003;37:2647–52.
65. Valkiūnas G, Bensch S, Iezhova TA, Križanauskienė A, Hellgren O, Bolshakov CV. Nested cytochrome b polymerase chain reaction diagnostics underestimate mixed infections of avian blood haemosporidian parasites: microscopy is still essential. J Parasitol. 2006;92:418–22.
66. Merino S, Moreno J, Vásquez RA, Martínez J, Sánchez-Monsálvez I, Estades CF, et al. Haematozoa in forest birds from southern Chile: latitudinal gradients in prevalence and parasite lineage richness. Austral Ecol. 2008;33:329–40.
67. Marzal A, Ricklefs RE, Valkiūnas G, Albayrak T, Arriero E, Bonneaud C, et al. Diversity, loss, and gain of malaria parasites in a globally invasive bird. PLoS One. 2011;6:e21905.
68. Chagas CR, Valkiūnas G, Nery CV, Henrique PC, Gonzalez IH, Monteiro EF, et al. *Plasmodium* (*Novyella*) *nucleophilum* from an Egyptian goose in São Paulo Zoo, Brazil: microscopic confirmation and molecular characterization. Int J Parasitol Parasites Wildl. 2013;2:286–91.
69. Palinauskas V, Valkiūnas G, Bolshakov CV, Bensch S. *Plasmodium relictum* (lineage SGS1) and *Plasmodium ashfordi* (lineage GRW2): the effects of the co-infection on experimentally infected passerine birds. Exp Parasitol. 2011; 127:527–33.
70. Martinez J, Martinez-De La Puente J, Herrero J, Del Cerro S, Lobato E, Rivero-De Aguilar J, et al. A restriction site to differentiate *Plasmodium* and *Haemoproteus* infections in birds: on the inefficiency of general primers for detection of mixed infections. Parasitology. 2009;136:713–22.
71. Bernotienė R, Palinauskas V, Iezhova T, Murauskaitė D, Valkiūnas G. Avian haemosporidian parasites (Haemosporida): a comparative analysis of different polymerase chain reaction assays in detection of mixed infections. Exp Parasitol. 2016;163:31–7.
72. Pacheco MA, Cepeda AS, Bernotienė R, Lotta IA, Matta NE, Valkiūnas G, et al. Primers targeting mitochondrial genes of avian haemosporidians: PCR detection and differential DNA amplification of parasites belonging to different genera. Int J Parasitol. 2018;48:657–70.
73. Dimitrov D, Ilieva M, Ivanova K, Brlík V, Zehtindjiev P. Detecting local transmission of avian malaria and related haemosporidian parasites (Apicomlexa, Haemosporida) at a Special Protection Area of Natura 2000 network. Parasitol Res. 2018;117:2187–99.
74. Ivanova K, Zehtindjiev P, Mariaux J, Dimitrov D, Georgiev BB. Avian haemosporidians from rain forests in Madagascar: molecular and morphological data of the genera *Plasmodium*, *Haemoproteus* and *Leucocytozoon*. Infect Genet Evol. 2018;58:115–24.

7

Epidemiology of *Taenia saginata* taeniosis/cysticercosis: a systematic review of the distribution in southern and eastern Africa

Veronique Dermauw[1*], Pierre Dorny[1,2], Uffe Christian Braae[3], Brecht Devleesschauwer[4,5], Lucy J. Robertson[6], Anastasios Saratsis[7] and Lian F. Thomas[8,9]

Abstract

Background: The beef tapeworm, *Taenia saginata*, causing cysticercosis in bovines and taeniosis in humans, is thought to have a global distribution. In eastern and southern Africa, cattle production plays a crucial role in the economy, but a clear overview of the prevalence of *T. saginata* in the region is still lacking. This review aims to summarize existing knowledge on *T. saginata* taeniosis and bovine cysticercosis distribution in eastern and southern Africa.

Methods: A systematic review was conducted, that gathered published and grey literature, including OIE reports, concerning *T. saginata* taeniosis and bovine cysticercosis in eastern and southern Africa published between January 1st, 1990 and December 31st, 2017.

Results: A total of 1232 records were initially retrieved, with 78 full text articles retained for inclusion in the database. Unspecified taeniosis cases were reported for Angola, Ethiopia, Kenya, Madagascar, Malawi, South Africa, Tanzania, Uganda and Zambia, whereas *T. saginata* taeniosis cases were found for Ethiopia, Kenya, South Africa, Tanzania, Zambia and Zimbabwe. The prevalence of taeniosis ranged between 0.2–8.1% based on microscopy, and between 0.12–19.7% based on coproAg-ELISA. In Ethiopia, the percentage of tapeworm self-reporting was high (45.0–64.2%), and a substantial number of anthelmintic treatments were reported to be sold in towns. The presence of bovine cysticercosis was reported in all 27 countries/territories included in the study, except for Rwanda and Somalia, Comoros, Madagascar, Mauritius, Mayotte, Seychelles and Socotra. The prevalence of cysticercosis ranged between 0.02–26.3% based on meat inspection, and between 6.1–34.9% based on Ag-ELISA.

Conclusions: Although *T. saginata* has been reported in the majority of countries/territories of the study area, *T. saginata* taeniosis/cysticercosis remains a largely ignored condition, probably due to the absence of symptoms in cattle, the lack of data on its economic impact, and the fact that human taeniosis is considered a minor health problem. However, the occurrence of bovine cysticercosis is a clear sign of inadequate sanitation, insufficient meat inspection, and culinary habits that may favour transmission. Measures to reduce transmission of *T. saginata* are therefore warranted and the infection should be properly monitored.

Keywords: *Taenia saginata*, Cestode, Beef tapeworm, Taeniosis, Bovine cysticercosis, Eastern Africa, Southern Africa

* Correspondence: vdermauw@itg.be
[1]Department of Biomedical Sciences, Institute of Tropical Medicine, Antwerp, Belgium
Full list of author information is available at the end of the article

Background

The beef tapeworm, *Taenia saginata*, utilizes bovines as intermediate hosts and humans as final hosts. Although tapeworm infections have been reported since ancient times [1], it was not until 1782 [2] that differentiation of *T. saginata* from the other well-known meat-transmitted human tapeworm, *Taenia solium*, was established. Furthermore, it was not until 1871 that the role of cattle as intermediate hosts for the parasite was established, with "measly" beef being reported as the source of infection in patients [3].

Ingestion of raw or undercooked infected beef is indeed the mode of transmission of this zoonotic parasite to humans, in whom it develops to its adult form, a several metres long segmented worm consisting of a scolex with four suckers, neck and strobila, i.e. a chain of proglottids [4]. In contrast to *T. solium*, the gravid proglottids of *T. saginata*, which contain thousands of embryonated eggs, are mobile and can migrate from the anus independently of, as well as during, defaecation [5]. Eggs are then shed into the environment, and cattle become infected through grazing contaminated pastures, or ingesting contaminated fodder or water. After hatching, and penetration of the intestinal wall, the oncospheres reach the general circulation, distributing them throughout the body where they develop into cysticerci [4]. Common predilection sites for *T. saginata* cysticerci include the heart and masseter muscles [6].

In both intermediate and definitive hosts, *T. saginata* causes few symptoms. In humans, infection is usually characterized by anal pruritus due the active migration of *T. saginata* proglottids and some mild abdominal pain [7]. Nevertheless, the (potential) presence of a tapeworm in the body can cause distress [8], and some people even suffer from a pathological fear of tapeworms, often encouraged by horror stories circulating in popular media or books [9, 10]. Moreover, although rare, complications due to taeniosis, such as appendicitis, have been reported [11]. In cattle, the infection is generally asymptomatic but nevertheless may incur great economic losses for the meat sector due to carcass condemnation or treatment upon detection of cysticerci during meat inspection, as well as related insurance costs [12, 13].

Taenia saginata is distributed globally, with the parasite occurring in both developed and developing countries, although less frequently in countries where cultural preferences limit consumption of bovids or where adequate sanitary infrastructure reduces the likelihood of bovids ingesting human faecal matter. Thus, the prevalence of human taeniosis and bovine cysticercosis are considered particularly high in Africa, Latin America and some parts of Asia [4].

In eastern and southern Africa, the cattle population was estimated at a massive 20.6 million in 2016 [14], so the parasite is thought to be of particular relevance here. In the area, bovines are essential for the livelihoods of smallholders, serving as a source of food, draft power and manure, as well as acting as a financial buffer for challenging times. Although there are indications of the widespread presence of the parasite in at least some countries in this region (e.g. Ethiopia: [15–17]), an extensive overview of its distribution in this region, along with epidemiological considerations regarding its presence, is still lacking. Our aim was therefore to gather recent information on the presence of *T. saginata* in eastern and southern Africa.

Methods

Search strategy

A systematic review of published literature was conducted to collect data on the occurrence, prevalence, and geographical distribution of bovine cysticercosis and human taeniosis in eastern and southern Africa, published between January 1st, 1990 and December 31st, 2017. For the purpose of this study, eastern and southern Africa was defined as the area covered by the following countries/territories: Angola, Botswana, Burundi, Comoros, Djibouti, Eritrea, Ethiopia, Kenya, Lesotho, Madagascar, Malawi, Mauritius, Mayotte (French), Mozambique, Namibia, Réunion (French), Rwanda, Seychelles, Socotra (Yemini), Somalia (including the autonomous regions Puntland and Somaliland), South Africa, Swaziland, Tanzania (including the semi-autonomous region of Zanzibar), Uganda, Zambia and Zimbabwe. The PRISMA guidelines were followed whilst conducting the review [18] (Additional file 1). The search protocol can be found in Additional file 2.

The international bibliographic databases PubMed (http://www.ncbi.nlm.nih.gov/pubmed) and Web of Science (http://ipscience.thomsonreuters.com/product/web-of-science/) were searched using the following search phrase: (cysticerc* OR cisticerc* OR "C. bovis" OR taenia* OR tenia* OR saginata OR taeniosis OR teniosis OR taeniasis OR ténia OR taeniid OR cysticerque) AND (Angola OR Botswana OR Burundi OR Comoros OR Djibouti OR Eritrea OR Ethiopia OR Kenya OR Lesotho OR Madagascar OR Malawi OR Mauritius OR Mayotte OR Mozambique OR Namibia OR Réunion OR Rwanda OR Seychelles OR Socotra OR Somalia OR South Africa OR Swaziland OR Tanzania OR Uganda OR Zanzibar OR Zambia OR Zimbabwe OR "East Africa" OR "Horn of Africa" OR "Southern Africa" OR Puntland OR Somaliland).

Furthermore, a range of databases for grey literature and MSc/PhD thesis documents were searched using keywords from the above search phrase (the full list of databases is presented in Additional file 3). Data on bovine cysticercosis from the different scientific databases were complemented with data from OIE databases "Handistatius" (1996–2004) and "WAHIS" (2005) [19, 20]. Finally, reference lists of reviews on the topic were screened and additional relevant records were added to the database.

Selection criteria

Upon compilation of search results from the different databases, duplicate records were removed. Thereafter, titles and abstracts were screened for relevance, applying the following exclusion criteria: (i) studies concerning a parasite other than *T. saginata*; (ii) studies conducted outside the study area; (iii) studies published outside the study period; (iv) studies reporting results outside the scope of the review question (e.g. review, experiment, intervention trial); and (v) duplicated data. After the screening process, full text articles were evaluated using the same criteria listed above (Additional file 4).

Data extraction and generation

Data from included records were extracted. In reports where the numerator and denominator of the study sample were available, prevalence data were calculated, if not already provided. When not presented in the manuscript, the 95% exact confidence intervals (CI) were calculated, using the "binom.test" function ("*stats*" package) in R 3.5.1 [21].

Results

Search results

A total of 1228 records were obtained from the database search, and four additional records were added through screening of the reference lists of relevant reviews (Additional file 4). After removal of duplicate records (n = 71), 1161 records were screened based on title and, thereafter, abstract. During title screening, 987 records were excluded, and a further 85 records were removed upon abstract screening; three of these were remaining duplicate records, whereas the other removed records focussed on a different parasite (n = 32) or study area (n = 18), were published outside the study period (n = 1), or had a different scope (e.g. laboratory experiments, review) (n = 31). Thus, 89 full text articles (n = 89) fulfilled the eligibility criteria for evaluation, but three of these were unavailable. During the evaluation of the remaining 86 records, eight were excluded due to having a different scope.

Thus, 78 records were included in the qualitative synthesis (journal articles: 73, online data repositories: 2, MSc thesis: 2, PhD thesis: 1). Apart from the two OIE sources describing the occurrence of bovine cysticercosis throughout the study area, the majority of records presented data from Ethiopia (n = 37). The others included data from Kenya (n = 11), Tanzania (n = 7), South Africa (n = 7), Zambia (n = 4), Zimbabwe (n = 2), Angola (n = 2), Uganda (n = 1), Swaziland (n = 1), Namibia (n = 1), Malawi (n = 1), Madagascar (n = 1) or Botswana (n = 1).

Human taeniosis occurrence

A total of 48 records reported the presence of human taeniosis cases (excluding those with confirmed *T. solium* taeniosis). Unspecified taeniosis cases were reported from Angola, Ethiopia, Kenya, Madagascar, Malawi, South Africa, Tanzania, Uganda and Zambia, whereas known *T. saginata* taeniosis cases were reported from Ethiopia, Kenya, South Africa, Tanzania, Zambia and Zimbabwe (Fig. 1). Microscopy results were included in 32 reports, most of which presented data from Ethiopia (18) (Table 1). Taeniosis

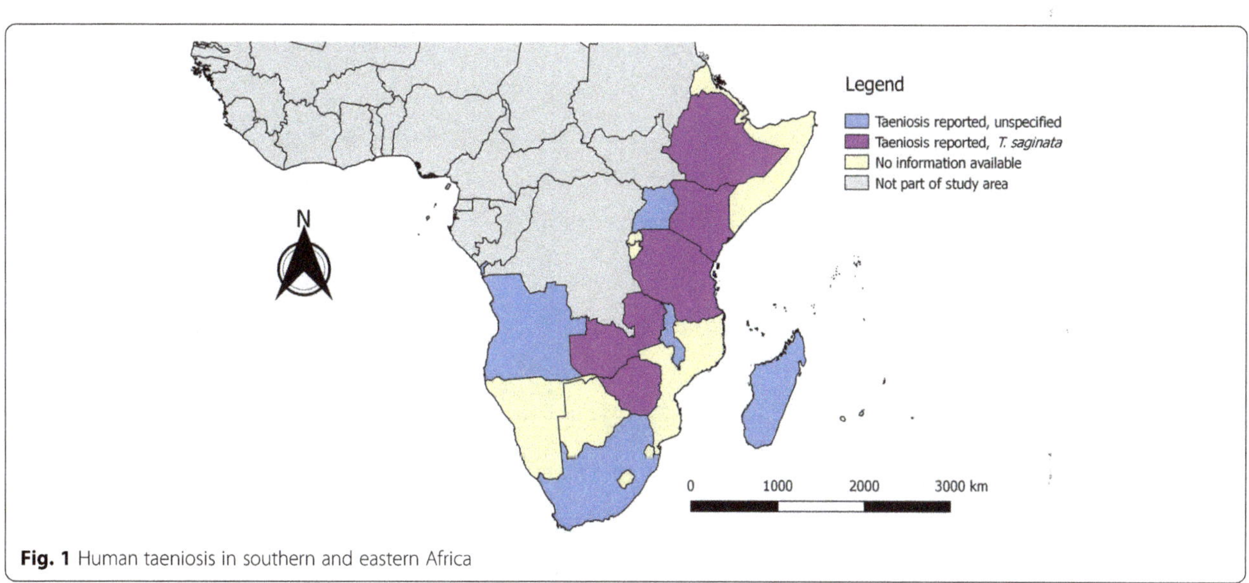

Fig. 1 Human taeniosis in southern and eastern Africa

Table 1 Reported occurrence of taeniosis in southern and eastern Africa: microscopy studies

Country	Period	People tested	People positive	Prevalence (%) (95% CI)	Species identification	Group studied	Reference
Angola	9/2012-12/2013	344	2	0.58 (0.07–2.1)	N	Children below 5 with diarrhea	[50]
Angola	1/2015-5/2015	230	2	0.87 (0.10–3.1)	N	School children in 16 schools	[51]
Ethiopia	11/1995-4/1996; 6-9/1996	1750	79	4.5 (3.6–5.6)	Y[a]	Sugar-estate residents	[52]
Ethiopia	3-4/1999; 2/2002	3167	na	< 4 (na)	N	Schoolchildren, peasants and teachers	[53]
Ethiopia	1/2002-2/2002	104	1	0.96 (0.02–5.2)	Y[a]	HIV/AIDS and HIV-seronegative individuals in a teaching hospital	[54]
Ethiopia	2007–2012	32191	322	1.0 (0.9–1.1)	N	Rural hospital visiters	[55]
Ethiopia	5/2007-6/2007	419	na	1.4 (na)	N	na	[56]
Ethiopia	12/2007-2/2008	7171	23	0.32 (0.20–0.48)	N	Visitors of health centers	[57]
Ethiopia	8/2008-12/2008	343	14	4.1 (2.2–6.8)	N	HIV patients recruited at hospital	[58]
Ethiopia	11/2008	121	5	4.1 (1.4–9.4)	N	Prison inmates	[59]
Ethiopia	11/2008	115	1	0.87 (0.02–4.7)	N	Tobacco farm workers	[59]
Ethiopia	4/2009	384	5	1.3 (0.4–3.0)	N	Food handlers	[60]
Ethiopia	9/2010-7/2011	858	18	2.1 (1.2–3.3)	N	Highland and lowland dwellers	[61]
Ethiopia	1/2011-6/2011	200	1	0.5 (0.01–2.8)	N	Food handlers	[62]
Ethiopia	3/2012-11/2012	260	1	0.38 (0.01–2.12)	N	Children recruited in Health Center	[63]
Ethiopia	1/2013-5/2013	172	5	2.9 (1.0–6.7)	N	Asymptomatic food handlers	[64]
Ethiopia	8/2013-11/2013	180	2	1.1 (0.13–4.0)	N	HAART initiated and naive paediatric HIV patients	[65]
Ethiopia	1/2015-2/2015	503	13	2.6 (1.4–4.4)	N	School children from 5 schools	[66]
Ethiopia	1/2016-8/2016	213	5	2.3 (0.8–5.4)	N	Active pulmonary TB patients	[67]
Ethiopia	na	1537	na	8.1 (na)	Y[a]	Participants from 19 communities, includes children and adults	[23]
Ethiopia	na	491	12	2.4 (1.3–4.2)	N	Villagers	[68]
Kenya	2000–2009	31	1	3.2 (0.08–16.7)	N	Sleeping sickness patients	[69]
Kenya	7/2010-7/2012	2057	na	0.20 (na)	N	na	[22]
Kenya	8/2010-7/2012	2113	na	0.30 (0–0.5)	N	Mixed-farming community	[26]
Kenya	na	285	na	5.3 (na)	N	HIV-positive patients	[70]
Kenya	na	151	0	0 (0–2.4)	N	Geophagous pregnant women	[24]
Madagascar	11/1996-1/1997	401	3	0.75 (0.15–2.2)	N	Patients referred for parasitological examination	[71]
South Africa	2009	na	2	na	N	Laboratory results	[72]
South Africa	2009	na	4	na	Y	Laboratory results	[72]
South Africa	4/2009-9/2009	162	3	1.9 (0.4–5.3)	N	School children	[73]
South Africa	2010	na	11	na	Y	Laboratory results	[72]
South Africa	2010	na	1	na	N	Laboratory results	[72]
South Africa	na	183	3	1.6 (0.3–4.7)	N	Rural black preschool children	[74]
Tanzania	2008–2009	1057	3	0.30 (0.06–0.8)	Y[b]	Villagers, after treatment with niclosamide/praziquantel and purgation	[75]
Uganda	na	5313	36	0.70 (0.5–0.9)	N	Primary school children	[76]
Zambia	6/2007-8/2007	403	na	0.90 (na)	N	School children	[77]

[a]Reported as *T. saginata*, yet unclear from methodology
[b]Confirmed by PCR
Abbreviations: CI, confidence interval; na, not available; HAART, highly active antiretroviral therapy

Table 2 Reported occurrence of taeniosis in southern and eastern Africa: coproAg-ELISA studies

Country	Study period	People tested	People positive	Prevalence (%) 95% CI	Species identification	Group studied	Reference
Kenya	1/2007-4/2007	204	12	5.9 (3.1–10.0)	Y[a]	District inhabitants	[78]
Kenya	8/2010-7/2012	2113	na	19.7 (16.7–22.7)	N	Mixed-farming community	[26]
Kenya	na	691	na	1.9 (na)	N	Slaughterhouse workers	[79]
Zambia	2006	190	5	2.6 (0.9–6.0)	Y[a]	Pupils primary schools	[78]
Zambia	8/2009;10/2010	817	1	0.12 (0.003–0.68)	Y[b]	Consenting villagers	[25]

[a]Results based on coproAg-ELISA, specific for *T. saginata*
[b]Results based on coproAg-ELISA with coproPCR (*T. saginata* specific) confirmation
Abbreviations: CI, confidence interval; na, not available

prevalence based on microscopy alone ranged between 0.2–8.1% (villagers in Kenya [22] and Ethiopia [23], respectively), and one study reported the absence of taeniosis (in geophagous pregnant women in Kenya [24]). Four records presented data from coproAg-ELISA studies conducted in Kenya and/or Zambia, with a prevalence ranging between 0.12–19.7% (villagers in Zambia [25] and Kenya [26], respectively) (Table 2), two of which involved confirmed *T. saginata* cases. Overall, common study groups were school-children, patients suffering from other diseases [e.g. HIV infection, sleeping sickness and active pulmonary tuberculosis (TB)], as well as occupational groups (e.g. tobacco farm workers, food handlers). Furthermore, eight studies reported taeniosis prevalence in communities based on self-reporting by questionnaire respondents (prevalence range: 45.5–64.2%) (Table 3), and five records presented data on anthelmintic sales in towns (Table 4), both in Ethiopia. Another two records contained data on household latrine sampling, thus presenting prevalence at the household level (Malawi: 40.4% [27]; South Africa: 18.0% [28]). Finally, one report discussed a case of intestinal obstruction due to impaction of a *T. saginata* tapeworm in Zimbabwe, requiring enterotomy with bolus removal as well as appendectomy [29].

Bovine cysticercosis

Based on the retrieved data sources (both OIE databases and manuscripts/reports), the presence of bovine cysticercosis was reported in all of the 27 countries/territories studied, except for Comoros, Madagascar, Mauritius, Mayotte and Seychelles. In addition, no information was available for Rwanda, Somalia, Mayotte and Socotra (Fig. 2). Data from the two OIE data sources indicating the occurrence and/or number of cases are presented in Table 5. Apart from the OIE data sources, a total of 39 records were found to document results on bovine cysticercosis in the study region. Meat inspection results were included in 35 records (Table 6), with prevalence estimates ranging between 0.02–26.3%, while two records reported the absence of positive animals (Tanzania: 2011 [30], Zambia: 2001 [31]). Seven records provided serological data, mostly based on Ag-ELISA results (prevalence range: 6.1–53.5%), while one presented Ab-ELISA data (prevalence: 10.0%) [32] and another IHAT results (prevalence: 25.7%) [33] (Table 7). One study estimated the town level costs due to condemnation caused by bovine cysticercosis [Mekelle, abattoir level: 31,952 ETB/6 months (991 EUR, according to July 2018 exchange rates; 1 ETB = 0.0310 EUR) [34]], and another five studies provided data on total economic losses due to condemnation for a wide variety of conditions [17, 30, 35–37]. Overall, the

Table 3 Reported occurrence of taeniosis: questionnaire studies in Ethiopia

Town	Study period	People interviewed	People reporting infection	Prevalence (%) 95% CI	Reference
Awassa	10/2005-4/2006	120	77	64.2 (54.9–72.7)	[44]
Soddo	11/2007-4/2008	79	40	50.6 (39.1–62.1)	[45]
Jimma	11/2008-3/2009	60	34	56.7 (43.2–69.4)	[46]
Yirgalem	11/2009-3/2011	170	119	70.0 (62.5–76.8)	[47]
Sebeta, Tulu Bolo, Weliso	na	392	na	55.1 (na)	[48]
Harar	na	300	182	60.7 (54.9–66.2)	[16]
Adama	11/2013-4/2014	200	91	45.5 (38.5–52.7)	[15]
Batu	12/2014-4/2015	100	59	59.0 (48.7–68.7)	[49]

Abbreviations: CI, confidence interval; na, not available

Table 4 Reported town level taeniicidal sales in Ethiopia

Town	Year	Number	Value (ETB)	Value (EUR)[a]	Reference
Awassa	2002	1,582,254	1,880,330	58,290	[44]
Awassa	2003	1,221,004	1,746,585	54,144	[44]
Awassa	2004	946,330	1,803,300	55,902	[44]
Awassa	2005	889,759	1,788,776	55,452	[44]
Soddo	2004	74,747	192,979	5982	[45]
Soddo	2005	77,705	203,675	6342	[45]
Soddo	2006	79,230	210,133	6314	[45]
Soddo	2007	105,090	279,660	8669	[45]
Jimma	2007	51,462	na	na	[46]
Jimma	2008	52,134	na	na	[46]
Yirgalem	2005	95,712	na	na	[47]
Yirgalem	2006	93,059	na	na	[47]
Yirgalem	2007	95,093	na	na	[47]
Yirgalem	2008	95,121	na	na	[47]
Yirgalem	2009	93,028	na	na	[47]
Batu	2013	42,557	148,100	4591	[49]
Batu	2014	29,049	97,492	3022	[49]

[a]Based on July 2018 exchange rates (1 ETB = 0.0310 EUR)
Abbreviation: na, not available

majority of records presented data from Ethiopia (21/41), followed by Tanzania (8/41) and Kenya (7/41).

Taeniosis and bovine cysticercosis occurrence

The co-occurrence of both bovine cysticercosis and taeniosis during the study period was reported in Angola, Ethiopia, Malawi, South Africa, Tanzania, Uganda, Zambia and Zimbabwe, but this was not the case for the other countries/territories studied. The occurrence of bovine cysticercosis or taeniosis was reported for all the countries/territories studied, except for Somalia, Rwanda and the Comoros, Mauritius, Mayotte, Seychelles, Mayotte and Socotra islands.

Discussion

The present study aimed at describing the epidemiology of *T. saginata* taeniosis/cysticercosis in eastern and southern Africa (1990–2017). Based on our findings, both human taeniosis and bovine cysticercosis were widespread in the 27 countries/territories studied, except for Somalia, Rwanda and six island states/territories, indicating that *T. saginata* is present in most countries of the study area. However, lack of diagnosis and reporting, particularly in rural areas, mean that the data accrued are likely to underestimate occurrence. The absence of data for some countries does not exclude the possibility that this parasite is present there as well. For example, given that of the three countries bordering Rwanda that are included in this review (Burundi, Tanzania and Uganda) all report the presence of this parasite, it seems unlikely that Rwanda is free from *T. saginata*. On the other hand, one potential hypothesis for the lack of reported *T. saginata* in Rwanda is the remarkably higher rate of access to improved sanitation services, at 60.8% in comparison to neighbouring Burundi at 35.5% [38]. The Rwandan civil war, during 1990–1994, culminating in the genocide of 1994, may have impacted reporting during that period, but does not explain the more recent lack of reporting. For Somalia, the ongoing civil war might explain the lack of reported data for the country, whereas for the six island states and territories, governmental or scientific interest in reporting cases may be lacking.

Cases of taeniosis were reported for Angola, Ethiopia, Kenya, Madagascar, Malawi, South Africa, Tanzania,

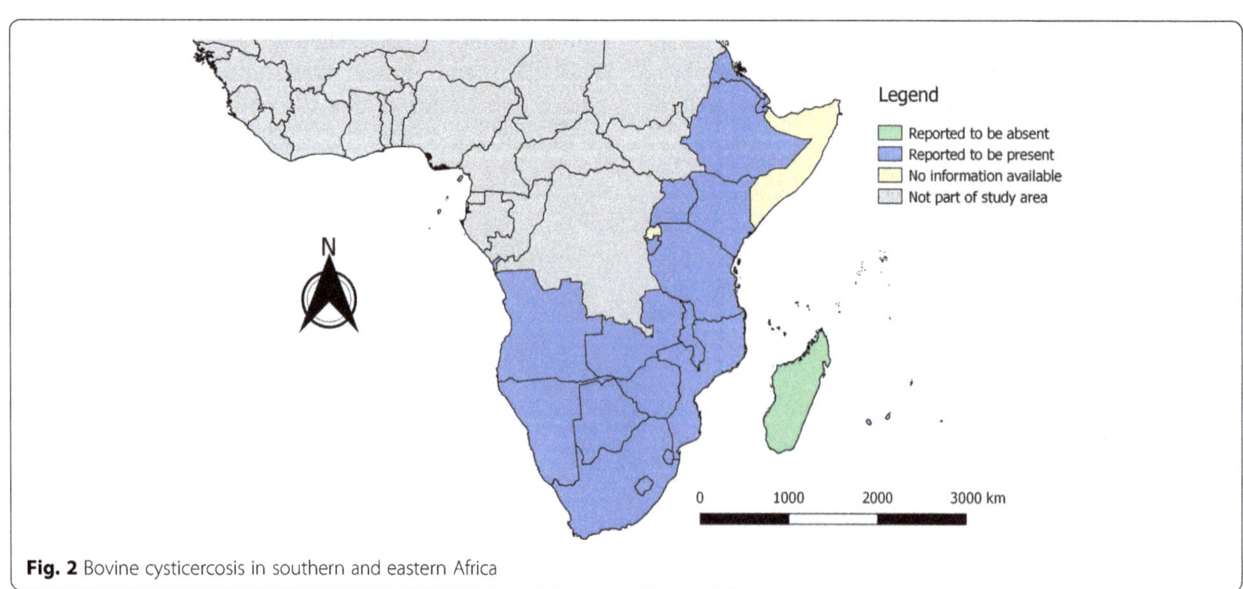

Fig. 2 Bovine cysticercosis in southern and eastern Africa

Table 5 OIE data on occurrence of bovine cysticercosis in the southern and eastern Africa (1996–2005) [19, 20]

Country	Year									
	1996	1997	1998	1999	2000	2001	2002	2003	2004	2005
Angola	6	11	na	na	na	na	na	na	4	+
Botswana	na	53	4356	12,863	14,000	14,000	10,181	15,363	na	+
Burundi	na	na	na	na	na	+	na	na	na	na
Comoros	na	na	-	na	na	na	na	na	na	na
Djibouti	na	na	na	na	na	na	+	+	+	+
Eritrea	+	+	+	2	+	+	na	+	370	-
Ethiopia	+	na	na	na	na	+	+	+	+	+
Kenya	+	+	+	+	+	+	+	+	3999	na
Lesotho	56	38	139	na	na	na	68	na	na	-
Madagascar	na	na	na	na	na	na	-	na	na	-
Malawi	+	+	+	+	+	+	+	+	6	+
Mauritius	na	na	na	na	na	-	-	-	-	na
Mozambique	+	+	+	na	na	na	na	na	na	-
Namibia	+	3833	3118	+	2852	2226	2399	54	1616	+
Réunion	+	na	na	-	-	-	-	-	na	-
Rwanda	na	na	na	na	na	na	na	na	na	na
Seychelles	-	-	-	na	-	na	-	na	-	na
Somalia	na	na	na	na	na	na	na	na	na	na
South Africa	+	+	+	+	+	+	+	+	+	+
Swaziland	969	+	+	+	1419	530	245	1909	561	+
Tanzania	+	+	+	+	na	na	+	6	na	+
Uganda	+	24	152	+	+	+	+	na	na	+
Zambia	na	na	na	na	+	na	2	248	na	na
Zimbabwe	244	1744	2062	1988	160	1447	+	na	na	na

Abbreviations: na, not available; +, occurrence of the disease; -, absence of the disease

Uganda, Zambia and Zimbabwe, yet the majority of reports on human taeniosis cases did not, unfortunately, provide species determination. Thus, cases of *T. saginata* taeniosis were not differentiated from infections caused by other *Taenia* spp. The pork tapeworm, *T. solium*, for instance, is presumed to also be widely distributed throughout eastern and southern Africa [39] and therefore we cannot conclude that all reported, unspecified taeniosis cases are due to *T. saginata*. *Taenia solium* is known to be the causative agent of the severe condition neurocysticercosis, associated with epilepsy, severe headaches, cognitive deficits [40] and a major cause of deaths among the food-borne diseases [41]. The presence of a single *T. solium* tapeworm carrier poses a major risk for his/her surroundings, as humans acquire neurocysticercosis through the ingestion of *T. solium* eggs transmitted through poor hygiene practices resulting in faecal-oral transmission [42]. Although tapeworm infections usually have an asymptomatic course [7] apart from some sporadic complications (e.g. intestinal obstruction in the Zimbabwean patient [29]), it is thus paramount to register cases as well as to differentiate case species, to allow precise prevalence estimates, and to guide appropriate control measures. Species determination, however, is hampered by the fact that *Taenia* spp. eggs cannot be differentiated upon coprological examination. Expelled proglottids of *T. solium* and *T. saginata* can be distinguished on the basis of the number of uterine branches, but such material is not always available. Moreover, more advanced diagnostic tools (e.g. copro-PCR) to differentiate species are often lacking in resource poor settings [43], and even in developed countries are not often performed due to lack of awareness about neurocysticercosis [12].

In certain countries in the study area, specific culinary habits put the consumers at great risk of contracting *T. saginata* taeniosis. For instance, in Ethiopia, "*kitfo*" is a very popular beef dish, in which the meat is usually consumed raw or lightly cooked, while "*tibs*" is another dish often containing undercooked beef. Furthermore, "*kurt*"

Table 6 Reported occurrence of bovine cysticercosis in southern and eastern Africa: meat inspection studies

Country	Period	Animals tested	Animals positive	Prevalence (%) (95% CI)	Reference
Botswana	1995	na	na	na (9.1–12.6)	[80]
Ethiopia	9/2004-8/2005	11,227	842	7.5 (7.0–8.0)	[81]
Ethiopia	9/2005-2/2007	4456	824	18.5 (17.4–19.7)	[82]
Ethiopia	10/2005-4/2006	400	105	26.3 (22.0–30.9)	[83]
Ethiopia	12/2006-7/2007	3711	308	8.3 (7.4–9.2)	[34]
Ethiopia	10/2007-3/2008	512	15	2.9 (1.6–4.8)	[84]
Ethiopia	11/2007-4/2008	415	47	11.3 (8.4–14.8)	[45]
Ethiopia	12/2007-2/2008	1023	74	7.2 (5.7–9.0)	[57]
Ethiopia	11/2008-3/2009	500	22	4.4 (2.8–6.6)	[46]
Ethiopia	10/2009-9/2010	898	177	19.7 (17.2–22.5)	[16]
Ethiopia	11/2009-3/2011	400	48	12 (9.0–15.6)	[47]
Ethiopia	2010	12,708	669	5.3 (4.9–5.7)	[37]
Ethiopia	9/2010-9/2012	3055	126 organs	na	[35]
Ethiopia	2011	34,674	3259	9.4 (9.1–9.7)	[37]
Ethiopia	2012	10,363	803	7.7 (7.2–8.3)	[37]
Ethiopia	10/2012-4/2013	745	21 organs	na	[35]
Ethiopia	2013	5172	247	4.8 (4.2–5.4)	[37]
Ethiopia	11/2013-4/2014	384	10	2.6 (1.3–4.7)	[15]
Ethiopia	11/2013-5/2014	3675	40 organs	na	[36]
Ethiopia	05/2014-6/2014	439	23	5.2 (3.3–7.8)	[85]
Ethiopia	12/2014-4/2015	384	10	2.6 (1.3–4.7)	[49]
Ethiopia	na	522	39	7.4 (5.4–10.1)	[33]
Ethiopia	na	1022	64	6.3 (4.9–7.9)	[17]
Ethiopia	na	1216	na	4.6 (na)	[48]
Kenya	1974	77,810	6784	8.8 (8.5–8.9)	[86]
Kenya	1975–1978	na	na	< 6.0 (na)	[86]
Kenya	1979–1983	na	na	< 4.0 (na)	[86]
Kenya	1984	na	na	1.8 (na)	[86]
Kenya	1985–1990	na	na	< 2.0 (na)	[86]
Kenya	1991	315,801	3457	1.1 (1.06–1.13)	[86]
Kenya	9/2006-1/2007	188	6	3.2 (1.2–6.8)	[87]
Kenya	na	511	39	7.6 (5.5–10.3)	[88]
Kenya	na	1184	189	16.0 (13.9–18.2)	[32]
Namibia	2000	12,204	973	8.0 (7.5–8.5)	[89]
Namibia	2001	7888	713	9.0 (8.4–9.7)	[89]
Namibia	2002	10,561	798	7.6 (7.1–8.1)	[89]
Namibia	2003	4411	347	7.9 (7.1–8.7)	[89]
Namibia	2004	5309	401	7.6 (6.9–8.3)	[89]
Namibia	2006	7085	435	6.1 (5.6–6.7)	[89]
Namibia	2006	71,388	243	0.34 (0.30–0.39)	[89]
South Africa	2009–2011	1,022,556	24,443	2.39 (2.36–2.42)	[90]
South Africa	2010	356,006	2169	0.61 (0.58–0.64)	[91]
South Africa	2011	349,458	2389	0.68 (0.66–071)	[91]

Table 6 Reported occurrence of bovine cysticercosis in southern and eastern Africa: meat inspection studies *(Continued)*

Country	Period	Animals tested	Animals positive	Prevalence (%) (95% CI)	Reference
South Africa	2012	348,309	1980	0.57 (0.54–0.59)	[91]
South Africa	2013	361,232	3382	0.94 (0.91–0.97)	[91]
Tanzania	1987–1989	42,434	na	16.4 (na)	[92]
Tanzania	1/2002-4/2004	12,444	185	1.5 (1.3–1.7)	[93]
Tanzania	2005	na	19	0.06 (na)	[94]
Tanzania	2006	na	24	0.06 (na)	[94]
Tanzania	2007	na	16	0.04 (na)	[94]
Tanzania	2010	27,444	20 organs	na	[30]
Tanzania	2/2010-1/2011	30,713	18 organs	na	[95]
Tanzania	2011	30,671	0 organs	na	[30]
Tanzania	2012	27,865	6 organs	na	[30]
Tanzania	12/2013	2438	1 and 0.1% organs	na	[30]
Tanzania	na	na	21	na	[96]
Zambia	2000	4629	1	0.02 (0.0005–0.12)	[31]
Zambia	2001	9422	0	0 (0–0.04)	[31]
Zambia	2002	10,147	2	0.02 (0.002–0.07)	[31]
Zambia	2003	11,519	2	0.02 (0.002–0.06)	[31]
Zimbabwe	1/2006-12/2007	86,080	1364	1.6 (1.5–1.7)	[97]

Abbreviations: CI, confidence interval; na, not available

refers to the habit of eating cubes of raw beef, finished off with local spices. Unsurprisingly, a high proportion of the Ethiopian population reports having had a tapeworm, and sales of taeniicidal drugs in Ethiopia are high [15, 16, 44–49].

Access to adequate clean water and sanitation services (WASH) is notoriously poor across the whole of sub-Saharan Africa, including the region of interest to this paper. There are large between and within-country disparities, but overall sub-Saharan Africa lags far behind the goals set out by the international community in both the millennium development and the sustainable development goals with only 25.7% (23.1–28.6%) of the population having access to improved sanitation [38]. This lack of WASH capacity is strongly reflected by the presence of parasites such as *T. saginata* which requires ingestion of eggs passed in faecal material for the propagation of its life-cycle.

In eastern and southern Africa the cattle population is large, and bovine products, including meat, are an

Table 7 Reported occurrence of bovine cysticercosis in southern and eastern Africa: serological studies

Country	Period	Diagnostic tool	Animals tested	Animals positive	Prevalence (%) 95% CI	Reference
Ethiopia	na	IHAT	743	190	25.6 (22.4–28.9)	[33]
Kenya	9/2006-1/2007	Ag-ELISA	188	44	23.4 (17.8–30.1)	[87]
Kenya	10/2006-11/2006	Ag-ELISA	792	143	18.1 (15.4–20.9)	[87]
Kenya	8/2010-7/2012	Ag-ELISA	983	na	53.5 (48.7–58.3)	[26]
Kenya	na	Ag-ELISA	511	117	22.9 (19.3–26.8)	[88]
Kenya	na	Ag-ELISA	1184	413	34.9 (32.2–37.7)	[32]
Kenya	na	Ab-ELISA	1184	118	10.0 (8.3–11.8)	[32]
South Africa	na	Ag-ELISA	1315	300	22.8 (20.6–25.2)	[98]
South Africa	na	Ag-ELISA	1159	174	15.0 (13.0–17.2)	[98]
Swaziland	na	Ag-ELISA	600	na	28.0 (na)	[99]
Zambia	12/1999-9/2000	Ag-ELISA	628	38	6.1 (4.3–8.2)	[100]

Abbreviations: CI, confidence interval; na, not available; IHAT, indirect hemagglutination test

important protein source for humans, as well as a source of draft power and form of investment. Beef cattle are typically kept in an extensive manner; animals are basically free-ranging. The presence of human *T. saginata* carriers shedding eggs into the environment puts these cattle at risk of bovine cysticercosis, and this presumably occurs widely in the study area. In developed countries, the condition is known to cause economic losses due to freezing or condemnation of the carcass as well as related insurance costs (e.g. Belgium: 3,408,455 EUR/year [13]). Studies investigating the magnitude of this economic loss in the study area are, however, limited, with data available from only one abattoir in Ethiopia [34]. Furthermore, reporting of bovine cysticercosis to OIE appeared to be inconsistent, with large variations in number of cases reported even within the same country, and gaps in the annual reporting (e.g. no data available after 2005).

Conclusions

Taenia saginata taeniosis/cysticercosis is a widespread, yet largely ignored, condition in southern and eastern Africa. This is probably due to the lack of symptoms in cattle, the lack of good data on its economic impact, and because human taeniosis is considered a minor health problem. Nevertheless, the presence of bovine cysticercosis is a clear sign of inadequate sanitation, insufficient meat inspection, and culinary habits that may favour transmission. Measures to reduce transmission of *T. saginata* are therefore warranted, and the infection should be properly monitored, in both humans and cattle. It should also be noted that as cattle are an important source of human protein and livelihoods in the area, ensuring optimal health and productivity of cattle is of indirect importance to human health and welfare as well as any direct impact. Species identification in tapeworm carriers is paramount to gain detailed insights in the distribution of the different *Taenia* spp. in the area, as well to avoid the development of the severe condition neurocysticercosis within communities due to ingestion of eggs shed by a *T. solium* tapeworm carrier. We conclude that in order to ensure both the safety of beef consumed in the southern and eastern Africa, and to improve the underlying sanitary conditions perpetuating the parasitic life-cycle, concerted, co-ordinated efforts must be made by integrating public, animal and environmental health in a One Health approach.

Abbreviations

ETB: Ethiopian Birr; EUR: Euro; HAART: Highly active antiretroviral therapy; IHAT: Indirect hemagglutination test; OIE: World Organisation for Animal Health/Office International des Epizooties

Acknowledgments

This work was performed within the framework of CYSTINET, the European network on taeniosis/cysticercosis, COST ACTION TD1302.

Funding

Not applicable.

Authors' contributions

VD conducted the systematic review of literature, extracted and analysed the data and drafted the first version of the manuscript. All authors contributed to the design of the study, interpretation of the data and writing the paper. All authors read and approved the final manuscript.

Competing interests

The authors declare that they have no competing interests.

Author details

[1]Department of Biomedical Sciences, Institute of Tropical Medicine, Antwerp, Belgium. [2]Department of Virology, Parasitology and Immunology, Faculty of Veterinary Medicine, Ghent University, Merelbeke, Belgium. [3]One Health Center for Zoonoses and Tropical Veterinary Medicine, Ross University School of Veterinary Medicine, Basseterre, Saint Kitts, Trinidad and Tobago. [4]Department of Epidemiology and Public Health, Sciensano, Brussels, Belgium. [5]Department of Veterinary Public Health and Food Safety, Faculty of Veterinary Medicine, Ghent University, Merelbeke, Belgium. [6]Parasitology, Department of Food Safety and Infection Biology, Faculty of Veterinary Medicine, Norwegian University of Life Sciences, Adamstuen Campus, Oslo, Norway. [7]Laboratory of Parasitology, Veterinary Research Institute, Hellenic Agricultural Organization Demeter, Thermi, 57001 Thessaloniki, Greece. [8]International Livestock Research Institute (ILRI), P.O. Box 30709, Nairobi, Kenya. [9]Institute for Infection and Global Health, University of Liverpool, Neston, UK.

References

1. Del Brutto OH, García HH. *Taenia solium* cysticercosis - the lessons of history. J Neurol Sci. 2015;359:392–5.
2. Goeze J. Versuch einer Naturgeschichte der Eingeweidewürmer thierischer Körper. Blankenburg, Germany: Philipp Adam Pape; 1782.
3. Oliver J. Seventh annual report of the sanitary commissioner (1870) of the Government of India. Calcutta, India: Government Printing House; 1871.
4. Murrell KD. Epidemiology of taeniosis and cysticercosis. In: Murrell KD, editor. WHO/FAO/OIE guidelines for the surveillance, prevention and control of taeniosis/cysticercosis. Paris: Office International des Epizooties (OIE); 2005. p. 27–43.
5. Dorny P, Praet N. *Taenia saginata* in Europe. Vet Parasitol. 2007;149:22–4.

6. Scandrett B, Parker S, Forbes L, Gajadhar A, Dekumyoy P, Waikagul J, et al. Distribution of *Taenia saginata* cysticerci in tissues of experimentally infected cattle. Vet Parasitol. 2009;164:223–31.
7. Tembo A, Craig PS. *Taenia saginata* taeniosis: copro-antigen time-course in a voluntary self-infection. J Helminthol. 2015;89:612–9.
8. Craig P, Ito A. Intestinal cestodes. Curr Opin Infect Dis. 2007;20:524–32.
9. Bryce A. I have a pathological fear of tapeworms. Tonic. 2017. https://tonic.vice.com/en_us/article/wj8x5z/i-have-a-pathological-fear-of-tapeworms. Accessed 26 Apr 2018.
10. Butcher N. The strange case of the walking corpse: a chronicle of medical mysteries, curious remedies, and bizarre but true healing folklore. New York, USA: Avery; 2004.
11. Karatepe O, Adas G, Tukenmez M, Battal M, Altiok M, Karahan S. Parasitic infestation as cause of acute appendicitis. G Chir. 2009;30:426–8.
12. Laranjo-González M, Devleesschauwer B, Trevisan C, Allepuz A, Sotiraki S, Abraham A, et al. Epidemiology of taeniosis/cysticercosis in Europe, a systematic review: Western Europe. Parasit Vectors. 2017;10:349.
13. Jansen F, Dorny P, Trevisan C, Dermauw V, Laranjo-González M, Allepuz A, et al. Economic impact of bovine cysticercosis and taeniosis caused by *Taenia saginata* in Belgium. Parasit Vectors. 2018;11:241.
14. FAO. Food and Agriculture Organization of the United Nations Statistical Databases. 2016. http://faostat3.fao.org. Accessed 26 Apr 2018.
15. Tolossa Y, Taha A, Terefe G, Jibat T. Bovine cysticercosis and human taeniosis in Adama town, Oromia region, Ethiopia. J Vet Sci Technol. 2015;S10:003.
16. Terefe Y, Redwan F, Zewdu E. Bovine cysticercosis and its food safety implications in Harari People's National Regional State, eastern Ethiopia. Onderstepoort J Vet Res. 2014;81:676.
17. Shiferaw S, Kumar A, Amssalu K. Organs condemnation and economic loss at Mekelle municipal abattoir. Ethiopia. Haryana Vet. 2009;48:17–22.
18. Moher D, Liberati A, Tetzlaff J, Altman DG, Grp P. Preferred reporting tems for systematic reviews and meta-analyses: The PRISMA Statement (Reprinted from Annals of Internal Medicine). Phys Ther. 2009;89:873–80.
19. Office International des Epizooties. OIE Handistatus II. 2018. http://web.oie.int/hs2/report.asp?lang=en. Accessed 1 Apr 2018.
20. Office International des Epizooties. OIE World Animal Health Information Database (WAHIS). 2018. http://www.oie.int/wahis_2/public/wahid.php/Wahidhome/Home/indexcontent/newlang/en. Accessed 1 Apr 2018.
21. R Core Team. R: A language and environment for statistical computing. Vienna: R Foundation for Statistical Computing; 2018.
22. Wardrop NA, Thomas LF, Atkinson PM, de Glanville WA, Cook EAJ, Wamae CN, et al. The influence of socio-economic, behavioural and environmental factors on *Taenia* spp. transmission in western Kenya: evidence from a cross-sectional survey in humans and pigs. PLoS Negl Trop Dis. 2015;9:e0004223.
23. Birrie H, Erko B, Tedla S. Intestinal helminthic infections in the southern Rift Valley of Ethiopia with special reference to schistosomiasis. East Afr Med J. 1994;71:447–52.
24. Odongo AO, Moturi WN, Mbuthia EK. Heavy metals and parasitic geohelminths toxicity among geophagous pregnant women: a case study of Nakuru Municipality, Kenya. Environ Geochem Health. 2016;38:123–31.
25. Praet N, Verweij JJ, Mwape KE, Phiri IK, Muma JB, Zulu G, et al. Bayesian modelling to estimate the test characteristics of coprology, coproantigen ELISA and a novel real-time PCR for the diagnosis of taeniasis. Trop Med Int Heal. 2013;18:608–14.
26. Fèvre EM, de Glanville WA, Thomas LF, Cook EAJ, Kariuki S, Wamae CN. An integrated study of human and animal infectious disease in the Lake Victoria crescent small-holder crop-livestock production system, Kenya. BMC Infect Dis. 2017;17:457.
27. Kumwenda S, Msefula C, Kadewa W, Diness Y, Kato C, Morse T, et al. Is there a difference in prevalence of helminths between households using ecological sanitation and those using traditional pit latrines? A latrine based cross sectional comparative study in Malawi. BMC Res Notes. 2017;10:200.
28. Trönnberg L, Hawksworth D, Hansen A, Archer C, Stenström TA. Household-based prevalence of helminths and parasitic protozoa in rural KwaZulu-Natal, South Africa, assessed from faecal vault sampling. Trans R Soc Trop Med Hyg. 2010;104:646–52.
29. Bordon L. Intestinal obstruction due to *Taenia saginata* infection: a case report. J Trop Med Hyg. 1990;95:352–3.
30. Tembo W, Nonga HE. A survey of the causes of cattle organs and/or carcass condemnation, financial losses and magnitude of foetal wastage at an abattoir in Dodoma, Tanzania. Onderstepoort J Vet Res. 2015;82:a855.
31. Phiri A. Common conditions leading to cattle carcass and offal condemnations at 3 abattoirs in the Western Province of Zambia and their zoonotic implications to consumers. J S Afr Vet Assoc. 2006;77:28–32.
32. Onyango-Abuje JA, Nginyi JM, Rugutt MK, Wright SH, Lumumba P, Hughes G, et al. Seroepidemiological survey of *Taenia saginata* cysticercosis in Kenya. Vet Parasitol. 1996;64:177–85.
33. Kebede N, Tilahun G, Hailu A. Development and evaluation of indirect hemagglutination antibody test (IHAT) for serological diagnosis and screening of bovine cysticercosis in Ethiopia. Ethiop J Sci. 2008;31:135–40.
34. Kumar A, Berhe G. Occurrence of cysticercosis in cattle of parts of Tigray region of Ethiopia. Haryana Vet. 2008;47:88–90.
35. Assefa A, Tesfay H. Major causes of organ condemnation and economic loss in cattle slaughtered at Adigrat municipal abattoir, northern Ethiopia. Vet World. 2013;6:734–8.
36. Edo JJ, P M, Rahman MT. Investigation into major causes of organs condemnation in bovine slaughtered at Adama municipal abattoir and their economical importance. Haryana Vet. 2014;53:139–43.
37. Mummed Y. Beef carcass quality, yield and causes of condemnations in Ethiopia. PhD thesis, University of Pretoria; 2015.
38. Roche R, Bain R, Cumming O. A long way to go - estimates of combined water, sanitation and hygiene coverage for 25 sub-Saharan African countries. PLoS One. 2017;12:e0171783.
39. Braae UC, Saarnak CFL, Mukaratirwa S, Devleesschauwer B, Magnussen P, Johansen MV. *Taenia solium* taeniosis/cysticercosis and the co-distribution with schistosomiasis in Africa. Parasit Vectors. 2015;8:323.
40. Garcia HH, Nash TE, Del Brutto OH. The tapeworm that turned. Lancet Neurol. 2014;13:1173.
41. Havelaar A, Kirk M, Torgerson P, Gibb H, Hald T, Lake R, et al. World Health Organization global estimates and regional comparisons of the burden of foodborne disease in 2010. PLoS Med. 2015;12:e1001923.
42. Nash TE, Mahanty S, Garcia HH. Neurocysticercosis - more than a neglected disease. PLoS Negl Trop Dis. 2013;7:e1964.
43. WHO. *Taenia solium* taeniasis/cysticercosis diagnostic tools. Report of a stakeholder meeting. Geneva, 17-18 December 2015. Geneva: World Health Organization; 2016.
44. Abunna F, Tilahun G, Megersa B, Regassa A. Taeniasis and its socio-economic implication in Awassa town and its surroundings, southern Ethiopia. East Afr J Public Health. 2007;4:73–9.
45. Regassa A, Abunna F, Mulugeta A, Megersa B. Major metacestodes in cattle slaughtered at Wolaita Soddo municipal abattoir, southern Ethiopia: prevalence, cyst viability, organ distribution and socioeconomic implications. Trop Anim Health Prod. 2009;41:1495–502.
46. Megersa B, Tesfaye E, Regassa A, Abebe R, Abunna F. Bovine cysticercosis in cattle slaughtered at Jimma municipal abattoir, South Western Ethiopia: prevalence, cyst viability and its socio-economic importance. Vet World. 2010;3:257–62.
47. Abunna F. Prevalence, orgain distribution, viability and socioeconomic implication of bovine cysticercosis/teniasis, Ethiopia. Rev Elev Med Vet Pays Trop. 2013;66:25–30.
48. Tadesse A, Tolossa YH, Ayana D, Terefe G. Bovine cysticercosis and human taeniosis in south-west Shoa zone of Oromia Region, Ethiopia. Ethiop Vet J. 2013;17:121–33.
49. Teklemariam AD, Debash W. Prevalence of *Taenia saginata*/cysticercosis and community knowledge about zoonotic cestodes in and around Batu, Ethiopia. J Vet Sci Technol. 2015;6:273.
50. Gasparinho C, Mirante MC, Centeno-Lima S, Istrate C, Mayer AC, Tavira L, et al. Etiology of diarrhea in children younger than 5 years attending the Bengo general hospital in Angola. Pediatr Infect Dis J. 2016;35:e28–34.
51. Nindia A, Moreno M, Salvador F, Amor A, de Alegría MLAR, Kanjala J, et al. Prevalence of *Strongyloides stercoralis* and other intestinal parasite infections in school children in a rural area of Angola: a cross-sectional study. Am J Trop Med Hyg. 2017;97:1226–31.
52. Fontanet A, Sahlu T, Rinke de Wit T, Messele T, Masho W, Woldemichael T, et al. Epidemiology of infections with intestinal parasites and human immunodeficiency virus (HIV) among sugar-estate residents in Ethiopia. Ann Trop Med Parasitol. 2000;94:269–78.
53. Berhanu M, Girmay E. Human helminthiasis in Wondo Genet Southern Ethiopia with emphasis on geohelminthiasis. Ethiop Med J. 2003;41:333–46.
54. Hailemariam G, Kassu A, Abebe G, Abate E, Damte D, Mekonnen E, et al. Intestinal parasitic infections in HIV/AIDS and HIV seronegative individuals in a teaching hospital, Ethiopa. Jpn J Infect Dis. 2004;57:41–3.

55. Ramos JM, Rodríguez-Valero N, Tisiano G, Fano H, Yohannes T, Gosa A, et al. Different profile of intestinal protozoa and helminthic infections among patients with diarrhoea according to age attending a rural hospital in southern Ethiopia. Trop Biomed. 2014;31:392–7.
56. Terefe A, Shimelis T, Mengistu M, Hailu A, Erko B. *Schistosomiasis mansoni* and soil-transmitted helminthiasis in Bushulo Village, southern Ethiopia. Ethiop J Heal Dev. 2011;25:46–50.
57. Abay G, Kumar A. Cysticercosis in cattle and its public health implications in Mekelle City and surrounding areas, Ethiopia. Ethiop Vet J. 2013;17:31–40.
58. Fekadu S, Taye K, Teshome W, Asnake S. Prevalence of parasitic infections in HIV-positive patients in southern Ethiopia: a cross-sectional study. J Infect Dev Ctries. 2013;7:868–72.
59. Mamo H. Intestinal parasitic infections among prison inmates and tobacco farm workers in Shewa Robit, north-central Ethiopia. PLoS One. 2014;9:e99559.
60. Abera B, Biadegelgen F, Bezabih B. Prevalence of *Salmonella typhi* and intestinal parasites among food handlers in Bahir Dar Town, northwest Ethiopia. Ethiop J Heal Dev. 2010;24:46–50.
61. Wegayehu T, Tsalla T, Seifu B, Teklu T. Prevalence of intestinal parasitic infections among highland and lowland dwellers in Gamo area, South Ethiopia. BMC Public Health. 2013;13:151.
62. Dagnew M, Tiruneh M, Moges F, Tekeste Z. Survey of nasal carriage of *Staphylococcus aureus* and intestinal parasites among food handlers working at Gondar University, northwest Ethiopia. BMC Public Health. 2012;12:837.
63. Beyene G, Tasew H. Prevalence of intestinal parasite, *Shigella* and *Salmonella* species among diarrheal children in Jimma health center. Jimma southwest Ethiopia: a cross sectional study. Ann Clin Microbiol Antimicrob. 2014;13:10.
64. Aklilu A, Kahase D, Dessalegn M, Tarekegn N, Gebremichael S, Zenebe S, et al. Prevalence of intestinal parasites, *Salmonella* and *Shigella* among apparently health food handlers of Addis Ababa University student's cafeteria, Addis Ababa, Ethiopia. BMC Res Notes. 2015;8:17.
65. Mengist HM, Taye B, Tsegaye A. Intestinal parasitosis in relation to CD4+T cells levels and anemia among HAART initiated and HAART naive pediatric HIV patients in a model ART center in Addis Ababa, Ethiopia. PLoS One. 2015;10:e0117715.
66. Alemayehu B, Tomass Z, Wadilo F, Leja D, Liang S, Erko B. Epidemiology of intestinal helminthiasis among school children with emphasis on *Schistosoma mansoni* infection in Wolaita zone, southern Ethiopia. BMC Public Health. 2017;17:587.
67. Alemu G, Mama M. Intestinal helminth co-infection and associated factors among tuberculosis patients in Arba Minch, Ethiopia. BMC Infect Dis. 2017; 17:68.
68. Nyantekyi L, Legesse M, Medhin G, Animut A, Tadesse K, Macias C, et al. Community awareness of intestinal parasites and the prevalence of infection among community members of rural Abaye Deneba area, Ethiopia. Asian Pac J Trop Biomed. 2014;4:S152–7.
69. Kagira JM, Maina N, Njenga J, Karanja SM, Karori SM, Ngotho JM. Prevalence and types of coinfections in sleeping sickness patients in Kenya (2000/2009). J Trop Med. 2011;2011:248914.
70. Kipyegen CK, Shivairo RS, Odhiambo RO. Prevalence of intestinal parasites among HIV patients in Baringo, Kenya. Pan Afr Med J. 2012;13:37.
71. Buchy P. Les parasitoses digestives dans la région de Mahajanga, côte Ouest de Madagascar. Bull La Soc Pathol Exot. 2003;96:41–5.
72. Du Plooy I. Results of routine examinations for parasitic infections of humans from laboratory-submitted samples in Gauteng, North West and Mpumalanga provinces between 2009 and 2010. MSc thesis: University of Pretoria; 2014.
73. Nxasana N, Baba K, Bhat V, Vasaikar S. Prevalence of intestinal parasites in primary school children of Mthatha, Eastern Cape Province, South Africa. Ann Med Health Sci Res. 2013;3:511–6.
74. Taylor M, Pillai G, Kvalsvig JD. Targeted chemotherapy for parasite infestations in rural black preschool children. South African Med J. 1995;85:870–4.
75. Eom KS, Chai JY, Yong TS, Min DY, Rim HJ, Kihamia C, et al. Morphologic and genetic identification of *Taenia* tapeworms in Tanzania and DNA genotyping of *Taenia solium*. Korean J Parasitol. 2011;49:399–403.
76. Kabatereine N, Kemijumbi J, Kazibwe F, Onapa A. Human intestinal parasites in primary school children in Kampala, Uganda. East Afr Med J. 1997;74:311–4.
77. Siwila J, Phiri IGK, Enemark HL, Nchito M, Olsen A. Intestinal helminths and protozoa in children in pre-schools in Kafue district, Zambia. Trans R Soc Trop Med Hyg. 2010;104:122–8.
78. Tembo A. Detection and diagnosis of *Taenia saginata* taeniosis. PhD thesis, University of Salford, UK; 2010.
79. Cook EA. Epidemiology of zoonoses in slaughterhouse workers in western Kenya. PhD thesis, University of Edinburgh, UK; 2014.
80. Skjerve E. Possible increase of human *Taenia saginata* infections through import of beef to Norway from a high prevalence area. J Food Prot. 1999; 62:1314–9.
81. Kebede N, Tilahun G, Hailu A. Current status of bovine cysticercosis of slaughtered cattle in Addis Ababa abattoir, Ethiopia. Trop Anim Health Prod. 2009;41:291–4.
82. Kebede N. Cysticercosis of slaughtered cattle in northwestern Ethiopia. Res Vet Sci. 2008;85:522–6.
83. Abunna F, Tilahun G, Megersa B, Regassa A, Kumsa B. Bovine cysticercosis in cattle slaughtered at Awassa municipal abattoir, Ethiopia: prevalence, cyst viability, distribution and its public health implication. Zoonoses Public Health. 2008;55:82–8.
84. Tolosa T, Tigre W, Teka G, Dorny P. Prevalence of bovine cysticercosis and hydatidosis in Jimma municipal abattoir, South West Ethiopia. Onderstepoort J Vet Res. 2009;76:323–6.
85. Belay S. Prevalence of *Cysticercus bovis* in cattle at municipal abbatoir of Shire. J Vet Sci Technol. 2014;5:196.
86. Kang'ethe EK. The impact of meat inspection on the control of bovine hydatidosis in Kenya. Bull Anim Heal Prod Africa. 1995;63:261–8.
87. Asaava LL, Kitala PM, Gathura PB, Nanyingi MO, Muchemi G, Schelling E. A survey of bovine cysticercosis/human taeniosis in Northern Turkana District, Kenya. Prev Vet Med. 2009;89:197–204.
88. Onyango-Abuje JA, Hughes G, Opicha M, Nginyi KM, Rugutt MK, Wright SH, et al. Diagnosis of *Taenia saginata* cysticercosis in Kenyan cattle by antibody and antigen ELISA. Vet Parasitol. 1996;61:221–30.
89. Shikongo-Kuvare LT. Development of risk communication strategies to improve control of *Cysticercosis bovis* in north-central Namibia. MSc thesis: University of Pretoria, South Africa; 2007.
90. Ndou R, Dlamini M. The control of measles (bovine cysticercosis (*Taenia saginata*)) from South African feedlot cattle: where do we come from, where are we now and where are we going with control and prevention programmes against this zoonosis. Proceedings of the 10th Annual Congress of the Southern African Society for Veterinary Epidemiology and Preventive Medicine, Pretoria, South Africa; 2012.
91. Qekwana DN, Oguttu JW, Venter D, Odoi A. Disparities in beef tapeworm identification rates in the abattoirs of Gauteng Province, South Africa: a descriptive epidemiologic study. PLoS One. 2016;11:e0151725.
92. Kambarage DM, Kimera SI, Kazwala RR, Mafwere BM. Disease conditions responsible for condemnation of carcasses and organs in short-horn Zebu cattle slaughtered in Tanzania. Prev Vet Med. 1995;22:249–55.
93. Swai ES, Schoonman L. A survey of zoonotic diseases in trade cattle slaughtered at Tanga city abattoir: a cause of public health concern. Asian Pac J Trop Biomed. 2012;2:55–60.
94. Mellau BL, Nonga HE, Karimuribo ED. Slaughter stock abattoir survey of carcasses and organ/offal condemnations in Arusha region, northern Tanzania. Trop Anim Health Prod. 2011;43:857–64.
95. Komba EVG, Komba EV, Mkupasi EM, Mbyuzi AO, Mshamu S, Luwumba D, et al. Sanitary practices and occurrence of zoonotic conditions in cattle at slaughter in Morogoro municipality, Tanzania: implications for public health. Tanzan J Health Res. 2012;14:131–8.
96. Maeda GE, Kyvsgaard NC, Nansen P, Bøgh HO. Distribution of *Taenia saginata* cysts by muscle group in naturally infected cattle in Tanzania. Prev Vet Med. 1996;28:81–9.
97. Sungirai M, Masaka L, Mbiba C. The prevalence of *Taenia saginata* cysticercosis in the Matabeleland provinces of Zimbabwe. Trop Anim Health Prod. 2014;46:623–7.
98. Tsotetsi-Khambule AM, Njiro S, Katsande TC, Thekisoe OMM, Harrison LJS. Sero-prevalence of *Taenia* spp. infections in cattle and pigs in rural farming communities in Free State and Gauteng provinces, South Africa. Acta Trop. 2017;172:91–6.
99. Hughes G, Hoque M, Tewes MS, Wright SH, Harrison LJS. Seroepidemiological study of *Taenia saginata* cysticercosis in Swaziland. Res Vet Sci. 1993;55:287–91.
100. Dorny P, Phiri I, Gabriël S, Speybroeck N, Vercruysse J. A sero-epidemiological study of bovine cysticercosis in Zambia. Vet Parasitol. 2002;104:211–5.

8

Topical or oral fluralaner efficacy against flea (*Ctenocephalides felis*) transmission of *Dipylidium caninum* infection to dogs

Deepa Gopinath[1], Leon Meyer[2], Jehane Smith[2] and Rob Armstrong[3*]

Abstract

Background: *Dipylidium caninum* is a common tapeworm of dogs contracted from ingestion of fleas containing the infective cysticercoid stage. Fluralaner is a systemically distributed isoxazoline class insecticide that delivers highly effective activity against fleas and ticks for up to 12 weeks after a single oral or topical treatment. This study evaluated the impact of this flea insecticidal efficacy on the transmission of *D. caninum* to dogs.

Methods: Dogs were weighed and treated with a cestocide and then randomly assigned to 3 groups of 8. Fluralaner was administered topically (at the commercial dose) to one group and orally to another group while the third received topically administered sterile water. All dogs were subsequently infested with about 100 *D. caninum* infected *Ctenocephalides felis* at 7, 14, 21, 28, 35, 42, 49, 56, 63, 70, 77 and 83 days after treatment. Visual proglottid inspections and counts were conducted daily from 35 to 113 days post-treatment. Post-treatment *D. caninum* incidence was calculated for each group and compared between treated and untreated groups.

Results: All 8 dogs in the placebo-treated group became infected with *D. caninum* while no shed proglottids were observed at any point during the post-treatment period from any dog in either fluralaner treated group.

Conclusions: The insecticidal efficacy of a single treatment of either orally or topically administered fluralaner prevented *D. caninum* transmission from infected fleas to susceptible dogs for up to 12 weeks following administration.

Keywords: *Dipylidium caninum*, Dogs, Fluralaner, Flea control, Flea-borne disease

Background

Dipylidium caninum, commonly known as the flea tapeworm, is a frequently diagnosed intestinal cestode parasite of dogs and cats, although occasionally humans have become infected following ingestion of the saliva of infected pets [1]. *Ctenocephalides* spp. fleas, of which *C. felis* is the most prevalent on domestic dogs and cats [2, 3], are intermediate hosts in the life-cycle of *D. caninum*. In brief, *D. caninum* eggs passed in the feces of infected animals are ingested by flea larvae in the environment and the flea larvae then develop into pupae while hosting tapeworm embryos. The adult flea then emerges and infests a host, and within 2–3 days the hexacanth cestode embryo develops into an infective cysticercoid stage within the flea. The cysticercoid larvae require at least 24–36 hours before they are infective for the definitive host [4–6], a development period that is temperature-dependent [5]. Dogs and cats become infected when they ingest fleas containing the infective cysticercoid larvae during grooming. Adult *D. caninum* develop in the small intestine and within 2–3 weeks begin to shed egg packets called proglottids [7]. The overall pre-patent period can be as short as two weeks [6].

Clinical signs in *D. caninum* infected dogs generally consist of mild gastrointestinal manifestations and anal pruritus, which may cause the animal to exhibit 'scooting' behavior [8]. In addition, slowly motile proglottids may be observed on the animals' feces and the combination of this behavior and the sight of proglottids can be distressing for owners [9]. The potential zoonotic transmission of this parasite [6, 10, 11] and wide geographical range [12] underline the value of protecting dogs and cats from *D. caninum*. Routine cestocidal treatment of household dog(s) and cat(s) is one option for managing this tapeworm [9]; however, the

* Correspondence: robert.armstrong@merck.com
[3]Merck Animal Health, 2 Giralda Farms, Madison, NJ 07940, USA
Full list of author information is available at the end of the article

brief pre-patent period means that exposure to infective stages between cestocidal treatments can lead to infection and development of adult tapeworms in dogs. Dog owners easily underestimate the required frequency of cestocidal re-treatment administration needed to prevent *D. caninum* infections from reaching the egg shedding stage. Re-infection of pets can occur very quickly following cestocidal treatment, which has no residual effect [9].

Effective and persistent flea control can control the environmental proglottid load and prevent *D. caninum* infection, provided that fleas are killed sufficiently quickly before animals with fleas become tapeworm infected [4]. This is an additional benefit from an effective flea control regimen, adding to the control of other flea-related disorders such as flea-bite dermatitis and flea hypersensitivity dermatitis [2, 9]. PCR assessment found that 2.2% of *C. felis* from client-owned cats and 5.2% of *C. felis* from client-owned dogs in Europe were *D. caninum* infected [7]. These results show that the prevalence of *D. caninum* in Europe is sufficient to ensure that appropriate measures are routinely needed to prevent this tapeworm infection of domestic dogs and cats.

Fluralaner (Bravecto Chews and Bravecto Spot-On, Merck Animal Health, Madison, NJ, USA) is a highly effective flea insecticide that is systemically distributed in dogs following either topical or oral administration [13–15]. This active ingredient kills fleas following ingestion of a blood meal, with an onset of activity within two hours of initial oral administration [13]. Flea insecticidal efficacy following oral fluralaner administration reaches 98–100% at 8–24 hours after flea infestation [13] and efficacy of ≥ 99% has been demonstrated for 12 weeks following application of a single topical dose of fluralaner [13, 16, 17]. The hypothesis in this study is that fluralaner treatment will provide flea insecticidal efficacy that is sufficiently rapid to prevent *D. caninum* transmission to dogs infested with infected fleas. This result was previously reported in dogs treated orally with a combination of another isoxazoline class molecule, afoxolaner, and milbemycin against challenges with infected fleas over a 28-day study period [18]. The current study evaluated both orally and topically administered fluralaner at the recommended clinical dose (25–56 mg/kg) with flea challenges over the 12 week period following a single treatment. Fluralaner does not have a label indication against cestodes.

Methods

This study was a parallel group designed, blinded, randomized, single center, placebo controlled efficacy study [19]. The study consisted of 24 dogs within 3 groups of 8 dogs each from an initial enrolled group of 28 dogs. Dogs were either beagles or mongrels (mixed-breed), and body weight ranged between 12.0–27.6 kg, with a mean body weight of 17.7 kg prior to commencement of the study (Day -3). Mean body weight within the groups was 17.7 kg in Group 1, 17.1 kg in Group 2 and 17.6 kg in Group 3. No statistically significant differences were recorded with respect to the body weights ($P = 0.9640$) measured in different groups, indicating homogeneity at the time of inclusion. There were four male and four female dogs within each group ranging from 12 to 85 months-old at the time of inclusion. To be included in the study, dogs had to have been clinically healthy on physical examination by a veterinarian on Day -7, older than 6 months of age at the time of inclusion, not clinically pregnant and not of an excessively fractious temperament which makes handling overtly difficult. The four dogs with the lowest body measurements on Day -2 were excluded from the study. Dogs included in the study had not been treated with a long-acting acaricide/insecticide during the 12 weeks preceding Day 0, and were also not treated with a macrocyclic lactone or other long acting anthelmintic during the three weeks preceding Day 0 (with the exception of deworming with a short-acting anthelmintic (a combination of praziquantel, pyrantel pamoate and febantel) during the study preparation phase prior to Day -7). None of the dogs were removed from the study prior to scheduled study termination and after inclusion on Day -3 (with the exception of the dogs that were infected with *D. caninum*).

Study dogs were acclimatized to conditions for 21 days before treatment and a centrifuged fecal parasite examination was run on all dogs on the first day of acclimatization to ensure the dogs were free of resident enteric parasites. The centrifuged fecal examination was conducted by thoroughly mixing the entire fecal sample of each dog to ensure a homogenized sample after collection. One gram of the homogenized sample was mixed with 10 ml of sugar solution and strained through a double layer of gauze. A 15 ml centrifuge tube was filled with the suspension and placed into the centrifuge and the tube was filled with sugar solution to a slight positive meniscus. A coverslip was placed on top of each tube, simultaneously ensuring that a small bubble was present under the coverslip. Samples were centrifuged in a swinging-head centrifuge at 1250× *rpm* for 5 min. After centrifugation, the tubes were removed and placed in a test tube rack and let stand for 10 min, then coverslips were removed and examined. All dogs were weighed and treated with a cestocide, a combination of milbemycin oxime and praziquantel (Milbemax®, Elanco, Greenfield, IN, USA). Their cages were screened daily for proglottids over the following 20-day acclimation period to detect any resident tapeworm infections persisting despite treatment.

Two days before treatment administration, dogs were ranked within sex in descending order of individual body weights, and blocked into 3 groups of 8 dogs each. One group was treated topically with sterile water, another group received orally administered fluralaner and the third received topically administered fluralaner. Fluralaner was dosed according to the product label, at a dose of 25–56 mg/kg body weight. Dogs treated with oral fluralaner were also treated with topical sterile water to maintain blinding. On treatment day, all dogs received half of their daily food ration approximately 20 min before treatment and the second half directly after treatment. All dogs were observed hourly for 6 h after treatment administration.

Thirty fleas per batch were sampled from at least three batches of fleas and examined microscopically for the presence of *D. caninum* metacestodes (Table 1) to determine the proportion containing the infective stage [20]. Approximately 100 *D. caninum*-infected *C. felis* fleas were placed on every dog in the study at 7, 14, 21, 28, 35, 42, 49, 56, 63, 70, 77 and 83 days after treatment.

Visual proglottid inspections and counts were conducted daily on cage floors, sleeping areas and dog feces of all dogs from 35 to 113 days post-treatment to detect cestode-infected dogs. All dogs observed to have shed proglottids, and all dogs at the end of the study period, were removed from the study, dewormed and treated with a flea adulticide.

The experimental unit was the individual dog and the *D. caninum* infection incidence at the end of the study period was calculated for each group using the formula:

Infection incidence (%) = (No. of dogs infected in each group / No. of dogs enrolled in each group) × 100.

Significance was determined by comparing the infection incidence in each of the treated groups with the sterile water-treated control group (SAS Version 9.3 TS Level 1M2). Proportions were compared between the groups using a Fisher's exact test. Significance of the two sided significance test was set at 5%.

Results

All 8 dogs in the placebo treated control group were observed to be shedding *D. caninum* proglottids: there were 3 positive control dogs at 35 days after treatment, 1 positive control dog at 38 days after treatment, and 4 positive control dogs at 43 days after treatment. Transmission of *D. caninum* to all control dogs confirms that the challenge is adequate. No dog in either of the fluralaner-treated groups shed *D. caninum* proglottids at any time during the post-treatment observation period between 35 and 113 days post-treatment. Therefore, both oral and topically administered fluralaner were 100% effective for prevention of transmission of *D. caninum* tapeworms to dogs in this natural flea infestation model. This difference between the proportion of *D. caninum*-infected dogs in the control and treated groups was significant (Fisher's exact test, $P < 0.0001$) (Table 2).

Discussion

These results show that treatment with either topically or orally administered fluralaner kills fleas with sufficient rapidity to prevent transmission of *D. caninum* to dogs throughout the 84-day period following administration of a single dose. The overall study period extended to 113 days to allow maturation of any *D. caninum* possibly infecting the intestinal tracts of dogs. This result is consistent with the flea control observed following oral fluralaner administration to dogs in field challenge situations [16, 21, 22] and in laboratory challenges [13, 22]. The fluralaner onset of activity following oral

Table 1 *Dipylidium caninum* infection in flea batches used to infest dogs using a natural challenge model

Time post-treatment (days)	Flea age (days)	Metacestode infection prevalence (%)[a]	Metacestode intensity per infected flea[b]	Metacestode abundance[c]
7	12	23.3	3.1	0.7
14	14	66.7	8.8	5.8
21	13	33.3	3.3	1.1
28	18	40.0	2.8	1.1
35	14	13.3	6.8	0.9
42	14	13.3	5.0	0.7
49	14	16.7	2.0	0.3
56	12	13.3	1.0	0.1
63	14	13.3	1.3	0.2
70	14	26.7	5.1	1.4
77	16	13.3	9.3	1.2
84	13	13.3	3.5	0.5

[a]No. infected fleas / total no. fleas examined
[b]Total no. metacestodes recovered / no. infected fleas
[c]Total no. metacestodes recovered / total no. of fleas examined

Table 2 *Dipylidium caninum* infection incidence for dogs treated and subsequently challenged with *D. caninum* infected *Ctenocephalides felis*

Treatment	Sterile water	Topical fluralaner	Oral fluralaner	*P*-value[a]
No. of proglottid-shedding dogs per 8 dog group	8	0	0	< 0.0001
Dipylidium caninum infection prevention efficacy	na	100%	100%	

[a]For each treated group compared to the placebo-treated control using Fisher's exact test
Abbreviation: na - not applicable

administration to dogs is rapid, with mortality observed at 1 hour after dosing; significant flea mortality compared with untreated control dogs at 2 hours; and 99.4% mortality of adult fleas by 8 hours of dosing [13].

The *D. caninum* challenge presented to dogs in this study was greater than might be encountered under natural conditions. Field survey data in Europe indicate that 5.2% of fleas infesting client-owned dogs are infected with *D. caninum* [7], while in this study, all dogs were experimentally infested with approximately 100 fleas at weekly intervals, with 13 to 68% of the challenge fleas estimated to be *D. caninum*-infected (Table 1). *Dipylidium caninum* can also be transmitted by biting lice (*Trichodectes canis*), a transmission mechanism not addressed in the present study [23] although field efficacy has been shown for fluralaner against the sucking louse, *Linognathus setosus* [24].

Flea challenges began 7 days after treatment and continued until 83 days after treatment. Housing and dog feces were examined daily for *D. caninum* proglottids from 35 days until 113 days (30 days after the final flea challenge) after treatment. The intervals between the initial flea challenge on day 7, the start of the observation period on day 35, the final flea challenge (day 83) and the end of the study (day 113) provided time to allow the parasite to complete its pre-patent period in any infected dog and begin shedding proglottids. No proglottids were seen in the feces of any fluralaner treated dog, regardless of the route of administration, at any time point. Detection of *D. caninum* proglottids in feces, cage floor and bedding is sufficiently sensitive to detect infected dogs [18].

The cysticercoid larvae of *D. caninum* require 24–36 hours following arrival of the flea on the dog to become infective for the definitive host. These results confirm that either oral or topical administration of fluralaner effectively kills fleas before this *D. caninum* development time has elapsed and is consistent with the reported speed of kill times for orally administered fluralaner over the recommended retreatment interval [13].

Conclusions

The insecticidal efficacy of a single treatment of either orally or topically administered fluralaner prevented *D. caninum* transmission from infected fleas to susceptible dogs for up to 12 weeks following administration.

Abbreviation

PCR: polymerase chain reaction

Acknowledgements

The authors are sincerely grateful to the Research Operations team and to all the monitors who ensured adherence to GCP standards.

Funding

This study was funded by MSD Animal Health (Madison NJ, USA).

Authors' contributions

All authors assisted in the study design, monitoring, interpretation of results, manuscript preparation and data analysis. All authors read and approved the final manuscript.

Competing interests

DG is currently employed by MSD Animal Health, Sydney, Australia and RA is currently employed by Merck Animal Health, Madison, NJ, USA. LM and JS worked on this project under contract with Merck Animal Health.

Author details

[1]MSD Animal Health, 26 Talavera Rd, Macquarie Park, NSW 2113, Australia. [2]Clinvet International, Uitzich Road, Bainsvlei, Bloemfontein 9338, South Africa. [3]Merck Animal Health, 2 Giralda Farms, Madison, NJ 07940, USA.

References

1. Guzman RF. A survey of cats and dogs for fleas: with particular reference to their role as intermediate hosts of *Dipylidium caninum*. N Z Vet J. 1984;32:71–3.
2. Dryden MW, Rust MK. The cat flea: biology, ecology and control. Vet Parasit. 1994;52:1–19.
3. Rust M. The biology and ecology of cat fleas and advancements in their pest management: a review. Insects. 2017;8:118.
4. Beugnet F, Delport P, Luus H, Crafford D, Fourie J. Preventive efficacy of Frontline® Combo and Certifect® against *Dipylidium caninum* infestation of cats and dogs using a natural flea (*Ctenocephalides felis*) infestation model. Parasite. 2013;20:7.
5. Pugh RE, Moorhouse DE. Factors affecting the development of *Dipylidium caninum* in *Ctenocephalides felis* felis (Bouché, 1835). Parasitol Res. 1985;71:765–75.
6. Pugh RE. Effects on the development of *Dipylidium caninum* and on the host reaction to this parasite in the adult flea (*Ctenocephalides felis* felis). Parasitol Res. 1987;73:171–7.
7. Beugnet F, Labuschagne M, Fourie J, Jacques G, Farkas R, Cozma V, et al. Occurrence of *Dipylidium caninum* in fleas from client-owned cats and dogs in Europe using a new PCR detection assay. Vet Parasit. 2014;205:300–6.
8. Mani I, Maguire JH. Small animal zoonoses and immuncompromised pet owners. Top Companion Anim Med. 2009;24:164–74.
9. Fourie JJ, Crafford D, Horak IG, Stanneck D. Prophylactic treatment of flea-infested dogs with an imidacloprid / flumethrin collar (Seresto®, Bayer) to preempt infection with *Dipylidium caninum*. Parasitol Res. 2013;112:33–46.
10. Chappell C, Enos JP, Pen HM. *Dipylidium caninum*, an underrecognised infection in infants and children. Pediatr Infect Dis J. 1990;9:745–7.
11. Raitiere CR. Tapeworm (*Dipylidium caninum*) infestation in a 6-month-old infant. J Fam Prac. 1992;34:101–2.
12. de Avelar DM, Bussolotti AS, Ramos M, Linardi PM. Endosymbionts of *Ctenocephalides felis felis* (Siphonaptera: Pulicidae) obtained from dogs captured in Belo Horizonte, Minas Gerais, Brazil. J Invertebr Pathol. 2007;94:149–52.

13. Taenzler J, Wengenmayer C, Williams H, Fourie J, Zschiesche E, Roepke RK, et al. Onset of activity of fluralaner (BRAVECTO™) against *Ctenocephalides felis* on dogs. Parasit Vectors. 2014;7:567.
14. Kilp S, Ramirez D, Allan MJ, Roepke RK, Nuernberger MC. Pharmacokinetics of fluralaner in dogs following a single oral or intravenous administration. Parasit Vectors. 2014;7:85.
15. Kilp S, Ramirez D, Allan MJ, Roepke RK. Comparative pharmacokinetics of fluralaner in dogs and cats following single topical or intravenous administration. Parasit Vectors. 2016;9:296.
16. Meadows C, Guerino F, Sun F. A randomized, blinded, controlled USA field study to assess the use of fluralaner topical solution in controlling canine flea infestations. Parasit Vectors. 2017;10:36.
17. Taenzler J, Gale B, Zschiesche E, Roepke RKA, Heckeroth AR. The effect of water and shampooing on the efficacy of fluralaner spot-on solution against *Ixodes ricinus* and *Ctenocephalides felis* infestations in dogs. Parasit Vectors. 2016;9:233.
18. Beugnet F, Meyer L, Fourie J, Larsen D. Preventive efficacy of NexGard Spectra® against *Dipylidium caninum* infection in dogs using a natural flea (*Ctenocephalides felis*) infestation model. Parasite. 2017;24:16.
19. Marchiondo AA, Holdsworth PA, Fourie LJ, Rugga D, Hellmannd K, Snyder DE, et al. World Association for the Advancement of Veterinary Parasitology (W.A.A.V.P.) second edition: Guidelines for evaluating the efficacy of parasiticides for the treatment, prevention and control of flea and tick infestations on dogs and cats. Vet Parasit. 2013;194:84–97.
20. Venard CE. Morphology, bionomics, and taxonomy of the cestode *Dipylidium caninum*. Ann N Y Acad Sci. 1937;3:273–328.
21. Rohdich N, Roepke RK, Zschiesche E. A randomized, blinded, controlled and multi-centered field study comparing the efficacy and safety of Bravecto™ (fluralaner) against Frontline™ (fipronil) in flea- and tick-infested dogs. Parasit Vectors. 2014;7:83.
22. Williams H, Young DR, Qureshi T, Zoller H, Heckeroth AR. Fluralaner, a novel isoxazoline, prevents flea (*Ctenocephalides felis*) reproduction *in vitro* and in a simulated home environment. Parasit Vectors. 2014;7:275.
23. Saini VK, Gupta S, Kasondra A, Rakesh RL, Latchumikanthan A. Diagnosis and therapeutic management of *Dipylidium caninum* in dogs: a case report. J Parasit Dis. 2016;40:1426–8.
24. Kohler-Aanesen H, Saari S, Armstrong R, Péré K, Taenzler J, Zschiesche E, et al. Efficacy of fluralaner (Bravecto™ chewable tablets) for the treatment of naturally acquired *Linognathus setosus* infestations on dogs. Parasit Vectors. 2017;10:426.

Babesia bovis RON2 contains conserved B-cell epitopes that induce an invasion-blocking humoral immune response in immunized cattle

Mario Hidalgo-Ruiz[1], Carlos E. Suarez[2], Miguel A. Mercado-Uriostegui[1], Ruben Hernandez-Ortiz[3], Juan Alberto Ramos[3], Edelmira Galindo-Velasco[4], Gloria León-Ávila[5], José Manuel Hernández[6] and Juan Mosqueda[1*]

Abstract

Background: *Babesia bovis* belongs to the phylum Apicomplexa and is the major causal agent of bovine babesiosis, the most important veterinary disease transmitted by arthropods. In apicomplexan parasites, the interaction between AMA1 and RON2 is necessary for the invasion process, and it is a target for vaccine development. In *B. bovis*, the existence of AMA1 has already been reported; however, the presence of a homolog of RON2 is unknown. The aim of this study was to characterize RON2 in *B. bovis*.

Results: The *B. bovis ron2* gene has a similar synteny with the orthologous gene in the *B. bigemina* genome. The entire *ron2* gene was sequenced from different *B. bovis* strains showing > 99% similarity at the amino acid and nucleotide level among all the sequences obtained, including the characteristic CLAG domain for cytoadherence in the amino acid sequence, as is described in other Apicomplexa. The *in silico* transcription analysis showed similar levels of transcription between attenuated and virulent *B. bovis* strains, and expression of RON2 was confirmed by western blot in the *B. bovis* T3Bo virulent strain. Four conserved peptides, containing predicted B-cell epitopes in hydrophilic regions of the protein, were designed and chemically synthesized. The humoral immune response generated by the synthetic peptides was characterized in bovines, showing that anti-RON2 antibodies against peptides recognized intraerythrocytic merozoites of *B. bovis*. Only peptides P2 and P3 generated partially neutralizing antibodies that had an inhibitory effect of 28.10% and 21.42%, respectively, on the invasion process of *B. bovis* in bovine erythrocytes. Consistently, this effect is additive since inhibition increased to 42.09% when the antibodies were evaluated together. Finally, P2 and P3 peptides were also recognized by 83.33% and 87.77%, respectively, of naturally infected cattle from endemic areas.

Conclusions: The data support RON2 as a novel *B. bovis* vaccine candidate antigen that contains conserved B-cell epitopes that elicit partially neutralizing antibodies.

Keywords: Bovine babesiosis, *Babesia bovis*, Tight junction, Invasion process, CLAG domain

* Correspondence: joel.mosqueda@uaq.mx
[1]Immunology and Vaccines Laboratory, C. A. Facultad de Ciencias Naturales, Universidad Autónoma de Querétaro, Carretera a Chichimequillas, Ejido Bolaños, 76140 Queretaro, Queretaro, Mexico
Full list of author information is available at the end of the article

Background

The intraerythrocytic protozoan *Babesia bovis* is the major causal agent of bovine babesiosis, which is one of the most important veterinary diseases transmitted by arthropods. *B. bovis* belongs to the phylum Apicomplexa, which includes *Plasmodium* spp., and *Toxoplasma gondii*, two examples of pathogens within this phylum with medical importance. The parasites of this phylum are characterized by apical organelles such as rhoptries, micronemes and spherical bodies. The proteins related to these organelles are implicated in the invasion and egression of host target cells [1–3]. Importantly, most apicomplexan parasites share four basic steps in the invasion process: (i) attachment to the target host cell; (ii) parasite reorientation to align the apical organelles in close contact with the membrane surface of the target cell; (iii) target cell surface membrane invagination, involving several molecular interactions between protozoan ligands and host receptors so as to make tight junctions; and (iv) parasite internalization, a process that also occurs continuously in the blood of *Babesia* infected bovines. Thus, *B. bovis* merozoites invade red blood cells (RBC), while secreting proteins from the apical organelles and forming close junctions between the membrane of the parasite and the RBC membrane. Once inside the RBC, the parasite multiplies by binary fission in two merozoites, which, upon egression from their original host erythrocyte, go to invade other RBCs to perpetuate this cycle of asexual replication [4–6]. In *Plasmodium falciparum*, the "tight junction" is also known as the "moving junction", and it was described as a specific and irreversible interaction between two proteins: the apical membrane antigen-1 (AMA-1) located on the merozoite surface and the rhoptry neck protein 2 (RON2), which is integrated to the RBC membrane after its secretion from the rhoptries in a complex formed with other RON proteins [7–9]. The disruption of AMA-1-RON2 interaction ceases the merozoite invasion, making these proteins vaccine candidates [10]. Expression of the neutralization-sensitive AMA-1 was already reported in *B. bovis*; however, there are no previous reports describing the conservation and functional role of RON2 in this parasite despite being recently described in *B. divergens* and *B. microti* [11, 12]. Therefore, the purpose of the present study was to identify a *B. bovis* homolog gene of RON2 and define its pattern of expression and functional relevance.

Results

The *B. bovis* genome encodes for a *ron2* orthologous gene

A BLAST search against the *B. bovis* T2Bo reference genome using the nucleotide (KU696964.1) and amino acid (AQU42588.1) sequences as a query identified an orthologous gene (BBOV_I001630) in the chromosome 1 contig_1104837696198 (NW_001820854.1). The *ron2* gene does not contain introns and has a very similar synteny between the genome of *B. bovis* and *B. bigemina* (Fig. 1a). The nucleotide sequence has an identity of 70% and the amino acid sequence identity is 64%. Employing eight different pairs of primers (see Table 1), which were designed based using the BBOV_I001630 reference sequence, it was possible to obtain the full sequence of *ron2* in four isolates of *B. bovis*: Chiapas, Colima, Nayarit and Veracruz. The sequence of each isolate was submitted to the GenBank database under the accession numbers

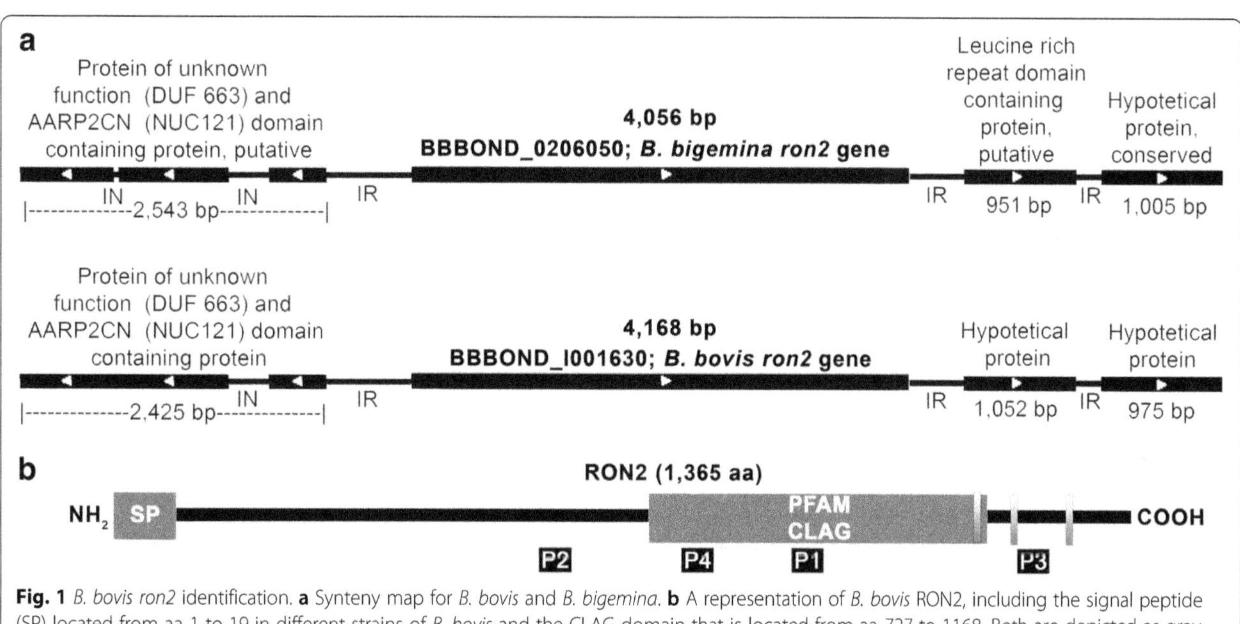

Fig. 1 *B. bovis ron2* identification. **a** Synteny map for *B. bovis* and *B. bigemina*. **b** A representation of *B. bovis* RON2, including the signal peptide (SP) located from aa 1 to 19 in different strains of *B. bovis* and the CLAG domain that is located from aa 727 to 1168. Both are depicted as gray boxes. Shaded boxes represent the transmembrane regions and black boxes represent the sequences of the selected peptides

Table 1 *Babesia bovis ron2* designed primers

Primer	Sequence (5'-3')
Fw0 RON2Bo	CACCTCACCGATATGCGTAC
RvI0 RON2Bo	GAGTCACTGACACCTTGCC
FwI0 RON2Bo	GTCAGTGACTCCCCTCTTCAAG
Rv0 RON2Bo	GGAATCACCGCCTAGTAGC
Fw1 RON2Bo	GCTACTAGGCGGTGATTCC
RvI1 RON2Bo	GCGTCAATAGAGATAAGCAGG
FwI1 RON2Bo	CCTGCTTATCTCTATTGACGC
Rv1 RON2Bo	CAACCCATTGCTTGATTCCC
Fw2 RON2Bo	GGGAATCAAGCAATGGGTTG
RvI2 RON2Bo	CTTTCTTAGCAATAGCGTCGG
FwI2 RON2Bo	CTTCGTTGCTGGAGGCTACATC
Rv2 RON2Bo	CGTTGGATATTCGGTTGAGC
Fw3 RON2Bo	GCTCAACCGAATATCCAACG
Rv3 RON2Bo	CCGTACTTGATTGCTCTGAG
Fw4 RON2Bo	CTCAGAGCAATCAAGTACGG
Rv4 RON2Bo	CACGGATGGCTATGACAATG

Note: Eight pairs of primers were designed to get the amplification and sequencing of 4169 bp under the same PCR protocol

MG944401, MG944402, MG944403 and MG944404, respectively. All nucleotide sequences obtained from *ron2* (T2Bo, Chiapas, Colima, Nayarit and Veracruz) have a consensus identity of 99.56%; all RON2 amino acid sequences have a consensus identity of 99.78% and the same predicted physicochemical features: a length of 1365 aa, a signal peptide located in the first 19 aa, a CLAG domain for cytoadherence between the amino acids 176 and 1168, three transmembrane domains, an isoelectric point of 8.9 and a molecular weight of 150 kDa (Fig. 1b and Additional files 1:Table S1, Additional file 2: Table S2, Additional file 3: Table S3). When compared with other species of *Babesia*, RON2 showed an identity of 64% with *B. bigemina* (query cover 98%), 81% with *Babesia* sp. Xinjiang (query cover 73%), 60% with *B. divergens* (query cover 99%), 39% with *B. microti* strain RI (query cover 74%), 42% with the hypothetical protein BEWA 034640 of *Theileria equi* (query cover 89%) and finally 26% with the related Apicomplexa *P. falciparum* (query cover 74%).

The *ron2* gene is transcribed in *B. bovis* virulent and attenuated strains

The *in silico* transcription profiling database available from the whole genome microarray at the PiroplasmaDB portal, shows that the genes *ron2* (BBOV_I001630) and *ama-1* (BBOV_IV011230) of attenuated and virulent strains of *B. bovis* have equivalent transcription levels in both strains, suggesting that the expression levels of *ama-1* and *ron2* genes are similar among both strains (Fig. 2a). To validate the results obtained with this analysis, *sbp-tc9* (spherical body protein truncated copy 9) was also included in the analysis, showing upregulation in the attenuated strain, confirming the results reported previously for this gene [13].

RON2 is expressed in *B. bovis* and contains immunogenic peptides

To identify conserved, antigenic and immunogenic regions in the RON2 sequence, a bioinformatics strategy was employed. A total of four peptides containing predicted B-cell epitopes were designed (Fig. 1b and

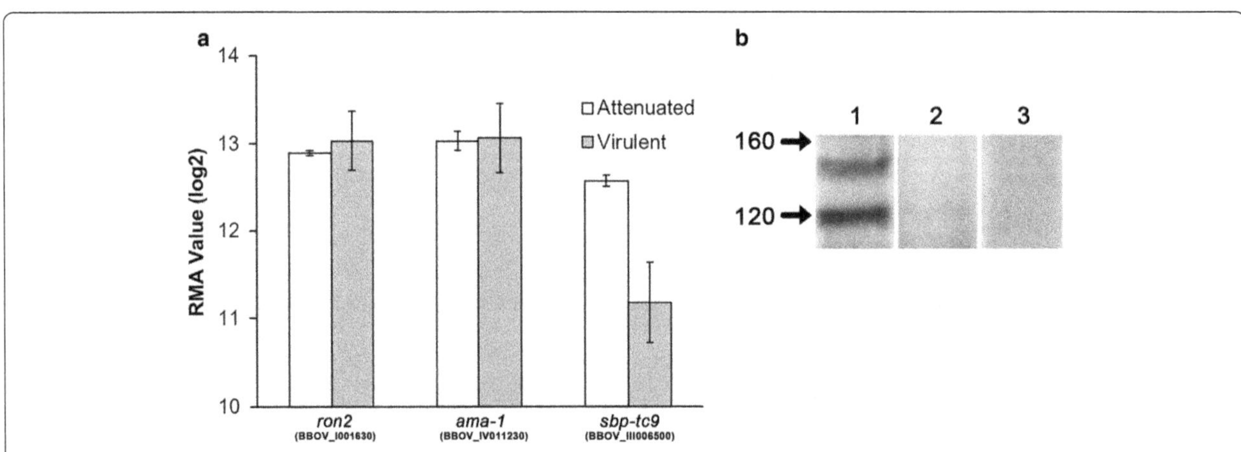

Fig. 2 Transcription and expression analysis of *B. bovis ron2*. **a** Bioinformatics transcription analysis. The results on the y-axis are shown by robust multi-array average (RMA) normalized values ($\log_2$). The comparison of the expression level of *ron2*, *ama-1* and *sbp-tc9* (spherical body protein 2 truncated copy 9) genes between attenuated (white) and virulent (gray) strains is shown on the x-axis. **b** WB expression analysis of RON2. Lane 1: proteins of *B. bovis* iRBC incubated with post-immunization sera anti-RON2; Lane 2: proteins of *B. bovis* iRBC incubated with pre-immunization sera anti-RON2; Lane 3: proteins of nRBC incubated with post-immunization sera anti-RON2. The molecular weight marker is shown in kDa

Additional file 4: Table S4). The four peptides have the capacity to elicit an immune response, confirming the *in silico* prediction of antigenicity and immunogenicity. The bovine anti-RON2 antisera reacted in western blots with antigens sized between 120 and 160 kDa, which are present only in the iRBC lysate (Fig. 2b, Lane 1). However, these antigens were not recognized by pre-immune sera (Fig. 2b, Lane 2), nor was their reactivity detected with nRBC lysates in immunoblots by anti RON2 antisera (Fig. 2b, Lane 3). The estimated molecular weight of *B. bovis* RON2 is ~150 kDa, which is consistent with the size of the antigen recognized by the anti RON2 peptide antisera. In addition, the immune serum against the selected RON2 peptides reacts with a 120 kDa band present in the sample containing the iRBC lysate (Fig. 2b, Lane 1). These results showed that the bovine anti-peptide antibodies were able to recognize the native *B. bovis* RON2 in immunoblots confirming the antigenicity of the predicted B-cell epitopes included in the synthetic peptides.

Recognition of *B. bovis* blood stages by anti-RON2 sera

We then analyzed the pattern of reaction of the bovine antibodies against the selected RON2 peptides with *B. bovis* blood stages by IFAT. All the post-immunization sera samples tested showed a very similar staining pattern, consisting of defined and strongly marked dots (Fig. 3a, c). This pattern of reactivity was comparable to the signals observed when smears of *B. bovis*-infected red blood cells were incubated with the serum of naturally infected cattle, employed as a positive control (Fig. 3e). This signal was not observed when *B. bovis*-infected red blood cells were incubated with the pre-immunization sera or with serum from cattle immunized only with adjuvant (Fig. 3b, d, f). Additionally, it was verified by confocal microscopy, that the observed signal corresponds to intraerythrocytic merozoites (see Additional file 5: Figure S1).

In vitro neutralization assay

We then tested the capacity of anti-RON2 antibodies to block merozoite invasion in an *in vitro* neutralization assay. The results, shown in Fig. 4, demonstrate a statistically significant difference in the percentage of parasitemia between the culture supplemented with the post-immunization serum and the culture supplemented with the pre-immunization serum only for P2 and P3 (P2: $t_{(4)}= 19.81$, $P < 0.0001$; P3: $t_{(4)}= 33.64$, $P < 0.0008$). In addition, combination of the anti-P2 and P3 anti-sera in the *in vitro* neutralization assay resulted in a significant ($t_{(4)}= -10.6$, $P < 0.0004$) increase of parasite inhibition (42.09%).

Neutralization-sensitive peptides are implicated in a natural immune response

We used an indirect ELISA to evaluate whether antibodies in 90 serum samples from cattle naturally infected with *B. bovis* developed antibodies against the neutralization-sensitive epitopes present in the selected RON2 peptides. The results are shown in Table 2: peptide 2 was recognized by 75 sera (83.33%), and peptide 3 was recognized by 79 sera (87.77%). Thus, both peptides were recognized by all positive controls and the 11 negative serum samples analyzed did not recognize any of the peptides evaluated.

Discussion

In the present study we demonstrated the conservation of a single copy gene encoding for RON2 in the *Babesia bovis* genome, which is highly conserved among four distinct strains isolated in Mexico and the reference strain T2Bo. The synteny of *ron2* between *B. bovis* and *B. bigemina*, as well as the high identity of this gene among all the compared species, suggest an implication of RON2 in a well conserved, likely essential, parasite function in the genus *Babesia*, which is also maintained in other related Apicomplexa parasites through the presence of the CLAG domain. Importantly, the implication of this domain in cytoadherence during the erythrocyte invasion process has been previously demonstrated in *P. falciparum* [14, 15]. Additionally, the transcription analysis showed a similar level of transcripts in both attenuated and virulent strains, implying that the levels of expression of this gene are not critical for the modulation of a virulent phenotype of *B. bovis*, as previously demonstrated for the *sbp2t-11* gene [16]. Furthermore, the transcription level of *ron2* was similar to that observed for *ama-1*, a gene involved in the same invasion step, as is described in other apicomplexan parasites [17]. Taking together, the data showing similarity between the level of expression of these proteins among virulent and attenuated strains may support the notion that the mechanism of invasion is highly conserved because it is required for the maintenance of the parasite inside the host. Moreover, similar levels of expression of the *ama-1* and *ron2* genes suggests a concerted function among these two proteins in *Babesia* parasites, as already described for *Plasmodium*. Since AMA-1 was also shown to be neutralization sensitive [11], this would support the evaluation of these two proteins in a single vaccine formulation. Specific bovine anti-RON2 antibodies were produced and used to detect RON2 in *B. bovis* protein extracts, showing a band of approximately 150 kDa in the western blot, which correlates with the expected molecular weight of the protein. Additionally, a band of a lower molecular weight was observed in the same protein extracts but was not present in the extracts

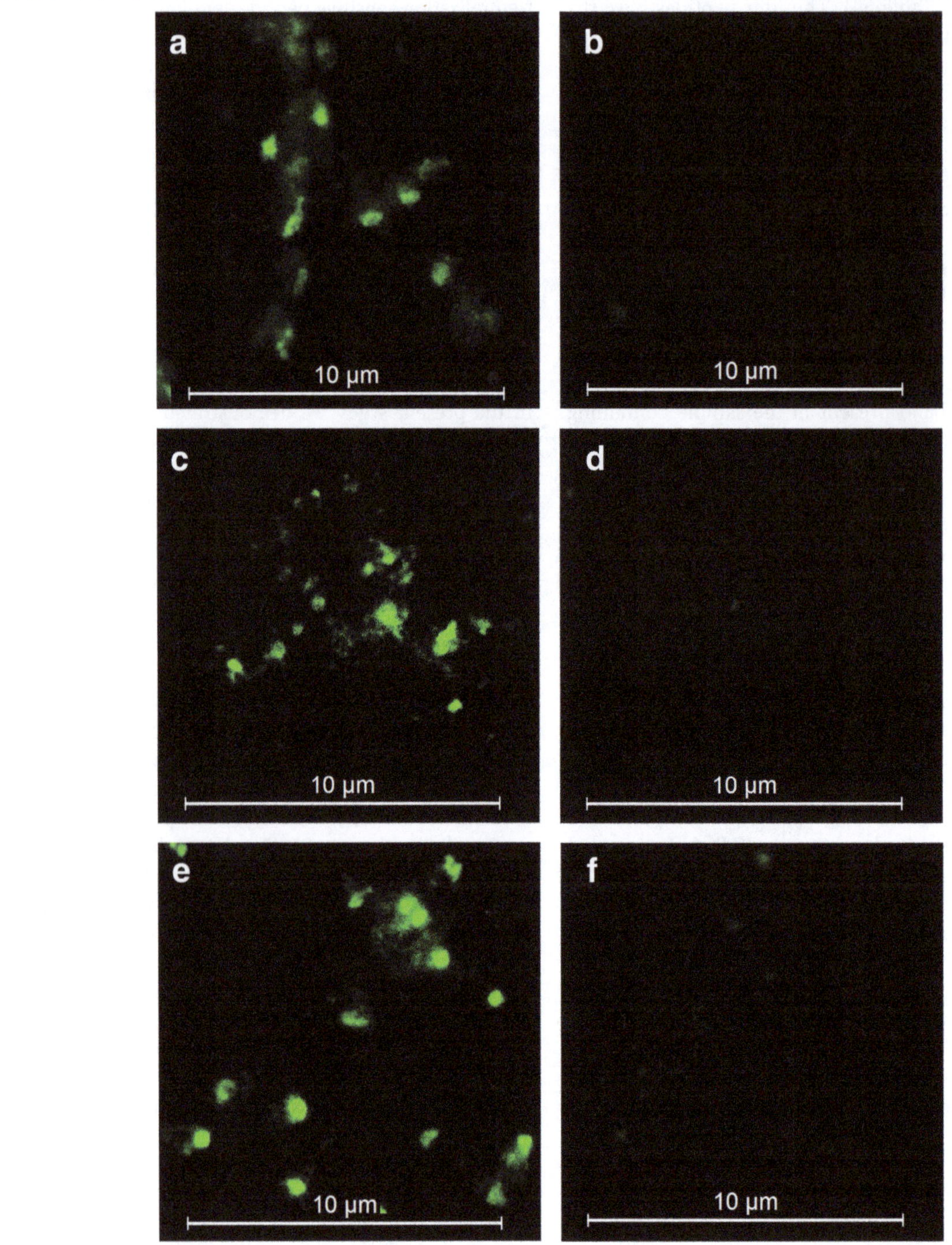

Fig. 3 Indirect immunofluorescence of *B. bovis* blood stages detected with antibodies against RON2. Smears of *B. bovis*-infected merozoites were incubated with bovine antiserum against P2 (**a**), P3 (**c**) or serum from naturally infected cattle (**e**). No signal was observed in the pre-immunization serum of cattle immunized with P2 (**b**), P3 (**d**) or cattle immunized only with adjuvant (**f**) used as the negative control. *Scale-bars*: 10 μm

of uninfected erythrocytes. Since the peptide used to generate the RON2 antibodies was analyzed by bioinformatics in the *B. bovis* genome and proved to be specific to RON2, the *in silico* analysis supports that this band is not another protein from the parasite, suggesting that this lower band could be generated due to a RON2 proteolysis process. This proteolysis event on RON2 has also been observed in other *Babesia* species [12].

Although peptide design remains a challenge due to paradoxically inconsistent results obtained with bioinformatics tools [18], in the present study we successfully designed four immunogenic peptides that generated antibodies in

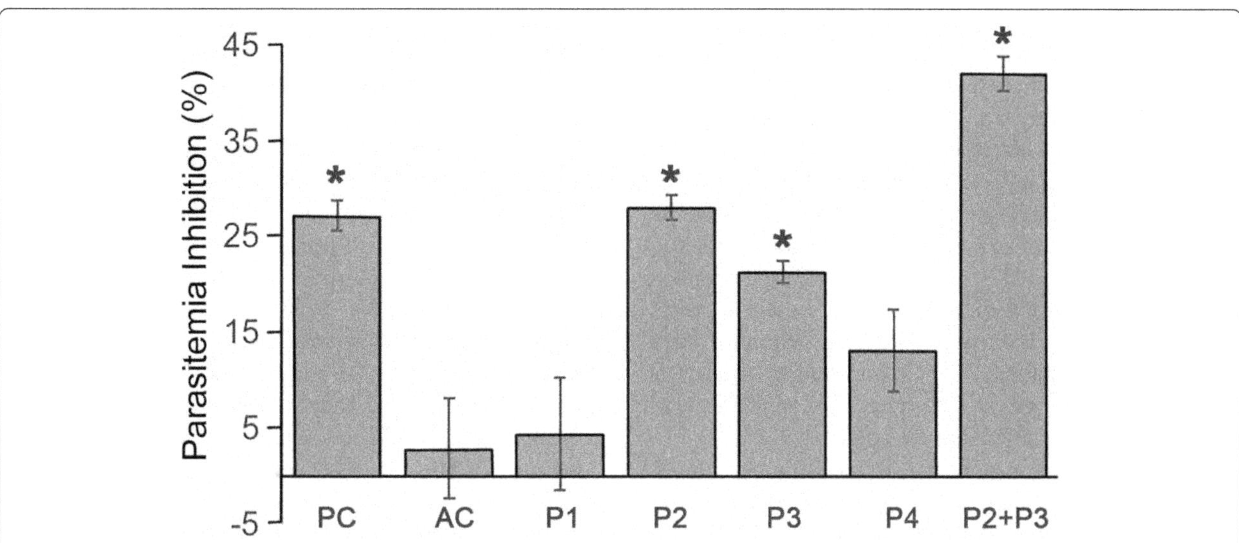

Fig. 4 Neutralization assay. The results on the y-axis are shown as percentages of the parasitemia inhibition. The evaluation of the inhibition generated by different antibodies is shown on the x-axis. *Abbreviations*: PC, positive control; AC, adjuvant control (PBS + ADJ); P1, anti-Peptide1 antibodies; P2, anti-Peptide2 antibodies; P3, anti-Peptide3 antibodies; P4, anti-Peptide4 antibodies; P2+P3, a mix of the anti-Peptide2 and anti-Peptide3 antibodies. There were significant differences between the pre- and post-immunization serum samples (*$P < 0.05$)

Table 2 RON2 peptides are recognized by sera of naturally infected cattle

State	Farm	Peptide 2			Peptide 3		
		Positive	Negative	Total	Positive	Negative	Total
Jalisco	A	6	1	12	6	1	12
	B	2	0		2	0	
	C	3	0		2	1	
Veracruz	A	20	3	36	18	5	36
	B	10	2		11	1	
	C	1	0		1	0	
Querétaro	A	1	1	12	2	0	12
	B	1	0		1	0	
	C	2	1		3	0	
	D	1	0		1	0	
	E	3	1		4	0	
	F	1	0		1	0	
Guanajuato	A	2	0	2	2	0	2
Chiapas	A	1	0	7	1	0	7
	B	6	0		5	1	
Chihuahua	A	1	2	16	3	0	16
	B	1	0		1	0	
	C	2	1		3	0	
	D	1	0		1	0	
	E	6	2		7	1	
Sinaloa	A	1	0	5	1	0	5
	B	0	1		1	0	
	C	3	0		2	1	
Total positive/negative		75	15		79	11	

Key: Positive, *B. bovis* positive serum samples that recognized the peptide; Negative, *B. bovis* positive serum samples that did not recognize the peptide

immunized bovines and that were able to recognize blood stage parasites. The anti-RON2 antibodies were also able to identify the native protein expressed in blood stage parasites demonstrated by IFAT and confocal microscopy. This is significant as the selected B-cell epitopes used for the generation of these antibodies were predicted on the linear sequence of RON2, suggesting that this part of the sequence is accessible to antibodies in the native protein. It has been demonstrated that RON2 localizes specifically to the neck region of the rhoptries, which possess a protein repertoire conserved across the phylum and involved in tight-junction formation [17]. Co-localization or electron microscopy studies are necessary to determine the exact subcellular location of RON2 in *B. bovis*.

Interestingly, only antibodies produced by peptides P2 and P3 were able to block the invasion process, as observed in the *in vitro* neutralization assays. A higher inhibition of parasitemia was observed when antibodies anti-P2 and anti-P3 were used together, suggesting a synergic effect. This type of synergy can be used to improve the inhibition effect, for example by mixing antibodies against other proteins, but it also demonstrates that the antibodies can act independently in their inhibitory activity, and no allosteric inhibitory effects are present. In *Plasmodium yoelii*, for example, it was described that a mix of antibodies against a complex of AMA-1 and RON2L completely inhibited the invasion process through the disruption of the specific interaction between these two peptides, and this complex elicited protective immunity in *Aotus* monkeys against a virulent strain of *P. falciparum* [19, 20]. RON2L is a peptide located between the second and third predicted transmembrane region in *P. falciparum* RON2. This location is the same for the P3 designed in this study, highlighting the importance of this peptide as a blocking vaccine candidate. These data demonstrate that targeting epitopes in RON2 with specific antibodies significantly impairs the ability of the parasite to invade erythrocytes. Importantly, the effect is additive, suggesting that the epitopes recognized at least by antibodies reactive with two predicted B-cell epitopes work independently and are accessible to interact with the antigen. The data is also strongly suggestive of a possible role of RON2 in erythrocyte invasion.

Finally, we demonstrated that RON2 generates antibodies in cattle naturally infected with *B. bovis*. These findings indicate that the predicted B-cell epitopes contained in the peptides have a role in the humoral immune response under natural conditions and that these B-cell epitopes are conserved among strains from different geographical locations, which have been reported to have high antigenic variation [21, 22], demonstrating that the selected neutralization-sensitive RON2 peptides are implicated in immune responses in bovines naturally infected with *B. bovis*. Another important implication emerging from these results is that the antibodies against RON2 epitopes may help the chronically infected animals to prevent emergence of clinical signs on the face of parasite persistence, suggesting a direct role of RON2 in the development of protective immunity, and supporting the use of this antigen as a potential vaccine candidate. Although we presented evidence of the conservation of RON2 in different Mexican strains of *B. bovis* and showed the biological effect of conserved anti-RON2 antibodies against a USA strain (T3Bo), and the identity between the amino acid sequences is very high (99.78%), the fact that 15 sera for peptide 2 and 11 sera for peptide 3 did not recognize the respective peptides (out of 90 in total), suggests that some degree of variation may occur between strains. It is, therefore, necessary to evaluate a worldwide conservation of RON2 by obtaining sequences or testing sera samples from other countries. The fact that antibodies against two RON2 peptides were unable to completely block the parasite growth *in vitro*, suggests that antibodies against peptides from additional antigens are necessary for vaccine development against this pathogen.

Conclusions

In summary, *ron2* is a functional gene in *B. bovis* that codes for a protein with a characteristic CLAG domain. RON2 has highly conserved B-cell epitopes that elicit neutralizing antibodies in bovines and are recognized by protective antibodies in naturally infected cattle. All these data together emphasize the importance of RON2 as a vaccine candidate to prevent bovine babesiosis.

Methods

Babesia bovis DNA extraction from field isolates

Rhipicephalus (*Boophilus*) *microplus* ticks were manually collected from bovines from four different states in Mexico: Chiapas, Colima, Nayarit and Veracruz. They were individually incubated for oviposition and then tested for *Babesia* spp. infection by microscopic examination of hemolymph for kinete detection [23]. DNA was purified from the infected ticks [24] and was used for specific nPCR-diagnosis of *B. bovis* [25]. Larvae from ticks infected only with *B. bovis* were used to infest one splenectomized calf for each isolate. Additionally, each calf was treated with an acaricide five days after infestation to avoid transmission of *B. bigemina* by infected nymphs and the parasitemia was monitored daily by examination of blood smears stained with Giemsa. When the parasitemia exceeded 1%, infected blood from the jugular vein was collected in transfusion bags with ACD anticoagulant solution (375 Blorecep, Industrias Plasticas Medicas, Ayala, Morelos, Mexico). Genomic DNA was extracted using the illustra blood genomicPrep

Mini Spin kit (GE Healthcare, Piscataway, NJ, USA) and was stored at -20 °C.

Identification and sequencing of *ron2* in *Babesia bovis*

The *B. bigemina ron2* nucleotide (KU696964.1) and amino acid (AQU42588.1) sequences were used as a query in a BLAST search of the SANGER institute database [26] against the *B. bovis* T2Bo reference genome. The synteny of the chromosomal region of the *ron2* gene was determined and compared between *B. bovis* and *B. bigemina* through PiroplasmaDB at the EuPathDB portal [27, 28]. Eight pairs of primers (see Table 1) were designed based on the *B. bovis* T2Bo *ron2* gene using Oligoanalyzer 3.1 [29]. These primers were designed to amplify the whole *ron2* sequence using a common PCR protocol: an initial denaturation at 94 °C for 4 min, followed by 30 cycles of denaturation at 94 °C for 30 s, annealing at 56 °C for 45 s, and extension at 72 °C for 45 s, followed by a final extension at 72 °C for 7 min. DNA from four field isolates of *B. bovis*, each from a different state in Mexico (Chiapas, Colima, Nayarit and Veracruz), were used for the amplification and sequencing of 4169 bp of the *B. bovis ron2* gene. All of the amplifications were cloned into a pCR™ 4-TOPO® vector using a TOPO® TA Cloning® kit (Invitrogen, Carlsbad, CA, USA), and *E. coli* strain TOP10 cells were transformed with the vector following the manufacturer's instructions (Invitrogen). For each amplification, two positive colonies determined by PCR were selected to be sequenced with the dideoxy chain-termination method by the Biotechnology Institute of Universidad Nacional Autonoma de Mexico (UNAM, Cuernavaca, Mexico). The assembly and obtaining of consensus sequences was undertaken using BioEdit 7.2.6 and CLC Genomics Workbench 7.5.

The sequences obtained were compared against *B. bigemina* (AQU42588.1), *Babesia* sp. Xinjiang (ORM40446.1), *B. divergens* (ADM34975.2), *B. microti* strain RI (XP_021338832.1), *Theileria equi* (XP_004830272.1) and *P. falciparum* (BAH22613.1). The *B. bovis* sequences were analyzed with bioinformatics programs to: (i) identify open reading frames using the ORF finder program [30]; (ii) determine the signal peptide with the programs SignalP 4.0 [31] and SMART [32]; (iii) find conserved domains and their localization with SMART [32]; (iv) assess the presence of transmembrane helices using the TMHMM program [33]; and (v) determine the isoelectric point and the molecular weight using CLC Genomics Workbench 7.5.

In silico transcription analysis

RMA values from transcriptomic analyses of biological replicate (BR) sample pairs were obtained from previously published data deposited in PiroplasmaDB in the EuPathDB portal [27]. The transcription of the *ron2* gene (BBOV_I001630) was evaluated among the attenuated and virulent strains, and the level of transcription of the *ama-1* gene (BBOV_IV011230) was also evaluated. These results were validated with the transcript expression level of the *spherical body protein 2 truncated copy 9* gene (*sbp2-tc9*, BBOV_III006500). This analysis was performed in the PiroplasmaDB portal [13, 27].

Expression analysis

To produce anti-RON2 antibodies, a conserved region among all the isolates was analyzed to find predicted linear B-cell epitopes using different programs: ABCpred [34], BCEpred [35] and antibody epitope prediction IEDB-AR [36]. The conserved regions were located with multiple sequence alignments using Clustal Omega [37]. The peptide was synthesized in a Multiple Antigen Peptide System of 8 branches (MAPS-8) by GL Biochem (Shanghai, China). The synthetic peptide (see Additional file 4: Table S4) was solubilized in PBS (pH 7.4) and emulsified v/v with the adjuvant Montanide ISA 71vg (Seppic, Puteaux, Paris, France) at a final concentration of 100 μg/ml. Finally, two cattle born in a tick-free area and free of antibodies against *B. bovis* and *B. bigemina* by IFAT were immunized four times at 21-day intervals with the peptide/adjuvant emulsions described above. Additionally, two control cattle were immunized just with the same adjuvant emulsified with PBS (1:1) under identical conditions. The immunizations were performed *via* subcutaneous injection in the scapular region with 1 ml of the corresponding emulsion mixes in each bovine. Sera samples were collected from each animal before the first immunization and 15 days after the last immunization.

The bovine sera containing specific anti-RON2 antibodies and control sera were diluted at 1:20 with PBS containing non-infected erythrocyte (nRBC) lysate and 5% skim milk to evaluate the expression of RON2 in a western blot analysis (WB). Briefly, *Babesia bovis*-infected erythrocytes (iRBC) were obtained from an *in vitro* culture with 42% parasitemia; lysates were prepared by washing the cells several times with ice-cold PBS containing protease inhibitor (Roche-Applied Science, Penzberg, Upper Bavaria, Germany) until the supernatant was clear. Then, the pellet was frozen at -80 °C, thawed on ice and washed again three times. All the centrifugations between washes were performed at 2500× *g* for 10 min. After washes, the parasite pellet was suspended in 2× lysis buffer v/v (100 mM Tris, 10 mM EDTA, 2% NP-40) containing protease inhibitor (Roche-Applied Science). The suspended pellet was kept at -80 °C until used. Finally, when the pellet was thawed, it was maintained on ice; the loading buffer was then added and the sample sonicated and then centrifuged briefly. The supernatant was used in an SDS-PAGE (4–20%) and was run at 100 V for 1 h employing Mini-PROTEAN TGX precast gels (Bio-Rad Laboratories, Richmond, CA, USA). The proteins were transferred to a nitrocellulose membrane at 100 V, for 1 h. The membrane was blocked overnight at 4 °C with PBS containing 5% skim milk (PBS-M). The membrane was incubated for 1 h at room temperature with each diluted antiserum and washed five times with agitation at room temperature in PBS and 0.1% Tween (PBS-T). The membrane was incubated under the same conditions employing a donkey anti-bovine IgG antibody conjugated with HRP (Jackson ImmunoResearch, West Grove, PA, USA), diluted at 1:500 in TBS-T (0.1%), and followed by a final wash. Finally, the reaction was visualized with LumiFlash Prime Chemiluminescent Spray (Visual Protein, Taiwan, China).

Generation of anti-RON2 antibodies

Four peptides (see Additional file 4: Table S4) were designed and each peptide was emulsified and immunized into two bovines using the methodology described above. Pre- and post-immunization sera samples were collected and analyzed for the presence of antibodies against the specific RON2 peptide by an indirect ELISA test as it was described elsewhere [38]. Briefly, each serum sample was added at a dilution of 1:3000 in PBS, and the secondary antibody, a donkey anti-bovine IgG antibody conjugated with HRP (Jackson ImmunoResearch), was added at 100 µl/well, diluted 1:500 in PBS. The reaction was detected in an iMark™ Microplate Absorbance Reader (Bio-Rad Laboratories) at 450 nm and analyzed with Microplate Manager 6 software (Bio-Rad Laboratories). All samples were tested in triplicate, and the cut-off values were determined as the average of the pre-immunization OD value for each bovine plus 3 standard deviations.

Parasite recognition by anti-RON2 antibodies using an indirect immunofluorescence antibody test (IFAT)

To determine if the anti-RON2 antibodies against each peptide recognize the native protein in the parasite, an indirect immunofluorescence antibody test (IFAT) was performed [39]. Smears of bovine blood infected with *B. bovis* (Chiapas isolate) were permeated at 4 °C for 15 min with acetone (90%) diluted in ethanol. The bovine RON2 antisera were tested at a dilution of 1:100 and detected with Alexa Fluor-488 conjugated with Protein G (Molecular Probes®, Eugene, OR, USA). All the incubations were performed at 37 °C in a humidity chamber for 1 h. Between each incubation, three washes were performed in PBS-T (0.1% Tween20); each wash was done for 5 min with agitation, with the final step in distilled water as described elsewhere [39]. Serum from a bovine naturally infected with *B. bovis* was used as a positive control, and the serum of a bovine immunized with PBS and adjuvant was used as a negative control.

Neutralization assay

To determine if the invasion process could be blocked by the anti-RON2 antibodies, a neutralization assay (NA) was carried out as previously described [40, 41], using an *in vitro* culture of *B. bovis*. The *B. bovis* T3Bo strain (provided by the ADRU-USDA lab at Washington State University) was cultured in a 96-well plate using 200 µl per well with 5% hematocrit. First, an incubation step was done in an atmosphere of 5% CO_2 for 30 min at 37 °C with a mix containing 60% HL-1 medium (pH 7.2), 40% sera and 1% iRBC with 1% parasitemia. Then, culture medium with 4% nRBC was added and, after a gentle mix, 200 µl of sample was split into three wells. The culture was maintained at 37 °C in a 5% CO_2 atmosphere for 72 h with changes of media (120 µl media plus 30 µl sera) every 24 h. Serum from a non-infected steer (c1537) born in a tick-free area was used as a negative control (NC) and the serum from a steer (C168) inoculated with *B. bovis* T2Bo and challenged with *B. bovis* T3Bo was used as positive control (PC). As a control for the effect of the adjuvant (AC), pre- and post-immunization serum from a heifer immunized only with PBS plus adjuvant was used. At the end of the incubation, the percentage of parasitized erythrocytes (PPE) was determined by flow cytometry [42]. For statistical analysis, an independent Student's t-test was used, where *P*-values < 0.05 were considered significant. The percentages of parasitemia inhibition (% pi) for the anti-RON2 antibodies and the AC were calculated with the following formula: % pi = 100 – ([(PPE Post) / (PPE Pre)] × 100). The formula for the PC was: % pi = 100 – ([(PPE PC) / (PPE NC)] × 100).

Babesia bovis RON2 recognition by naturally infected bovines

A total of 112 bovine serum samples were tested against peptides P2 and P3 using the indirect ELISA protocol described above: all of the 90 serum samples collected from cattle living in regions of Mexico where babesiosis is endemic were positive to *B. bovis* infection as determined by IFAT; 11 bovine serum samples previously confirmed positive to *B. bovis* antibodies, were used as positive controls. Eleven serum samples were from cattle born and maintained in a tick-free area and they were used as negative controls. All serum samples were tested in triplicate at a 1:50 dilution in PBS and incubated for 1 h at 37 °C. As a secondary antibody, a goat anti-bovine IgG (H+L) conjugated with HRP (Jackson ImmunoResearch) was used at a 1:1500 dilution in PBS. The ELISA plates were incubated for 1 h at 37 °C. The cut-off value was determined by adding the average of the negative control OD values plus 3 standard deviations.

Additional files

Additional file 1: Table S1. Percent nucleotide identity matrix. Comparison of the *ron2* nucleotide sequences obtained. (XLSX 9 kb)

Additional file 2: Table S2. Percent amino acid identity matrix. Comparison of the RON2 amino acid sequences obtained. (XLSX 9 kb)

Additional file 3: Table S3. RON2 physicochemical features. (XLSX 10 kb)

Additional file 4: Table S4. Peptides designed in conserved regions with predicted B-cell epitopes. Sequence of the peptides designed, length and position in the RON2 amino acid sequence. (XLSX 9 kb)

Additional file 5: Figure S1. Intraerythrocytic *Babesia bovis* merozoites express RON2. Merozoites were incubated with bovine antiserum against RON2 (**a-c**), bovine pre-immune serum (**d-f**), or bovine antiserum against *B. bovis* (**g-i**), then with an Alexa Fluor-488 conjugated with protein G (green fluorescence) and DAPI for DNA staining (blue fluorescence). The smears were analyzed by confocal microscopy using the following channels: individual channel for Alexa Fluor-488 (**a**, **d** and **g**), individual channel for DAPI (**b**, **e** and **h**) or merged channels for Alexa Fluor-488 and DAPI (**c**, **f** and **i**). *Scale-bars*: 10 μm. (TIF 17380 kb)

Abbreviations

nRBC: non-infected erythrocyte; iRBC: *Babesia bovis*-infected erythrocytes; NC: Negative control; PC: Positive control; AC: Adjuvant control; PPE: Percentage of parasitized erythrocytes; % pi: Percentages of parasitemia inhibition

Acknowledgements

We greatly appreciate the technical support provided by Paul Lacy and Jacob Laughery. Martín Andrés López Padilla provided the necessary facilities to work with the cattle.

Funding

Mario Hidalgo-Ruiz and Miguel Angel Mercado Uriostegui received a fellowship from CONACyT-Mexico. The research was funded by FOPER-UAQ, PRODEP-REDES and CONACyT-Ciencia Basica (167129).

Authors' contributions

MHR wrote the manuscript, identified *ron2* by bioinformatics, designed primers, cloned and sequence the Chiapas strain of *ron2*, generated antibodies, and performed the WB, IFAT and neutralization assays. CS contributed reagents and materials and helped design and interpret neutralization assays and the Western blot. MAMU contributed to the indirect ELISA analysis. JAR and RHO obtained the field serum samples and performed the IFAT test. EG obtained the Colima *B. bovis* strain. GLA and JMH helped with confocal microscopy. JM conceived and supervised the project and edited the manuscript. All authors read and approved the final manuscript.

Competing interests

The authors declare that they have no competing interests

Author details

[1]Immunology and Vaccines Laboratory, C. A. Facultad de Ciencias Naturales, Universidad Autónoma de Querétaro, Carretera a Chichimequillas, Ejido Bolaños, 76140 Queretaro, Queretaro, Mexico. [2]Animal Disease Research Unit, USDA-ARS, 3003 ADBF, WSU, P. O. Box 647030, Pullman, WA 99164-6630, USA. [3]CENID-Parasitologia Veterinaria / INIFAP, Carretera federal Cuernavaca-Cuautla #8534, Col. Progreso, 62550 Jiutepec, Morelos, Mexico. [4]Facultad de Medicina Veterinaria y Zootecnia, Universidad de Colima, Km. 40 carretera Colima-Manzanillo, 28100 Tecoman, Colima, Mexico. [5]Departamento de Zoología, Escuela Nacional de Ciencias Biológicas, Instituto Politécnico Nacional, Carpio y Plan de Ayala, Col. Casco de Santo Tomás, 11340 Mexico City, Mexico. [6]Departamento de Biología Celular, Centro de Investigación y Estudios Avanzados del Instituto Politécnico Nacional, Av. IPN 2508, Col. San Pedro Zacatenco, 07360 Mexico City, Mexico.

References

1. Bock R, Jackson L, De Vos A, Jorgensen W. Babesiosis of cattle. Parasitology. 2004;129:S247–69.
2. Schnittger L, Rodriguez AE, Florin-Christensen M, Morrison DA. *Babesia*: a world emerging. Infect Genet Evol. 2012;12:1788–809.
3. Yabsley MJ, Shock BC. Natural history of zoonotic *Babesia*: role of wildlife reservoirs. Int J Parasitol Parasites Wildl. 2013;2:18–31.
4. Dubremetz JF, Garcia-Réguet N, Conseil V, Fourmaux MN. Apical organelles and host-cell invasion by *Apicomplexa*. Int J Parasitol. 1998;28:1007–13.
5. Soldati D, Dubremetz JF, Lebrun M. Microneme proteins: structural and functional requirements to promote adhesion and invasion by the apicomplexan parasite *Toxoplasma gondii*. Int J Parasitol. 2001;31:1293–302.
6. Yokoyama N, Okamura M, Igarashi I. Erythrocyte invasion by *Babesia* parasites: current advances in the elucidation of the molecular interactions between the protozoan ligands and host receptors in the invasion stage. Vet Parasitol. 2006;138:22–32.
7. Alexander DL, Mital J, Ward GE, Bradley P, Boothroyd JC. Identification of the moving junction complex of *Toxoplasma gondii*: a collaboration between distinct secretory organelles. PLoS Pathog. 2005;1:e17.
8. Besteiro S, Dubremetz J-F, Lebrun M. The moving junction of apicomplexan parasites: a key structure for invasion. Cell Microbiol. 2011;13:797–805.
9. Shen B, Sibley LD. The moving junction, a key portal to host cell invasion by apicomplexan parasites. Curr Opin Microbiol. 2012;15:449–55.
10. Srinivasan P, Yasgar A, Luci DK, Beatty WL, Hu X, Andersen J, et al. Disrupting malaria parasite AMA1-RON2 interaction with a small molecule prevents erythrocyte invasion. Nat Commun. 2013;4:2261.
11. Gaffar FR, Yatsuda AP, Franssen FFJ, de Vries E. Erythrocyte invasion by *Babesia bovis* merozoites is inhibited by polyclonal antisera directed against peptides derived from a homologue of *Plasmodium falciparum* apical membrane antigen 1. Infect Immun. 2004;72:2947–55.
12. Ord RL, Rodriguez M, Cursino-Santos JR, Hong H, Singh M, Gray J, et al. Identification and characterization of the Rhoptry Neck Protein 2 in *Babesia divergens* and *B. microti*. Infect Immun. 2016;84:1574–84.
13. Pedroni MJ, Sondgeroth KS, Gallego-Lopez GM, Echaide I, Lau AO. Comparative transcriptome analysis of geographically distinct virulent and attenuated *Babesia bovis* strains reveals similar gene expression changes through attenuation. BMC Genomics. 2013;14:763.
14. Cao J, Kaneko O, Thongkukiatkul A, Tachibana M, Otsuki H, Gao Q, et al. Rhoptry neck protein RON2 forms a complex with microneme protein AMA1 in *Plasmodium falciparum* merozoites. Parasitol Int. 2009;58:29–35.
15. Holt DC, Gardiner DL, Thomas EA, Mayo M, Bourke PF, Sutherland CJ, et al. The cytoadherence linked asexual gene family of *Plasmodium falciparum*: are there roles other than cytoadherence? Int J Parasitol. 1999;29:939–44.
16. Gallego-Lopez GM, Lau AOT, Brown WC, Johnson WC, Ueti MW, Suarez CE. Spherical Body Protein 2 truncated copy 11 as a specific *Babesia bovis* attenuation marker. Parasit Vectors. 2018;11:169.
17. Proellocks NI, Coppel RL, Waller KL. Dissecting the apicomplexan rhoptry neck proteins. Trends Parasitol. 2010;26:297–304.
18. Flower DR. Towards *in silico* prediction of immunogenic epitopes. Trends Immunol. 2003;24:667–74.
19. Srinivasan P, Baldeviano GC, Miura K, Diouf A, Ventocilla JA, Leiva KP, et al. A malaria vaccine protects *Aotus monkeys* against virulent *Plasmodium falciparum* infection. NPJ Vaccines. 2017;2:14.

20. Srinivasan P, Ekanem E, Diouf A, Tonkin ML, Miura K, Boulanger MJ, et al. Immunization with a functional protein complex required for erythrocyte invasion protects against lethal malaria. Proc Natl Acad Sci USA. 2014;111: 10311–6.
21. Borgonio V, Mosqueda J, Genis AD, Falcon A, Alvarez JA, Camacho M, et al. msa-1 and msa-2c gene analysis and common epitopes assessment in Mexican *Babesia bovis* isolates. Ann N Y Acad Sci. 2008;1149:145–8.
22. Genis AD, Mosqueda JJ, Borgonio VM, Falcón A, Alvarez A, Camacho M, et al. Phylogenetic analysis of Mexican *Babesia bovis* isolates using msa and ssrRNA gene sequences. Ann N Y Acad Sci. 2008;1149:121–5.
23. Riek R. The life cycle of *Babesia bigemina* (Smith and Kilborne, 1893) in the tick vector *Boophilus microplus* (Canestrini). Aust J Agric Res. 1964;15:802–21.
24. Mosqueda J. Extracción de ADN de hemoparásitos. In: Bautista-Garfias CR, editor. Diagnóstico de enfermedades parasitarias selectas de rumiantes. Mexico City, Mexico: INIFAP; 2010. p. 178–91.
25. Figueroa JV, Chieves LP, Johnson GS, Buening GM. Multiplex polymerase chain reaction based assay for the detection of *Babesia bigemina*, *Babesia bovis* and *Anaplasma marginale* DNA in bovine blood. Vet Parasitol. 1993;50:69–81.
26. Altschul SF, Gish W, Miller W, Myers EW, Lipman DJ. Basic local alignment search tool. J Mol Biol. 1990;215:403–10.
27. Aurrecoechea C, Brestelli J, Brunk BP, Fischer S, Gajria B, Gao X, et al. EuPathDB: a portal to eukaryotic pathogen databases. Nucleic Acids Res. 2010;38:D415–9.
28. Chen F, Mackey AJ, Stoeckert CJ, Roos DS. OrthoMCL-DB: querying a comprehensive multi-species collection of ortholog groups. Nucleic Acids Res. 2006;34:D363–8.
29. Owczarzy R, Tataurov AV, Wu Y, Manthey JA, McQuisten KA, Almabrazi HG, et al. IDT SciTools: a suite for analysis and design of nucleic acid oligomers. Nucleic Acids Res. 2008;36:W163–9.
30. Rombel IT, Sykes KF, Rayner S, Johnston SA. ORF-FINDER: a vector for high-throughput gene identification. Gene. 2002;282:33–41.
31. Petersen TN, Brunak S, von Heijne G, Nielsen H. SignalP 4.0: discriminating signal peptides from transmembrane regions. Nat Methods. 2011;8:785–6.
32. Schultz J, Milpetz F, Bork P, Ponting CP. SMART, a simple modular architecture research tool: identification of signaling domains. Proc Natl Acad Sci USA. 1998;95:5857–64.
33. Krogh A, Larsson B, von Heijne G, Sonnhammer ELL. Predicting transmembrane protein topology with a hidden markov model: application to complete genomes. J Mol Biol. 2001;305:567–80.
34. Saha S, Raghava GPS. Prediction of continuous B-cell epitopes in an antigen using recurrent neural network. Proteins. 2006;65:40–8.
35. Saha S, BcePred RGPS. Prediction of continuous B-cell epitopes in antigenic sequences using physico-chemical properties. In: Nicosia G, Cutello V, Bentley PJ, Timmis J, editors. Artificial Immune Systems. Berlin-Heidelberg: Springer; 2004. p. 197–204.
36. Zhang Q, Wang P, Kim Y, Haste-Andersen P, Beaver J, Bourne PE, et al. Immune epitope database analysis resource (IEDB-AR). Nucleic Acids Res. 2008;36:W513–8.
37. Sievers F, Wilm A, Dineen D, Gibson TJ, Karplus K, Li W, Lopez R, McWilliam H, Remmert M, Söding J, Thompson JD, Higgins DG. Fast, scalable generation of high-quality protein multiple sequence alignments using Clustal Omega. Mol Syst Biol. 2011;7:539.
38. Hernández-Silva DJ, Valdez-Espinoza UM, Mercado-Uriostegui MA, Aguilar-Tipacamú G, Ramos-Aragón JA, Hernández-Ortiz R, et al. Immunomolecular characterization of MIC-1, a novel antigen in *Babesia bigemina*, which contains conserved and immunodominant B-cell epitopes that induce neutralizing antibodies. Vet Sci. 2018;5:32.
39. OIE - World Organization for Animal Health. Manual of diagnostic test and vaccines for terrestrial animals. 2018. http://www.oie.int/en/standard-setting/terrestrial-manual/access-online/. Accessed 30 Aug 2018.
40. Hines SA, Palmer GH, Jasmer DP, Goff WL, McElwain TF. Immunization of cattle with recombinant *Babesia bovis* merozoite surface antigen-1. Infect Immun. 1995;63:349–52.
41. Suarez CE, Florin-Christensen M, Hines SA, Palmer GH, Brown WC, McElwain TF. Characterization of allelic variation in the *Babesia bovis* merozoite surface antigen 1 (MSA-1) locus and identification of a cross-reactive inhibition-sensitive MSA-1 epitope. Infect Immun. 2000;68:6865–70.
42. Wyatt CR, Goff W, Davis WC. A flow cytometric method for assessing viability of intraerythrocytic hemoparasites. J Immunol Methods. 1991;140:23–30.

10

Impact of indoor residual spraying on malaria parasitaemia in the Bunkpurugu-Yunyoo District in northern Ghana

Benjamin Abuaku[1*], Collins Ahorlu[1], Paul Psychas[2], Philip Ricks[3], Samuel Oppong[4], Sedzro Mensah[1], William Sackey[1] and Kwadwo A Koram[1]

Abstract

Background: Since 2008 indoor residual spraying (IRS) has become one of the interventions for malaria control in Ghana. Key partners in the scale-up of IRS have been the US President's Malaria Initiative (PMI) and AngloGold Ashanti (AGA). This study was designed to assess the impact of IRS on malaria parasitaemia among children less than 5 years-old in Bunkpurugu-Yunyoo, one of PMI-sponsored districts in northern Ghana, where rates of parasitaemia significantly exceeded the national average.

Methods: Two pre-IRS cross-sectional surveys using microscopy were conducted in November 2010 and April 2011 to provide baseline estimates of malaria parasitaemia for the high and low transmission seasons, respectively. IRS for the entire district was conducted in May/June to coincide with the beginning of the rains. Alpha-cypermethrin was used in 2011 and 2012, and changed to pirimiphos-methyl in 2013 and 2014 following declining susceptibility of local vectors to pyrethroids. Post-IRS cross-sectional surveys were conducted between 2011 and 2014 to provide estimates for the end of high (2011–2014) and the end of low (2012–2013) transmission seasons.

Results: The end of high transmission season prevalence of asexual parasitaemia declined marginally from 52.4% (95% CI: 50.0–54.7%) to 47.7% (95% CI: 45.5–49.9%) following 2 years of IRS with alpha-cypermethrin. Prevalence declined substantially to 20.6% (95% CI: 18.4–22.9%) following one year of IRS with pirimiphos-methyl.

Conclusions: The use of a more efficacious insecticide for IRS can reduce malaria parasitaemia among children less than 5 years-old in northern Ghana.

Keywords: Indoor residual spraying, Malaria parasitaemia, Northern Ghana

Background

Indoor residual spraying (IRS) remains one of the two main vector control interventions for malaria prevention, along with long-lasting insecticidal nets (LLINs). Several studies in sub-Saharan Africa and Asia have shown that IRS is associated with reduced malaria transmission in young children and protects all age groups, particularly in combination with LLINs and other control interventions, such as artemisinin-based combination therapy (ACT) and intermittent preventive treatment of pregnant women (IPTp) [1–12]. Following a scale-up of IRS in Africa, it is estimated that the number of Africans protected by IRS increased from 10 million in 2005 to 124 million in 2013 [2]. However, the proportion of the population at risk protected by IRS declined from 10.5% in 2010 to 5.7% in 2015 following a decline in funding between 2013 and 2015 [13].

In 2008, the Ghana National Strategic Plan for malaria control included a scale-up of IRS to cover at least a third of districts in the country by 2015 [14]. Key partners in the scale-up exercise were the US President's Malaria Initiative (PMI) and AngloGold Ashanti (AGA) [14]. The US PMI's IRS program focused on selected districts in the northern savannah zone whilst AGA's program focused on selected districts in the northern

* Correspondence: babuaku@noguchi.ug.edu.gh
[1]Epidemiology Department, Noguchi Memorial Institute for Medical Research, College of Health Sciences, University of Ghana, Legon, P. O. Box LG581, Legon, Ghana
Full list of author information is available at the end of the article

savannah zone as well as the forest zone of the country. To monitor the effectiveness of IRS within PMI catchment districts, a study was designed in 2010 to assess the impact of IRS on malaria parasitaemia in one district in the northern savannah zone, which was about to receive IRS in 2011. Data from that study are presented in this paper.

Methods

Study site

The study was conducted in the Bunkpurugu-Yunyoo District (10.4846°N, 0.1121°W) located in the northern region of Ghana, where malaria transmission markedly peaks with seasonal rains lasting 3–4 months (August to November) [15]. The district lies within the northern savannah zone with mean annual rainfall of 100–115 mm, and has an estimated population of 122,591, 50.9% of which being female. The district, which is bounded to the east by Togo, west by the East Mamprusi District of Ghana, north by the Garu-Tempane District of Ghana and south by the Gushegu and Chereponi districts of Ghana, is made up of 5 sub-districts: Nasuan, Binde, Nakpanduri, Bunkpurgu and Yunyoo (Fig. 1) [16, 17]. As many as 94.1% of households in the district are engaged in agriculture [16].

The district benefitted from two mass LLIN campaigns implemented by the Ghana Health Service in May 2010 and August 2012. The district was sprayed in 2011 and 2012 using alpha-cypermethrin (0.4% WP) at a rate of 25 mg/m^2. The declining susceptibility of local vectors [predominantly *Anopheles gambiae* (*s.l.*)] to pyrethroids necessitated the switch of insecticide to pirimiphos-methyl (an organophosophate) at an application rate of 1 g/m^2 in 2013 and 2014. Generally, IRS operations in the district were conducted in May/June to coincide with the beginning of the rains. In November 2011 and 2012 two of the

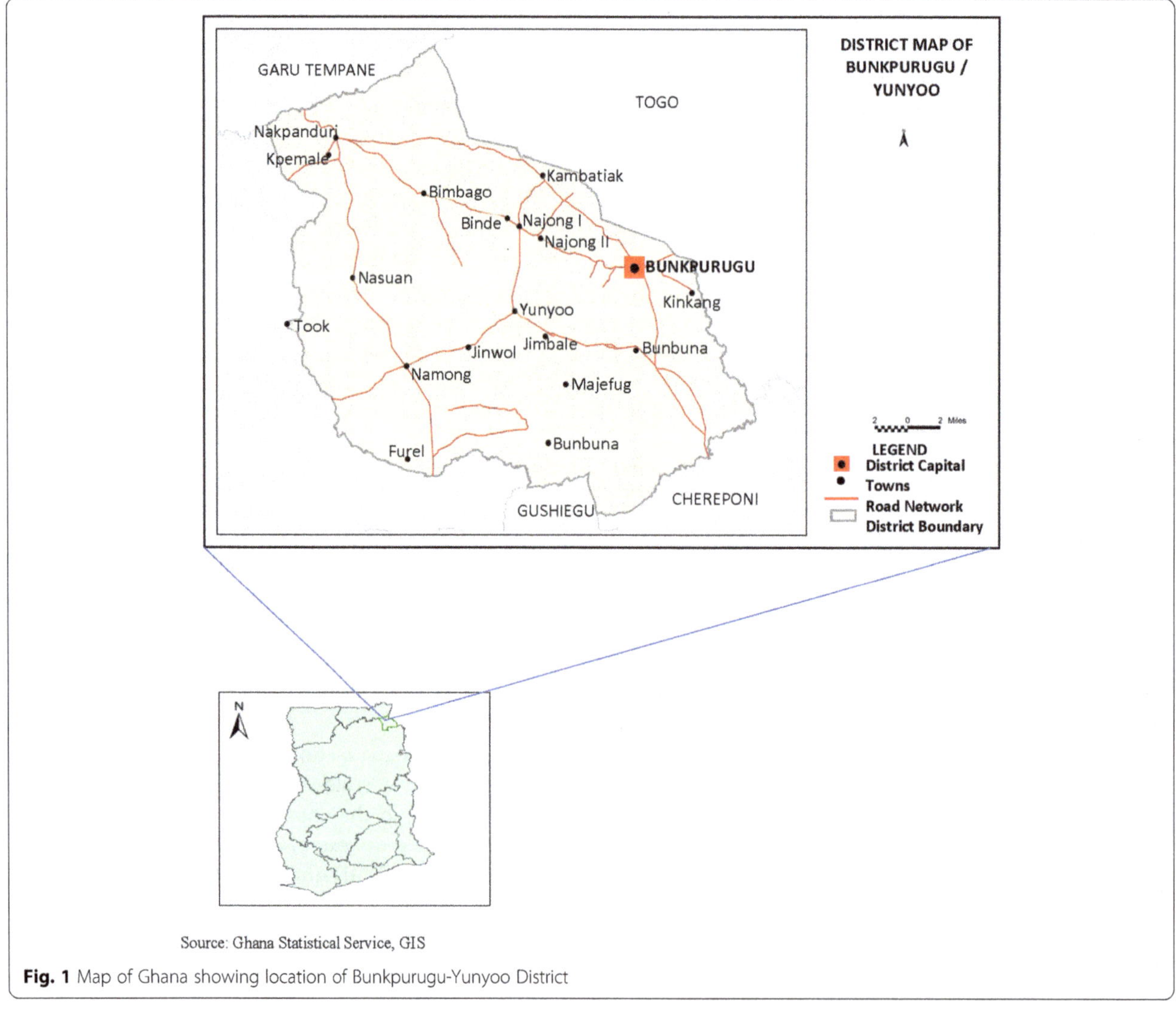

Fig. 1 Map of Ghana showing location of Bunkpurugu-Yunyoo District

five sub-districts (Bunkpurugu and Yunyoo) received a second IRS in a design comparing the impact of one-round of IRS per year *vs* two-rounds of IRS per year. This design did not show any superiority of two-round IRS over one-round IRS: malaria prevalence declined from 49.4 to 44.4% in the area with one-round IRS ($P = 0.037$) and from 55.1 to 50.9% in the area with two-round IRS ($P = 0.071$) (unpublished data).

Study design

Two cross-sectional surveys were conducted in November 2010 and April 2011 to provide pre-IRS baseline estimates for the high and low malaria transmission seasons, respectively. Six post-IRS cross-sectional surveys were subsequently conducted between 2011 and 2014 to assess the impact of IRS within the district. Detailed schedules of IRS activities and cross-sectional surveys are shown in Fig. 2. During each survey, probability proportional to size estimates (PPSE) was used to sample 50 communities in the district, followed by a random selection of 17 compounds with children less than five years-old in each selected community. All children less than five years-old within the selected compounds were eligible to participate in the study.

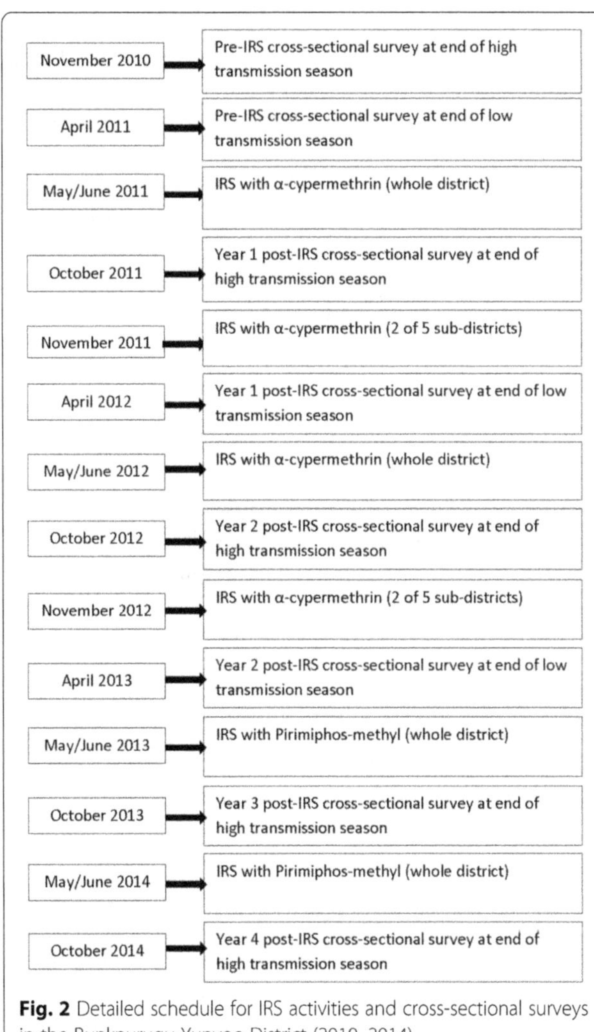

Fig. 2 Detailed schedule for IRS activities and cross-sectional surveys in the Bunkpurugu-Yunyoo District (2010–2014)

Data collection

A standard questionnaire was used to obtain data from mothers/caregivers of children less than five years-old in all selected compounds. Data collected included demographic characteristics of mother and child, bednet ownership and use, recent history of fever and recent intake of an antimalarial. Teams comprising an Interviewer, a Prescriber and a laboratory Technician were deployed to specific communities on the basis of the Interviewer's fluency in the local language. This was to ensure accurate data collection.

Clinical evaluation

Clinical evaluation by the Prescriber in the team included the measurement of axillary temperature using a digital thermometer (Omron digital, Omron Healthcare Inc., Hoofddorp, the Netherlands). All children were tested for the presence of malaria parasites using the CareStart^{TM} Malaria HRP2/pLDH (pf/PAN) Combo (AccessBio, New Jersey, USA) rapid diagnostic test (mRDT). Children with a history of fever during the 48 h period preceding the day of survey or with an axillary temperature ≥ 37.5 °C at the time of examination and a positive mRDT result were considered as having malaria and treated with artesunate-amodiaquine (AS-AQ) combination as per national treatment guidelines [18]. Children with fever but a negative mRDT result were given an antipyretic and referred to the nearest health centre. Severely ill children were sent to the Baptist Medical Centre, the primary referral hospital in that part of the northern region, for further management at the expense of the project.

Parasitological evaluation

Samples of blood were obtained through a finger prick, using a sterile lancet, to perform mRDT and prepare thick and thin blood smears for microscopy. The thin smears were fixed in methanol and both thick and thin smears stained with 3% Giemsa stain for 30–45 min. Stained slides were rinsed, dried, and stored in slide boxes for later reading in the research laboratory. For quality control purposes, all blood slides were read by two independent senior microscopists, and discordant slides read by a third senior microscopist. Discordance was related to presence of asexual/sexual parasites as well as plasmodial species identified. For all discordant results, the reading of the third microscopist was considered final. Thick smears were used for parasite quantification whilst thin smears were used for species identification. Parasite quantification was done per 200 white blood cell counts and converted to counts per µl of blood assuming 8000 cells per µl of blood. At least 200 fields of the thick film were examined before declaring a blood slide negative.

Hematological evaluation

Hemoglobin concentration was determined using a portable automated Hemocue® photometer (Hemocue AB, Ängelholm, Sweden). Anaemia was defined as Hb < 11 g/dl using the 2014 Ghana Demographic and Health Survey (GDHS) definitions [19]. Children with Hb < 6 g/dl were considered as having severe anaemia, and were referred to the Baptist Medical Centre.

Data analysis

The minimum sample size for each survey was 1229, and was based on an estimated prevalence of not more than 60% with 3% precision and 20% non-response rate. Data entries for all surveys were validated by two independent operators using Epidata 3.1. Analysis of validated data was done using SPSS version 21. The outcome variable was malaria parasitaemia by microscopy among children tested. Explanatory variables were gender, age-group, sleeping under a net the night preceding survey, history of fever 48 h prior to survey, and antimalarial intake two weeks prior to survey. Other explanatory variables were caregiver's age-group, educational status, and occupation as well as bednet availability in the home. Univariate analyses (Chi-square and Fisher's exact tests) were used to determine significant associations between parasitaemia and the explanatory variables for the high and low transmission seasons.

All variables showing significant association with parasitaemia were used in a multivariate logistic regression to determine their independent effects on parasitaemia in each transmission season adjusting for gender of child and history of IRS. Variables included in the logistic regression for the high transmission season were gender, history of IRS, child's age-group (months), caregiver's age-group (years), caregiver's education, caregiver's occupation, child sleeping under net night prior to survey, reported fever 48 h prior to survey, and reported antimalarial intake two weeks prior to survey. Variables included in the logistic regression for the low transmission season were gender, time of survey, child's age-group (months), caregiver's age-group (years), caregiver's education, caregiver's occupation, child sleeping under net night prior to survey, reported fever 48 h prior to survey, and reported antimalarial intake two weeks prior to survey.

Results

General characteristics of children tested

Generally, the male to female ratio of children tested in all surveys was approximately 1:1, with approximately 20% of the children aged less than 12 months. In all surveys, over 50% of caregivers of the children tested were 25–34 years-old, had never been to school and practiced farming as an occupation (Tables 1 and 2). Pre-IRS bednet availability in homes visited at the end of the high transmission season was 98.5%, and ranged between 91.1–98.6% during post-IRS surveys in the same season; pre-IRS bednet use among children tested was 95%, and ranged between 82.2–93.7% during post-IRS surveys following application of a pyrethroid, and between 68.1–68.5% following application of an organophosphate (Table 1). At the end of the low transmission season pre-IRS bednet availability was 96.6%, and ranged between 86.9–97.4% during post-IRS surveys following application of a pyrethroid; pre-IRS bednet use among children tested was 62.6% and post-IRS bednet use ranged between 47.7–69.7% (Table 2). The proportion of children who were reported to have had fever within 48 h prior to the pre-IRS survey at the end of the high transmission season was 47.0%, and ranged between 37.3–40.9% during post-IRS surveys following application of a pyrethroid and between 21.3–25.0% during post-IRS surveys following application with an organophosphate (Table 1). The proportion of children who were reported to have had fever within 48 h prior to the pre-IRS survey at the end of the low transmission season was 23.9%, and ranged between 18.7–25.2% during post-IRS surveys following application of a pyrethroid (Table 2). The proportion of children reported to have taken an antimalarial within two weeks prior to each survey conducted at the end of the high transmission season ranged between 2.4–13.8% (Table 1). The proportion of children with anaemia (Hb < 11 g/dl) at the end of the high transmission season pre-IRS survey was 77.7%, and ranged between 67.8–72.5% during post-IRS surveys following application with a pyrethroid, and between 48.3–57.0% during post-IRS surveys following application with an organophosphate (Table 1).

Prevalence of parasitaemia among children tested

Prevalence of asexual parasitaemia among children tested at the end of the high transmission season declined from 52.4% (95% CI: 50.0–54.7%) in November 2010 to 47.7% (95% CI: 45.5–49.9%) in October 2012 (a difference of 4.7%; 95% CI: 1.5–10.0%) following two years of alpha-cypermethrin application. Prevalence further declined from 47.7% in October 2012 to 20.6% (95% CI: 18.4–22.9%) in October 2013 (a difference of 27.1%; 95% CI: 24.0–30.3%) following the application of pirimiphos-methyl, and remained stable in October 2014 at 22.2% (95% CI: 20.1–24.5%) following the second year application of pirimiphos-methyl (Fig. 3). Prevalence of asexual parasitaemia among children tested at the end of the low transmission season significantly declined from 35.6% (95% CI: 33.5–37.8%) in April 2011 to 25.2% (95% CI: 23.4–27.2%) in April 2013 (a difference

Table 1 Background characteristics of children tested in Bunkpurugu-Yunyoo District at the end of the high malaria transmission season (2010–2014)

Characteristic	November 2010 (*n* = 1919)[a]		October 2011 (*n* = 2040)[b]		October 2012 (*n* = 2026)[b]		October 2013 (*n* = 1311)[c]		October 2014 (*n* = 1408)[c]	
	%	95% CI	%	95% CI	%	95% CI	%	95% CI	%	95% CI
Gender										
Male	51.2	48.9–53.5	51.4	49.2–53.6	49.8	47.6–52.0	51.0	48.3–53.7	51.3	48.7–53.9
Female	48.8	46.5–51.1	48.6	46.4–50.8	50.2	48.0–52.4	49.0	46.3–51.7	48.7	46.1–51.4
Age-group (months)										
< 12	19.6	17.9–21.5	20.8	19.1–22.6	20.5	18.8–22.3	22.0	19.8–24.4	21.6	19.5–23.9
12–23	18.6	16.9–20.4	19.6	17.9–21.4	22.4	20.6–24.3	21.6	19.4–24.0	20.5	18.4–22.7
24–35	20.4	18.6–22.3	20.3	18.6–22.1	19.3	17.6–21.1	19.1	17.0–21.4	22.5	20.4–24.8
36–47	20.8	19.0–22.7	19.1	17.4–20.9	18.4	16.8–20.2	18.1	16.1–20.3	20.3	18.3–22.5
48–59	20.6	18.8–22.5	20.2	18.5–22.0	19.3	17.6–21.1	19.2	17.1–21.5	15.1	13.3–17.1
Caregiver's age-group (years)										
< 25	16.8	15.0–18.8	19.2	17.5–21.0	20.8	19.1–22.7	19.0	16.9–21.3	19.6	17.6–21.8
25–34	52.9	50.4–55.4	54.2	52.0–56.4	52.5	50.3–54.7	53.1	50.4–55.8	53.8	51.2–56.4
35–44	24.7	22.6–26.9	22.3	20.5–24.2	23.1	21.3–25.0	23.7	21.4–26.1	22.9	20.8–25.2
45 and above	5.7	4.6–7.0	4.3	3.5–5.3	3.6	2.9–4.5	4.2	3.2–5.5	3.6	2.7–4.8
Caregiver's education										
Never attended school	84.2	82.5–85.8	80.7	78.9–82.4	80.6	78.8–82.3	74.4	71.9–76.7	75.3	72.9–77.5
Ever attended school	15.8	14.2–17.5	19.3	17.6–21.1	19.4	17.7–21.2	25.6	23.3–28.1	24.7	22.5–27.1
Caregiver's occupation										
Non-farming	15.2	13.6–16.9	21.8	20.0–23.7	17.6	16.0–19.3	21.1	18.9–23.4	20.1	18.1–22.3
Farming	84.8	83.1–86.4	78.2	76.3–80.0	82.4	80.7–84.0	78.9	76.6–81.1	79.9	77.7–82.0
Bednet availability in the home										
None	1.5	1.0–2.2	3.7	2.9–4.7	1.4	1.0–2.0	8.9	7.4–10.6	6.8	5.6–8.3
At least one	98.5	97.8–99.0	96.3	95.3–97.1	98.6	98.0–99.1	91.1	89.4–92.6	93.2	91.7–94.5
Child slept under net night prior to survey										
No	5.0	4.1–6.1	17.8	16.2–19.6	6.3	5.3–7.5	31.5	29.0–34.1	31.9	29.5–34.4
Yes	95.0	93.9–95.9	82.2	80.5–83.8	93.7	92.5–94.7	68.5	65.9–71.0	68.1	65.6–70.5
Reported fever 48 h prior to survey										
No	53.0	50.7–55.3	62.8	60.7–64.9	59.1	56.9–61.3	78.7	76.4–80.9	75.0	72.6–77.2
Yes	47.0	44.8–49.3	37.2	35.1–39.4	40.9	38.8–43.1	21.3	19.1–23.6	25.0	22.8–27.4
Antimalarial intake 2 weeks prior to survey										
No	84.6	82.9–86.2	86.2	84.6–87.6	94.1	93.0–95.1	97.6	96.6–98.4	94.8	93.5–95.9
Yes	15.4	13.9–17.1	13.8	12.4–15.4	5.9	4.9–7.0	2.4	1.6–3.4	5.2	4.1–6.5
Anaemia (Hb <11g/dl)										
No	22.3	20.5–24.3	27.5	25.6–29.5	32.2	30.2–34.3	51.7	49.0, 54.4	43.0	40.4–45.6
Yes	77.7	75.6–79.5	72.5	70.5–74.4	67.8	65.7–69.8	48.3	45.6–51.1	57.0	54.4–59.6

[a]Pre-IRS
[b]Post-IRS with pyrethorid
[c]Post-IRS with organophosphate

of 10.4%; 95% CI: 7.5–13.3%) following two years of alpha-cypermethrin application (Fig. 3). Prevalence of gametocytaemia at the end of the high transmission season significantly declined from 15.9% (95% CI: 14.2–17.7%) in November 2010 to 5.3% (95% CI: 4.2–6.6%) in October 2014 (a difference of 10.6%; 95% CI: 8.5–12.7%) following two years of alpha-cypermethrin application and two years of organophosphate application. Gametocytaemia at the end of the low transmission season significantly declined from 10.4% (95% CI: 9.1–11.9%) in

Table 2 Background characteristics of children tested in Bunkpurugu-Yunyoo District at the end of the low malaria transmission season (2011–2013)

Characteristic	April 2011 (*n* = 1967)[a]		April 2012 (*n* = 1984)[b]		April 2013 (*n* = 1998)[b]	
	%	95% CI	%	95% CI	%	95% CI
Gender						
Male	52.2	50.0–54.4	50.3	48.1–52.5	50.2	48.0–52.4
Female	47.8	45.6–50.0	49.7	47.5–51.9	49.8	47.6–52.0
Age-group (months)						
< 12	17.9	16.2–19.7	18.3	16.6–20.1	20.4	18.7–22.3
12–23	20.6	18.9–22.5	21.6	19.8–23.5	22.2	20.4–24.1
24–35	22.2	20.4–24.1	20.3	18.6–22.2	21.1	19.3–23.0
36–47	20.3	18.6–22.2	20.3	18.6–22.2	17.7	16.1–19.5
48–59	19.1	17.4–20.9	19.5	17.8–21.3	18.7	17.0–20.5
Caregiver's age-group (years)						
< 25	19.2	17.4–21.1	14.4	12.9–16.1	20.4	18.7–22.3
25–34	53.0	50.7–55.3	52.2	50.0–54.4	54.5	52.3–56.7
35–44	24.1	22.2–26.2	28.7	26.7–30.8	22.2	20.4–24.1
45 and above	3.7	2.9–4.7	4.6	3.7–5.7	2.9	2.2–3.8
Caregiver's education						
Never attended school	83.0	81.3–84.6	83.2	81.5–84.8	77.9	76.0–79.7
Ever attended school	17.0	15.4–18.8	16.8	15.2–18.5	22.1	20.3–24.0
Caregiver's occupation						
Non-farming	17.1	15.5–18.9	22.4	20.6–24.3	21.7	19.9–23.6
Farming	82.9	81.1–84.5	77.6	75.7–79.4	78.3	76.4–80.1
Bednet availability in the home						
None	3.4	2.7–4.3	13.1	11.7–14.7	2.6	2.0–3.4
At least one	96.6	95.7–97.4	86.9	85.3–88.3	97.4	96.6–98.0
Child slept under net night prior to survey						
No	37.4	35.2–39.6	52.3	50.1–54.5	30.3	28.3–32.4
Yes	62.6	60.4–64.8	47.7	45.5–49.9	69.7	67.6–71.7
Reported fever 48 h prior to survey						
No	76.1	74.1–78.0	74.8	72.8–76.7	81.3	79.5–83.0
Yes	23.9	22.0–25.9	25.2	23.3–27.2	18.7	17.0–20.5
Antimalarial intake 2 weeks prior to survey						
No	96.7	95.8–97.5	97.5	96.7–98.1	98.9	98.4–99.3
Yes	3.3	2.5–4.2	2.5	1.9–3.3	1.1	0.7–1.6
Anaemia (Hb <11g/dl)						
No	57.6	55.3–59.8	53.9	51.7–56.1	53.4	51.2–55.6
Yes	42.4	40.2–44.7	46.1	43.9–48.4	46.6	44.4–48.8

[a]Pre-IRS
[b]Post-IRS with pyrethorid

April 2011 to 6.9% (95% CI: 5.9–8.1%) in April 2013 (a difference of 3.5%; 95% CI: 1.7–5.3%) following two years of alpha-cypermethrin application (Fig. 3). Most infections were *Plasmodium falciparum*, either alone (87–96.5% in surveys conducted at the end of the high transmission season and 83.1–87.7% in surveys conducted at the end of the low transmission season), mixed with *Plasmosium malariae* (1.5–4.9% in surveys conducted at the end of the high transmission season and 6.1–9.7% in surveys conducted at the end of the low transmission season) or mixed with *Plasmodium ovale* (0.2–2.3% in surveys conducted at

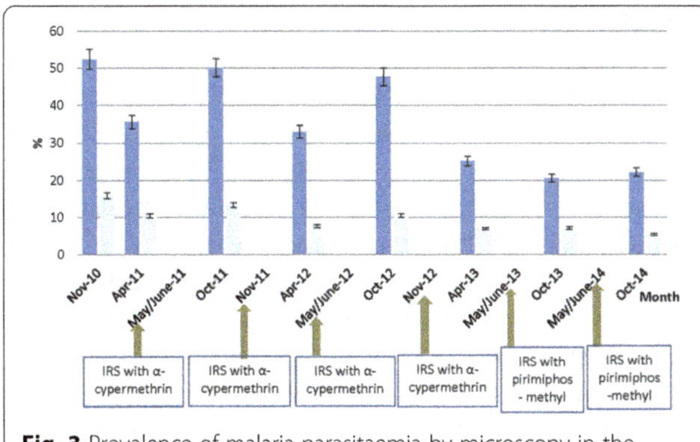

Fig. 3 Prevalence of malaria parasitaemia by microscopy in the Bunkpurugu-Yunyoo District. Blue bars represent asexual parasitaemia whilst aqua bars represent gametocytaemia

the end of the high transmission season and 0–0.4% in surveys conducted at the end of the low transmission season). Geometric mean parasite density ranged between 2022–4373/μl at the end of the high transmission season, and between 1577–2230/μl at the end of the low transmission season.

Univariate analyses of indicators associated with malaria parasitaemia

Univariate analyses showed that the prevalence of malaria parasitaemia at the end of both high and low transmission seasons was significantly associated with: (i) age of child tested; (ii) age, educational status, and occupation of caregiver; (iii) child reported to have had fever within 48 h prior to survey; and (iv) child reported to have taken an antimalarial within two weeks prior to survey (Table 3). Additionally, parasitaemia at the end of the high transmission season was significantly associated with child sleeping under a net the night prior to survey (Table 3).

Prevalence of malaria parasitaemia at the end of the high transmission season was: (i) significantly increased with increasing age of child (from 23.4% among children aged less than 12 months to 52.0% among children aged 48–59 months); (ii) increased with increasing age of caregiver (from 35.1% among caregivers aged less than 25 years to 44.8% among caregivers aged 45 years and above); (iii) higher among caregivers who never attended school compared with those who attended school (45.7 *vs* 22.2%); (iv) higher among caregivers who were farmers compared with non-farmers (44.3 *vs* 26.0%); (v) higher among children who were reported to have slept under a net night preceding the survey compared with those who did not sleep under a net (42.0 *vs* 34.8%); (vi) higher among children reported to have had fever 48 h prior to survey compared with those without fever (59.8 *vs* 30.4%); and (vii) higher among children reported not to have taken an antimalarial two weeks prior to survey compared with those who had taken an antimalarial (42.0 *vs* 29.5%) (Table 3).

Table 3 Association between selected indicators and malaria asexual parasitaemia at the end of the high and low transmission seasons in Bunkpurugu-Yunyoo District (2010–2014)

Characteristic	High season			Low season		
	Total	%	*P*-value	Total	%	*P*-value
Gender						
Male	4323	40.6	0.825	3008	31.8	0.312
Female	4158	40.9		2900	30.6	
Age-group (months)						
< 12	1767	23.4	<0.001	1113	8.4	<0.001
12-23	1754	37.3		1268	23.5	
24–35	1716	43.5		1257	34.8	
36–47	1642	49.2		1144	43.1	
48–59	1615	52.0		1127	46.4	
Caregiver's age-group (years)						
< 25	1569	35.1	<0.001	1032	25.9	<0.001
25–34	4389	39.0		3055	29.2	
35–44	1901	45.9		1436	36.2	
45 and above	348	44.8		215	35.3	
Caregiver's education						
Never attended school	6770	45.7	<0.001	4810	35.3	<0.001
Ever attended school	1742	22.2		1103	13.5	
Caregiver's occupation						
Non-farming	1614	26.0	<0.001	1200	16.5	<0.001
Farming	6866	44.3		4705	34.9	
Child slept under net night prior to survey						
No	1432	34.8	<0.001	2340	31.7	0.545
Yes	7020	42.0		3511	30.9	
Reported fever 48 h prior to survey						
No	5467	30.4	<0.001	4532	24.1	<0.001
Yes	3020	59.8		1323	55.4	
Antimalarial intake 2 weeks prior to survey						
No	7741	42.0	<0.001	5779	31.6	<0.001
Yes	772	29.5		134	16.4	

Prevalence of malaria parasitaemia at the end of the low transmission season was: (i) significantly increased with increasing age of child (from 8.4% among children aged less than 12 months to 46.4% among children aged 48–59 months); (ii) increased with increasing age of caregiver (from 25.9% among caregivers aged less than 25 years to 35.3% among caregivers aged 45 years and above); (iii) higher among caregivers who never attended school compared with those who attended school (35.3 *vs* 13.5%); higher among caregivers who were farmers compared with non-farmers (34.9 *vs* 16.5%); (iv) higher among children reported to have had fever 48 h prior to survey compared with those without fever (55.4 *vs* 24.1%); and (v) higher among children reported not to have taken an antimalarial two weeks prior to survey compared with those who had taken an antimalarial (31.6 *vs* 16.4%) (Table 3).

Multivariate analyses of indicators associated with malaria parasitaemia

When all indicators significantly associated with asexual parasitaemia in the univariate analyses were included in a logistic regression analysis, adjusting for gender and history of IRS, asexual parasitaemia was not associated with caregiver's age-group or child sleeping under a net night prior to survey at the end of either transmission season. The odds of parasitaemia significantly increased with age in both transmission seasons: (i) from 1.9 (95% CI: 1.6–2.2) among children aged 12–23 months to 3.5 (95% CI: 2.9–4.1) among children aged 48–59 months at the end of the high transmission season; and (ii) from 3.3 (95% CI: 2.5–4.3) among children aged 12–23 months to 10.7 (95% CI: 8.2–13.9) among children aged 48–59 months at the end of the low transmission season (Table 4). Odds of parasitaemia at the end of both transmission seasons were significantly lower among caregivers who indicated they had ever attended school compared with those who had never attended school (OR = 0.4, 95% CI: 0.4–0.5 for the high transmission season and OR = 0.4, 95% CI: 0.3–0.5 for the low transmission season). Caregivers who were farmers had higher odds of parasitaemia compared with non-farmers for both transmission seasons (OR = 1.7, 95% CI: 1.5–2.0 for the high transmission season and OR = 2.2, 95% CI: 1.8–2.7 for the low transmission season). Odds of parasitaemia at the end of both transmission seasons were significantly higher among children who were reported to have had fever within 48 h prior to survey compared with those who had no fever (OR = 3.2, 95% CI: 2.9–3.6 for the high transmission season and OR = 4.4, 95% CI: 3.8–5.1 for the low transmission season). Children who were reported to have taken an antimalarial within two weeks prior to survey had lower odds of parasitaemia compared with those who had not taken any antimalarial (OR = 0.3, 95% CI: 0.3–0.4 for the high season and OR = 0.3, 95% CI: 0.2–0.5 for the low season) (Table 4). History of IRS was significantly associated with parasitaemia in both transmission seasons. The association observed in the high transmission season was not evident until the third year when pyrethroid was replaced with organophosphate. The odds of parasitaemia was significantly lower after the application of an organophosphate compared with the pre-IRS survey (OR = 0.3, 95% CI: 0.2–0.3), and remained stable after another round of IRS with an organophosphate (OR = 0.3, 95% CI: 0.2–0.3) (Table 4).

Discussion

A series of cross-sectional surveys conducted between 2010 and 2014 showed a positive impact of IRS on malaria parasitaemia in the Bunkpurugu-Yunyoo District in northern Ghana. Malaria parasitaemia was found to be significantly associated with similar characteristics in both the high and low transmission seasons. The factors that associated with asexual parasitaemia during both transmission seasons were: increasing age of child; reported fever within 48 h prior to survey; reported intake of an antimalarial within two weeks prior to survey; caregiver's educational status; and caregiver's occupation.

Prevalence of malaria asexual parasitaemia declined by 9.0 and 29.2% at the end of the high and low transmission seasons, respectively, after 2 years of IRS with alpha-cypermethrin. The quantum of decline does not agree with findings from Sao Tome and Principe, another sub-Saharan African country, where malaria parasitaemia reduced by 97% [from 20.1% (95% CI: 18.0–22.4%) to 0.6% (95% CI: 0.2–1.6%)] after two years of annual IRS with alpha-cypermethrin [20]. Prevalence of malaria asexual parasitaemia, however, declined by almost 57% at the end of the peak transmission season of 2013 after using pirimiphos-methyl. The better performance of pirimiphos-methyl, compared with alpha-cypermethrin, can be explained by the high levels of pyrethroid resistance reported in the district (60–90% mosquito susceptibility to pyrethroids and 98–100% susceptibility to organophosphates) (unpublished 2012 data) and other parts of the country [21, 22]. The decision to change insecticide in Bunkpurugu-Yunyoo District in 2013 was therefore appropriate for achieving better impact on malaria parasitaemia. After the second year application of pirimiphos-methyl in 2014, prevalence of asexual parasitaemia remained stable at 22.2% compared with the 2013 prevalence of 20.6%. This finding of stable malaria prevalence or no further decline in prevalence after two consecutive applications of an alternative insecticide suggests that other interventions will be critical in achieving consistent decline in parasitaemia in areas where IRS is deployed. Although LLIN ownership at the end of the high transmission season in the Bunkpurugu-Yunyoo District ranged between 91.1–98.6% over the 5 year period of this study, net-use declined over the years from 95% to 68.1%. However, high transmission seasons of 2010 and 2012 experienced over 90% LLIN usage rate following mass campaigns. This observation suggests that promoting LLIN use, during the high transmission season in particular, is necessary to benefit from the contributing effect of LLINs on the reduction of malaria prevalence.

Risk of parasitemia increased with increasing age group, irrespective of transmission season. Odds of parasitaemia almost doubled from 1.9 among children aged 12–23 months to 3.5 among children aged 48–59 months at the

Table 4 Multivariate logistic regression analysis of indicators associated with malaria asexual parasitaemia by transmission season in Bunkpurugu-Yunyoo District

Characteristic	High season			Low season		
	OR	95% CI	*P*-value	OR	95% CI	*P*-value
Gender						
Male[a]						
Female	1.1	1.0–1.2	0.070	1.0	0.8–1.1	0.521
History of IRS (high season)						
None[a]						
Year 1 IRS with α-cypermethrin	1.1	0.9–1.3	0.190	–	–	–
Year 2 IRS with α-cypermethrin	0.9	0.7–1.0	0.058	–	–	–
Year 3 IRS with pirimiphos-methyl	0.3	0.2–0.3	<0.001	–	–	–
Year 4 IRS with pirimiphos-methyl	0.3	0.2–0.3	<0.001	–	–	–
History of IRS (low season)						
None[a]						
Year 1 IRS with α-cypermethrin	–	–	–	0.9	0.8–1.1	0.352
Year 2 IRS with α-cypermethrin	–	–	–	0.7	0.6–0.8	<0.001
Age-group (months)						
< 12[a]						
12–23	1.9	1.6–2.2	<0.001	3.3	2.5–4.3	<0.001
24–35	2.4	2.0–2.8	<0.001	6.1	4.7–8.0	<0.001
36–47	3.1	2.6–3.6	<0.001	9.3	7.2–12.2	<0.001
48–59	3.5	2.9–4.1	<0.001	10.7	8.2–13.9	<0.001
Caregiver's age-group (years)						
< 25[a]						
25–34	0.9	0.8–1.0	0.144	0.8	0.7–1.0	0.059
35–44	1.0	0.9–1.2	0.732	0.9	0.8–1.2	0.572
45 and above	0.9	0.7–1.1	0.224	0.8	0.5–1.1	0.130
Caregiver's education						
Never attended school[a]						
Ever attended school	0.4	0.4–0.5	<0.001	0.4	0.3–0.5	<0.001
Caregiver's occupation						
Non-farming[a]						
Farming	1.7	1.5–2.0	<0.001	2.2	1.8–2.7	<0.001
Child slept under net night prior to survey						
No[a]						
Yes	0.9	0.8–1.1	0.181	1.0	0.9–1.2	0.864
Reported fever 48 h prior to survey						
No[a]						
Yes	3.2	2.9–3.6	<0.001	4.4	3.8–5.1	<0.001
Antimalarial intake 2 weeks prior to survey						
No[a]						
Yes	0.3	0.3–0.4	<0.001	0.3	0.2–0.5	<0.001

[a]Reference category

end of the high transmission season and almost tripled from 3.3 among children aged 12–23 months to 10.7 among children aged 48–59 months at the end of the low transmission season. This finding compares well with findings from the 2011 multiple indicator cluster survey in Ghana, suggesting that older child age-groups within children less than five years bear the highest burden of malaria infection [23]. Malaria interventions for children less than five year-old should therefore be designed to take care of the vulnerabilities of children within the older age-groups, particularly those aged 3 years and above.

As expected, the risk of parasitaemia was higher among children with reported history of fever and children reported not to have taken an antimalarial within two weeks prior to surveys at the end of either transmission season. This finding suggests that fever remains a predictor of malaria infection in the study district, and therefore supports global and national guidelines for case management of malaria [18, 24, 25]. Use of antimalarials is primarily aimed at both parasitological and clinical cure, and therefore a good predictor of absence of parasitaemia, particularly in the era of artemisinin-based combination therapy [24].

For both transmission seasons, the odds of parasitaemia were higher among children with caregivers who had never attended school. This finding compares well with the 2011 multiple indicator survey, which showed that malaria parasitaemia was highest among children with caregivers who had never attended school [23]. Mother's education has generally been associated with child health inequalities, and so empowering women with education could go a long way to impact on childhood malaria prevalence reduction, among others [26]. Children with caregivers who engaged in farming as an occupation had almost a double odds of parasitaemia compared with children with non-farming caregivers. Farming in Ghana is largely practiced by persons with low levels of education, and therefore it is not surprising to see the two characteristics showing a similar effect on parasitaemia in the Bunkpurugu-Yunyoo District. Also, compound farming, a home garden-type of agroforestry system, is one of the major types of farming practiced in northern Ghana, and so increases exposure to outdoor mosquito bites [27, 28].

Our study has a couple of limitations. Our evidence of a positive impact of IRS on malaria parasitaemia would have been stronger if we had a comparison area. Our study was designed in a period when IRS was being scaled-up in the northern region of Ghana, and therefore there was limited opportunity to have a comparison area. Nevertheless, our study provides useful insight into the impact of IRS on parasitaemia and other indicators such as fever and anaemia. Another limitation is our inability to control for migration; we did not consider movement of persons in and out of the district to be able to estimate different levels of exposure to mosquito vectors. Although we cannot conclude that living within the district adequately protects against malaria infection, several studies have shown that IRS is associated with reduced malaria transmission. Our entomological monitoring in the district over a period of two years showed entomological inoculation rates (EIRs) declining from pre-IRS level of 0.350 infective bites/person/year to post-IRS level of 0.021 infective bites/person/year (unpublished data).

Conclusions

Following a 2-year application of alpha-cypermethrin at the beginning of the high malaria transmission season in the Bunkpurugu-Yunyoo District, the end of high transmission season prevalence of malaria parasitaemia declined by only 9%, whilst a change of insecticide to pirimiphos-methyl yielded a decline of 57% after one year of application. We conclude that the use of a more efficacious insecticide for IRS can reduce malaria parasitaemia among children less than five years-old in northern Ghana.

Abbreviations

ACT: Artemisinin-based combination therapy; AGA: AngloGold Ashanti; AS-AQ: Artesunate-amodiaquine combination; IPTp: Intermittent preventive treatment of pregnant women; IRS: Indoor residual spraying; LLINs: Long-lasting insecticidal nets; mRDT: Malaria rapid diagnostic test; PMI: President's Malaria Initiative

Acknowledgements

We are grateful to the staff of Research Triangle Institute (RTI) and Africa IRS project (Abt Associates) in Accra and Tamale for their administrative and field support. We thank the experienced field staff who helped with data collection for the different cross-sectional surveys. We also want to thank Supervisors from the National Malaria Control Programme, Noguchi Memorial Institute for Medical Research, United States Agency for International Development (Ghana), Centers for Disease Control and Prevention (Atlanta) for ensuring quality data collection. We thank all caregivers and families for their consent to participate in the study. We are indebted to the political, health, and traditional authorities in the Bunpkurugu-Yunyoo District as well as the Management of Baptist Medical Centre (Nalerigu) for their support.

Funding

The study received funding from the US President's Malaria Initiative (PMI).

Authors' contributions

BA, CA, PP, PR and KK conceived and designed the study. BA, CA, SM, WS and SO analysed the data. BA and CA prepared the first draft of manuscript. All authors read and approved the final manuscript.

Competing interests

The authors declare that they have no competing interests.

Author details
[1]Epidemiology Department, Noguchi Memorial Institute for Medical Research, College of Health Sciences, University of Ghana, Legon, P. O. Box LG581, Legon, Ghana. [2]University of Florida, 410 NE Waldo Rd, Gainesville, FL 32641, USA. [3]President's Malaria Initiative/Malaria Branch, Centers for Disease Control and Prevention, Atlanta, GA, USA. [4]National Malaria Control Programme, Public Health Division, Ghana Health Service, Accra, Ghana.

References

1. Mabaso ML, Sharp B, Lengeler C. Historical review of malarial control in southern African with emphasis on the use of indoor residual house-spraying. Trop Med Int Health. 2004;9:846–56.
2. WHO. Indoor Residual Spraying: An Operational Manual for Indoor Residual Spraying (IRS) for Malaria Transmission Control and Elimination. 2nd ed. Geneva: World Health Organization; 2015.
3. Sharp BL, Ridl FC, Govender D, Kuklinski J, Kleinschmidt I. Malaria vector control by indoor residual insecticide spraying on the tropical Island of Bioko, Equatorial Guinea. Malar J. 2007;6:52.
4. Misra SP, Webber R, Lines J, Jaffar S, Bradley DJ. Malaria control: bednets or spraying? Spray *versus* treated nets using deltamethrin - a community randomized trial in India. Trans R Soc Trop Med Hyg. 1999;93:456–7.
5. Rowland M, Mahmood P, Igbal J, Carneiro I, Chavasse D. Indoor residual spraying with alphacypermethrin controls malaria in Pakistan: a community randomized trial. Trop Med Int Health. 2000;5:472–81.
6. Curtis CF, Maxwell CA, Finch RJ, Njunwa KJ. A comparison of use of a pyrethroid either for house spraying of for bednet treatment against malaria vectors. Trop Med Int Health. 1998;3:619–31.
7. Kleinschmidt I, Sharp B, Benavente LE, Schwabe C, Torrez M, Kuklinski J, et al. Reduction in infection with *Plasmodium falciparum* one year after the introduction of malaria control interventions on Bioko Island, Equatorial Guinea. Am J Trop Med Hyg. 2006;74:972–8.
8. WHO. World Malaria Report, vol. 2011. Geneva: World Health Organization; 2011.
9. Barnes KI, Durrheim DN, Little F, Jackson A, Mehta U, Allen E, et al. Effect of artemether-lumefantrine policy and improved vector control on malaria burden in KwaZulu-Natal, South Africa. PLoS Med. 2005;2:e330.
10. Kleinschmidt I, Scwabe C, Shiva M, Segura JL, Sima V, Mabunda SJA, et al. Combining indoor residual spraying and insecticide-treated net interventions. Am J Trop Med Hyg. 2009;81:519–24.
11. Korenromp EL, Armstrong-Schellenberg RM, Williams BG, Nahlen BL, Snow RW. Impact of malaria control on childhood anaemia in Africa - a quantitative review. Trop Med Int Health. 2004;9:1050–65.
12. Kim D, Fedak K, Kramer R. Reduction of malaria prevalence by indoor residual spraying: a meta-regression analysis. Am J Trop Med Hyg. 2012;87:117–24.
13. WHO. World Malaria Report, vol. 2016. Geneva: World Health Organization; 2016.
14. Ministry of Health, Ghana. Strategic Plan for Malaria Control in Ghana 2008–2015. Accra: Ministry of Health; 2009.
15. Baird JK, Owusu Agyei S, Utz GC, Koram K, Barcus MJ, Jones TR, et al. Seasonal malaria attack rates in infants and young children in northern Ghana. Am J Trop Med Hyg. 2002;66:280–6.
16. Ghana Statistical Service. 2010 Population & Housing Census. District Analytical Report. Bunkpurugu Yunyoo District. Accra: Ghana Statistical Service; 2014.
17. Composite Budget for 2018-2021. Programme based budget Estimates for 2018. Bunkpurugu/Yunyoo District Assembly. https://www.mofep.gov.gh/sites/default/files/composite-budget/2018/NR/Bunkpurugu.pdf. Accessed 10 Oct 2018.
18. Ministry of Health, Ghana. Guidelines for Case Management of Malaria in Ghana. 3rd ed. Accra: Ministry of Health; 2014.
19. Ghana Statistical Service, Ghana Health Service, and ICF International. Ghana Demographic and Health Survey 2014. Rockville: Ghana Statistical Service, Ghana Health Service, and ICF International; 2015.
20. Tseng LF, Chang WC, Ferreira MC, Wu CH, Rampao HS, Lien JC. Rapid control of malaria by means of indoor residual spraying of alphacypermethrin in the Democratic Republic of Sao Tome and Principe. Am J Trop Med Hyg. 2008;78:248–50.
21. Baffour-Awuah S, Annan AA, Maiga-Ascofare O, Dieudonné SD, Adjei-Kusi P, Owusu-Dabo E, et al. Insecticide resistance in malaria vectors in Kumasi, Ghana. Parasit Vectors. 2016;9:633.
22. Hunt RH, Fuseini G, Knowles S, Stiles-Ocran J, Verster R, Kaiser ML, et al. Insecticide resistance in malaria vector mosquitoes at four localities in Ghana, West Africa. Parasit Vectors. 2011;4:107.
23. Ghana Statistical Service. Ghana Multiple Indicator Cluster Survey with an Enhanced Malaria Module and Biomarker, 2011, Final Report. Accra: Ghana Statistical Service; 2011.
24. WHO. Guidelines for the Treatment of Malaria. Geneva: World Health Organization; 2010.
25. Okiro EA, Snow RW. The relationship between reported fever and *Plasmodium falciparum* infection in African children. Malar J. 2010;9:99.
26. Wamani H, Tylleskar T, Astrom AN, Tumwine JK, Peterson S. Mothers' education but not fathers' education, household assets or land ownership is the best predictor of child health inequalities in Uganda. Int J Equity Health. 2004;3:9.
27. Govella NJ, Ferguson H. Why use of interventions targeting outdoor biting mosquitoes will be necessary to achieve malaria elimination. Front Physiol. 2012;3:199.
28. Reddy MR, Overgaard HJ, Abaga S, Reddy VP, Caccone A, Kiszewski AE, et al. Outdoor host seeking behavior of *Anopheles gambiae* mosquitoes following initiation of malaria vector control on Bioko Island, Equatorial Guinea. Malar J. 2011;10:184.

11

Triatominae: does the shape change of non-viable eggs compromise species recognition?

Soledad Santillán-Guayasamín[1], Anita G. Villacís[1*], Mario J. Grijalva[1,2] and Jean-Pierre Dujardin[1,3]

Abstract

Background: Eggs have epidemiological and taxonomic importance in the subfamily Triatominae, which contains Chagas disease vectors. The metric properties (size and shape) of eggs are useful for distinguishing between close species, or different geographical populations of the same species.

Methods: We examined the effects of egg viability on its metric properties, and the possible consequences on species recognition. Four species were considered: *Panstrongylus chinai*, *P. howardi* and *Triatoma carrioni* (tribe Triatomini), and *Rhodnius ecuadoriensis* (tribe Rhodniini). Digitization was performed on pictures taken when the viability of the egg could not clearly be predicted by visual inspection. We then followed development to separate viable from non-viable eggs, and the metric changes associated with viability status of the eggs were tested for species discrimination (interspecific difference).

Results: The shape of the complete contour of the egg provided satisfactory species classification (95% of correct assignments, on average), with improved scores (98%) when discarding non-viable eggs from the comparisons. Using only non-viable eggs, the scores dropped to 90%. The morphometric differences between viable and non-viable eggs were also explored (intraspecific comparison). A constant metric change observed was a larger variance of size and shape in non-viable eggs. For all species, larger eggs, or eggs with larger operculum, were more frequently non-viable. However, these differences did not allow for an accurate prediction regarding egg viability.

Conclusions: The strong taxonomic signal present in egg morphology was affected by the level of viability of the eggs. The metric properties as modified in non-viable eggs presented some general trends which could suggest the existence of an optimum phenotype for size and for shape. Globally, viable eggs tended to have intermediate or small sizes, and presented a less globular shape in the Triatomini, or a relatively wider neck in *Rhodnius ecuadoriensis*.

Keywords: Ecuador, Egg contour, Egg viability, Operculum landmarks, Triatominae

Background

The species of the subfamily Triatominae (Hemiptera: Reduviidae) are blood-sucking vectors of *Trypanosoma cruzi*, the causative agent of Chagas disease. Currently, more than 150 species have been recognized as potential vectors of the parasite to mammals; however, only a few have significant importance in transmission to humans [1–3]. In Ecuador, 16 species of the Triatominae have been reported, distributed in 20 of the 24 provinces [4, 5]. The infestation index in this country is variable among provinces, ranging between 0.2–29%, with a national average of 2.6% according to the complete analysis of records from the Ministry of Public Health from 2004–2014 [6]. *Rhodnius ecuadoriensis* (Lent & León, 1958) and *Triatoma dimidiata* (Latreille, 1811) are considered the main vectors in this country. However, other species belonging to the genera *Triatoma* and *Panstrongylus* are increasingly reported as secondary vectors [4].

Triatoma carrioni (Larrousse, 1926) is distributed in the southern Andean region of Ecuador (Loja and El Oro) and northern Peru. It occupies a wide range of ecological zones, either arid or humid areas, between 800

* Correspondence: agvillacis@puce.edu.ec
[1]Center for Research on Health in Latin America (CISeAL), School of Biological Sciences, Pontifical Catholic University of Ecuador, Calle Pambahacienda s/n y San Pedro del Valle, Campus Nayón, Quito, Ecuador
Full list of author information is available at the end of the article

and 2242 m above sea level (masl). It is the only species in Ecuador that has been found up to 2242 masl [7]. It may infest human dwellings, primarily in bedrooms as well as peridomestic environments such as chicken nests, guinea pig pens, dog houses, piles of wood, bricks, and firewood [7]. Thus far, the species has not been reported in sylvatic environment (Padilla et al., unpublished data).

Panstrongylus chinai (Del Ponte, 1929) is more widely distributed in Ecuador and Peru [4, 8]. In Peru, this species is reported to be the primary household vector in the Department of Piura [9]. In Ecuador, it is reported at altitudes ranging from 175 to 2003 masl, in peridomestic environments (chicken nests, guinea pig pens) as well as in human dwellings (bedrooms) in the southern provinces of Loja and El Oro [4, 7, 10]. Despite considerable sampling efforts, there are no reports of sylvatic populations of *P. chinai* in Ecuador [11].

Panstrongylus howardi (Neiva, 1911) is an endemic species restricted to Ecuador in the Manabí Province (central coast region) [12]. It has been associated with rodent nests located between brick piles. Abundant colonies of this species can be found also in wood piles, as well as in the "piñuelas" plant *Aechmea magdalenae*, again in association with nesting places of rodents or of marsupials [13]. Sylvatic specimens have also been reported [14].

Populations of *R. ecuadoriensis* are widely distributed in the southern Andean regions (Loja and el Oro provinces) of Ecuador, and in the central coast, Santo Domingo de los Tsáchilas and Manabí provinces [7, 15]. The species is found also in northern Peru [16]. In Ecuador it occupies domestic, peridomestic and sylvatic habitats [14, 15]. In both countries, abundant sylvatic populations can be found in nests of the Guayaquil squirrel (*Sciurus stramineus*) and the fasciated wren bird (*Campylorhynchus fasciatus*) [5, 14, 17, 18].

The taxonomic classification of the Triatominae was historically based on qualitative morphological descriptions. To introduce more quantitative data and open the field more widely to the study of biological diversity, species in the Triatominae have been studied using quantitative, morphometric techniques. During the last two decades, the geometric approach to morphometrics has become a popular and useful tool in quantifying shape and size variation [19, 20]. This approach has been put into practice in various fields of ecology, evolution, and medicine [21, 22].

Triatomine eggs are oval, elliptical, cylindrical or spherical, slightly asymmetrical forms, and present a smooth convex or ornamented operculum [23, 24]. Egg morphology has been examined mainly on the basis of qualitative characters such as color pattern and structural traits (shape, texture of shell and operculum, exochorial architecture). The quantitative traits of eggs usually were based on traditional morphometric techniques [25–30], while geometric techniques have only recently been introduced [31, 32]. In dwellings, eggs could be found in the cracks of walls, boards of the beds, clothes, chicken nests, and any material accumulated in the domicile and peridomicile [10, 33]. In general, eggs are important to consider because the presence of eggs of some species of the Triatominae in the domicile could be related to its capacity to colonize human dwellings [34], suggesting its importance as a vector. It is therefore relevant to develop egg-based species identification techniques [32].

Many factors could cause artefactual morphometric differences between groups [35]; for the eggs it is important to consider the impact of position, developmental stage, and some other parameters related to the mother and/or the environment [32]. The physiological status of females could influence indeed some traits of their eggs. This possible effect was hereby taken into account by comparing eggs coming from newly-molted females.

The primary justification of our study was to explore the possible interference of egg viability in species distinction. It is a relevant issue because, in some cases, only eggs are collected in the field and some of them could be non-viable eggs. The causes of non-viability are many: eggs could be unfertilized, or even if they are fertilized, they could fail to develop into viable nymph because of unknown genetic or environmental reasons.

As previously shown, geometric techniques of morphometrics applied to viable eggs allow for a very accurate recognition of species or even geographical populations within-species [32, 36]. In four species of Ecuadorian Triatominae, we verified whether the egg-based species morphometric discrimination was affected by the viability of the eggs. We then examined within each species the metric differences between viable (V) and non-viable (NV) eggs.

Methods

Insect collection

Specimens were collected in two separate provinces of Ecuador: Loja and Manabí (Fig. 1). In Loja, the houses have roofs of clay tiles, dusty floors, and adobe walls, which provide hiding places and breeding sites for bugs [37]. The houses of Manabí are elevated by wooden stilts and the walls and floors are made of guadúa cane (*Guadua angustifolia*), which allows passage by insects but does not offer hiding places for the bugs [38]. Therefore, in Manabí Province, bugs are usually found in the peridomestic environment.

The peridomestic environment is characterized by chicken and pigeon coops, guinea pig pens, agricultural and household waste, plants used as natural fences, piles of construction materials (stones, wood, bricks), and accumulations of palm fronds (only in Manabí) [15, 38]. In

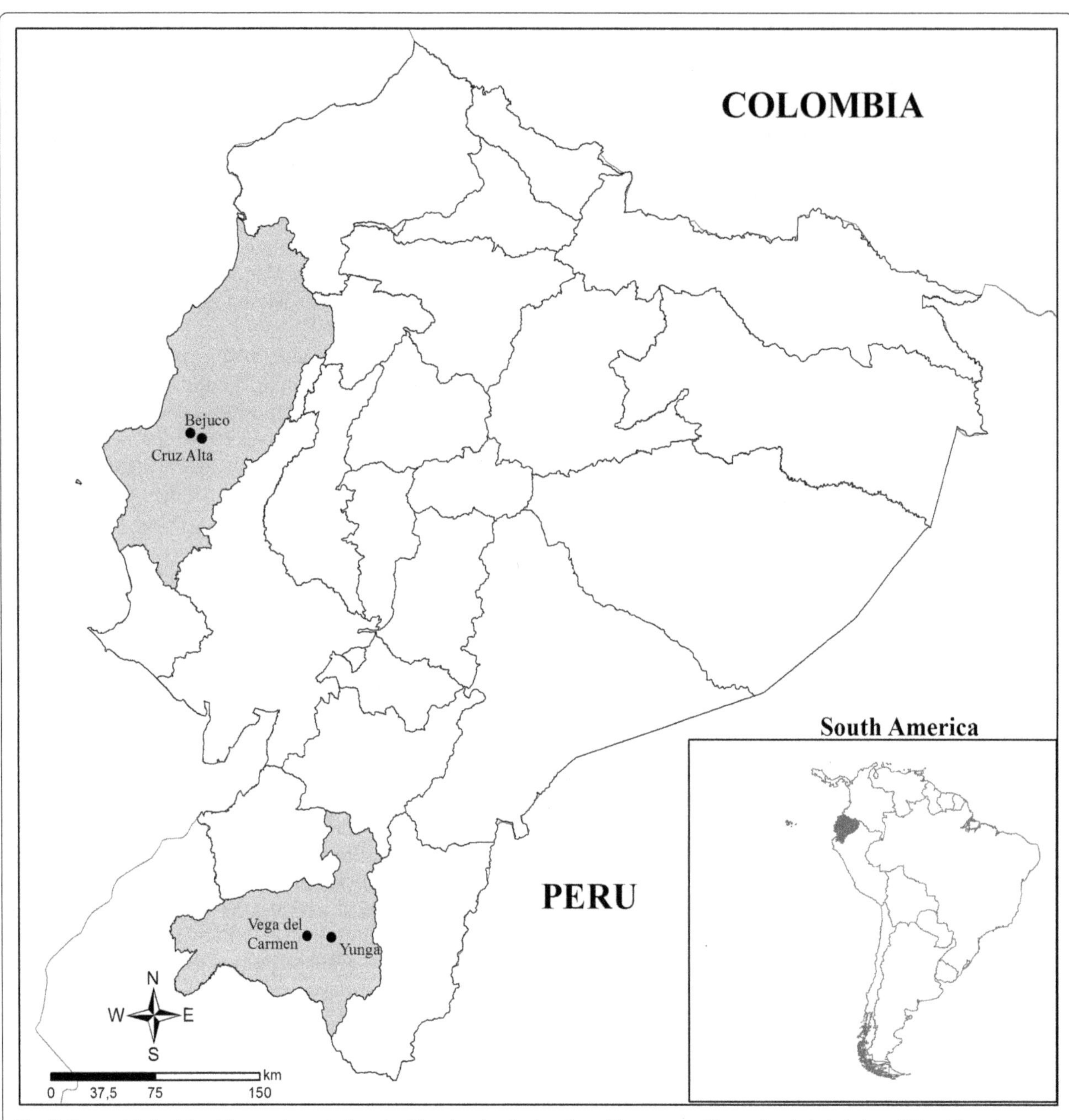

Fig. 1 Geographical origin of the specimens in Ecuador. Map showing the location of the communities under study in Loja and Manabí provinces

the sylvatic environment in Manabí Province, an abundance of *Phytelephas aequatorialis* is typical, which is cultivated for its nuts used in manufacturing and its leaves for the construction of roofs [38].

The four Ecuadorian species were chosen because of their epidemiological importance for the country. *Rhodnius ecuadoriensis* is one of the most important vectors of Chagas disease in Ecuador, while *T. carrioni*, *P. chinai* and *P. howardi* are considered secondary vectors in their respective provinces [4, 11, 12].

Panstrongylus chinai and *T. carrioni* were collected in Loja Province, while *P. howardi* and *R. ecuadoriensis* were collected in the Manabi Province (Table 1). The eggs were obtained from females that had spent various generations (from 4 to 10) in the laboratory. In the case of *T. carrioni*, the eggs were obtained directly from field females collected from domestic habitat. The colonies of *Panstrongylus* spp. and *R. ecuadoriensis* were maintained in the insectary of the Center for Research on Health in Latin America (CISeAL), Pontifical Catholic University

Table 1 Geographical location and year of collection in communities from which parents were used for egg production

Spp.	Province, community	E	Latitude	Longitude	Altitude	Year	Parents' origin[a]	Group	*n*
P. c.	Loja, Vega del Carmen	P	-4.1137	-79.5928	1086	2009	Laboratory colony (6th generation)	V	34
								NV	22
T. c.	Loja, Yunga	I	-4.1225	-79.4284	1622	2015	Field colony (1st generation)	V	21
								NV	12
P. h.	Manabí, Bejuco	P	-0.99007	-80.3475	134	2007	Laboratory colony (8th generation)	V	67
								NV	55
R. e.	Manabí, Cruz Alta	S	-1.00149	-80.2705	971	2013	Laboratory colony (4th generation)	V	19
								NV	14

Abbreviations: *P.c. Panstrongylus chinai*, *P.h. P. howardi*, *T.c. Triatoma carrioni*, *R.e. Rhodnius ecuadoriensis*, *E* ecotopes, *P* peridomicile, *I* intradomicile, *S* sylvatic, *V* viable eggs, *NV* non-viable eggs, *n* number of eggs analyzed by group per species. A total of 244 eggs were analyzed

[a]Provenance of the parents which were used for obtaining the eggs (estimated number of generations according to the life-cycle)

of Ecuador (PUCE), under controlled conditions of 25 ± 6 °C, 70 ± 5% relative humidity (RH) for Loja specimens, 27 ± 5 °C, 75 ± 5% RH for Manabí specimens, and a photoperiod of 12:12 h (L:D) for specimens of both provinces. Blood meals were offered every 15 days for 30 min, using immobilized pigeon (*Columba livia*).

For *P. chinai*, *P. howardi* and *R. ecuadoriensis*, four crosses were conducted and inspected everyday (looking for eggs). Each cross was composed of two females and three males. The eggs of *T. carrioni* came from two field-collected females; they were laid in the collection vials during the transportation of females from the field to the insectary of the center at Quito. Therefore, the eggs came from eight females per species, except for *T. carrioni*. A total of 244 eggs were analyzed: 56 *P. chinai*, 122 *P. howardi*, 33 *T. carrioni* and 33 *R. ecuadoriensis* (Table 1). For each species, the bugs used as genitors came from a single collection (i.e. one house in one locality).

Egg viability

The eggs were considered as non-viable (NV) if no hatching occurred after 45 days of development. Egg viability (%) was assessed for each species as the ratio of total hatched eggs over total laid eggs. We also estimated the average number of eggs obtained by female per day, and the development time of the four species.

Morphometric analyses of eggs

As described in Santillán-Guayasamín et al. [32], the eggs were photographed one by one at the same developmental stage and exactly the same position using a MiScope-MIP (www.zarbeco.com) on a platform. The developmental stage was identified by (i) the number of days of embryonic development at photography day and (ii) the presence of visible, darker eye-spots in the anterior operculum zone. The photography day is different between species because of the genus-specific development time. *Panstrongylus* eggs were photographed at the 25 days of development, *Triatoma* eggs at 20–23 days, and *Rhodnius* eggs at 10 days of development [32].

Eggs of the Triatomini tribe were photographed in ventral position while those of the Rhodniini tribe were photographed in lateral position [32]. The viability status of the eggs was checked after the photographs were taken (days 20–25 for Triatomini, or day 10 for Rhodniini). After this step the NV eggs could be observed developing a progressive deflation-like deformation and/or lacking some obvious development signals (i.e. eye-spots) (Fig. 2).

Morphometric approaches

We applied two different geometric approaches: the outline-based morphometrics for the complete contour of the egg, and the landmark/semilandmark-based morphometrics for the contour of the operculum (Additional file 1: Table S1) [32]. Both approaches included two main steps: (i) extraction of size and shape variables, which is specific to the technique used, and (ii) discrimination using final shape variables.

Egg contour

For shape variable definition, we exclusively used the elliptic Fourier analysis (EFA) [39]. Briefly, the observed contour is decomposed in terms of sine and cosine curves of successive frequencies called harmonics, and each harmonic is described by four coefficients. With this method, the first harmonic ellipse parameters are used to normalize the elliptic Fourier (NEF) coefficients so that they are invariant to size, rotation, and the starting position of the outline trace. By doing this, the three first coefficients become constant (1, 0 and 0) and are not used in the remaining analyses. The fourth coefficient, the one related to the width-on-length ratio of the outline, has been used in our study. The EFA algorithm does not require the points to be equidistant, nor does it require them to be in the same number [40]. The square root of the internal area of the contour (sqrA) and the perimeter of the contour (Per) were computed to estimate the size of the complete egg. For

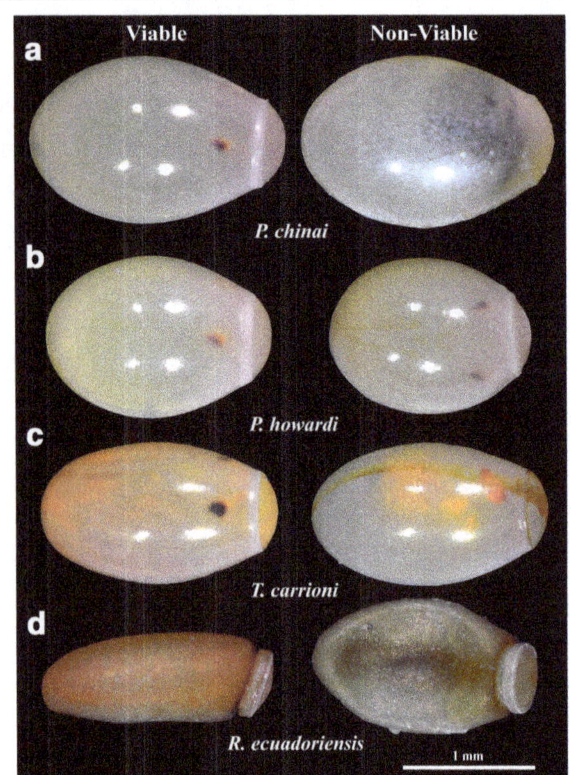

Fig. 2 Egg viability. Examples of viable (left) and non-viable (right) eggs of *Panstrongylus chinai*, *P. howardi*, *Triatoma carrioni* and *Rhodnius ecuadoriensis*. The non-viable eggs show eggs with yolk only (lacking of obvious development signals, as in *P. chinai*) (**a**); embryo in normal development (as in *P. howardi*) (**b**); embryo with malformations (development alteration, as in *T. carrioni*) (**c**) or a deflation-like deformation after 25 days of development (as in *R. ecuadoriensis*) (**d**). *Abbreviations*: *P*, *Panstrongylus*; *T*, *Triatoma*; *R*, *Rhodnius*

each species, the linear correlation coefficient (r) was computed between these two estimates of size (sqrA and Per).

To accurately represent a closed curve, many harmonics are needed, each one with four coefficients, so that the number of variables would be too numerous relative to the number of individuals. The normalized coefficients (NEF) were thus submitted to a principal component analysis (PCA), and the principal components (PC) or a reduced set of first PC were the final shape variables. This procedure allows for reducing the number of input variables (PC) where necessary.

Operculum shape

We used 2 unambiguous landmarks for the Triatomini eggs and 4 unambiguous landmarks for the *Rhodnius* eggs. Between landmarks, we additionally used 8 semilandmarks to capture the external, curved line of the operculum, and 4 to trace the curved boundary between egg and operculum in both types of eggs.

All landmarks and semilandmarks were submitted to partial Procrustes superimposition [41] and semilandmarks then subjected to a sliding procedure [42, 43]. The tangent space orthogonal projections [44] of the aligned configurations were used as input for a principal components analysis (PCA), and the principal components (PC) or a set of first PC were retained as final shape variables. The centroid size (CS) was estimated as the square root of the sum of the squared distances between the center of the landmarks configuration and each individual landmark [45].

Statistical comparisons

We compared the different species using either the V eggs, NV eggs, or both, and within each species we also compared V and NV eggs. All statistical comparisons considered separately the metric properties (size and shape) of the complete egg and those of the operculum only.

Size comparisons

Statistical comparisons of sizes were based on non-parametric, permutation-based tests (1000 cycles) with statistical significance estimated after Bonferroni correction. Using estimates of size, a validated classification procedure was applied based on the maximum likelihood method [36] between either different species or between V eggs and NV eggs.

Shape-based discrimination

For the egg contour, each pairwise Mahalanobis distance between groups was computed using the first 32 principal components (PC) of the normalized elliptic Fourier coefficients. For the operculum, Mahalanobis distance was computed using the PC of the tangent space variables. Statistical significance was based on non-parametric, permutation-based tests (1000 cycles), and submitted to the Bonferroni correction. The validated reclassification derived from shape was based on the Mahalanobis distances using PC as input. The latter were used to build an unweighted pair-group method with arithmetic average (UPGMA) tree, using as operating taxonomic units (OTUs) the four species subdivided according to V eggs and NV eggs.

We compared the variance of shape (also called metric disparity, MD) between species as well as between V eggs and NV eggs. It was computed as the trace of the variance-covariance matrix of the final shape variables of each group. Statistical significance of comparisons between MD was based on bootstrap tests (5000 runs) as described by Zelditch et al. [20].

Contribution of size to shape-based discrimination

The contribution of size variation to shape variation was estimated through the determination coefficient between the estimator of size and the first shape-derived discriminant factor.

Software

Collection of landmarks/semilandmarks and pseudolandmarks on eggs, as well as image digitalization and statistical methods (EFA, Procrustes superposition, multivariate analyses) were performed using the CLIC package (http://xyom-clic.eu/). The UPGMA tree was constructed using the *ape* R package (http://ape-package.ird.fr/).

Results

The primary aim of our study was to evaluate the possible effects of egg viability on the morphometric discrimination between species. The results of this study were divided into: (i) interspecific discriminations, where we checked the influence of NV eggs on species discrimination; and (ii) intraspecific comparison, where we explored possible morphometric differences between viable (V) and non-viable (NV) eggs of the four species.

Egg viability

The highest developmental time of the eggs was observed in *P. chinai* (30.15 ± 1.13 days), while the lowest time was scored for *R. ecuadoriensis* (18.22 ± 0.94 days). The eggs laid per female varied from 83 (*P. howardi*) to 144 (*P. chinai*) depending on the species. The percentage of V eggs from females reared in the laboratory was lower (from 42 to 79%) than for the field collected eggs (88% for *T. carrioni*) (Table 2).

Interspecific discrimination by size

Since the contour of the egg is smooth, the estimations of size such as the perimeter and the square root of area were correlated with generally high scores (r = 92%, r = 88% and r = 75% for *Panstrongylus* spp., *T carrioni* and *R. ecuadoriensis*, respectively; $P < 0.001$), we thus restricted our size estimator to the square root of the egg area (sqrA).

For all comparisons (V, NV and both), *R. ecuadoriensis* was the species with smallest eggs, while *P. chinai* harbored the largest ones. The size of the operculum did not show a strict parallelism with the whole egg, since the largest operculum was observed for *P. howardi*, not for *P. chinai* (Table 3, Fig. 3). Almost all the pairwise comparisons of size between species were found to be significant ($P < 0.001$).

For the complete egg contour, the variance of size did not show any significant difference between species (P ranging between 0.994–0.100). However, for the operculum, in three pairwise comparisons the variance of size showed significant interspecific difference: (i) between *P. chinai* and *P. howardi* for the total sample and for the NV eggs (P = 0.004 and P = 0.007, respectively); (ii) between V eggs of *P. chinai* and *T. carrioni* (P = 0.002); and (iii) between NV eggs of *P. howardi* and *T. carrioni* (P = 0.015) (Table 4).

On average, mixing V eggs and NV eggs, species were weakly separated by the size of the egg contour (72%) or by the size of the operculum (65%). Opposite trends between the egg contour and the operculum could be observed when taking into account egg viability to distinguish species (Table 5).

Interspecific discrimination by shape

All pairwise interspecific comparisons of shape (of either eggs or operculum) were highly significant (permutation test, 1000 cycles, $P < 0.001$). For the egg contour, the values of Mahalanobis distances between V eggs were higher than between NV eggs, with an increase going from 42 up to 85%. An opposite trend was observed for the distances derived from the operculum shape. When considering the total sample mixing V eggs and NV eggs, the Mahalanobis distances showed intermediate values.

For all the interspecific comparisons (using V, NV or both kinds of eggs), the reclassification scores obtained from the contour of the whole egg (95%, on average) were better than those obtained from the operculum (71%, on average) (Table 5).

As for size, opposite results between egg contour and operculum shape were observed when distinguishing species using either V eggs or NV eggs. For the egg contour, reclassification scores and Mahalanobis distances were negatively affected when we included the NV eggs in the analysis; for the operculum, however, the reclassification improved when we included NV eggs (Table 5).

The UPGMA tree based on the external contour of the eggs showed (i) complete separation between tribes (Rhodniini and Triatomini); (ii) notable difference between genera of the tribe Triatomini (*Panstrongylus*

Table 2 For each species: time of development in days, average number of eggs per female per day, number of hatched eggs per female per month, and percentage of viable eggs

Species	Developmental time (days)	Eggs laid/female/day[a]	Eggs hatched	% Viability
P. c.	30.15 ± 1.13	4.79 (144)	114	79.17
P. h.	28.99 ± 1.38	2.78 (83)	35	42.17
T. c.	25.00 ± 0.79	3.77 (113)	99	87.61
R. e.	18.22 ± 0.94	3.71 (111)	81	72.97

Abbreviations: *P.c. Panstrongylus chinai, P.h. P. howardi, T.c. Triatoma carrioni, R.e. Rhodnius ecuadoriensis*

[a]Average number of eggs per female per day, computed from the monthly record of eggs (value in parentheses)

Table 3 Mean values of size and standard deviation of the complete egg contour (square root of the area within the egg boundary) and of its operculum (centroid size of the operculum) for viable eggs (V), non-viable eggs (NV) and both

Species		V	NV	*P*-value*	V + NV
P. c.	Egg	1.34 ± 0.04^{a}	1.36 ± 0.05^{a}	0.089	1.35 ± 0.04^{a}
	Operculum	0.74 ± 0.03^{e}	0.74 ± 0.03^{d}	0.834	0.74 ± 0.03^{d}
P. h.	Egg	1.27 ± 0.03^{b}	1.27 ± 0.04^{b}	0.722	1.26 ± 0.04^{b}
	Operculum	0.77 ± 0.03^{f}	0.80 ± 0.05^{e}	<0.001	0.78 ± 0.04^{e}
T. c.	Egg	1.21 ± 0.03^{c}	1.26 ± 0.04^{b}	0.000	1.22 ± 0.04^{c}
	Operculum	0.70 ± 0.02^{g}	0.71 ± 0.03^{f}	0.219	0.70 ± 0.02^{f}
R. e.	Egg	1.09 ± 0.03^{d}	1.09 ± 0.04^{c}	0.605	1.09 ± 0.04^{d}
	Operculum	0.74 ± 0.02^{h}	0.73 ± 0.03	0.678	–

Abbreviations: *P. c. Panstrongylus chinai*, *P. h. P. howardi*, *T. c. Triatoma carrioni*, *R. e. Rhodnius ecuadoriensis*

**P*-values, statistical significance for the comparison of mean sizes between V eggs and NV eggs. If means are different between species, the superscripts (a-h) show different letters. These letters must be read within each column, not between columns. Mean and standard deviation are expressed in millimeters

and *Triatoma*); (iii) distinction between species, either for V eggs or NV eggs; and (iv) a constant clustering of V eggs and NV eggs together. On the other hand, the UPGMA tree based on the operculum shape could not produce interspecific relationships in accordance with known phylogenetic relationships when NV eggs were included. For the operculum, the viability status of eggs could affect the representation of interspecific relatedness (Fig. 4).

Comparisons of size between viable (V) and non-viable (NV) eggs

The sqrA for NV eggs of *P. chinai* or *T. carrioni* showed larger values than observed for V eggs, while no such difference was observed for the eggs of *P. howardi* or *R. ecuadoriensis*. These differences in size

Table 4 Variance of size and variance of shape for the egg contour and for the operculum

Species	Viability	Egg, variance		Operculum, variance	
		Size	Shape	Size	Shape
P. c.	V	0.0015^{a}	0.00017^{a,b}	0.0010^{a}	0.0016^{a}
	NV	0.0022^{b}	0.00062^{d}	0.0008^{c}	0.0040^{c}
	*P**	0.4360	0.00000	0.427	0.0000
	V + NV	0.0018^{c}	0.00035^{f}	0.0009^{e}	0.0026^{e}
P. h.	V	0.0008^{a}	0.00017^{a}	0.0012^{a}	0.0025^{a}
	NV	0.0019^{b}	0.00026^{e}	0.0023^{d}	0.0024^{d}
	*P**	0.0010	0.02900	0.046	0.4160
	V + NV	0.0013^{c}	0.00021^{e}	0.0019^{f}	0.0025^{f}
T. c.	V	0.0008^{a}	0.00012^{b}	0.0004^{b}	0.0010^{b}
	NV	0.0019^{b}	0.00029^{e}	0.0007^{c}	0.0028^{c,d}
	*P**	0.1480	0.00200	0.157	0.0000
	V + NV	0.0017^{c}	0.00019^{e}	0.0005^{e}	0.0022^{g}
R. e.	V	0.0011^{a}	0.00034^{c}	0.0004	0.0009
	NV	0.0014^{b}	0.00045^{d}	0.0008	0.0011
	*P**	0.6120	0.03800	0.2370	0.1430
	V + NV	0.0012^{c}	0.00037^{f}		

Abbreviations: *P. c. Panstrongylus chinai*, *P. h. P. howardi*, *T. c. Triatoma carrioni*, *R. e. Rhodnius ecuadoriensis*, *V* viable, *NV* non-viable

**P*, statistical significance of the comparison between V eggs and NV eggs for either the variance of size or the variance of shape. Except for *P*, values are variances of either size or shape, for either the egg contour or the operculum. For the egg contour, size was the square root of the area within the egg boundary and shape was the normalized elliptic Fourier coefficients. For the operculum, size was the centroid size and shape was estimated by the tangent space orthogonal projections (see Methods). The variance of shape was computed as the trace of the variance-covariance matrix (see Methods). Different superscripts (a-f) between species indicate significant difference between species. These letters must be read within each column, not between columns. Variance of size is expressed in millimeters

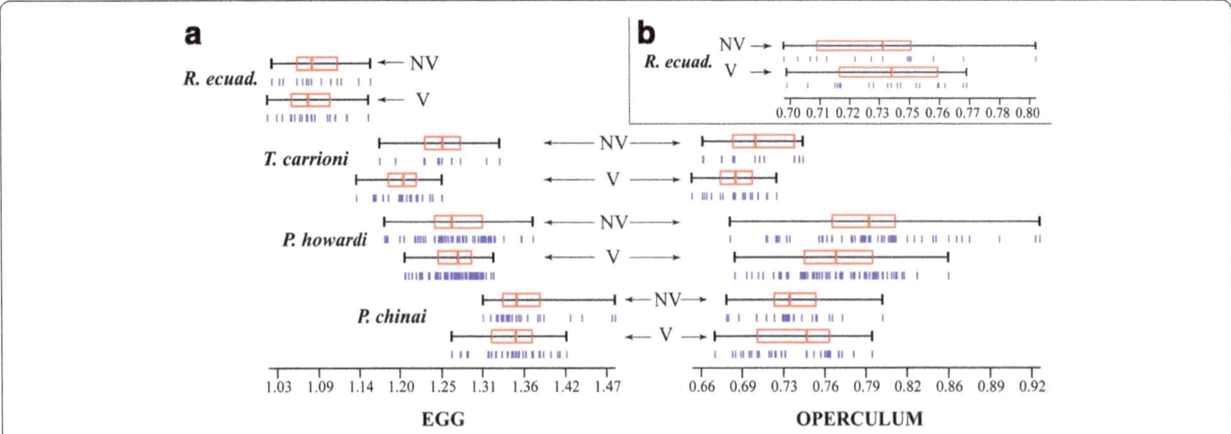

Fig. 3 Size variation of egg and operculum. **a** Differences between *Panstrongylus chinai, P. howardi, Triatoma carrioni* and *Rhodnius ecuadoriensis*. **b** Differences in operculum size between V eggs and NV eggs of *R. ecuadoriensis*. All values are expressed in millimeters. *Abbreviations*: *P*, *Panstrongylus*; *T*, *Triatoma*; *R. ecuad.*, *Rhodnius ecuadoriensis*; V, viable; NV, non-viable

Table 5 Percentages of correctly assigned species (ratios between parentheses) for viable eggs (V), non-viable eggs (NV) and both, using either size or shape, egg contour or operculum

Species		Egg			Operculum		
		% V	% NV	% V + NV	% V	% NV	% V + NV
P. c.	Si	82 (28/34)	95 (21/22)	87 (49/56)	35 (12/34)	59 (13/22)	45 (25/56)
	Sh	100 (34/34)	73 (16/22)	87 (49/56)	56 (19/34)	64 (14/22)	62 (35/56)
P. h.	Si	72 (48/67)	38 (21/55)	61 (74/122)	64 (43/67)	84 (46/55)	71 (87/122)
	Sh	96 (64/67)	93 (51/55)	98 (119/122)	66 (44/67)	80 (44/55)	75 (92/122)
T. c.	Si	81 (17/21)	50 (6/12)	70 (23/33)	76 (16/21)	75 (9/12)	76 (25/33)
	Sh	100 (21/21)	100 (12/12)	97 (32/33)	76 (16/21)	42 (5/12)	70 (23/33)
R. e.	Si	95 (18/19)	93 (13/14)	91 (30/33)	–	–	–
	Sh	100 (19/19)	100 (14/14)	100 (33/33)	–	–	–
Global	Si	79 (111/141)	59 (61/103)	72 (176/244)	58 (71/122)	76 (68/89)	65 (137/211)
	Sh	98 (138/141)	90 (93/103)	95 (233/244)	65 (79/122)	71 (63/89)	71 (150/211)

Abbreviations: *P. c. Panstrongylus chinai*, *P. h. P. howardi*, *T. c. Triatoma carrioni*, *R. e. Rhodnius ecuadoriensis*, *Si* size, *Sh* shape, *Global* total scores across species

between V eggs and NV eggs were generally not statistically significant, except for *T. carrioni* ($P < 0.001$). Considering the operculum only, the size did not significantly vary between groups, except for *P. howardi* where the NV eggs showed larger values ($P < 0.001$) (Table 3). Thus, larger eggs, or eggs with larger operculum, were found more frequently in NV groups, although this trend was not systematically significant.

On the other hand, the variance of egg size showed larger values in NV eggs, although it was significant only for *P. howardi* ($P = 0.001$) (Table 4). Looking at the distribution of sizes (Fig. 3), NV eggs tended to have extreme sizes, either very small or very large, a pattern particularly obvious for *P. howardi*. Similar trends (excepting *P. chinai*, Table 4) which were not significant and less apparent, were observed also for the operculum (Fig. 3).

The validated reclassification of V eggs and NV eggs, based on egg or operculum size, showed relatively low scores on average (between 42–76% and 39–64%, respectively) (Table 6).

Comparisons of shape between viable (V) and non-viable (NV) eggs

In Triatomini ("neck-less eggs"), the V eggs tended to be more slender (Fig. 5); this trend was statistically significant only in *P. howardi* ($P = 0.008$). For *R. ecuadoriensis*, the V eggs did not necessarily present a narrower form, but they showed a relatively wider neck than NV eggs (Fig. 5).

The operculum exhibited significant shape difference between V eggs and NV eggs. The shape change was located at the curved limit between the egg and the operculum (Fig. 5). It was statistically significant in *P. chinai*, *P. howardi* and *T. carrioni* ($P = 0.012$, $P = 0.014$ and $P = 0.013$, respectively); however, it was not significant for the Rhodniini ($P = 0.165$).

The reclassification scores between V eggs and NV eggs based on the contour of the whole eggs were lower (between 45–67%) than the ones based on the operculum (between 59–73%) (Table 6). In all species, the metric disparity (MD, variance of shape) of the NV egg contour was significantly larger (1.5 to 3.7 times larger) than the one of V eggs (*P* ranging

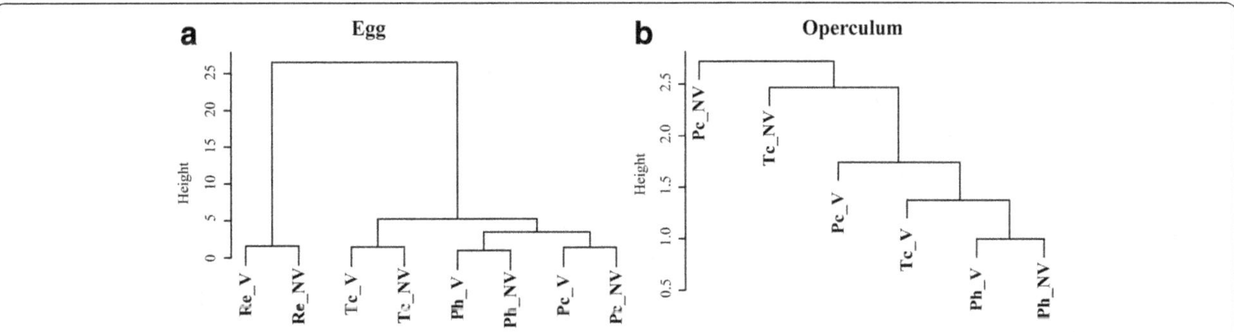

Fig. 4 UPGMA phenogram based on shape variation. **a** UPGMA tree inferred from shape of the contour of the complete egg of *Panstrongylus chinai*, *P. howardi*, *Triatoma carrioni* and *Rhodnius ecuadoriensis*. **b** UPGMA tree derived from operculum shape of *P. chinai*, *P. howardi*, and *T. carrioni*. *Abbreviations*: Re, *Rhodnius ecuadoriensis*; Tc, *Triatoma carrioni*; Ph, *Panstrongylus howardi*; Pc, *P. chinai*; V, viable eggs; NV, non-viable eggs

Table 6 For each species, validated reclassification scores between viable (V) and non-viable eggs (NV)

Species		Egg			Operculum		
		% V	% NV	Global (%)	% V	% NV	Global (%)
P. c.	Si	56 (19/34)	45 (10/22)	52	85 (29/34)	32 (7/22)	64
	Sh	67 (23/34)	59 (13/22)	64	72 (24/34)	55 (12/22)	64
P. h.	Si	8 (5/67)	95 (52/55)	47	55 (37/67)	73 (40/55)	63
	Sh	70 (47/67)	64 (35/55)	67	60 (40/67)	58 (32/55)	59
T. c.	Si	71 (15/21)	83 (10/12)	76	33 (7/21)	50 (6/12)	39
	Sh	71 (15/21)	50 (6/12)	64	86 (18/21)	50 (6/12)	73
R. e.	Si	47 (9/19)	36 (5/14)	42	21 (4/19)	71 (10/14)	42
	Sh	42 (8/19)	50 (7/14)	45	68 (13/19)	50 (7/14)	61
Total	Si	34 (48/141)	75 (77/103)	54	55 (77/141)	61 (63/103)	57
	Sh	66 (93/141)	59 (61/103)	62	67 (95/141)	55 (56/103)	63

The reclassification method was based on either size (Si) or shape (Sh), separately. Validated classification, i.e. the percent of correctly assigned individuals (ratio in parentheses)

Abbreviations: *Si* size, *Sh* shape, *P. c. Panstrongylus chinai*, *P. h. P. howardi*, *T. c. Triatoma carrioni*, *R. e. Rhodnius ecuadoriensis*, *Global* total scores

between 0.038– < 0.001). For the operculum, the MD of NV eggs was larger, although statistically significant only in *P. chinai* and *T. carrioni* ($P < 0.001$ for both species) (Table 4).

Except for the operculum of *P. howardi* (20%), the influence of size variation on shape distinction was low, both for the egg and the operculum (from 0.3 to 6.9%).

Discussion

This study is motivated by the need for a more precise taxonomic identification of some potential vectors whatever the stage of development available, either adult, nymph or egg. We focused here on the taxonomic interest of eggs according to their viability. The use of eggs is relevant because, in some cases, only eggs (and nymphs) are found in human dwellings [46], and eggs were recently shown to be highly discriminant between species and populations [32, 36].

The diversification of egg morphology among species of the Triatominae is likely to be primarily under genetic determinism. However, various environmental and artefactual causes could interfere with species divergence. Among them, in addition to the developmental stages and the position of the egg [32], we could cite the sampling conditions (time and place of collection), the mother age, the source of blood of the genitors and their feeding frequency, and the origin of the colonies (parents from laboratory colonies or from the field) [47–52]. These factors primarily affect the size of organisms; for this reason the morphometric distinction between taxa was based on shape variation, not on size variation, even if shape distinction was not completely free of some residual size influence (allometric residue). Moreover, these confusing factors were tentatively ruled out here by selecting controlled laboratory conditions (except for *T. carrioni*) and, for each species, by selecting new-molted genitors coming not only from the same locality, but also from the same house.

In these conditions, we could focus better on another possible interference: egg viability. At the time of development as selected by Santillán-Guayasamín et al. [32] to capture egg morphometric data in the best conditions, it is not possible to predict the future of each egg: viable (V) and non-viable (NV) eggs are mixed. Our study tries to estimate the effect of egg viability on its metric properties. Even with a relatively low number of female genitors (eight per species), it was possible to detect some trends.

We observed the highest percentage of viability for the eggs laid by field females (see *T. carrioni*, Table 2). The eggs of females that spent a few generations in the laboratory showed lower viability scores, especially for the females transported from a very different natural environment (see *P. howardi*, Table 2).

The hatching success scores used in this study provided only a partial indication of fitness. However, our study was not designed to understand the causes of egg viability, rather its protocol was set up to describe, and possibly to understand, any association with modified metric properties. Our main question was: could the viability status of the egg affect its morphology to such an extent that species distinction was compromised? We also checked whether there was any typical difference in the size and in the shape of V eggs and NV eggs.

Using V eggs only, the shape of the complete contour could recognize almost perfectly (98%) the four species, while the interspecific comparisons limited to NV eggs or mixing both kinds of eggs reached a consistently lower score (90 and 95%, respectively). For the operculum, the shape was not highly discriminant between species. Unexpectedly, the inclusion of NV eggs in the

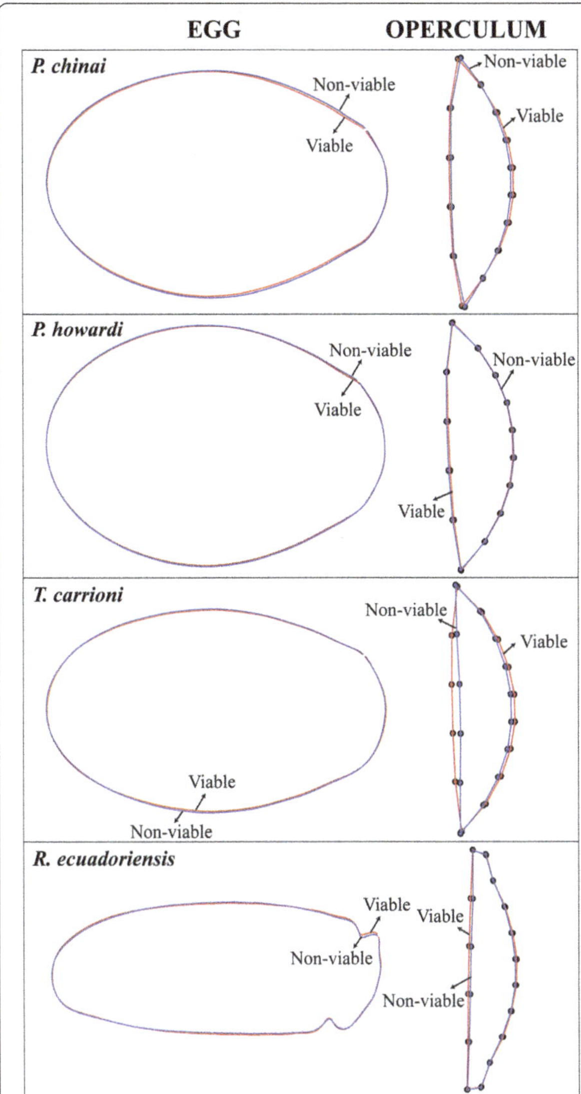

Fig. 5 Egg and operculum shape. On the left: egg shape differences between outlines of V eggs and NV eggs of *Panstrongylus chinai*, *P. howardi*, *Triatoma carrioni* and *Rhodnius ecuadoriensis*. In the tribe Triatomini, the shape of V eggs tend to be more slender. On the right: difference in operculum shape between V eggs and NV eggs of *P. chinai*, *P. howardi*, *T. carrioni* and *R. ecuadoriensis*. *Abbreviations*: *P*, *Panstrongylus*; *T*, *Triatoma*; *R*, *Rhodnius*

discrimination increased the classification scores between species.

Thus, in spite of variation according to species, our data suggest that the viability of eggs could modify the interspecific discrimination. Although there were differences in egg shape and size between V eggs and NV eggs, it was not possible to accurately recognize them. When based on shape, the operculum or the complete egg contour produced similar but low reclassification scores between V and NV eggs (62 and 63%, respectively; see Table 6). When based on size, the reclassification scores were lower than those based on shape (54 and 57%, respectively, on average).

The difference in size between V eggs and NV eggs could be related to the consumption of yolk during the development [53, 54], or to an insufficient amount of yolk provided by the mother [49]. In that case, size modification would be the consequence of pathological changes in the egg development. However, physical properties of eggs may also influence their viability by altering resistance to tensile stresses and thus to breakage [55], or by modifying gas exchange (O_2, CO_2 and water vapor) between the environment and the developing embryo [56].

The variation in egg size probably reflects adaptive processes for each species in response to environmental heterogeneity [57, 58]. In this regard, our observations could suggest that there is an optimal phenotype for the size. Indeed, the distribution of operculum and egg size between V eggs and NV eggs supported the idea that the eggs of *P. chinai*, *T. carrioni* and *R. ecuadoriensis* could be subject to directional selection in which smaller individuals had a higher probability of surviving than larger ones. However, the eggs of *P. howardi* were apparently subject to stabilizing selection, where either large or small eggs suffered a higher risk of death than eggs of intermediate size [59, 60]. If confirmed, these features would represent another distinction between the very close species *P. chinai* and *P. howardi* (Villacís et al., in prep.).

Conclusions

To distinguish between species, size did not prove to be a good discriminant character for either the operculum or complete egg. Regarding shape, using either V eggs or NV eggs, the operculum did not appear to be a reliable source for interspecific recognition (65 and 71% of correct assignments, respectively). The complete contour of the egg provided much more satisfactory species classification (95% of correct assignments, on average), with better scores comparing V (98%) than NV (90%) eggs. Thus, species recognition by the complete contour of the egg was very high. We showed that it was affected by the viability status of the egg. A constant metric change from V to NV eggs observed for all species was a larger variance of size and shape in the NV group. For all species, larger eggs, or eggs with larger operculum, were found more frequently in the NV group, suggesting that an optimum phenotype could be found preferably among intermediate or small sizes, presenting a less globular shape in the Triatomini, or a relatively wider neck in *R. ecuadoriensis*. However, it was not possible to use the metric properties to perform an accurate prediction about egg viability.

Abbreviations

CS: Centroid size; EFA: Elliptic Fourier analysis; MD: Metric disparity; NEF: Normalized elliptic Fourier; NV: Non-viable; OTUs: Operating taxonomic units; PC: Principal component; PCA: Principal components analysis; sqrA: Square root of the internal area of the contour; UPGMA: Unweighted pair-group method with arithmetic average; V: Viable

Acknowledgments

Special thanks to the inhabitants of the visited communities and the personnel of the National Chagas Control Program from the Ministry of Health of Ecuador who participated in the collection of the triatomines. Technical assistance was provided by Julio Sánchez-Otero and César Yumiseva from the Pontifical Catholic University of Ecuador (PUCE). English editing was provided by Lori Lammert.

Funding

Financial support was received from the Pontifical Catholic University of Ecuador (E13037, G13042, J13066, L13254 and M13480), the National Institutes of Health, Fogarty International Center, Global Infectious Disease Training Grant (1D43TW008261-01A1), and the National Institute of Allergy and Infectious Diseases, Division of Microbiology and Infectious Diseases, Academic Research Enhancement Award (1R15AI077896-01).

Authors' contributions

SSG participated in the conception and design of the study, the collection of field specimens in 2015, the acquisition and digitization of pictures, the making and design of the figures, the analysis and interpretation of data and the writing of the paper. AGV participated in the conception and design of the study, the collection of field specimens between 2005 and 2015, and the writing of the manuscript. MJG participated in the collection of field specimens between 2005 and 2015, and the revision of the manuscript. JPD participated in the design of the study, the development of the computer software, the analysis and interpretation of data and the writing of the paper. All authors read and approved the final manuscript.

Competing interests

The authors declare that they have no competing interests.

Author details

[1]Center for Research on Health in Latin America (CISeAL), School of Biological Sciences, Pontifical Catholic University of Ecuador, Calle Pambahacienda s/n y San Pedro del Valle, Campus Nayón, Quito, Ecuador. [2]Infectious and Tropical Disease Institute, Department of Biomedical Sciences, Heritage College of Osteopathic Medicine, Ohio University, Athens, OH 45701, USA. [3]IRD, UMR 177 IRD-CIRAD INTERTRYP, Campus international de Baillarguet, Montpellier, France.

References

1. Mendonça VJ, Alevi KCC, Pinotti H, Gurgel-Gonçalves R, Pita S, Guerra AL, et al. Revalidation of *Triatoma bahiensis* Sherlock & Serafim, 1967 (Hemiptera: Reduviidae) and phylogeny of the *T. brasiliensis* species complex. Zootaxa. 2016;4107:239–54.
2. Souza dos SE, Von Atzingen NCB, Furtado MB, de Oliveira J, Nascimento JD, Vendrami DP, et al. Description of *Rhodnius marabaensis* sp. n. (Hemiptera, Reduviidade, Triatominae) from Pará State, Brazil. ZooKeys. 2016;621:45–62.
3. de Oliveira J, Ayala JM, Justi SA, de Rosa JA, Galvão C. Description of a new species of *Nesotriatoma* Usinger, 1944 from Cuba and revalidation of synonymy between *Nesotriatoma bruneri* (Usinger, 1944) and *N. flavida* (Neiva, 1911). J Vector Ecol. 2018;43:148–57.
4. Abad-Franch F, Paucar A, Carpio C, Cuba CA, Aguilar HM, Miles MA. Biogeography of Triatominae (Hemiptera: Reduviidae) in Ecuador: Implications for the design of control strategies. Mem Inst Oswaldo Cruz. 2001;96:611–20.
5. Grijalva MJ, Villacís AG. Presence of *Rhodnius ecuadoriensis* in sylvatic habitats in the southern highlands (Loja Province) of Ecuador. J Med Entomol. 2009;46:708–11.
6. Quinde-Calderón L, Rios-Quituizaca P, Solorzano L, Dumonteil E. Ten years (2004–2014) of Chagas disease surveillance and vector control in Ecuador: successes and challenges. Trop Med Int Health. 2016;21:84–92.
7. Grijalva MJ, Villacís AG, Ocaña-Mayorga S, Yumiseva CA, Moncayo AL, Baus EG. Comprehensive survey of domiciliary triatomine species capable of transmitting Chagas disease in southern Ecuador. PLoS Negl Trop Dis. 2015; 9:e0004142.
8. Patterson JS, Barbosa SE, Feliciangeli MD. On the genus *Panstrongylus* Berg 1879: evolution, ecology and epidemiological significance. Acta Trop. 2009; 110:187–99.
9. Barrett TV. Advances in triatomine bug ecology in relation to Chagas disease. In: Harris KF, editor. Advances in Disease Vector Research. New York: Springer-Verlag; 1991. p. 143–76.
10. Grijalva MJ, Palomeque-Rodríguez F, Costales JA, Davila S, Arcos-Teran L. High household infestation rates by synanthropic vectors of Chagas disease in southern Ecuador. J Med Entomol. 2005;42:68–74.
11. Mosquera KD, Villacís AG, Grijalva MJ. Life cycle, feeding, and defecation patterns of *Panstrongylus chinai* (Hemiptera: Reduviidae: Triatominae) under laboratory conditions. J Med Entomol. 2016;53:776–81.
12. Villacís AG, Ocaña-Mayorga S, Lascano MS, Yumiseva CA, Baus EG, Grijalva MJ. Abundance, natural infection with trypanosomes, and food source of an endemic species of triatomine, *Panstrongylus howardi* (Neiva 1911), on the Ecuadorian Central Coast. Am J Trop Med Hyg. 2015;92:187–92.
13. Pinto CM, Ocaña-Mayorga S, Lascano MS, Grijalva MJ. Infection by trypanosomes in marsupials and rodents associated with human dwellings in Ecuador. J Parasitol. 2006;92:1251–5.
14. Suarez-Davalos V, Dangles O, Villacís AG, Grijalva MJ. Microdistribution of sylvatic triatomine populations in central-coastal Ecuador. J Med Entomol. 2010;47:80–8.
15. Villacís AG, Grijalva MJ, Catalá SS. Phenotypic variability of *Rhodnius ecuadoriensis* populations at the ecuadorian central and southern Andean region. J Med Entomol. 2010;47:1034–43.
16. Cuba CA, Abad-Franch F, Roldán Rodríguez J, Vargas Vásquez F, Pollack Velasquez L, Miles MA. The triatomines of northern Peru, with emphasis on the ecology and infection by trypanosomes of *Rhodnius ecuadoriensis* (Triatominae). Mem Inst Oswaldo Cruz. 2002;97:175–83.
17. Grijalva MJ, Palomeque-Rodríguez F, Villacís AG, Black CL, Arcos-Teran L. Absence of domestic triatomine colonies in an area of the coastal region of Ecuador where Chagas disease is endemic. Mem Inst Oswaldo Cruz. 2010; 105:677–81.
18. Grijalva MJ, Suarez-Davalos V, Villacís AG, Ocaña-Mayorga S, Dangles O. Ecological factors related to the widespread distribution of sylvatic *Rhodnius ecuadoriensis* populations in southern Ecuador. Parasit Vectors. 2012;5:17.
19. Bookstein FL. A hundred years of morphometrics. Acta Zool Acad Sci Hung. 1998;44:7–59.
20. Adams DC, Rohlf FJ, Slice DE. Geometric morphometrics: ten years of progress following the "revolution". Ital J Zool. 2004;71:5–16.
21. Zelditch ML, Swiderski DL, Sheets HD, Fink WL. Geometric Morphometrics for Biologists: A Primer. New York: Elsevier Academic Press; 2004.

22. Murray CM, Piller KR, Merchant M, Cooper A, Easter ME. Salinity and egg shape variation: a geometric morphometric analysis. J Herpetol. 2013;47:15–23.
23. Lent H, Wygodzinsky P. Revision of the Triatominae (Hemiptera, Reduviidae), and their significance as vectors of Chagas' disease. Bull Am Mus Nat Hist. 1979;163:123–520.
24. Galvão C. Vectors of Chagas' disease in Brazil. Curitiba: Sociedade Brasileira de Zoologia; 2014.
25. Barata JMS. Aspectos morfológicos de ovos de Triatominae. Rev Saude Publica. 1981;15:490–542.
26. Monte Gonçalves TC, Jurberg J, Costa J, de Souza W. Estudio morfológico comparativo de ovos e ninfas de *Triatoma maculata* (Erichson, 1848) e *Triatoma pseudomaculata* Correa & Espinola, 1964 (Hemiptera, Reduviidae, Triatominae). Mem Inst Oswaldo Cruz. 1985;80:263–76.
27. Costa J, Barth OM, Marchon-Silva V, de Almeida CE, Freitas-Sibajev MGR, Panzera F. Morphological studies on the *Triatoma brasiliensis* Neiva, 1911 (Hemiptera, Reduviidae, Triatominae) genital structures and eggs of different chromatic forms. Mem Inst Oswaldo Cruz. 1997;92:493–8.
28. Barbosa SE, Dujardin J-P, Soares RP, Pires HH, Margonari C, Romanha AJ, et al. Interpopulation variability among *Panstrongylus megistus* (Hemiptera: Reduviidae) from Brazil. J Med Entomol. 2003;40:411–20.
29. Obara MT, Barata JMS, da Silva NN, Ceretti Júnior W, Urbinatti PR, da Rosa JA, et al. Morphologic, morphometrical, and histological aspects of the eggs of four species of the genera *Meccus* (Hemiptera, Reduviidae, Triatominae). Mem Inst Oswaldo Cruz. 2007;102:13–9.
30. Obara MT, da Rosa JA, da Silva N, Ceretti Júnior W, Urbinatti PR, Barata JMS, et al. Morphological and histological study of eggs of six species of the *Triatoma* genus (Hemiptera: Reduviidae). Neotrop Entomol. 2007;36:798–806.
31. Páez-Colasante X, Aldana E. Geometric morphometrics of the chorial rim and the collar of the eggs of five species of the *Rhodnius* genus (Heteroptera, Reduviidae, Triatominae). EntomoBrasilis. 2008;1:57–61.
32. Santillán-Guayasamín S, Villacís AG, Grijalva MJ, Dujardin J. The modern morphometric approach to identify eggs of Triatominae. Parasit Vectors. 2017;10:55.
33. Evangelista-Martínez Z, Imbert-Palafox JL, Becerril-Flores MA, Gómez-Gómez JV. Análisis morfológico de huevos de *Triatoma barberi* Usinger (Hemiptera: Reduviidae). Neotrop Entomol. 2010;39:207–13.
34. Forattini OP, Ferreira OA, da Rocha e Silva E, Rabello EX. Ecological aspects of trypanosomiasis americana. VIII. The domicile of *Panstrongylus megitus* and itsextradomiciliary presence. Rev Saude Publica. 1977;11:73–86.
35. Dujardin J-P, Slice DE. Contributions of morphometrics to medical entomology. In: Tibayrenc M, editor. Encyclopedia of Infectious Diseases: Modern Methodologies. New Jersey: Wiley & Sons, Inc.; 2007. p. 435–47.
36. Dujardin J-P, Dujardin S, Kaba D, Santillán-Guayasamín S, Villacís AG, Piyaselakul S, et al. The maximum likelihood identification method applied to insect morphometric data. Zool Syst. 2017;42:46–58.
37. Black CL, Ocaña-Mayorga S, Riner D, Costales JA, Lascano MS, Davila S, et al. Household risk factors for *Trypanosoma cruzi* seropositivity in two geographic regions of Ecuador. J Parasitol. 2007;93:12–6.
38. Grijalva MJ, Villacís AG, Ocaña-Mayorga S, Yumiseva CA, Baus EG. Limitations of selective deltamethrin application for triatomine control in central coastal Ecuador. Parasit Vectors. 2011;4:20.
39. Kuhl FP, Giardina CR. Elliptic Fourier features of a closed contour. Comput Graphics Image Process. 1982;18:236–58.
40. Rohlf FJ, Archie JW. A comparison of Fourier methods for the desciption of wing shape in mosquitoes (Diptera: Culicidae). Syst Zool. 1984;33:302–17.
41. Rohlf FJ, Slice DE. Extensions of the Procrustes method for the optimal superimposition of landmarks. Syst Zool. 1990;39:40–59.
42. Bookstein FL. Landmark methods for forms without landmarks: morphometrics of group differences in outline shape. Med Image Anal. 1997;1:225–43.
43. Gunz P, Mitteroecker P. Semilandmarks: a method for quantifying curves and surfaces. Hystrix, Ital J Mammal. 2013;24:103–9.
44. Rohlf FJ. Rotational fit (Procrustes) methods. In: Rohlf F, Bookstein F, editors. Proceedings of the Michigan Morphometrics Workshop. Ann Arbor: The University of Michigan Museum of Zoology; 1990. p. 227–36.
45. Bookstein FL. Morphometric Tools for Landmark Data: Geometry and Biology. 1st ed. New York: Cambridge University Press; 1991.
46. dos Santos CM, Jurberg J, Galvão C, da Rosa JA, Júnior WC, Barata JMS, et al. Comparative descriptions of eggs from three species of *Rhodnius* (Hemiptera: Reduviidae: Triatominae). Mem Inst Oswaldo Cruz. 2009;104:1012–8.
47. Rabinovich JE. Vital statistics of Triatominae (Hemiptera: Reduviidae) under laboratory conditions. I. *Triatoma infestans* Klug. J Med Entomol. 1972;9:351–70.
48. Karlsson B, Wiklund C. Egg weight variation in relation to egg mortality and starvation endurance of newly hatched larvae in some satyrid butterflies. Ecol Entomol. 1985;10:205–11.
49. Begon M, Parker GA. Should egg size and clutch size decrease with age? Oikos. 1986;47:293–302.
50. Crailsheim K. Trophallactic interactions in the adult honeybee (*Apis mellifera* L.). Apidologie. 1998;29:97–112.
51. Pirk CW, Neumann P, Hepburn R, Moritz RFA, Tautz J. Egg viability and worker policing in honey bees. Proc Natl Acad Sci USA. 2004;101:8649–51.
52. da Rosa JA, Justino HHG, Barata JMS. Differences in the size of eggshells among three *Pangstrongylus megistus* colonies. Rev Saude Publica. 2003;37: 528–30.
53. Atella GC, Gondim KC, Machado EA, Medeiros MN, Silva-Neto MA, Masuda H. Oogenesis and egg development in triatomines: a biochemical approach. An Acad Bras Cienc. 2005;77:405–23.
54. Santos R, Rosas-Oliveira R, Saraiva FB, Majerowicz D, Gondim KC. Lipid accumulation and utilization by oocytes and eggs of *Rhodnius prolixus*. Arch Insect Biochem Physiol. 2011;77:1–16.
55. Srivastava DP, Yu EJ, Kennedy K, Chatwin H, Reale V, Hamon M, et al. Rapid, nongenomic responses to ecdysteroids and catecholamines mediated by a novel *Drosophila* G-protein-coupled receptor. J Neurosci. 2005;25:6145–55.
56. Van Schalkwyk SJ, Brown CR, Cloete SWP. Gas exchange of the ostrich embryo during peak metabolism in relation to incubator design. South African J Anim Sci. 2002;32:122–9.
57. Einum S, Fleming IA. Maternal effects of egg size in brown trout (*Salmo trutta*): norms of reaction to environmental quality. Proc R Soc B. 1999;266: 2095–100.
58. Einum S, Fleming IA. Does within-population variation in fish egg size reflect maternal influences on optimal values? Am Nat. 2002;160:756–65.
59. Johnston RF, Niles DM, Rohwer SA. Hermon bumpus and natural selection in the house sparrow *Passer domesticus*. Evolution. 1972;26:20–31.
60. Bumpus HC. The elimination of the unfit as illustrated by the introduced sparrow, *Passer domesticus*. Biol Lect Deliv Mar Biol Lab Woods Hole. 1989; 47:209–26.

12

Zoonotic *Cryptosporidium* species and subtypes in lambs and goat kids in Algeria

Djamel Baroudi[1,2], Ahcene Hakem[3], Haileeyesus Adamu[4], Said Amer[5], Djamel Khelef[1], Karim Adjou[6], Hichem Dahmani[7], Xiaohua Chen[8], Dawn Roellig[2], Yaoyu Feng[9] and Lihua Xiao[9*]

Abstract

Background: Little is known on the occurrence and identity of *Cryptosporidium* species in sheep and goats in Algeria. This study aimed at investigating the occurrence of *Cryptosporidium* species in lambs and goat kids younger than 4 weeks.

Methods: A total of 154 fecal samples (62 from lambs and 92 from kid goats) were collected from 13 sheep flocks in Médea, Algeria and 18 goat flocks across Algiers and Boumerdes. They were screened for *Cryptosporidium* spp. by nested-PCR analysis of a fragment of the small subunit (*SSU*) rRNA gene, followed by restriction fragment length polymorphism and sequence analyses to determine the *Cryptosporidium* species present. *Cryptosporidium parvum* and *C. ubiquitum* were further subtyped by sequence analysis of the 60 kDa glycoprotein gene.

Results: *Cryptosporidium* spp. were detected in 17 fecal samples (11.0%): 9 from lambs (14.5%) and 8 from goat kids (8.7%). The species identified included *C. parvum* in 3 lambs, *C. xiaoi* in 6 lambs and 6 goat kids, and *C. ubiquitum* in 2 goat kids. *Cryptosporidium* infections were detected mostly in animals during the first two weeks of life (7/8 for goat kids and 7/9 for lambs) and in association with diarrhea occurrence (7/17 or 41.2% goat kids and 7/10 or 70.0% lambs with diarrhea were positive for *Cryptosporidium* spp.). Subtyping of *C. parvum* and *C. ubiquitum* isolates identified the zoonotic IIaA13G2R1 and XIIa subtype families, respectively. Minor differences in the *SSU* rRNA gene sequences were observed between *C. xiaoi* from sheep and goats.

Conclusions: Results of this study indicate that three *Cryptosporidium* species occur in lambs and goat kids in Algeria, including zoonotic *C. parvum* and *C. ubiquitum*. They are associated with the occurrence of neonatal diarrhea.

Keywords: *Cryptosporidium parvum*, *Cryptosporidium ubiquitum*, *Cryptosporidium xiaoi*, Goat, Sheep, Algeria

Background

Cryptosporidium spp. are common enteric protozoa of humans and a wide range of animals [1]. They are involved in numerous outbreaks of diarrheal illness in humans and pre-weaned calves [2, 3]. However, studies of *Cryptosporidium* spp. in small ruminants are much smaller in numbers compared to those in cattle, especially from developing countries [4–6]. Data accumulated thus far indicate that cryptosporidiosis in small ruminants can lead to severe diarrhea, anorexia and weight loss in goat kids and lambs [5, 7–9]. Considerably high infection rates have been reported in these animals in some areas [10–14].

Currently, over 30 *Cryptosporidium* species have been recognized based on morphological, biological and molecular characteristics (reviewed in [1]). Among them, *C. parvum*, *C. ubiquitum* and *C. xiaoi* are common species in small ruminants, although a small number of animals were reportedly infected with other *Cryptosporidium* species such as *C. andersoni* and *C. hominis* [4, 5, 14–18]. Geographical variations in the distribution of these *Cryptosporidium* spp. in small ruminants, however, have been described among the small number of studies conducted [19]. The common occurrence of zoonotic *C. parvum* and *C. ubiquitum* in goats and sheep has raised public health concerns over cryptosporidiosis. While *C.*

* Correspondence: lxiao1961@gmail.com
[9]Key Laboratory of Zoonosis of Ministry of Agriculture, College of Veterinary Medicine, South China Agricultural University, Guangzhou 510642, China
Full list of author information is available at the end of the article

parvum is well known for causing diarrhea in small ruminants, the pathogenicity of *C. ubiquitum* and *C. xiaoi* remains unclear [2].

Algeria is adopting intensive farming of small ruminants to cope with the high demand for meat and milk. A recent estimate from the Ministère De L'Agriculture et du Développement Rural indicates that the country has approximately 2,800,000 sheep and 490,000 goats (http://www.minagri.dz/contacts.html). Although *Cryptosporidium* spp. from cattle, horses, camels and chickens have been recently characterized using molecular biological tools [20–23], little information is available on the identity of *Cryptosporidium* spp. in goats and sheep. In the present study we therefore generated some preliminary data on the occurrence of *Cryptosporidium* species in goat kids and lambs in Algeria.

Methods

Collection of samples

This study was conducted between January 2012 and January 2014 on 13 sheep flocks in Ksar el Boukhari of Médea Province (No. 1), and 18 goat flocks from seven localities in the provinces of Algiers (Nos 2, 3, 4, 5) and Boumerdes (Nos 6, 7, 8) (Fig. 1). A total of 92 and 62 fecal samples were collected directly from the rectum of goat kids and lambs, respectively. Only animals aged 4 weeks or younger were sampled. Fecal consistency and demographic data on the animals were recorded at the site of sample collection. The samples were transported to the laboratory in ice boxes and preserved in 2.5% potassium dichromate at 4 °C until molecular analysis.

DNA extraction and PCR analysis

Potassium dichromate was washed off fecal samples with distilled water by centrifugation. Genomic DNA was extracted from 0.2 ml of fecal slurry without further pathogen concentration using the FastDNA SPIN Kit for Soil (BIO 101, MP Biomedicals, Carlsbad, CA, USA). DNA preparations were screened for *Cryptosporidium* spp. by using a small subunit (*SSU*) rRNA-based nested PCR, with DNA of *C. baileyi* as the positive control and reagent-grade water as the negative control. The detection limit of the approach was ~10 oocysts per gram of feces. *Cryptosporidium* species in positive PCR products were determined by restriction fragment length polymorphism (RFLP) analysis using restriction enzymes *Ssp*I and *Mbo*II as described [24] and by DNA sequencing. *Cryptosporidium parvum* and *C. ubiquitum* were subtyped by nested-PCR-sequence analysis of the *gp60* gene as previously described [25, 26].

DNA sequence analysis

To confirm the identification of *C. ubiquitum* and *C. xiaoi*, the secondary PCR products of the *SSU* rRNA gene from the two *Cryptosporidium* species were sequenced in both directions on an ABI 3130 Genetic Analyzer (Applied Biosystems, Foster City, CA, USA). The *SSU* rRNA gene products of *C. parvum* were not sequenced because it has a well-known *Ssp*I and *Mbo*II RFLP pattern. In addition, all PCR products of the *gp60* gene were sequenced to identify *C. parvum* and *C. ubiquitum* subtypes. The generated sequences were assembled using the

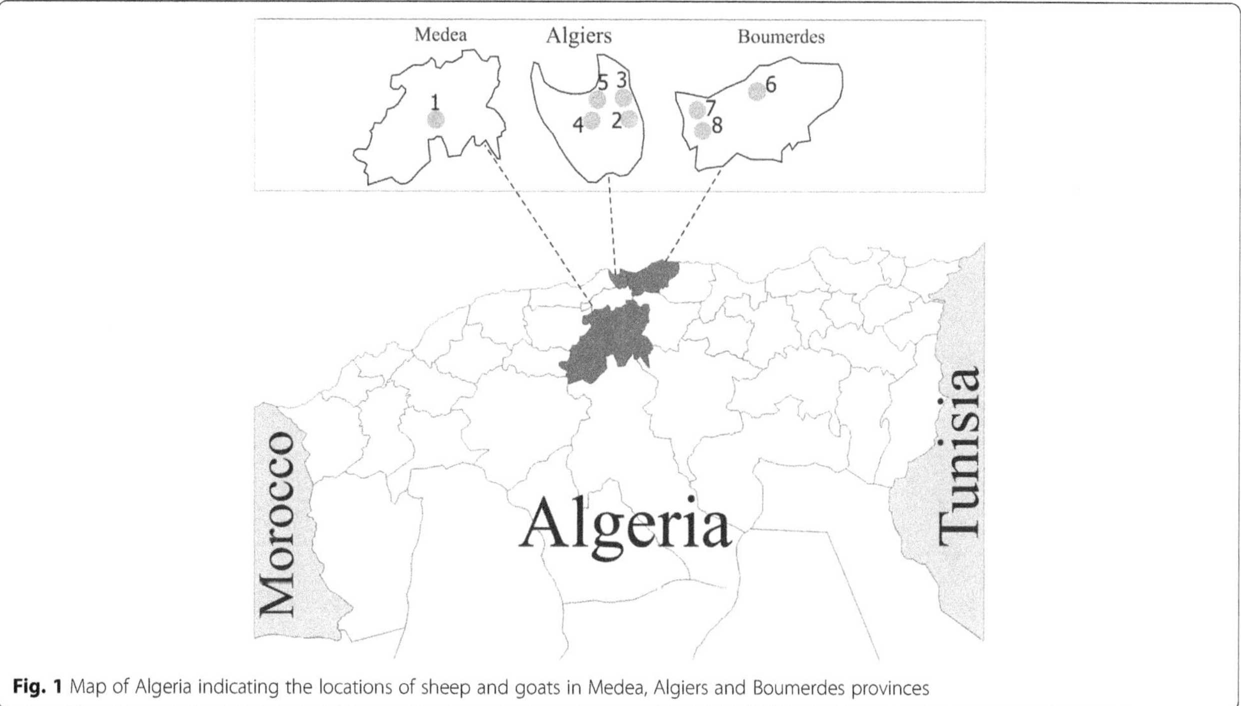

Fig. 1 Map of Algeria indicating the locations of sheep and goats in Medea, Algiers and Boumerdes provinces

ChromasPro v.1.5 software (http://www.technelysium.com.au/ChromasPro.html) and aligned with each other and reference sequences downloaded from GenBank using ClustalX (http://www.clustal.org/). Representative sequences generated in the study were submitted to GenBank under accession numbers LC414387-LC414393 for the *SSU* rRNA gene and LC414394 and JX412917 for the *gp60* gene of *C. parvum* and *C. ubiquitum*, respectively.

Statistical analysis

Cryptosporidium infection rates between diarrheic and non-diarrheic animals were compared statistically using Fisher's exact test implemented in the Statistical Package for the Social Sciences (SPSS version 22.0). Differences were considered significant at $P \leq 0.05$.

Results

Occurrence of *Cryptosporidium* spp. in goat kids and lambs

Cryptosporidium spp. were detected in 8/92 (8.7%) fecal samples from goat kids and in 9/62 (14.5%) fecal samples from lambs, with an overall infection rate of 11.0%. They were present on 3/18 goat farms and 4/9 sheep farms (Table 1). Most *Cryptosporidium*-positive samples were from animals up to 3 weeks of age with diarrhea for both goats and sheep (Table 2).

Cryptosporidium species and subtypes

The RFLP analysis of the *SSU* rDNA PCR products identified two *Cryptosporidium* species in goat kids, including *C. xiaoi* in 6 of 8 *Cryptosporidium*-positive samples and *C. ubiquitum* in 2 of 8 *Cryptosporidium*-positive samples (Fig. 2). *Cryptosporidium xiaoi* was detected in Rouiba (Algiers) and Zemouri (Boumerdes), while *C. ubiquitum* was seen in Khemis-elkhechna (Boumerdes). In lambs, *C. parvum* was present in 3 of 9 *Cryptosporidium*-positive and *C. xiaoi* was identified in the 6 of 9 *Cryptosporidium*-positive samples from Ksar-elBoukhri (Médea). DNA sequencing of *SSU* rDNA PCR products confirmed the detection of *C. ubiquitum* and *C. xiaoi* in these samples.

Data from 12 samples of *C. xiaoi* (six each from sheep and goats) generated two sequence types. The first type was represented by six sequences from sheep and was identical to one *C. xiaoi* sequence (DQ871346) first obtained from a yak in China [24]. The second sequence type was represented by six sequences from goats and was identical to one *C. xiaoi* sequence (EF362478) first obtained from a sheep in the USA [27]. There were two nucleotide differences in the partial *SSU* rRNA gene between the two sequence types (substitution of TT in the first type by CA in the second sequence type at position 420 and 421 of the reference sequence EF362478). The two sequences of the *SSU* rRNA gene fragment of *C. ubiquitum* were identical to each other and to AF442484 initially detected in lemurs in the USA [28].

Sequence analysis of the gp60 gene indicated that the three *C. parvum*-positive samples from lambs had the IIaA13G2R1 subtype, whereas the two *C. ubiquitum*-positive samples from goat kids had the XIIa subtype.

Occurrence of *Cryptosporidium* spp. by age

In goat kids, *Cryptosporidium* was detected in 2/22 (9.1%), 5/25 (20.0%), 1/27 (3.9%) and 0/18 (0%) of the animals sampled in the first, second, third and fourth week of age, respectively. In contrast, *Cryptosporidium* was detected in 3/15 (20.0%), 4/18 (22.2%), 1/13 (7.7%) and 1/16 (6.3%) lambs sampled in the first, second, third and fourth week of age, respectively. In goat kids, *C. xiaoi* was mostly seen during the first three weeks of age, with two cases (2/22; 9.1%) in the first week, three cases (3/25; 12.0%) in the second week, and one case in the third week (1/27; 3.7%). The two *C. ubiquitum* cases identified in goat kids were seen in the second week of age (2/25; 8.0%) (Table 2). In lambs, one *C. parvum* infection was detected in the first week of age (1/15; 6.7%) and the other two infections in the second week (2/18; 11.1%), while *C. xiaoi* was detected in four animals

Table 1 *Cryptosporidium* species in goat kids and lambs in Algiers, Boumerdes and Médea provinces, Algeria

Location	No. of farms	Host	No. of samples	No. positive for *Cryptosporidium* (no. of positive farms)	*Cryptosporidium* spp. (no. of samples)	Subtype (no. of samples)
Ksar-el Boukhari (Médea)	13	Sheep	62	9 (4)	*C. xiaoi* (6), *C. parvum* (3)	IIaA13G2R1(3)
Rouiba (Algiers)	3	Goats	16	3 (1)	*C. xiaoi* (3)	–
Bordj-El-Kiffan (Algiers)	2	Goats	11	0	0	–
Heraoua (Algiers)	2	Goats	9	0	0	–
Khemis-elkhechna (Boumerdes)	2	Goats	11	2 (1)	*C. ubiquitum* (2)	XIIa (2)
Hamadi (Boumerdes)	3	Goats	17	0	0	–
Zemouri (Boumerdes)	4	Goats	15	3 (1)	*C. xiaoi* (3)	–
Oued-smar (Algiers)	2	Goats	13	0	0	–
Total	31		154	17 (7)	3 species	2 subtypes

Table 2 Occurrence of *Cryptosporidium* spp. in goat kids by age and diarrhea status

Distribution	No. of samples	No. positive for *Cryptosporidium* (%)	*Cryptosporidium* spp. (no. of samples)
By age (days)			
1–7	22	2 (9.1)	*C. xiaoi* (2)
8–14	25	5 (20.0)	*C. xiaoi* (3), *C. ubiquitum* (2)
15–21	27	1 (3.7)	*C. xiaoi* (1)
22–28	18	0	
By age (days) and diarrhea status			
1–7			
Diarrheic	8	2 (25.0)	*C. xiaoi* (2)
Non-diarrheic	14	0 (0)	
8–14			
Diarrheic	9	5 (55.6)	*C. xiaoi* (3), *C. ubiquitum* (2)
Non-diarrheic	16	0 (0)	
15–21			
Diarrheic	4	1 (25.0)	*C. xiaoi* (1)
Non-diarrheic	23	0 (0)	
22–28			
Diarrheic	2	0 (0)	
Non-diarrheic	16	0 (0)	
Total	92	8 (8.7)	*C. xiaoi* (6), *C. ubiquitum* (2)

during the first two weeks (2/15; 13.3% and 2/18; 11.1, respectively) and two animals during the third and fourth weeks (1/13; 7.7% and 1/16; 6.3%, respectively) (Table 2).

Occurrence of *Cryptosporidium* spp. by diarrhea status

Altogether, 23 of the 92 fecal samples (25.0%) were collected from goat kids with diarrhea, including 8/92 (8.7%) in the first week, 9/92 (9.8%) in the second week, 4/92 (4.3 %) in the third week, and 2/92 (2.2 %) in the fourth week of age (Tables 2, 3). All *Cryptosporidium* infections in goat kids were detected in animals with diarrhea. At the first week of age, *Cryptosporidium* infection was detected in 2/8 (25.0 %) diarrheic kids, with *C. xiaoi* as the only *Cryptosporidium* species involved. At the second week of age, *Cryptosporidium* was observed in 5/9 (55.6 %) diarrheic animals, including *C. xiaoi* (3/5) and *C. ubiquitum* (2/5). At the third week of age, *Cryptosporidium* was present in 1/4 (25.0%) diarrheic ones, with the species being diagnosed as *C. xiaoi*. The occurrence of cryptosporidiosis in diarrheic goat kids (34.8%) was statistically higher compared to that in non-diarrheic (0.0%) ones (P = 0.0000001).

Among the 62 fecal samples collected from lambs, 13 (21.0 %) were from diarrheic animals, including 4 in the first week, 6 in the second week, and 3 in the third week of age. *Cryptosporidium* was detected in 3/4 (75.0%), 4/6 (66.7%) and 1/3 (33.3%) of the diarrheic lambs in the first, second and third weeks, respectively (Tables 2, 3). Among them, *C. parvum* was detected in 1/3 and 2/4 of the *Cryptosporidium*-positive samples in the first and second week, respectively. *C. xiaoi* was found in diarrheic animals up to 3 weeks of age and in non-diarrheic ones after that (Table 2). Thus, the overall infection rate in lambs was 14.5%, with the infection rate in diarrheic ones reaching 61.5% (8/13), compared with 2.0% (1/49) in non-diarrheic ones (P = 0.0000003).

Discussion

In the present study, the occurrence and genotype and subtype identity of *Cryptosporidium* spp. in goat kids and lambs in Algeria were examined. The overall infection rate of *Cryptosporidium* spp. was 11.0% (8.7% in goat kids and 14.5 % in lambs). Previous studies reported *Cryptosporidium* infection rates of 5.1–82.0% in sheep and 7.1–93.0% in goats in industrialized nations [4, 10, 14, 16, 29–35]. Few comparable data are available from

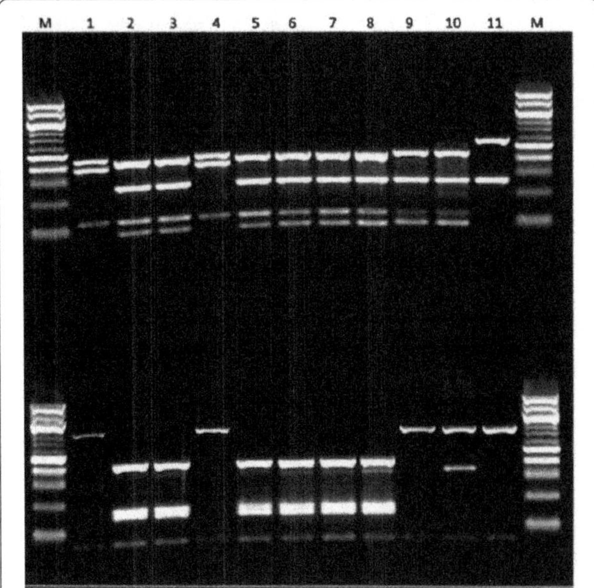

Fig. 2 Differentiation of *Cryptosporidium ubiquitum* (Lanes 1, 4), *C. xiaoi* (Lanes 2, 3, 5–8), and *C. parvum* (Lanes 9, 10) from lambs and goat kids by RFLP analysis of the *SSU* rDNA PCR products using restriction enzymes *Ssp*I (upper panel) and *Mbo*II (lower panel). Lane 11: positive control (*C. baileyi*); Lane M: 100 bp molecular markers. The extra *Mbo*II band in Lane 10 is due to the presence of a non-specific band in the PCR product

developing countries, but infection rates of 2.5–67.5 and 2.9–72.5% have been reported in sheep and goats, respectively, in Zambia, Egypt, China, Bangladesh, Iran, Argentina and México [11–13, 17, 36–41]. Variations in infection rates among studies could be attributed to the differences in animal age, diagnostic methods, sample sizes, animal management and climates.

In this study, three *Cryptosporidium* species were identified in small ruminants, including *C. parvum*, *C. xiaoi* and *C. ubiquitum*. In both goats and sheep *C. xiaoi* appeared to be the dominant species (6/8 in goats and 6/9 in sheep), with *C. ubiquitum* being detected only in two of the eight *Cryptosporidium*-positive goats and *C. parvum* in three of the nine *Cryptosporidium*-positive sheep. In concordance with this, *C. xiaoi* was detected as a dominant species in small ruminants in other African countries including Egypt [37] and Tanzania [42] as well as Asian countries such as Bangladesh [40] and China [11, 17, 41, 43]. Similarly, *C. xiaoi* was the major *Cryptosporidium* species in small ruminants in some developed countries such as France [34], Greece [18], Norway [44], Poland [14] and Australia [35, 45]. In the presence study, two types of *SSU* rDNA sequences were obtained from *C. xiaoi*, with sheep and goats having different types. Both sequence types, however, have been observed in both sheep and goats in previous studies based on BLAST analysis of GenBank sequences. As sheep and goat samples from the present study were collected from

Table 3 Occurrence of *Cryptosporidium* spp. in lambs by age and diarrhea status

Distribution	No. of samples	No. positive for *Cryptosporidium* (%)	*Cryptosporidium* spp. (no. of samples)
By age (days)			
1–7	15	3 (20.0)	*C. xiaoi* (2), *C. parvum* (1)
8–14	18	4 (22.2)	*C. xiaoi* (2), *C. parvum* (2)
15–21	13	1 (7.7)	*C. xiaoi* (1)
22–28	16	1 (6.3)	*C. xiaoi* (1)
By age (days) and diarrhea status			
1–7			
Diarrheic	4	3 (75.0)	*C. xiaoi* (2), *C. parvum* (1)
Non-diarrheic	11	0 (0)	
8–14			
Diarrheic	6	4 (66.7)	*C. xiaoi* (2), *C. parvum* (2)
Non-diarrheic	12	0 (0)	
15–21			
Diarrheic	3	1 (33.3)	*C. xiaoi* (1)
Non-diarrheic	10	0 (0)	
22–28			
Diarrheic	0	0 (0)	
Non-diarrheic	16	1 (6.25)	*C. xiaoi* (1)
Total	62	9 (14.5)	*C. xiaoi* (6), *C. parvum* (3)

different areas, it is unclear whether the two types represent different types of *C. xiaoi* circulating in different areas.

Cryptosporidium parvum was seen in three sheep among the small number of animals examined. These findings are in agreement with previous common findings of the pathogen in sheep in European countries and Australia [4, 10, 18, 31, 36, 46]. Among developing countries, a small number of *C. parvum* infections have been reported in goats and sheep from Asia, including China [17, 47, 48], India [49], Jordan [50] and Turkey [51]. Our results, however, are in contrast to those from studies conducted in most African countries including Egypt [37], Tunisia [52] and Ethiopia [53], where *C. parvum* has thus far not been reported in small ruminants. *Cryptosporidium parvum* was also absent in sheep and goats in other studies in China [38, 41].

The *C. parvum* identified in the study belonged to the IIaA13G2R1 subtype. Although IIaA13G2R1 subtype is not a common *C. parvum* subtype and has not reported previously in sheep, it was detected in some calves in Belgium and Algeria [54, 55], ponies in the USA [56], calves and goat kids in Turkey [51], and humans in Malaysia [57], indicating that it is likely a zoonotic pathogen in a broad range of areas. Similarly, the *C. ubiquitum* in goats in the present study was subtyped as XIIa, a well-known subtype family in goats elsewhere, including Greece [18], China [17, 38] and Australia [45]. It is also commonly reported in sheep in many countries [26, 35, 41]. It is responsible for zoonotic *C. ubiquitum* infection in humans in industrialized countries, especially the UK [26].

In this study, *C. parvum*, *C. xiaoi* and *C. ubiquitum* infections occurred mostly in animals younger than three weeks. This agrees with observations in previous studies [10, 17, 18, 34, 37–40, 47]. Currently, controversy exists on the clinical significance of *C. ubiquitum* and *C. xiaoi* [2]. In the present study, most *C. xiaoi* cases (11/12), the two *C. ubiquitum* and the three *C. parvum* cases all had diarrhea. *Cryptosporidium* infections in lambs and goat kids have been associated with the occurrence of diarrhea in some studies [10, 16, 32, 34, 39, 40]. Case-control studies are needed to confirm the role of *C. ubiquitum* and *C. xiaoi* in the induction of diarrhea in infected animals.

Conclusions

Results of this study showed a relatively common occurrence of *C. xiaoi* in lambs and goat kids in association with the occurrence of diarrhea. The additional presence of zoonotic *C. parvum* and *C. ubiquitum* indicates that cryptosporidiosis in small ruminants may have further public health implications. More extensive molecular epidemiological studies are needed to substantiate these observations and to improve our understanding of the epidemiology and public health significance of cryptosporidiosis in small ruminants in Algeria.

Acknowledgements

We thank Laathamna Abdelkarim of the University Ziane Achor of Djelfa for statistical analysis. The findings and conclusions in this report are those of the authors and do not necessarily represent the views of the Centers for Disease Control and Prevention.

Funding

This work was supported in part by the National Natural Science Foundation of China (31425025).

Authors' contributions

DB, AH, DK, YF and LX conceived the study. DB, AH, HA, SA, KA, HD, XC and DR conducted the experiments. DB, AH, SA and LX analyzed the data; DB, SA, AH and LX prepared the report. All authors read and approved the final manuscript.

Competing interests

The authors declare that they have no competing interests.

Author details

[1]École Nationale Supérieure Vétérinaire, Rue Issaad Abbes, El Alia, Alger, Algérie. [2]Division of Foodborne, Waterborne and Environmental Diseases, Centers for Disease Control and Prevention, 1600 Clifton Road, Atlanta, GA 30329, USA. [3]Laboratoire exploration et valorisation des écosystèmes steppique, Université Ziane Achor, 17000 Djelfa, Algérie. [4]Department of Biology, Addis Ababa University, Addis Ababa, Ethiopia. [5]Department of Zoology, Faculty of Science, Kafr El Sheikh University, Kafr El Sheikh 33516, Egypt. [6]UMR-BIPAR, ANSES-Ecole Nationale Vétérinaire d'Alfort, Maisons-Alfort, Paris, France. [7]Université Saad Dahleb Blida, Blida, Algérie. [8]Beijing Tropical Medicine Research Institute, Beijing Friendship Hospital, Beijing 100050, China. [9]Key Laboratory of Zoonosis of Ministry of Agriculture, College of Veterinary Medicine, South China Agricultural University, Guangzhou 510642, China.

References

1. Ryan U, Fayer R, Xiao L. *Cryptosporidium* species in humans and animals: current understanding and research needs. Parasitology. 2014;141:1667–85.
2. Xiao L. Molecular epidemiology of cryptosporidiosis: an update. Exp Parasitol. 2010;124:80–9.
3. Santin M. Clinical and subclinical infections with *Cryptosporidium* in animals. N Z Vet J. 2013;6:1–10.
4. Quílez J, Torres E, Chalmers R, Hadfield S, Del Cacho E, Sánchez-Acedo C. *Cryptosporidium* genotypes and subtypes in lambs and goat kids in Spain. Appl Environ Microbiol. 2008;74:6026–31.
5. Robertson L. *Giardia* and *Cryptosporidium* infections in sheep and goats: a review of the potential for transmission to humans via environmental contamination. Epidemiol Infect. 2009;137:913–21.

6. Kotkova M, Nemejc K, Sak B, Hanzal V, Kvetonova D, Hlaskova L, et al. *Cryptosporidium ubiquitum*, *C. muris* and *Cryptosporidium* deer genotype in wild cervids and caprines in the Czech Republic. Folia Parasitol (Praha). 2016;63:3.
7. Olson M, Ralston B, O'Handley R, Guselle N, Appelbee A. What is the clinical and zoonotic significance of cryptosporidiosis in domestic animals and wildlife. In: Thompson RC, Armson A, Ryan UM, editors. *Cryptosporidium*: From Molecules to Disease. Amsterdam: Elsevier B.V; 2003.
8. Noordeen F, Rajapakse R, Horadagoda N, Abdul-Careem M. *Cryptosporidium*, an important enteric pathogen in goats - a review. Small Rumin Res. 2012; 106:77–82.
9. Paraud C, Chartier C. Cryptosporidiosis in small ruminants. Small Rumin Res. 2012;103:93–7.
10. Díaz P, Quílez J, Prieto A, Navarro E, Pérez-Creo A, Fernández G, et al. *Cryptosporidium* species and subtype analysis in diarrhoeic preweaned lambs and goat kids from north-western Spain. Parasitol Res. 2015;114: 4099–105.
11. Peng XQ, Tian GR, Ren GJ, Yu ZQ, Lok JB, Zhang LX, et al. Infection rate of *Giardia duodenalis*, *Cryptosporidium* spp. and *Enterocytozoon bieneusi* in cashmere, dairy and meat goats in China. Infect Genet Evol. 2016;41:26–31.
12. Romero-Salas D, Alvarado-Esquivel C, Cruz-Romero A, Aguilar-Domínguez M, Ibarra-Priego N, Merino-Charrez JO, et al. Prevalence of *Cryptosporidium* in small ruminants from Veracruz, Mexico. BMC Vet Res. 2016;12:14.
13. Shafieyan H, Alborzi A, Hamidinejat H, Tabandeh M, Hajikolaei M. Prevalence of *Cryptosporidium* spp. in ruminants of Lorestan province, Iran. J Parasit Dis. 2016;40:1165–9.
14. Kaupke A, Michalski M, Rzeżutka A. Diversity of *Cryptosporidium* species occurring in sheep and goat breeds reared in Poland. Parasitol Res. 2017; 116:871–9.
15. Giles M, Chalmers R, Pritchard G, Elwin K, Mueller-Doblies D, Clifton-Hadley F. *Cryptosporidium hominis* in a goat and a sheep in the UK. Vet Rec. 2009; 164:24–5.
16. Díaz P, Quílez J, Robinson G, Chalmers R, Díez-Baños P, Morrondo P. Identification of *Cryptosporidium xiaoi* in diarrhoeic goat kids (*Capra hircus*) in Spain. Vet Parasitol. 2010;172:132–4.
17. Mi R, Wang X, Huang Y, Zhou P, Liu Y, Chen Y, et al. Prevalence and molecular characterization of *Cryptosporidium* in goats across four provincial level areas in China. PLoS One. 2014;9:e111164.
18. Tzanidakis N, Sotiraki S, Claerebout E, Ehsan A, Voutzourakis N, Kostopoulou D, et al. Occurrence and molecular characterization of *Giardia duodenalis* and *Cryptosporidium* spp. in sheep and goats reared under dairy husbandry systems in Greece. Parasite. 2014;21:45.
19. Xiao L, Feng Y. Molecular epidemiologic tools for waterborne pathogens *Cryptosporidium* spp. and *Giardia duodenalis*. Food Waterborne Parasitol. 2017;8–9:14–32.
20. Baroudi D, Khelef D, Goucem R, Adjou K, Adamu H, Zhang H, Xiao L. Common occurrence of zoonotic pathogen *Cryptosporidium meleagridis* in broiler chickens and turkeys in Algeria. Vet Parasitol. 2013;196:334–40.
21. Laatamna AE, Wagnerová P, Sak B, Květoňová D, Xiao L, Rost M, et al. Microsporidia and *Cryptosporidium* in horses and donkeys in Algeria: detection of a novel *Cryptosporidium hominis* subtype family (Ik) in a horse. Vet Parasitol. 2015;208:135–42.
22. Baroudi D, Khelef D, Hakem A, Abdelaziz A, Chen X, Lysen C, et al. Molecular characterization of zoonotic pathogens *Cryptosporidium* spp., *Giardia duodenalis* and *Enterocytozoon bieneusi* in calves in Algeria. Vet Parasitol Reg Stud Rep. 2017;8:66–9.
23. Baroudi D, Zhang H, Amer S, Khelef D, Roellig DM, Wang Y, et al. Divergent *Cryptosporidium parvum* subtype and *Enterocytozoon bieneusi* genotypes in dromedary camels in Algeria. Parasitol Res. 2018;117:905–10.
24. Feng Y, Ortega Y, He G, Das P, Xu M, Zhang X, et al. Wide geographic distribution of *Cryptosporidium bovis* and the deer like genotype in bovines. Vet Parasitol. 2007;144:1–9.
25. Alves M, Xiao L, Sulaiman I, Lal A, Matos O, Antunes F. Subgenotype analysis of *Cryptosporidium* isolates from humans, cattle, and zoo ruminants in Portugal. J Clin Microbiol. 2003;41:2744–7.
26. Li N, Xiao L, Alderisio K, Elwin K, Cebelinski E, Chalmers R, et al. Subtyping *Cryptosporidium ubiquitum*, a zoonotic pathogen emerging in humans. Emerg Infect Dis. 2014;20:217–4.
27. Fayer R, Santin M. *Cryptosporidium xiaoi* n. sp. (Apicomplexa: Cryptosporidiidae) in sheep (*Ovis aries*). Vet Parasitol. 2009;146:192 200.
28. da Silva AJ, Caccio S, Williams C, Won KY, Nace EK, Whittier C, et al. Molecular and morphologic characterization of a *Cryptosporidium* genotype identified in lemurs. Vet Parasitol. 2003;111:297–307.
29. Causapé AC, Quílez J, Sánchez-Acedo C, del Cacho E, López-Bernad F. Prevalence and analysis of potential risk factors for *Cryptosporidium parvum* infection in lambs in Zaragoza (northeastern Spain). Vet Parasitol. 2002;104: 287–98.
30. Santín M, Trou J, Fayer R. Prevalence and molecular characterization of *Cryptosporidium* and *Giardia* species and genotypes in sheep in Maryland. Vet Parasitol. 2007;146:17–24.
31. Mueller-Doblies D, Giles M, Elwin K, Smith RP, Clifton-Hadley FA, Chalmers R. Distribution of *Cryptosporidium* species in sheep in the UK. Vet Parasitol. 2008;154:214–9.
32. Imre K, Luca C, Costache M, Sala C, Morar A, Morariu S, et al. Zoonotic *Cryptosporidium parvum* in Romanian newborn lambs (*Ovis aries*). Vet Parasitol. 2013;191:119–22.
33. Cacciò SM, Sannella AR, Mariano V, Valentini S, Berti F, Tosini F. Pozio E. A rare *Cryptosporidium parvum* genotype associated with infection of lambs and zoonotic transmission in Italy. Vet Parasitol. 2013;191:128–31.
34. Rieux A, Paraud C, Pors I, Chartier C. Molecular characterization of *Cryptosporidium* spp. in pre-weaned kids in a dairy goat farm in western France. Vet Parasitol. 2013;192:268–72.
35. Yang R, Jacobson C, Gardner G, Carmichael I, Campbell AJ, Ng-Hublin J, Ryan U. Longitudinal prevalence, oocyst shedding and molecular characterisation of *Cryptosporidium* species in sheep across four states in Australia. Vet Parasitol. 2014;200:50–8.
36. Goma FY, Geurden T, Siwila J, Phiri I, Gabriel S, Claerebout E, Vercruysse J. The prevalence and molecular characterisation of *Cryptosporidium* spp. in small ruminants in Zambia. Small Rumin Res. 2007;72:77–80.
37. Mahfouz M, Mira N, Amer S. Prevalence and genotyping of *Cryptosporidium* spp. in farm animals in Egypt. J Vet Med Sci. 2014;76:1569–75.
38. Wang R, Li G, Cui B, Huang J, Cui Z, Zhang S, et al. Prevalence molecular characterization and zoonotic potential of *Cryptosporidium* spp. in goats in Henan and Chongqing, China. Exp Parasitol. 2014;142:11–6.
39. Zucatto A, Aquino M, Inácio S, Figueiredo R, Pierucci J, Perri S, et al. Molecular characterisation of *Cryptosporidium* spp. in lambs in the South Central region of the State of São Paulo. Arq Bras Med Vet Zootec. 2015;67: 441–6.
40. Siddiki A, Mina S, Farzana Z, Ayesa B, Das R, Hossain M. Molecular characterization of *Cryptosporidium xiaoi* in goat kids in Bangladesh by nested PCR amplification of 18S rRNA gene. Asian Pac J Trop Biomed. 2015; 5:202–7.
41. Li P, Cai J, Cai M, Wu W, Li C, Lei M, et al. Distribution of *Cryptosporidium* species in Tibetan sheep and yaks in Qinghai, China. Vet Parasitol. 2016;215: 58–62.
42. Parsons MB, Travis D, Lonsdorf EV, Lipende I, Roellig DM, Collins A, et al. Epidemiology and molecular characterization of *Cryptosporidium* spp. in humans, wild primates, and domesticated animals in the Greater Gombe Ecosystem, Tanzania. PLoS Negl Trop Dis. 2015;9:e0003529.
43. Wang Y, Feng Y, Cui B, Jian F, Ning C, Wang R, Zhang L, Xiao L. Cervine genotype is the major *Cryptosporidium* genotype in sheep in China. Parasitol Res. 2010;106:341–7.
44. Robertson L, Björkman C, Axén C, Fayer R. Cryptosporidiosis in farmed animals. In: Cacciò SM, Widmer G, editors. *Cryptosporidium*: Parasite and Disease. Vienna: Springer; 2014. p. 149–236.
45. Al-Habsi K, Yang R, Williams A, Miller D, Ryan U, Jacobson C. Zoonotic *Cryptosporidium* and *Giardia* shedding by captured rangeland goats. Vet Parasitol Reg Stud Rep. 2017;7:32–5.
46. Drumo R, Widmer G, Morrison LJ, Tait A, Grelloni V, D'Avino N, et al. Evidence of host-associated populations of *Cryptosporidium parvum* in Italy. Appl Environ Microbiol. 2012;78:3523–9.
47. Ye J, Xiao L, Wang Y, Wang L, Amer S, Roellig DM, et al. Periparturient transmission of *Cryptosporidium xiaoi* from ewes to lambs. Vet Parasitol. 2013;197:627–33.
48. Mi R, Wang X, Huang Y, Mu G, Zhang Y, Jia H, et al. Sheep as a potential source of cryptosporidiosis in China. Appl Environ Microbiol. 2018;84:17.
49. Maurya PS, Rakesh RL, Pradeep B, Kumar S, Kundu K, Garg R, et al. Prevalence and risk factors associated with *Cryptosporidium* spp. infection in young domestic livestock in India. Trop Anim Health Prod. 2013;45:941–6.

50. Hijjawi N, Mukbel R, Yang R, Ryan U. Genetic characterization of *Cryptosporidium* in animal and human isolates from Jordan. Vet Parasitol. 2016;228:116–20.
51. Taylan-Ozkan A, Yasa-Duru S, Usluca S, Lysen C, Ye J, Roellig DM, et al. *Cryptosporidium* species and *Cryptosporidium parvum* subtypes in dairy calves and goat kids reared under traditional farming systems in Turkey. Exp Parasitol. 2016;170:16–20.
52. Soltane R, Guyot K, Dei-Cas E, Ayadi A. Prevalence of *Cryptosporidium* spp. (Eucoccidiorida: Cryptosporiidae) in seven species of farm animals in Tunisia. Parasite. 2007;14:335–8.
53. Wegayehu T, Karim MR, Li J, Adamu H, Erko B, Zhang L, Tilahun G. Prevalence and genetic characterization of *Cryptosporidium* species and *Giardia duodenalis* in lambs in Oromia Special Zone, Central Ethiopia. BMC Vet Res. 2017;13:22.
54. Geurden T, Berkvens D, Martens C, Casaert S, Vercruysse J, Claerebout E. Molecular epidemiology with subtype analysis of *Cryptosporidium* in calves in Belgium. Parasitology. 2007;134:1981–7.
55. Benhouda D, Hakem A, Sannella AR, Benhouda A, Cacciò SM. First molecular investigation of *Cryptosporidium* spp. in young calves in Algeria. Parasite. 2017;24:15.
56. Wagnerová P, Sak B, McEvoy J, Rost M, Sherwood D, Holcomb K, Kváč M. *Cryptosporidium parvum* and *Enterocytozoon bieneusi* in American Mustangs and Chincoteague ponies. Exp Parasitol. 2016;162:24–7.
57. Iqbal A, Lim YA, Surin J, Sim BL. High diversity of *Cryptosporidium* subgenotypes identified in Malaysian HIV/AIDS individuals targeting gp60 gene. PLoS One. 2012;7:e31139.

13

The population genetics of parasitic nematodes of wild animals

Rebecca Cole* and Mark Viney

Abstract

Parasitic nematodes are highly diverse and common, infecting virtually all animal species, and the importance of their roles in natural ecosystems is increasingly becoming apparent. How genes flow within and among populations of these parasites - their population genetics - has profound implications for the epidemiology of host infection and disease, and for the response of parasite populations to selection pressures. The population genetics of nematode parasites of wild animals may have consequences for host conservation, or influence the risk of zoonotic disease. Host movement has long been recognised as an important determinant of parasitic nematode population genetic structure, and recent research has also highlighted the importance of nematode life histories, environmental conditions, and other aspects of host ecology. Commonly, factors influencing parasitic nematode population genetics have been studied in isolation, such that an integrated view of the drivers of population genetic structure of parasitic nematodes is still lacking. Here, we seek to provide a comprehensive, broad, and integrative picture of these factors in parasitic nematodes of wild animals that will be a useful resource for investigators studying non-model parasitic nematodes in natural ecosystems. Increasingly, new methods of analysing the population genetics of nematodes are becoming available, and we consider the opportunities that these afford in resolving hitherto inaccessible questions of the population genetics of these important animals.

Keywords: Helminths, Nematodes, Population genetics, Population genomics, Sequencing, Wild animals, Population structure, Conservation, Parasite ecology

Background

Parasitic nematode infection is ubiquitous in wild animals and can profoundly alter the physiology, behaviour and reproductive success of hosts [1, 2], and as such parasitic nematodes play key roles in ecosystem functioning [3, 4]. However, parasitic nematodes can raise conservation concerns - invasive parasitic nematodes may threaten naïve, native hosts [5], while environmental changes may render hosts more susceptible to pre-existing parasitic nematode species, resulting in more severe disease [6]. Furthermore, parasitic nematodes that normally infect wild animals can spill-over into human and domestic animal populations, acting as new sources of disease [7, 8].

Population genetic structure - the distribution of genetic variation in time and space - affects how a species responds to selection pressures, and so shapes its evolution [9]. Studying the population genetics of parasites in wild animals has several benefits. First, it provides an insight into the parasite's infection dynamics [9–11], with consequences for ecosystem functioning [3, 4]. Secondly, population genetic studies can reveal complexes of morphologically indistinguishable, but genetically very different, cryptic species, which are common among nematodes [12–14]. Thirdly, the patterning of population genetic structure of parasitic nematode species can inform on parasite phylogeography (see Table 1), and in so doing also clarify aspects of host phylogeography [15–19]. Finally, by studying the population genetics of parasitic nematodes in wild animals, ecological drivers of population genetic patterns in parasitic nematodes which may not be apparent in human- and livestock-infecting species can be identified.

The population genetics of metazoan parasites, including nematodes, has been reviewed extensively [9–11, 20–25], but much of this information is based on species that infect people and livestock. It is not clear how applicable these findings are to nematodes whose hosts

* Correspondence: rc16955@bristol.ac.uk
School of Biological Sciences, University of Bristol, Bristol BS8 1TQ, UK

Table 1 Glossary

Term	Definition
Census size (N)	The number of individuals in a population
Effective population size (Ne)	Effective population size (Ne): The number of individuals needed in an idealised population to explain the rate of change in allele frequency, or to explain the observed degree of inbreeding, observed in a real population [180]
Environmental DNA (eDNA)	DNA released by organisms into the environment [174]
Fixation	When only a single allele remains at a formerly-polymorphic locus
Gene flow	Movement of alleles among populations [181]. Tends to reduce genetic differentiation
Genetic drift	Stochastic change in allele frequencies within a population across generations [180]. Tends to increase genetic differentiation
Hardy-Weinberg equilibrium	The situation in which the number of heterozygotes observed matches the number of heterozygotes expected given the allele frequencies in the population [182]
Idealised population	A theoretical population in which each individual produces an infinite number of gametes, any gamete may fuse with any other of the opposite sex with equal probability, sex ratios are even, and there is no overlap in generations [180]
Infrapopulation	All the parasites of one species within one host individual [21]
Isozymes	Different, usually allelic, forms of an enzyme, which can be detected by differences in electrophoretic charge [183]
Linkage disequilibrium	The joint inheritance of particular alleles at different loci more often than would be expected by chance, usually due to their close physical proximity on a chromosome [184]
Phylogeography	Historical drivers of the current geographical distribution of a species [185]
Polymorphic	Sequence variation at a locus, classically with multiple alleles present at frequencies of 5% or greater [186]
Population (of a parasite)	A group of parasite infrapopulations that may exchange individuals freely [21]
Population bottleneck	Loss of a large, random portion of the population, resulting in reduced genetic diversity
Random amplified polymorphic DNA (RAPD)	DNA fragments amplified by a defined set of arbitrary PCR primers, polymorphic due to inter-individual differences in primer binding sites [187]
Ribosomal internal transcribed spacers (ITS)	Putatively non-functional stretches of DNA between the ribosomal RNA-encoding genes in eukaryotes. [188]. The first and second ITS are denoted ITS1 and ITS2 respectively
Selective sweep	An increase in the frequency of a set of alleles owing to their genetic linkage to an allele undergoing positive selection [189]

establish their populations naturally. Parasites' life histories, their hosts' life histories, and the extra-host environment will all contribute to parasites' population genetic structure [10, 11, 22, 23, 25], but little is known about the relative importance of these factors in natural ecosystems, and how they interact.

Here, we provide a resource that collates what is known about the population genetics of parasitic nematodes in natural ecosystems, that we envisage will be useful to researchers investigating the important, but little-understood, roles that parasitic nematodes play in such ecosystems. To this end, we comprehensively review the population genetics of parasitic nematodes in wild animals, including every relevant study of which we are aware. We take wild animals to be ones that establish populations without direct human management, even if they live commensally in human settlements (such as cities), or if their habitat is undergoing anthropogenic changes, since these host populations may nonetheless influence the population genetics of their parasitic nematodes in ways that hosts whose populations are managed by humans cannot. We consider the parasitic nematodes of terrestrial vertebrates, marine vertebrates, and arthropods, and draw together the evidence to present a synthesis on the factors determining the population genetics of parasitic nematodes in wild animals. We examine the population genetics of parasitic nematodes in wild animals that have undergone recent habitat change, asking how parasite populations respond to anthropogenic influences on natural systems. Finally, we assess future prospects in the study of parasitic nematode population genetics, discussing opportunities provided by high-throughput DNA-sequencing-based methods, and highlighting the importance of including extra-host stages in population genetics studies.

Parasitic nematodes of wild terrestrial vertebrates

Parasitic nematodes of marsupials

Commonly, population genetic studies of the parasitic nematodes that infect macropod marsupials reveal that what was previously classified as a single nematode species with a broad host range is actually a complex of cryptic species, each with a narrow host range (Table 2).

Table 2 Species complexes within strongylid nematode parasites of marsupials

Nominal species	Host(s) sampled	Genetic marker(s)	Remarks	Reference
Globocephaloides trifidospicularis	*Macropus rufogriseus*; *M. giganteus* (host numbers not given)	24 isozymes (see Table 1)	Two host-specific species, with 4 fixed differences. ITS1 and ITS2 sequencing later failed to detect these species [26]	[190]
Hypodontus macropi	3 *Macropus agilis*; 4 *M. dorsalis*; 1 *M. rufogriseus rufogriseus*; 1 *M. rufogriseus banksianus*; 2 *M. robustus robustus*; 1 *M. robustus erubescens*; 2 *M. rufus*; 3 *M. fuliginosus*; 2 *Wallabia bicolor*, 2 *Thylogale billardierii*	28 isozymes	Six species detected, with fixed differences at 20–50% of loci. One in *M. r. erubescens*, *M. r. robustus*, *M. rufus* and *M. fuliginosus*, one in *M. r. banksianus* and *M. r. rufogriseus*, and one in each other host. Species status of nematodes in *M. r. robustus*, *T. billardierii* and *M. bicolor* later supported in [191]	[27]
Rugopharynx omega	2 *Macropus rufogriseus*; 1 *Thylogale stigmatica*	23 isozymes	*R. omega* from each host species had fixed differences at 10 loci. *R. omega* from *T. stigmatica* named *Rugopharynx sigma*	[192]
Paramacropostrongylus typicus	4 *Macropus fuliginosus*; 2 *M. giganteus*	37 isozymes	*P. typicus* from each host species had fixed differences at 10 loci. *P. typicus* from *M. giganteus* named *Paramacropostrongylus iugalis*. Hybridisation later detected [193]	[194]
Macropostrongylus baylisi	2 *Macropus giganteus*; 15 *M. robustus robustus*; 4 *M. r. erubescens*; 15 *M. parryi*	27 isozymes	*M. baylisi* from *M. giganteus* had fixed differences at 9 loci compared with *M. baylisi* from other hosts examined	[195]
Rugopharynx zeta	1 *Petrogale assimilis*; 2 *Macropus dorsalis*	21 isozymes	*R. zeta* from *P. assimilis* had 10 fixed differences when compared with *R. zeta* from *M. dorsalis*. *M. dorsalis* parasite named *Rugopharynx mawsonae*	[196]
Rugopharynx australis	1 *Macropus eugenii*; 5 *M. fuliginosus*; 3 *M. giganteus*; 2 *M. robustus*, 2 *M. rufogriseus*, 3 *M. rufus*; 2 *Thylogale billardierii*; 1 *Wallabia bicolor*	17 isozymes	Six species found, with fixed differences at up to 50% of loci. One in *M. robustus* and *M. rufus*, one in *M. giganteus* and *M. fuliginosus*, 2 in *M. rufogriseus* and one each in the remaining hosts	[28]
Labiostrongylus uncinatus	1 *Macropus dorsalis*; 2 *M. parryi*	17 isozymes	*L. uncinatus* from each host species had fixed differences at 13 loci. *L. uncinatus* from *M. parryi* named *Labiostrongylus contiguus*	[197]
Labiostrongylus bancrofti	1 *Macropus dorsalis*; 1 *M. parryi*	18 isozymes	*L. bancrofti* from each host species had fixed differences at 15 loci. *L. bancrofti* from *M. parryi* named *Labiostrongylus turnbulli*	[198]
Zoniolaimus mawsonae	9 *Macropus rufus*	ITS2	Two sympatric taxa had fixed differences at 3 out of 230 nucleotides. One named *Zoniolaimus latebrosus*	[199]
Papillostrongylus labiatus	1 *Macropus dorsalis*; 1 *M. rufus*	ITS2	Two taxa, one in *M. dorsalis* and one in *M. rufus*, had fixed differences at 40 out of 240 nucleotides. Taxon in *M. rufus* named *Papillostrongylus barbatus*	[200]
Cloacina ernabella	1 *Petrogale purpureicollus*	ITS1 and ITS2	Geographically isolated taxa had fixed differences at 13 of 606 nucletides	[31]
Cloacina caenis	1 *Petrogale assimilis*; 1 *P. herberti*; 1 *P. inornata*; 1 *P. mareeba*; 1 *P. purpureicollis*	ITS1 and ITS2	Four taxa identifiable by 1–4 fixed differences. One each from *P. purpureicollis*, *P. herberti* and *P. mareeba*, and one in *P. assimilis* and *P. inornata*	[31]
Cloacina pearsoni	1 *Petrogale assimilis*; 1 *P. herberti*; 1 *P. inornata*; 1 *P. mareeba*; 1 *P. purpureicollis*	ITS1 and ITS2	Five taxa, identifiable by 2–9 fixed differences. One taxon in each host species	[31]

Table 2 Species complexes within strongylid nematode parasites of marsupials *(Continued)*

Nominal species	Host(s) sampled	Genetic marker(s)	Remarks	Reference
Cloacina robertsi	1 *Petrogale assimilis*; 1 *P. herberti*; 1 *P. inornata*; 1 *P. mareeba*; 1 *P. purpureicollis*; 1 *P. persephone*	ITS1 and ITS2	Two taxa, identifiable by 10 fixed differences. One taxon in *P. persephone*, the other in all other host species.	[31]
Globocephaloides macropodis	4 *Macropus dorsalis*; 1 *M. agilis*	ITS1 and ITS2	*G. macropodis* from each host species had fixed differences at 5.2% and 7.1% of nucleotides in ITS1 and ITS2, respectively	[26]

This highlights the ability of population genetic techniques to detect species complexes. In some cases, these studies also show whether, and if so, how, populations within these cryptic species are geographically structured. For example, geographical structuring of genetic diversity was not seen in populations of *Globocephaloides trifidospicularis* [26], nor in several species within the *Hypodontus macropi* complex [27], nor in *Rugopharynx australis* from *Macropus robustus* and *M. rufus* [28], nor in several *Capillaria* species [29], but was observed in populations of *H. macropi* from subspecies of *Macropus robustus*, *H. macropi* from subspecies of *Macropus rufogriseus* [27] and *Labiosimplex australis* from *M. rufogriseus* [30]. In some cases, studies have failed to detect any genetic variation within parasitic nematode species at all, such as in *H. macropi* from *Petrogale persephone* [27], *Globocephaloides affinis* from *Macropus dorsalis* [26], and several other *Cloacina* species [31], but this may be due to the very low numbers of hosts and parasites studied (Table 2).

Why do some of these parasite species have genetic population structuring while others do not? There was genetic differentiation between *L. australis* collected from Tasmania and Kangaroo Island, and between both of these populations and mainland Australia [30]. Similarly, Tasmanian populations of *H. macropi* in *M. rufogriseus* showed genetic differentiation from that on mainland Australia [27]. This suggests that marsupial hosts are ineffective at mediating nematode transmission across open water. However, a cryptic species of *R. australis* in *M. giganteus* and *M. fuliginosus* did not show population differentiation despite being sampled from both Kangaroo Island and mainland Australia [28], nor did *G. trifidospicularis* sampled from multiple macropod species [26]. This may indicate ongoing gene flow in these species between Kangaroo Island and the mainland, or alternatively, that one or both of these species only recently arrived on Kangaroo Island, and the island parasite populations have yet to differentiate detectably from their mainland counterparts.

Genetic differentiation is rarely detected within marsupial-infecting nematode species collected from only mainland Australia; it is apparently absent in three cryptic species of *H. macropi* in *Macropus dorsalis*, *M. agilis* and *Wallabia bicolor*, respectively [27], as well as in a single species within *R. australis* collected from *M. robustus* and *M. rufus* [28]. However, Queensland populations of a cryptic species of *H. macropi* recovered from *M. robustus* were found to be differentiated from those in South Australia [27]. This may simply reflect the size of the study area; sampling locations of *H. macropi* in *M. robustus* were over 1500 km apart, compared with up to 800 km in other species. Naturally, as distances between populations increase, host-mediated transmission between the populations becomes rarer, though the exact distances over which host-mediated transmission becomes inefficient will likely vary with the vagility of host species. It should be noted that in many cases these studies involved low numbers of hosts and parasites (Table 2), and so population genetic insights gleaned from them should be treated with caution. Further work using much larger sample sizes is needed to confirm the patterns of population genetic structure in the parasitic nematodes of marsupials that many existing studies suggest.

Parasitic nematodes of terrestrial carnivores: *Trichinella*

Trichinella spp. have broad geographical ranges and broad host species ranges, with each species parasitizing a variety of carnivorous vertebrates. *Trichinella* spp. share certain population genetic characteristics, such as differentiation among infrapopulations [32, 33] (see Table 1) and low intra-specific genetic diversity [32–39]. *Trichinella* spp. tend to show population genetic structuring among continents; for example, genetic differentiation was found among populations of *T. pseudospiralis* from Australia, North America, Europe and Asia [38, 40], and among *T. spiralis* populations from Asia and Europe [33]. *Trichinella nelsoni* from Kenya and Tanzania was differentiated from that in South Africa [37], but this parasite was recovered from only one host individual in each country, meaning that infrapopulation differentiation was not accounted for.

The apparent lack of population genetic differentiation in *Trichinella* spp. within continents matches observations made of other nematodes that parasitise large carnivorous mammals [41–43], and likely arises from long-distance dispersal of hosts, which promotes high parasite gene flow. For *Trichinella* spp., gene flow may also be promoted by smaller hosts (such as rats and foxes), facilitating parasite gene flow among otherwise discontiguous populations of very mobile hosts.

But what factors drive the among-host differentiation and low intra-specific diversity seen in *Trichinella* spp.? *Trichinella* transmission stages remain in the muscle of their parents' host and infection of a new host occurs by predation [44]. This life-cycle may lead to clumped transmission of siblings, potentially resulting in differentiation among infrapopulations and promoting inbreeding. Inbreeding tends to reduce effective population size (Ne, see Table 1), leading to stronger genetic drift (see Table 1), meaning that alleles are more readily lost from the population, reducing genetic diversity. Indeed, clumped transmission of related parasites has previously been suggested to promote low genetic variation and genetic differentiation among hosts in diverse parasite taxa (reviewed in [9, 10, 21]).

In summary, the population genetics of *Trichinella* spp. appears to be driven by (i) highly mobile hosts and a broad host range, promoting gene flow, and (ii) its life-cycle, promoting clumped transmission of sibling parasites and so lowering Ne.

Parasitic nematodes of rodents

The limited dispersal of wild rodent individuals [45–48] might be expected to limit gene flow in their nematode parasites, resulting in genetic structure over small geographical scales. Accordingly, populations of *Heligmosomoides polygyrus*, a parasite of the European woodmouse (*Apodemus sylvaticus*), show extensive population genetic structure across the host species' range [15, 49–51], with *H. polygyrus* populations being more strongly differentiated than those of *A. sylvaticus* according to mitochondrial sequence analysis of both species [15]. *Heligmosomoides polygyrus* has a faster mitochondrial mutation rate and generation time than its host [15, 52], likely meaning that mitochondrial genetic drift is faster in *H. polygyrus* compared with *A. sylvaticus* and so contributing to the comparatively stronger population genetic structure of *H. polygyrus*.

Trichuris muris infects rats and mice (including *A. sylvaticus*), while *T. arvicolae* infects arvicoline rodents (lemmings and voles), and both *Trichuris* spp. are found throughout Europe. Like *H. polygyrus*, *T. muris* and *T. arvicolae* both show extensive population genetic structure across their geographical range, as determined by analysis of both mitochondrial and nuclear loci [53–55]. Indeed, broadly similar patterns of population genetic structure were observed in *H. polygyrus* and both *Trichuris* spp., with a delineation between eastern and western populations, and greater diversity in southern populations, compared with northern. These patterns may reflect range expansion of the rodent hosts from southern refugia during the last ice age, at least 12,000 years ago [15, 53–55]. Stronger population genetic structuring and a smaller geographical range was observed in *H. polygyrus* than in *Trichuris* spp. [15, 53–55]. This may be partly due to faster genetic drift in *H. polygyrus* than in *Trichuris* spp., arising from a shorter generation time in the former compared with the latter (~14 days and 50–60 days, respectively) [56, 57], or may reflect the broader host range of *Trichuris* spp. A broader host range may allow a parasite to occupy and traverse a wider range of environments, potentially increasing gene flow rates and slowing genetic drift [23].

The population genetics of *Angiostrongylus cantonensis* and *A. malaysiensis*, parasites of rodents of the family Muridae [58], has been extensively studied, with genetic structure detected on both small and large geographical scales [59–69]. However, interpretation of these findings is made difficult by the recent discovery of at least two sympatric cryptic species within *A. cantonensis*, one of which may be conspecific with individuals identified as *A. malaysiensis* [70, 71]. It is now not clear whether the population genetic structure detected previously really represents the geographical distribution of genetic variants in a single species, or rather results from the accidental sampling of multiple reproductively isolated species. Nevertheless, if this cryptic speciation is taken into account, the population genetic data of *A. cantonensis* (*sensu stricto*) and *A. malaysiensis* can be examined. In both species, population genetic structure was detected among provinces in Thailand [70]. It is likely that limited vagility in both the definitive rodent host and the intermediate snail host limits gene flow in *Angiostrongylus* spp. over large distances.

Other studies have investigated parasitic nematode population genetic structure at finer geographical scales. For example, *Neoheligmonella granjoni*, a parasite of multimammate mice (*Mastomys* spp.), was sampled from *M. natalensis* and *M. erythroleucus* within a 70 km^2 rural area of Senegal, and genotyped at 10 microsatellite loci [72]. These data revealed an absence of genetic population structure, with alleles being distributed homogenously among sampling sites. This may be due to the relatively high dispersal of *M. erythroleucus*, which will promote gene flow across the study area, including among populations of the much more sedentary host, *M. natalensis* [72, 73]. A lack of population genetic structure over fine geographical scales (e.g. within a 100 km^2 area) was also seen in *Longistriata caudabullata*, a nematode that parasitises *Blarina* sp. shrews [74], showing that while parasitic nematodes of rodents and other small mammals show strong genetic structure at broad geographical scales, at finer scales, gene flow can be sufficient to genetically homogenise populations.

Strongyloides ratti is a parasite of brown rats, *Rattus norvegicus*, and shows little genetic differentiation among UK sampling sites ~20–250 km apart [75]. This may indicate that *R. norvegicus* dispersal is sufficient to genetically homogenise the *S. ratti* population at these scales. While *S. ratti* did not show genetic differentiation among host populations, there was differentiation among infrapopulations [75]. *Strongyloides* spp. are unusual because the parasitic adults reproduce clonally, so that all of a single parasite's offspring are genetically identical [76], and along with clumped transmission of clonal siblings [77], this may lead to the observed among-host differentiation.

Analysis of *Syphacia stroma* and *H. polygyrus* from the same *A. sylvaticus* host individuals showed that *S. stroma* has substantially lower genetic diversity and higher population differentiation than *H. polygyrus* [78]. *Syphacia stroma* has haplodiploid sex determination, in which haploid males develop from unfertilised eggs produced by diploid females, while in *H. polygyrus* males and females are both produced sexually. Mating system is recognised as an important factor in parasite population genetics [10, 11, 23], and so the different mating systems of *H. polygyrus* and *S. stroma* may explain their different population genetic structures. Haplodiploidy lowers Ne by reducing the number of individuals contributing to the next generation (because males are produced from the mother's genetic material only), and this may lead to greater genetic drift in *S. stroma* compared with *H. polygyrus*. *Syphacia stroma* and *H. polygyrus* have broadly similar generation times [79] and share a host, so their different mating systems emerge as likely important factors behind their different population genetics. Aspects of life history such as mating system have not been extensively studied in parasitic nematodes of wild animals, and further studies in this area may contribute to our understanding of population genetics in other parasitic nematode species.

In summary, the population genetics of parasitic nematodes in wild rodents appears to be defined largely by hosts' low dispersal ranges. However, different patterns of population genetic structure among parasite species sharing a host species suggest that parasite mating system and generation time are also influential.

Parasitic nematodes of ungulates

Ungulate (hoofed mammal) individuals travel over much greater distances than rodents, and so may facilitate comparatively greater gene flow of their parasitic nematodes. *Ostertagia gruehneri* and *Marshallagia marshalli*, both parasites of reindeer (*Rangifer tarandus*), show a lack of population genetic structuring [80, 81], a pattern similar to that of *Teladorsagia boreoarcticus* in muskoxen (*Ovibos moschatus*) [82]. In contrast, *Mazamastrongylus odocoilei*, a parasite of white-tailed deer (*Odocoileus virginianus*), showed genetically structured populations [83]. This difference may reflect the more rapid evolution of mtDNA, used to study *M. odocoilei*, compared with the internal transcribed spacer (ITS, see Table 1) sequences used for *O. gruehneri* and *M. marshalli*. However, species-specific differences in host ecology may also contribute to the different patterns of population genetic structure seen among *O. gruehneri*, *M. marshalli* and *M. odocoilei* - reindeer have large home ranges and are partially migratory [84], and so may provide more opportunities for gene flow in their parasitic nematodes compared with the more sedentary white-tailed deer [85].

Dictyocaulus eckerti is a parasite of several species of deer (*Cervus* spp. and *Dama* spp.). Analysis of mitochondrial sequence data found weak genetic structuring in *D. eckerti* [86], while *D. capreolus* (specific to roe deer, *Capreolus capreolus*), had comparatively lower genetic diversity and more strongly genetically structured populations when sampled sympatrically [86]. *Dictyocaulus capreolus* is susceptible to population bottlenecks if roe deer numbers fall, whereas *D. eckerti* can weather a crash in the population of any one host species by persisting in other host species, and thereby maintain a high census size (N, see Table 1). High genetic diversity and a genetically unstructured populations is also observed in *Trichostrongylus axei*, which parasitises diverse wild ungulate species [87], suggesting an association between these population genetic traits and broad host range. Differences in host behaviour may also contribute to the differences in the population genetics of *D. eckerti* and *D. capreolus*; specifically, *D. eckerti* may have higher gene flow than *D. capreolus* because of the territorial nature of roe deer, which limits the geographical distances they cover.

Parasitic nematodes of reptiles and amphibians

Spauligodon anolis infects anole lizards (*Anolis* spp.), while *Parapharyngodon cubensis* is a species complex (*P. cubensis* A, *P. cubensis* B and *P. cubensis* C) together infecting a broad range of lizards and snakes. Study of the population genetics of these nematodes, sampled from various Caribbean *Anolis* spp. hosts, found that genetic diversity was partitioned both among and within islands [88]. However, *S. anolis* populations were more strongly genetically differentiated than populations of *P. cubensis* A or *P. cubensis* B, likely because *S. anolis* has a narrow host species range made up of poor dispersers [89], while the species of the *P. cubensis* complex each make use of a wider range of hosts, among which may be more mobile host species [88]. In contrast, cryptic species within *Spauligodon atlanticus*, parasites of *Gallotia* spp. lizards, all showed strong genetic structuring within and among islands of the Canary Isles, despite differing in the extent of their host range [90]. This may be because the geographical ranges of the host species of *S. atlanticus* do not overlap, precluding nematode gene flow between them.

Population genetic analysis of *Rhabdias ranae*, a parasite of the northern leopard frog (*Lithobates pipiens*), revealed low microsatellite heterozygosity, differentiation among infrapopulations and population genetic structure at a very fine scale, with differentiation emerging among ponds less than 1 km apart [91]. *Rhabdias ranae* is a specific parasite of *L. pipiens* and lacks an intermediate host, so its dispersal is likely mediated almost entirely through *L. pipiens* movement. Hence, sibling extra-host stages are likely to remain clumped in the environment and infect a new host together, explaining infrapopulation differentiation. If *L. pipiens* habitually visit the same locations (e.g. show fidelity to a particular breeding pond), then they may even be re-infected with the offspring of their own parasites [91]. Such a habit might also explain differentiation among ponds, if the same cohort of frogs routinely utilise a particular pond [91]. Low heterozygosity is likely a product of inbreeding, arising from the life-cycle of *R. ranae*, which includes a self-fertilising hermaphroditic stage.

Parasitic nematodes of terrestrial birds: *Trichostrongylus tenuis*

Trichostrongylus tenuis is a strongylid parasite of galliform and anseriform birds, and is particularly prevalent in red grouse (*Lagopus lagopus scotica*). Population genetic analysis of *T. tenuis* in UK red grouse revealed high microsatellite diversity, and a lack of population genetic structure among host individuals and among geographically separated populations [92, 93]. This lack of population genetic structure is likely due to the very high prevalence and infection intensity of this parasite [94], presumably leading to a high Ne, so rendering genetic drift very slow. Population genetics can also be used to study parasite dispersal. For example, a lack of genetic differentiation between *T. tenuis* in a goose in Iceland and those in UK grouse suggests long distance *T. tenuis* gene flow. Some waterfowl species, such as the pink-footed goose (*Anser brachyrhynchus*), migrate between the UK and Iceland [95], presenting a possible avenue for *T. tenuis* gene flow between these countries.

Parasitic nematodes of aquatic vertebrates

Parasitic nematodes of marine mammals and birds

Most nematode parasites of marine mammals and birds are trophically transmitted among intermediate hosts before reaching the definitive host [96]. As hosts of each trophic level are likely to consume multiple infected hosts in the lower trophic levels, hosts will accumulate parasites from a variety of sources, and so definitive host individuals will probably sample widely from the parasite population. This may lead to genetically diverse parasite infrapopulations that obviate inbreeding and promote high Ne [11]. Because many marine fish, mammal and bird hosts travel large distances [97, 98], gene flow of their parasitic nematode populations is expected to be high, suggesting that these nematode populations will show little genetic structuring.

Many parasitic nematodes infecting marine vertebrates do indeed show little population genetic structure. *Anisakis simplex* is a complex of several cryptic species with different geographical and definitive host ranges [99–101]. Population genetic structure has rarely been observed within species of the *A. simplex* complex (Table 3), and it is likely that earlier reports of extensive genetic structure in *A. simplex* [102] resulted from inadvertent sampling of multiple species. A similar lack of population genetic structure has been observed in a variety of other nematodes with similar life histories, including other *Anisakis* spp. in pinnipeds and cetaceans, *Contracaecum* spp. from a variety of birds and mammals, and *Pseudoterranova* spp. from pinnipeds (Table 3). However, *Anisakis simplex* C may be an exception, with one study detecting genetic differentiation between northern and southern hemisphere populations [99]. Intra-taxon genetic diversity of parasitic nematodes of marine mammals in the southern hemisphere is generally greater than in the northern hemisphere, perhaps due to comparatively lower habitat disturbance (e.g. fishing, pollution) in the southern hemisphere [103].

Uncinaria sanguinis, a parasite of the Australian sea lion (*Neophoca cinerea*), requires adult female hosts on breeding beaches to complete its life-cycle [104], and female hosts always return to the beach they were born on to breed [105]. One might therefore expect *U. sanguinis* to show genetic differentiation among host breeding beaches, but in fact no population genetic structure was observed in *U. sanguinis* at all [106], and a similar situation is seen in *Uncinaria lucasi* infecting northern fur seals (*Callorhinus ursinus*) [107]. This may indicate that the life-cycle of *Uncinaria* spp. is not fully understood and that transmission also occurs in other ways - male sea lions do move among breeding beaches [105], so transmission involving males could homogenise parasite population genetic structure. Hence, population genetic studies can suggest hypotheses about transmission cycles of parasitic nematodes that might otherwise be unexpected.

Parasitic nematodes of fish

Some fish species travel around the globe, while others spend their whole lives in a small home patch, and this diversity in movement behaviour is likely to affect the population genetics of their parasitic nematodes. *Hysterothylacium aduncum* is a poorly-defined nematode

Table 3 Parasitic nematodes of marine mammals and birds that do not show population genetic structure

Species	Sampled non-definitive hosts	Sampled definitive hosts	Regions sampled	Genetic marker(s)	Reference
Anisakis pegreffii	Squid (*Todarodes* spp., *Tadaropsis eblanae*), teleosts (families Bramidae, Carangidae, Clupeidae, Congridae, Emmelycthidae, Engraulidae, Gadidae, Gempylidae, Lophiidae, Merlucciidae, Myctophidae, Ophidiidae, Scombridae, Scorpaenidae, Sparidae, Trachichtyidae, Trichiuridae, Xiphiidae)	Cuvier's beaked whale (*Ziphius cavirostris*), sperm whale (*Physeter microcephalus*), delphinid dolphins	Mediterranean, North-West Atlantic, Pacific off Falkland Islands, Madeira, New Zealand and South Africa	32 isozymes, ITS, mtDNA, RAPD	[99–101, 201–206]
Anisakis simplex (*sensu stricto*)	Squid (*Tadaropsis eblanae, Todarodes sagittus, Illex coindettii*), teleosts (families Carangidae, Clupeidae, Engraulidae, Gadidae, Merlucciidae, Pleuronectidae, Salmonidae, Scomberesocidae, Scombridae, Trichiuridae)	Beluga whale (*Delphinapterus leucas*), harbour porpoise (*Phocoena phocoena*), longfinned pilot whale (*Globicephala melas*), delphinid dolphins	North Sea, Norwegian Sea, Mediterranean Sea, Baltic Sea, Atlantic, North-West Pacific, off Japan and Madeira	32 isozymes, ITS1, 5.8S, ITS2, mtDNA, RAPD	[99–101, 202–209]
Anisakis simplex C	Teleosts (families Gadidae, Gempylidae, Myctophidae, Trachichtyidae)	Strap-toothed whale (*Mesoplodon layardii*), dolphins (*Pseudorca crassidens, Globicephala melas*)	Atlantic, Tasman Sea, North-West Pacific, off South Africa and New Zealand	24 isozymes, ITS1, 5.8S, ITS2, mtDNA, RAPD	[100, 101, 206]
Anisakis paggiae		Dolphins (*Delphinus delphis, Globicephala melas, Tursiops truncatus*), pygmy sperm whales (*Kogia breviceps, K. sima*)	Atlantic off Spain, off South Africa and USA	19 isozymes	[100]
Anisakis brevispiculata		Pygmy sperm whale (*Kogia breviceps*)	Off Spain and South Africa	22 isozymes	[210]
Anisakis physeteris	Teleosts (families Carangidae, Gadidae, Scombridae)	Sperm whale (*Physeter microcephalus*)	Mediterranean Sea, off Madeira	21 isozymes, ITS1, 5.8S, ITS2	[101, 210, 211]
Anisakis typica	Teleosts (families Carangidae, Coryphaenidae, Merlucciidae, Trichiuridae, Scombridae)	Delphinid dolphins, harbour porpoise (*Phocoena phocoena*) short-finned pilot whale (*Globicephala macrorhynchus*), La Plata dolphin (*Pontoporia blainvillei*)	Off Florida, Madeira, Somalia and Brazil, Mediterranean Sea	20 isozymes, ITS1, 5.8S, ITS2	[99, 101, 202]
Anisakis ziphidarum	Teleosts (families Carangidae, Scombridae, Trichiuridae)	Strap-toothed whale (*Mesoplodon layardii*) and Cuvier's beaked whale (*Ziphius cavirostris*)	Off Madeira	22 isozymes, ITS1, 5.8S, ITS2	[101, 212]
Anisakis nascettii	Black scabbardfish (*Aphanopus carbo*) and chub mackerel (*Scomber japonicus*)	Beaked whales (*Mesoplodon* spp.)	Off Madeira, Spain, New Zealand and South Africa	ITS1, 5.8S, ITS2 mtDNA	[101, 213–215]
Pseudoterranova decipiens A	Teleosts (families Gadidae, Pleuronectidae, Scopthalmidae)	Grey seal (*Halichoerus grypus*), harbour seal (*Phoca vitulina*)	North-East Atlantic	9 isozymes	[216]
Pseudoterranova decipiens B	Teleosts (Cottidae, Gadidae, Lotidae, Pleuronectidae)	Grey seal (*Halichoerus grypus*), harbour seal (*Phoca vitulina*) hooded seal (*Cystophora cristata*)	North Atlantic	9 isozymes	[216]
Pseudoterranova decipiens C	American plaice (*Hippoglossoides platessoides*)	Bearded seal (*Erignathus barbatus*)	North Atlantic	9 isozymes	[216]
Contracaecum spp.	Topminnows (*Poeciliopsis* spp.) and the cichlid *Cichlasoma beani*		Off Arroyo Aguajita (Mexico)	17 isozymes	[217]
Contracaecum osculatum A		Bearded seal (*Erignathus barbatus*), grey seal (*Halichoerus grypus*),	North Atlantic	17 isozymes	[218]
Contracaecum osculatum		Bearded seal (*Erignathus barbatus*), grey seal	North Atlantic	17 isozymes	[218]

Table 3 Parasitic nematodes of marine mammals and birds that do not show population genetic structure *(Continued)*

Species	Sampled non-definitive hosts	Sampled definitive hosts	Regions sampled	Genetic marker(s)	Reference
B		(*Halichoerus grypus*), harp seal (*Phoca groenlandica*), harbour seal (*Phoca vitulina*)			
Contracaecum osculatum C		Grey seal (*Halichoerus grypus*)	North-East Atlantic	17 isozymes	[218]
Contracaecum osculatum D	Teleosts (families Channichthyidae, Nototheniidae)	Weddel seal (*Leptonychotes weddellii*)	Antarctic Southern Ocean	24 isozymes, mtDNA	[219, 220]
Contracaecum osculatum E	Teleosts (families Channichthyidae, Nototheniidae)	Weddel seal (*Leptonychotes weddellii*)	Antarctic Southern Ocean	24 isozymes, mtDNA	[219, 220]
Contracaecum radiatum	Crocodile icefishes (*Chionodraco hamatus* and *Cryodraco antarcticus*)	Weddel seal (*Leptonychotes weddellii*)	Antarctic Southern Ocean	24 isozymes	[221]
Contracaecum ogmorhini		Fur seals (*Arctocephalus* spp.)	Off Australia, Argentina and South Africa	18 isozymes, ITS1, ITS2, mtDNA	[222, 223]
Contracaecum margolisi		Caliphornia seal lion (*Zalophus californianus*)	Pacific off Canada	18 isozymes, ITS1, ITS2, mtDNA	[222, 223]
Contracaecum rudolphii A		Cormorants (*Phalacrocorax* spp.)	Atlantic off Spain, off Poland and Italy	20 isozymes, ITS1, ITS2, mtDNA	[224, 225]
Contracaecum rudolphii B		Continental great cormorant (*Phalacrocorax carbo sinensis*)	Off Italy and Poland	20 isozymes, ITS1, ITS2, mtDNA	[224, 225]
Contracaecum septentrionale		Continental great cormorant (*Phalacrocorax carbo sinensis*)	Off Iceland and Norway	20 isozymes, mtDNA	[225]

species complex that infects a broad range of marine fish species [108]. ITS sequence data of *H. aduncum* from sprats (*Sprattus sprattus*) in western Europe showed two genetically distinct populations: one in the English Channel and the Bay of Biscay, and one in the Mediterranean and North Sea [109]. The geographical separation of the Mediterranean and North Sea (and that they are separated by the English Channel and Bay of Biscay), makes this parasite population genetic structure peculiar, and it contrasts with the population genetics of the sprats [110]. Potentially, another host species may be responsible for genetically homogenising the *H. aduncum* populations in the Mediterranean and North Sea *via* migration, and sampling of *H. aduncum* from other hosts is needed to test this hypothesis. In contrast with *H. aduncum*, there was no genetic structure in *Hysterothylacium fabri* within the Mediterranean, when considering either geography or host fish species [111].

Parasites of fish in discontiguous water bodies can become genetically distinct. For example, splitfin fishes (several genera within the Goodeidae) live in a series of unconnected lakes in Mexico, and their parasite, *Rhabdochona lichtenfelsi*, shows strong genetic differentiation among lakes, with the degree of differentiation correlating with the time since the lakes became separated [112]. In contrast, populations of the yellowhead catfish (*Pelteobagrus fulvidraco*) parasite *Procamallanus fulvidraconis* in isolated lakes were not significantly genetically different from each other [113]. These lakes were connected until the 1950s [114], so there may have been insufficient time for the parasite populations to diverge genetically. *Camallanus cotti* parasitizes a variety of freshwater fish species, and it showed no population genetic structure among the Yangtze and Minjiang river systems (geographically close and possibly occasionally connected by flood water), though populations from the Pearl River were distinct [115].

Collectively, studies of the population genetics of parasitic nematodes in aquatic environments reveal that their population genetic structures emerge at the scale over which hosts move, with genetically unstructured populations being common. Population genetic structure can emerge in these parasites when populations are restricted to isolated water bodies, or where host movement is constrained.

Nematode parasites of arthropods

Virtually all invertebrate taxa are infected by parasitic nematodes, but the life histories of these nematodes are often poorly understood, and their population genetics barely explored. The insect parasite *Heterorhabditis marelatus* has a low level of mitochondrial genetic diversity and shows extreme population genetic structuring among sample sites (7 to 890 km apart) [116]. This may arise from very low gene flow in *H. marelatus*, since the extreme pathogenicity of *H. marelatus* kills hosts before they can carry their parasites far, preventing host movement from contributing significantly to parasite dispersal [116]. The life-cycle of *H. marelatus* may also contribute to its strong population genetic structure; *Heterorhabditis* spp. infections are initiated by juveniles which, upon maturation into hermaphrodites, self-fertilise to produce males and further hermaphrodites that continue to reproduce on the host's cadaver [117]. This life-cycle promotes frequent founder effects (when an infective juvenile invades a host) and inbreeding (self-fertilisation and sib-mating), together driving low Ne. Low genetic diversity and population genetic structure was also observed in *Strelkovimermis spiculatus*, sampled from mosquito larvae (*Aedes* spp. and *Culex pipiens*), with genetic differentiation observed among ponds ~7 to 14 km apart [118]. In contrast, no population genetic structure was observed in *Isomermis lairdi*, a parasite of larval blackflies (*Simulium* spp.), when sampled from three rivers and multiple host species [119]. That the rivers were connected likely facilitates gene flow of *I. lairdi*, resulting in less structured populations compared with *S. spiculatus*.

Thaumamermis zealandica, a parasite of the sandhopper (*Bellorchestia quoyana*, a beach-dwelling amphipod), showed a complete absence of genetic diversity in three mitochondrial protein-coding genes when sampled from numerous hosts along an ~580 km stretch of New Zealand coast [120]. This could result from (i) panmixia among sampling sites and an extremely low Ne in the entire population, such that genetic drift affects *T. zealandica* at all sampling sites as a single population; (ii) a very recent population bottleneck; (iii) an extremely low mitochondrial mutation rate; or (iv) a combination of these factors [120]. Extremely low genetic variation in mitochondrial protein-coding genes was also seen in the woodlouse (*Armadillidium vulgare*) parasite *Thaumamermis cosgrovei* [121], suggesting that a low mutation rate in mitochondrial protein-coding genes may be a common feature of *Thaumamermis* spp.

RAPD (see Table 1) analysis of *Blatticola blattae*, a parasite of cockroaches (*Blattella germanica*), showed that the parasite population genetic structure closely mirrored that of the host, with both showing differentiation among buildings within cities, and among cities 900 km apart [122]. This strong genetic structuring likely reflects limited dispersal in cockroaches, promoting low gene flow in both parasite and host. Unlike *H. marelatus*, *B. blattae* is not markedly pathogenic and individuals form long-term associations with their hosts [123], so that there is time for host movement to mediate parasite gene flow.

Among parasitic nematodes of arthropods, then, pathogenicity to the host may influence the parasites' population genetic structure, as parasites that kill their hosts very quickly cannot rely on host movement for dispersal and gene flow. However, where the arthropod host has a very small home range and does not disperse far, even largely non-pathogenic parasites may have strongly structured populations, as seen in *B. blattae* [122]. Nevertheless, our knowledge of the population genetics of parasitic nematodes of arthropods is very incomplete, and future work analysing a broader range of both host and parasite life histories is needed if we are to better understand the factors influencing their population genetics.

Influence of anthropogenic disruption on parasitic nematode population genetics

Human activities have affected the geographical ranges of many host species, either shrinking a range through habitat loss, or increasing it through introduction of individuals into new regions. In many cases, the timing and extent of range changes are well documented, offering an opportunity to study how changes in host population size and connectivity shape parasitic nematode population genetics.

Baylisascaris schroederi is a nematode thought to be specific to giant pandas (*Ailuropoda melanoleuca*). Sequence analysis of both ITS and mtDNA have shown a lack of genetic differentiation among *B. schroederi* from geographically isolated panda populations [124–127], which is surprising because pandas do not migrate among populations, and pandas from each of these populations are themselves genetically differentiated [128]. The likely explanation for this difference between host and parasite population genetics is that *B. schroederi* has a much larger Ne than its host [129] and so undergoes population differentiation more slowly. Thus, while there may have been time for panda populations to differentiate through genetic drift in the 200 years since habitat fragmentation began [130], drift may not have been fast enough to yet differentiate *B. schroederi* populations. It has also been suggested that *B. schroederi* gene flow may occur among panda populations in the absence of panda movement, for example through association with a presently unknown paratenic host [127].

An analogous situation is seen in *Trypanoxyuris minutus* and *T. atelis*, parasites of the primates *Alouatta* spp. and *Ateles geoffroyi*, respectively, in Mexico. Since 1940, on-going forest fragmentation has created discontiguous host populations, among which host migration is very rare [131]. Despite this, mitochondrial sequence analysis of *Trypanoxyuris* spp. showed that parasite populations in different forest fragments were not genetically differentiated [132]. There are two non-mutually-exclusive explanations for this; unexpectedly high *Trypanoxyuris* gene flow among forest fragments, and/or the failure of *Trypanoxyuris* populations to detectably differentiate since becoming reproductively isolated. The latter explanation assumes that *Trypanoxyuris* populations were genetically unstructured prior to forest fragmentation, and this seems plausible as parasitic nematodes from a range of wild primates show limited population genetic structure when looking within host species [133–139].

The population genetics of *Baylisascaris procyonis* infecting raccoons (*Procyon lotor*) has been studied using both ribosomal and microsatellite loci in its native range [140, 141], with microsatellite loci revealing genetic differentiation across the Grand River (Michigan, USA). Among invasive *B. procyonis* populations in Germany, two well-differentiated clades have been detected by both ITS and mitochondrial sequence analysis, suggesting two independent introductions of *B. procyonis* into Germany [142]. Both German *B. procyonis* clades showed very low genetic diversity, likely the result of population bottlenecks (see Table 1) in the founding populations [142]. Low genetic diversity was seen also in *Rhabdias pseudosphaerocephala* in invasive cane toads (*Bufo marinus*) in Australia [143], and in *Passalurus ambiguus* in invasive rabbits (*Oryctolagus cuniculus*) in China [144], and is typical due to founder effects in these introduced species [145].

The nematode *Spirocamallanus istiblenni* was introduced to the Hawaiian archipelago with one of its hosts, the bluestripe snapper (*Lutjanus kasmira*). Population genetic analysis of *S. istiblenni* confirmed that the parasite originated from French Polynesia and showed that the introduced population was less genetically diverse than the native population [146]. Population genetic data also provided evidence that the introduced *S. istiblenni* has transmitted to native fish, shown by a lack of genetic differentiation between parasites from introduced and native hosts. Population genetic investigations into *Camallanus cotti*, invasive in Hawaiian stream fishes, revealed its probable invasion history, suggesting an initial introduction in O'ahu, where genetic diversity was highest, and subsequent migration to other islands in the archipelago [147]. Comparisons of the data in this study with data from *C. cotti* in its native range [115] showed that genetic diversity in introduced *C. cotti* was reduced compared with native populations, once again demonstrating the effects of population bottlenecks in introduced parasitic nematode populations.

Anguillicoloides crassus and its host, the Japanese eel (*Anguilla japonica*), were introduced from Asia to North America and Europe, and since then *A. crassus* has spread rapidly in European and American eels (*Anguilla anguilla* and *A. rostrata*, respectively), causing severe pathology in these naïve host species [148]. Population genetic studies have revealed multiple, distinct lineages of invasive *A. crassus*, suggesting multiple introduction events from different source populations [149, 150]. Furthermore, a southern to northern clinal decrease in its genetic diversity is seen in Europe, suggesting that *A. crassus* was introduced in southern Europe and has since spread northwards [150]. Hence, the population genetics of *A. crassus* has revealed its introduction history. Infrapopulation differentiation in *A. crassus* was studied in two European rivers, one of which was regularly artificially restocked with eels from a variety of sources and one in which eels had arrived by natural dispersal [151]. This showed that in the restocked river, *A. crassus* had high genetic diversity among hosts and a substantial deviation from Hardy-Weinberg equilibrium (see Table 1), while in the river with natural recruitment, there was no among-host structuring or deviation from Hardy-Weinberg equilibrium. These contrasting patterns were thought to be because the introduced eels had retained *A. crassus* infrapopulations reflective of their genetically distinct source populations, while *A. crassus* in the river with natural recruitment are derived from a single population that was already at Hardy-Weinberg equilibrium [151].

As environments continue to change, the ranges of parasitic nematodes will change too. The population genetics of parasitic nematodes currently undergoing such range changes show that (i) invasive parasitic nematodes are likely to have low genetic diversity (due to population bottlenecks); and (ii) that host populations are likely to lose diversity more rapidly following habitat fragmentation than parasitic nematode populations (due to the comparatively smaller Ne of hosts). This latter effect may have a consequence for parasite ecology, since hosts will differ in their genetic resistance to parasites, and genetic bottlenecks of host populations may therefore lead to altered degrees of parasitism. Supporting this, *Trypanoxyuris* spp. and *B. schroederi* all show genetic evidence of recent population expansion despite marked declines in host population size [127, 132], suggesting that prevalence and/or intensity of infection has increased since habitat fragmentation. Hence, population genetic analysis can inform on the biology of parasitic nematodes undergoing changes in range, and can be used to make predictions about how parasite populations might respond genetically to future range changes.

Prospects in nematode population genetics

Genome sequencing

Each of the methods routinely used to analyse parasitic nematode population genetics detects variation in a small number of loci [24], and it is often not clear how representative these loci are of a genome more widely. High-throughput sequencing techniques can be employed to interrogate large portions of the genome, thus reducing the effect of bias at any one genomic region. Other advantages include the ability to screen the genome for regions under selection, and the chance to analyse population genetic structure at several scales simultaneously. For example, highly polymorphic (see Table 1) genomic regions can inform on structure at very local scales, while more conserved regions will be appropriate for studying the relationships of more divergent populations. Genome-wide sequencing has been used to assess population genetics in non-nematode helminths, allowing detailed insight into parasite population genetic structure [152], and there is no reason why such insights should not be possible in parasitic nematodes. These techniques usually require a reference genome, which often will not be available *a priori* for non-model parasitic nematodes infecting wild animals. However, rapid advances in the sequencing and assembly of nematode genomes mean that it may often be feasible to generate a reference genome for the species in question [153].

In restriction-associated DNA sequencing (RADSeq) the genome of an individual is digested with a restriction endonuclease, and the resulting fragments are size-filtered and then sequenced [154]. Random distribution of restriction endonuclease sites across the genome ensures that the sequenced fragments are representative of the whole genome. Double-digest RADSeq (ddRADSeq) is a related technique that uses two restriction endonucleases [155]. While (dd)RADSeq data can be used without a reference genome assembly [156], having a reference means that non-target DNA can be detected and excluded. (dd)RADSeq approaches have not yet been used in the population genetic analysis of parasitic nematodes, but have been used in several other animal species [9, 157] including the free-living nematode *Caenorhabditis elegans* [158]. The study in *C. elegans* not only revealed the population genetics of this species, but also its recent evolutionary history, finding that the low genetic diversity of *C. elegans* likely arose from recent selective sweeps (see Table 1), in which a few beneficial alleles drove large swathes of the genome to near-fixation (see Table 1) due to extensive linkage disequilibrium (see Table 1) [158]. If (dd)RADSeq were used to study the population genetics of parasitic nematodes, we could expect similar insights into the biology and evolutionary history of these species.

In whole-genome sequencing, individuals are genotyped at virtually every locus polymorphic among samples. This allows the relationships among individuals, and hence the genetic structure of populations, to be resolved at the finest possible scale [159], and gives more power to make inferences about the evolutionary processes acting on a species [160, 161]. There are currently obstacles to routinely generating whole-genome sequence data. Firstly, sequencing the genomes of multiple individuals is often still expensive, such that there is a trade-off between the number of individuals sequenced and the genome coverage of each individual. However, population genetic techniques are robust to low genome coverage, with coverage of as little as two-fold having been applied [162]. Secondly, the small physical size of some nematodes can make it difficult to extract sufficient DNA for sequencing. Whole-genome amplification (WGA) prior to sequencing can ameliorate this difficulty [163], though not without some bias in genome coverage [164].

However, the difficulties of whole-genome sequencing are worth overcoming, due to the wealth of information it can provide. Of particular importance is the ability of whole-genome sequencing to identify genes that are under selection, and in the case of parasites, these genes may be relevant to pathogenicity, epidemiology and control. For example, whole-genome sequencing of the malaria parasite *Plasmodium falciparum* has found that genes that function in evasion of host immunity and in resistance to drugs show signs of selection [165]. Similar studies in parasitic nematodes are warranted, as anthelmintic resistance is an increasingly serious problem in both agricultural and medical settings, and the biochemical mechanisms of resistance are often poorly understood [20, 166]. Genes that show strong signatures of directional selection in anthelminthic-exposed populations are good candidates for genes conferring anthelmintic resistance [167].

Whole-genome sequencing has already been used to study the population genetics of parasitic nematodes that infect people, demonstrating among-host differentiation in *Wuchereria bancrofti* [168], and detecting differentiation in *Strongyloides stercoralis* among host individuals and populations [169]. However, these studies used small numbers of hosts and are limited in scope. Hence, there is now a need for studies on a comparatively larger scale that examine the distribution of polymorphisms within genomes as well as among them. In an intriguing recent study, whole-genome sequencing was used to interrogate the population genetics of the plant-parasitic nematode *Heterodera glycines* without the use of a reference genome [170]. This study, which made use of the UNEAK bioinformatics pipeline [171], was able to not only elucidate the population genetic structure of *H. glycines*, but also to identify genetic variants showing signatures of selection. Whether a reference assembly is used or not, whole-genome sequencing studies will improve our understanding of how parasitic nematodes respond to natural selection pressures. As the climate changes, parasitic nematodes will encounter novel selection pressures, and how they respond to these pressures may have important consequences, not only for host species but for the ecosystem as a whole.

Environmental DNA (eDNA) analysis

Parasitic nematodes typically have extra-host transmission stages in their life-cycle, and as these stages are the pool from which the next generation of parasites will arise, they contribute directly to Ne. Differences in the number, spatial distribution and temporal distribution of these stages may therefore influence the rate of genetic drift in a population, and hence the population genetic structure more widely. Despite their likely importance in both population genetics and epidemiology, very little is known about the ecology of extra-host stages, and what is known largely pertains to human or livestock pathogens [172, 173]. This knowledge gap is principally due to the difficulty in sampling and identifying extra-host nematode stages in the environment. Sequencing of environmental DNA (eDNA, see Table 1) may be a solution to this problem [174, 175]. DNA-based identification of parasitic nematodes stages in host faeces - in essence a form of eDNA - is often used to diagnose infection in livestock [176]. Adaptation of these techniques for the detection of parasitic nematode stages in soil and water (where target DNA concentrations will often be lower) would incorporate extra-host transmission stages into analysis of population genetics of parasitic nematodes infecting wild animals.

Synthesis and outstanding research questions

As with all species, the population genetics of parasitic nematodes in wild animals is ultimately determined by the (i) rate of gene flow among populations and (ii) strength of genetic drift within populations. Nematodes have very limited dispersal ability of their own, so that they are largely dependent on their hosts for dispersal. Therefore, in principle, nematode populations should ultimately come to be structured at the scale over which hosts move. Broadly speaking, this rule is largely followed - there is very limited population genetic structuring of parasitic nematodes infecting highly mobile hosts, such as ocean-going mammals [100], while the parasites of small, sedentary rodents, for example, generally have highly structured populations [15].

Nematode species that use more than one host species often have less structured populations than the movement of any one host species would predict. This has been observed in *Trichinella* spp., which shows gene flow at the continental scale [38], in *Dictyocaulus eckerti*, a generalist parasite of deer [86], and in *Neoheligmonella granjoni* [72, 73]. The use of multiple mobile host species allows nematodes to traverse or colonise a wider range of habitats than would be possible using only a single host, and this tends to promote parasite gene flow. In contrast, highly pathogenic parasitic nematodes, such as *Heterorhabditis marelatus*, may show reduced gene flow if they significantly hamper their host's movement [116].

In the absence of gene flow all populations will ultimately diverge genetically due to genetic drift, but this process takes time. How much time depends on the strength of genetic drift, in turn dictated by (among other things) Ne, and so Ne is a major determinant in population genetic structure. Ne is rarely measured directly but can be estimated from known aspects of parasite and host life history. For example, haploid males in *Syphacia stroma* likely reduce Ne in comparison with the fully diploid *Heligmosomoides polygyrus*, with which *S. stroma* shares a host [78], while the much lower infection prevalence and intensity of *Dictyocaulus viviparus* compared with *Ostertagia ostertagi* in domestic cattle means that the former likely has lower Ne [177, 178]. In both cases, the species presumed to have the lower Ne has stronger population genetic structuring. Naturally, parasites with a fast generation time will undergo more rapid genetic drift (and so faster population divergence) than parasites with a slow generation time. Indeed, the significantly faster generation time of *H. polygyrus* compared with *Trichuris muris* may contribute to the comparatively more strongly genetically structured populations of the former when both species are analysed from the same host individuals [15, 53, 54].

Parasite life history traits such as host range, reproductive strategy, generation time, and the prevalence, intensity and pathogenicity of infection in the host are therefore all important in determining the population genetics of parasitic nematodes. These factors interact with host ecology, and in particular, host movement behaviour, to establish patterns of parasite population genetic structure. However, the relative importance of parasite life history traits remains poorly understood. Animals are commonly infected by more than one species of nematode, and this fact could be exploited to better understand population genetics in nematodes infecting wild animals. For example, comparison of life history traits among co-infecting parasites would allow their effects on parasite populations genetics to be separated from host-dependent effects.

The abundance and spatial and temporal dynamics of extra-host stage parasitic nematodes in the environment remains almost entirely unknown. There have been some attempts to study the extra-host stages of nematodes infecting domestic livestock [179], but the findings may not be fully applicable to species infecting wild animals. Understanding the ecology of extra-host parasite stages is important for conservation of wild hosts, for monitoring the threat of zoonotic infection, and for our understanding of ecosystem processes. Particularly mysterious is the role of extra-host stages on the population genetics of parasitic nematodes, and future work must address this to complete our understanding of the population genetics of parasitic nematodes in wildlife. eDNA applications may be the only means of sampling extra-host nematode stages with sufficient rigour to understand their contribution to population genetics.

Looking to the future, the use of high-throughput sequencing-based methods (dd)RADSeq and whole-genome sequencing) will dramatically improve the resolution and accuracy with which population structure can be detected. Furthermore, whole-genome sequencing will allow other aspects of parasitic nematode genomes, such as the size and nature of selection, and the extent of linkage disequilibrium, to be interrogated, and this knowledge will improve our understanding of parasitic nematode biology.

Conclusions

The population genetics of parasitic nematodes in wild animals is determined by a combination of host ecology - especially host movement behaviour - and parasite life history. Studying the population genetics of parasitic nematodes of wild animals can reveal how their populations respond to selective pressures. With this information, we can assess the risk parasitic nematodes pose to natural ecosystems and to the health of humans and domestic animals, as anthropogenic activities drive environmental changes and changes in species' geographical ranges. Our understanding of the population genetics, biology and evolutionary history of parasitic nematodes will be improved if investigators incorporate extra-host transmission stages and take advantage of high-throughput DNA-sequencing technologies in future studies.

Abbreviations

ddRADSeq: Double-digest restriction-associated DNA sequencing; DNA: Deoxyribonucleic acid; eDNA: Environmental DNA; ITS: Internal transcribed spacer; mtDNA: Mitochondrial DNA; N: Census size; Ne: Effective population size; PCR: Polymerase chain reaction; RADSeq: Restriction-associated DNA sequencing; RAPD: Random amplified polymorphic DNA

Acknowledgments

RC is supported by a NERC studentship.

Funding

RC is supported by a NERC studentship.

Authors' contributions

RC wrote the manuscript, which was edited by MV and RC together. Both authors read and approved the final manuscript.

Competing interests

The authors declare that they have no competing interests.

References

1. Dobson AP. The population biology of parasite-induced changes in host behaviour. Q Rev Biol. 1988;63:139–65.
2. Hurd H. Physiological and behavioural interactions between parasites and invertebrate hosts. Adv Parasit. 1990;29:271–318.
3. Hudson PJ, Dobson AP, Lafferty KD. Is a healthy ecosystem one that is rich in parasites? Trends Ecol Evol. 2006;21:381–5.
4. Frainer A, McKie BG, Amundsen P-A, Lafferty KD. Parasitism and the biodiversity-functioning relationship. Trends Ecol Evol. 2018;33:260–8.
5. Kirk RS. The impact of *Anguillicola crassus* on European eels. Fisheries Manag Ecol. 2003;10:385–94.
6. Zhang J-S, Daszak P, Huang H-L, Yang G-Y, Kilpatrick AM, Zhang S. Parasite threat to panda conservation. EcoHealth. 2008;5:6–9.
7. Sakanari JA, McKerrow JH. Anisakiasis. Clin Micriobiol Rev. 1989;2:278–84.
8. Sorvillo F, Ash LR, Berlin OG, Yatabe J, Degiorgio MSA. *Baylisascaris procyonis*: an emerging helminthic zoonosis. Emerg Infect Dis. 2002;8:355–9.
9. Gilabert A, Wasmuth JD. Unravelling parasitic nematode natural history using population genetics. Trends Parasitol. 2013;29:438–48.
10. Gorton MJ, Kasl EL, Detwiller JT, Criscione CD. Testing local-scale panmixia provides insights into the cryptic ecology, evolution, and epidemiology of metazoan animal parasites. Parasitology. 2012;139:981–97.
11. Criscione CD, Poulin R, Blouin MS. Molecular ecology of parasites: elucidating ecological and microevolutionary processes. Mol Ecol. 2005;14: 2247–57.
12. Blouin MS. Molecular prospecting for cryptic species of nematodes: mitochondrial DNA *versus* internal transcribed spacer. Int J Parasitol. 2002;32: 527–31.
13. Nadler SA, Pérez-Ponce de León G. Integrating molecular and morphological approaches for characterizing parasite cryptic species: implications for parasitology. Parasitology. 2011;138:1688–709.
14. Pérez-Ponce de León G, Nadler SA. What we don't recognize can hurt us: a plea for awareness about cryptic species. J Parasitol. 2010;96:453–64.
15. Nieberding C, Morand S, Libois R, Michaux JR. A parasite reveals cryptic phylogeographic history of its host. P R Soc B. 2004;271:2559–68.
16. Galbreath KE, Hoberg EP. Return to Beringia: parasites reveal cryptic biogeographic history of North American pikas. Proc R Soc B Biol Sci. 2012; 279:371–8.
17. Wickström LM, Haukisalmi V, Varis S, Hantula J, Fedorov VB, Henttonen H. Phylogeography of the circumpolar *Paranoplocephala arctica* species complex (Cestoda: Anoplocephalidae) parasitizing collared lemmings (*Dicrostonyx* spp.). Mol Ecol. 2003;12:3359–71.
18. Wickström LM, Hantula J, Haukisalmi V, Hentonnen H. Genetic and morphometric variation in the Holarctic helminth parasite *Andrya arctica* (Cestoda, Anoplocephalidae) in relation to the divergence of its lemming hosts (*Dicrostonyx* spp.). Zool J Lind Soc-Lond. 2001;131:443–57.
19. Koehler AVA, Hoberg EP, Dokuchaev NE, Tranbenkova NA, Whitman JS, Nagorsen DW, Cook JA. Phylogeography of a Holarctic nematode, *Soboliphyme baturini*, among mustelids: climate change, episodic colonization, and diversification in a complex host-parasite system. Biol J Linn Soc. 96:651–63.
20. Gilleard JS, Redman E. Genetic diversity and population structure of *Haemonchus contortus*. Adv Parasitol. 2016;93:31–68.
21. Nadler SA. Microevolution and the genetic structure of parasite populations. J Parasitol. 1995;81:395–403.
22. Mazé-Guilmo E, Blanchet S, McCoy KD, Loot G. Host dispersal as the driver of parasite genetic structure: a paradigm lost? Ecol Lett. 2016;19:336–47.
23. Vázquez-Prieto S, Vilas R, Paniagua E, Ubeira FM. Influence of life history traits on the population genetic structure of parasitic helminths: a minireview. Folia Parasitol. 2015;62:060.
24. Anderson TJC, Blouin MS, Beech RN. Population biology of parasitic nematodes: applications of genetic markers. Adv Parsitol. 1998;41:219–83.
25. Barret LG, Thrall PH, Burdon JJ, Linde CC. Life history determines genetic structure and evolutionary potential of host-parasite interactions. Trends Ecol Evol. 2008;23:678–85.
26. Fazenda IP, Beveridge I, Chilton NB, Jex AR, Pangasa A, Campbell BE, et al. Analysis of genetic variation in *Globocephaloides* populations from macropodid marsupials using a mutation scanning-based approach. Electrophoresis. 2009;30:2758–64.
27. Chilton NB, Beveridge I, Andrews RH. Detection by allozyme electrophoresis of cryptic species of *Hypodontus macropi* (Nematoda: Strongyloidea) from macropodid marsupials. Int J Parasitol. 1992;22:271–9.
28. Chilton NB, Andrews RH, Beveridge I. Genetic evidence for a complex of species within *Rugopharynx australis* (Mönnig, 1926) (Nematoda: Strongyloidea) from macropodid marsupials. Syst Parasitol. 1996;34:125–33.
29. Zhu X, Spratt DM, Beveridge I, Haycock P, Gasser RB. Mitochondrial DNA polymorphism within and among species of *Capillaria sensu lato* from Australian marsupials and rodents. Int J Parasitol. 2000;30:933–8.
30. Chilton NB, Huby-Chilton F, Smales LR, Gasser RB, Beveridge I. Genetic divergence between island and continental populations of the parasitic nematode *Labiosimplex australis* in Australia. Parasitol Res. 2009;104:229–36.
31. Chilton NB, Huby-Chilton F, Johnson PM, Beveridge I, Gasser RM. Genetic variation within species of the nematode genus *Cloacina* (Strongyloidea: Cloacininae) parasitic in the stomachs of rock wallabies, *Petrogale* spp. (Marsupialia: Macropodidae) in Queensland. Aust J Zool. 2009;57(1):10.
32. Dunams-Morel DB, Reichard MV, Toretti L, Zarlenga DS, Rosenthal BM. Discernible but limited introgression has occurred where *Trichinella nativa* and the T6 genotype occur in sympatry. Infect Genet Evol. 2012;12:530–8.
33. La Rosa G, Marucci G, Rosenthal BM, Pozio E. Development of a single larva microsatellite analysis to investigate the population structure of *Trichinella spiralis*. Infect Genet Evol. 2012;12:369–76.
34. Dame JB, Murrel D, Worley DE, Schad GA. *Trichinella spiralis*: genetic evidence for synanthropic subspecies in sylvatic hosts. Exp Parasitol. 1987; 64:195–203.
35. La Rosa G, Pozio E, Rossi P. Biochemical resolution of European and African isolates of *Trichinella nelsoni* Britov and Boev, 1972. Parasitol Res. 1990;77: 173–6.
36. La Rosa G, Pozio E, Rossi P, Murrel KD. Allozyme analysis of *Trichinella* isolates from various host species and geographical regions. J Parasitol. 1992;78:641–6.
37. La Rosa G, Pozio E. Molecular investigation of African isolates of *Trichinella* reveals genetic polymorphism in *Trichinella nelsoni*. Int J Parasitol. 2000;(5): 663–7.
38. La Rosa G, Marucci G, Zarlenga DS, Pozio E. *Trichinella pseudospiralis* populations of the Palearctic region and their relationship with populations of the Nearctic and Australian regions. Int J Parasitol. 2001;31:297–305.
39. La Rosa G, Marucci G, Zarlenga DS, Casulli A, Zarnke RL, Pozio R. Molecular identification of natural hybrids between *Trichinella nativa* and *Trichinella* T6 provides evidence of gene flow and ongoing genetic divergence. Int J Parasitol. 2003;33:209–16.
40. Zarlenga DS, Aschenbrebber RA, Lechtenfels JR. Variations in microsatellite sequences provide evidence for population differences and multiple ribosomal gene repeats in *Trichinella pseudospiralis*. J Parasitol. 1996;82:534–8.
41. Otranto D, Testini G, De Luca F, Hu M, Shamsi S, Gasser RB. Analysis of genetic variability within *Thelazia callipaeda* (Nematoda: Thelazioidea) from Europe and Asia by sequencing and mutation scanning of the mitochondrial cytochrome c oxidase subunit 1 gene. Mol Cel Probe. 2005; 19:306–13.
42. Di Cisare A, Otranto D, Latrofa MS, Veronisi F, Perrucci S, Lalosevic D, et al. Genetic variability of *Eucoleus aerophilus* from domestic and wild hosts. Res Vet Sci. 2014;96:512–5.
43. Rothmann W, de Waal PJ. Diversity of *Spirocerca lupi* in domestic dogs and black-backed jackals (*Canis mesomelas*) from South Africa. Vet Parasitol. 2017;244:59–63.
44. Berntzen AK. Comparative growth and development of *Trichinella spiralis in vitro* and *in vivo*, with a redescription of the life cycle. Exp Parasitol. 1965;16: 74–106.
45. Montgomery WI, Wilson WL, Hamilton R, McCartney P. Dispersion in the wood mouse, *Apodemus sylvaticus*: variable resources in time and space. J Anim Ecol. 1991;60:179–92.
46. Mikesic DG, Drickamer LC. Factors affecting home-range size in house mice (*Mus musculus domesticus*) living in outdoor enclosures. Am Midl Nat. 1992; 127:31–40.
47. Pocock JO, Hauffe HC, Searle JB. Dispersal in house mice. Biol J Linn Soc. 2005;84:565–83.
48. Gardner-Santana LC, Norris DE, Fornadel CE, Hinson ER, Klein SL, Glass GE. Commensal ecology, urban landscapes, and their influence on the genetic characteristics of city-dwelling Norway rats (*Rattus norvegicus*). Mol Ecol. 2009;18:2766–78.

49. Nieberding C, Libois R, Douady CJ, Morand S, Michaux JR. Phylogeography of a nematode (*Heligmosomoides polygyrus*) in the western Palearctic region: persistence of northern cryptic populations during ice ages? Mol Ecol. 2005; 14:765–79.
50. Nieberding C, Morand S, Libois R, Michaux JR. Parasites and the island syndrome: the colonization of the western Mediterranean islands by *Heligmosomoides polygyrus* (Dujardin, 1845). J Biogeogr. 2006;33:1212–22.
51. Nieberding C, Durette-Desset M-C, Vanderpoorten A, Casanova JC, Ribas A, Deffontaine V, et al. Geography and host biogeography matter for understanding the phylogeography of a parasite. Mol Phylogenet Evol. 2008;47:538–54.
52. Monroy FG, Enriquez FJ. *Heligmosomoides polygyrus*: a model for chronic gastrointestinal helminthiasis. Parasitol Today. 1992;8:49–54.
53. Callejón R, de Rojas M, Nieberding C, Foronda P, Feliú C, Guevera D, Cutillas C. Molecular evolution of *Trichuris muris* isolated from different Muridae hosts in Europe. Parasitol Res. 2010;107:631–41.
54. Callejón R, de Rojas M, Feliú C, Balao F, Marrugal A, Henttonen H, et al. Phylogeography of *Trichuris* populations isolated from different Cricetidae rodents. Parasitology. 2012;139:1795–812.
55. Wasimuddin BJ, Ribas A, Baird SJE, Piálek J, Goüy de Bellocq J. Testing parasite 'intimacy': the whipworm *Trichuris muris* in the European house mouse hybrid zone. Ecol Evol. 2016;6:2688–701.
56. Fahmy MAM. An investigation on the life cycle of *Trichuris muris*. Parasitology. 1954;44:50–7.
57. Gregory RD, Keymer AE, Clarge JR. Genetics, sex and exposure: the ecology of *Heligmosomoides polygyrus* (Nematoda) in the wood mouse. J Anim Ecol. 1990;59:363–78.
58. Yong HS, Eamsobhana P. Definitive rodent hosts of the rat lungworm *Angiostrongylus cantonensis*. Raffles B Zool. 2013;29:111–5.
59. Liu CY, Zhang RL, Chen MX, Li J, Ai L, Wu CY, et al. Characterisation of *Angiostrongylus cantonensis* isolates from China by sequences of internal transcribed spacers of nuclear ribosomal DNA. J Anim Vet Adv. 2011;10: 593–6.
60. Thaenkham U, Pakdee W, Nuamtanong S, Maipannich W, Pubampen S, Sa-Nguankiat S, Komalamisra C. Population structure of *Angiostrongylus cantonensis* (Nematoda: Metastrongylidae) in Thailand based on PCR-RAPD markers. SE Asian J Trop Med. 2012;43:567–73.
61. Dusitsittipon S, Thaenkham D, Watthanakulpanich D, Adisakwattana P, Komalamisra C. Genetic differences in the rat lungworm, *Angiostrongylus cantonensis* (Nematoda: Angiostrongylidae), in Thailand. J Helminthol. 2015; 89:545–51.
62. Yong H-S, Eamsobhana P, Song S-L, Prasartvit A, Lim P-E. Molecular phylogeography of *Angiostrongylus cantonensis* (Nematoda: Angiostrongylidae) and genetic relationships with congeners using cytochrome b gene marker. Acta Trop. 2015;148:66–71.
63. Vitta A, Srisongcram N, Thiproaj J, Wongma A, Polsut W, Fukrusa C, et al. Phylogeny of *Angiostrongylus cantonensis* in Thailand based on cytochrome *c* oxidase subunit I gene sequence. SE Asian J Trop Med. 2016;47:377–86.
64. Eamsobhana P, Song S-L, Yong H-S, Prasartvit A, Boonyong S, Tungtrongchitr A. Cytochrome *c* oxidase subunit I haplotype diversity of *Angiostrongylus cantonensis* (Nematoda: Angiostrongylidae). Acta Trop. 2017; 171:141–5.
65. Tokiwa T, Harunari T, Tanikawa T, Komatsu N, Koizumi N, Tung K-C, et al. Phylogenetic relationships of rat lungworm, *Angiostrongylus cantonensis*, isolated from different geographical regions revealed widespread multiple lineages. Parasitol Int. 2012;61:431–6.
66. Monte TCC, Simões RO, Oliveira APM, Novaes CF, Thiengo SC, Silva AJ, et al. Phylogenetic relationship of the Brazilian isolates of the rat lungworm *Angiostrongylus cantonensis* (Nematoda: Metastrongylidae) employing mitochondrial COI gene sequence data. Parasit Vectors. 2012;5:248.
67. Eamsobhana P, Yong HS, Song SL, Prasartvit A, Boonyong S, Tungtongchitr A. Cytochrome *c* oxidase subunit I haplotype reveals high genetic diversity of *Angiostrongylus malaysiensis* (Nematoda: Angiostrongylidae). J Helminthol. 2018;92:254–9.
68. Rodpai R, Intapan PM, Thanchomnang T, Sanpool O, Sadaow L, Laymanivong S, et al. *Angiostrongylus cantonensis* and *A. malaysiensis* broadly overlap in Thailand, Lao PDR, Cambodia and Myanmar: a molecular survey of larvae in land snails. PLoS One. 2016;11:e0161128.
69. Yong HS, Song SL, Eamsobhana P, Goh SY, Lim PE. Complete mitochondrial genome reveals genetic diversity of *Angiostrongylus cantonensis* (Nematoda: Angiostrongylidae). Acta Trop. 2015;152:157–64.
70. Dusitsittipon S, Criscione CD, Morand S, Komalamisra C, Thaenkham U. Cryptic lineage diversity in the zoonotic pathogen *Angiostrongylus cantonensis*. Mol Phylogenet Evol. 2017;107:404–14.
71. Dusitsittipon S, Criscione CD, Morand S, Komalamisra C, Thaenkham U. Hurdles in the evolutionary epidemiology of *Angiostrongylus cantonensis*: pseudogenes, incongruence between taxonomy and DNA sequence variants, and cryptic lineages. Evol Appl. 2018;11:1257–69.
72. Brouat C, Tatard C, Machin A, Kane M, Diouf M, Bâ K, Duplantier JM. Comparative population genetics of a parasitic nematode and its host community: the trichostrongylid *Neoheligmonella granjoni* and *Mastomys* rodents in south-eastern Senegal. Int J Parasitol. 2011;41:1301–9.
73. Brouat C, Loiseau A, Kane M, Bâ K, Duplantier J-M. Population genetic structure of two ecologically distinct multimammate rats: the commensal *Mastomys natalensis* and the wild *M. erythroleucus* in south-eastern Senegal. Mol Ecol. 2007;16:2985–97.
74. Brant SV, Ortí G. Evidence for gene flow in parasitic nematodes between two host species of shrews. Mol Ecol. 2003;12:2853–9.
75. Fisher MC, Viney ME. The population genetic structure of the facultatively sexual parasitic nematode *Strongyloides ratti* in wild rats. Proc R Soc B Biol Sci. 1998;265:703–9.
76. Viney ME. A genetic analysis of reproduction in *Strongyloides ratti*. Parasitology. 1994;109:511–5.
77. Paterson S, Fisher MC, Viney ME. Inferring infection processes of a parasitic nematode using population genetics. Parasitology. 2000;120:185–94.
78. Müller-Graf CD, Durand P, Feliu C, Hugot J-P, O'Callaghan CJ, Renaud F, et al. Epidemiology and genetic variability of two species of nematodes (*Heligmosomoides polygyrus* and *Syphacia stroma*) of *Apodemus* spp. Parasitology. 1999;118:425–32.
79. Morand S. Life-history traits in parasitic nematodes: a comparative approach for the search of invariants. Funct Ecol. 1996;10:210–8.
80. Dallas JF, Irvine RJ, Halvorsen O. DNA evidence that *Ostertagia gruehneri* and *Ostertagia arctica* (Nematoda: Ostertagiinae) in reindeer from Norway and Svalbard are conspecific. Int J Parasitol. 2000;30:655–8.
81. Dallas JF, Irvine RJ, Halvorsen O. DNA evidence that *Marshallagia marshalli* Ransom, 1907 and *M. occidentalis* Ransom, 1907 (Nematoda: Ostertagiinae) from Svalbard reindeer are conspecific. Syst Parasitol. 2001;50:101–3.
82. Hoberg EP, Monsen KJ, Kutz S, Blouin MS. Structure, biodiversity, and historical biogeography of nematode faunas in Holarctic ruminants: morphological and molecular diagnoses for *Teladorsagia boreoarticus* n. sp. (Nemadota: Ostertagiinae), dimorphic cryptic species in muskoxen (*Ovibos moschatus*). J Parasitol. 1999;85:910–34.
83. Blouin MS, Yowell CA, Courtney CH, Dame JB. Host movement and the genetic structure of populations of parasitic nematodes. Genetics. 1995;141: 1007–14.
84. Tyler NJC, Øritsland NA. Home ranges in Svalbard reindeer. Rangifer. 1990; S3:147–8.
85. Long ES, Diefenbach DR, Rosenberry CS, Wallingford BD. Multiple proximate and ultimate causes of natal dispersal in white-tailed deer. Behav Ecol. 2008; 19:1235–42.
86. Ács Z, Hayward A, Sugár L. Genetic diversity and population genetics of large lungworms (*Dictyocaulus*, Nematoda) in wild deer in Hungary. Parasitol Res. 2016;115:3295–312.
87. Archie EA, Ezenwa VO. Population genetic structure and history of a generalist parasite infecting multiple sympatric host species. Int J Parasitol. 2011;41:89–98.
88. Falk BG, Perkins SL. Host specificity shapes population structure of pinworm parasites in Caribbean reptiles. Mol Ecol. 2013;22:4576–90.
89. Calsbeek R. Sex-specific adult dispersal and its selective consequences in the brown anole, *Anolis sagrei*. J Anim Ecol. 2009;78:617–24.
90. Jorge F, Roca V, Perera A, Harris DJ, Carretero MA. A phylogenetic assessment of the colonisation patterns in *Spauligodon atlanticus* Astasio-Arbiza et al., 1987 (Nematoda: Oxyurida: Pharyngodonidae), a parasite of lizards of the genus *Gallotia* Boulenger: no simple answers. Syst Parasitol. 2011;80:53–66.
91. Gustafson KD, Newman RA, Rhen T, Tkach W. Spatial and genetic structure of directly-transmitted parasites reflects the distribution of their specific amphibian hosts. Pop Ecol. 2018;60:261–73.
92. Johnson PCD, Webster LMI, Adam A, Buckland R, Dawson DA, Keller LF. Abundant variation in microsatellites of the parasitic nematode *Trichostrongylus tenuis* and linkage to a tandem repeat. Mol Biochem Parasit. 2006;148:210–8.

93. Webster LMI, Johnson PCD, Adam A, Mable BK, Keller MF. Macrogeographic population structure in a parasitic nematode with avian hosts. Vet Parasitol. 2007;144:93–103.
94. Seivwright LJ, Redpath SM, Mougeot F, Watt L, Hudson PJ. Faecal egg counts provide a reliable measure of *Trichostrongylus tenuis* intensities in free-living red grouse *Lagopus lagopus scoticus*. J Helminthol. 2004;78:69–76.
95. Wernham CV, Toms MP, Marchant JH, Clark JA, Siriwardena GM, Baillie SE. Migration Atlas: Movements of the Birds of Britain and Ireland. London: Poyser; 2002.
96. Nagasawa K. The life cycle of *Anisakis simplex*: a review. In: Ishikura H, Kikuchi K, editors. Intestinal Anisakiasis in Japan. Tokyo: Springer; 1990. p. 31–40.
97. Åkesson S, Weimerskirch H. Albatross long-distance navigation: comparing adults and juveniles. J Navigation. 2005;58:365–73.
98. Tsai Y-JJ, Mann J. Dispersal, philopatry, and the role of fission-fusion dynamics in bottlenose dolphins. Mar Mammal Sci. 2012;29:261–79.
99. Mattiucci S, Nascetti G, Cianchi R, Paggi L, Arduino P, Margolis L, et al. Genetic and ecological data on the *Anisakis simplex* complex, with evidence for a new species (Nematoda, Ascaridoidea, Anisakidae). J Parasitol. 1997;83: 401–16.
100. Mattiucci S, Nascetti G, Dailey M, Webb SC, Barros NB, Cianchi R, Bullini L. Evidence for a new species of *Anisakis* Dujardin, 1845: morphological description and genetic relationships between congeners (Nematoda: Anisakidae). Syst Parasitol. 2005;61:157–71.
101. Pontes T, D'Amelio S, Costa G, Paggi L. Molecular characterization of larval anisakid nematodes from marine fishes of Madeira by a PCR-based approach, with evidence for a new species. J Parasitol. 2005;91:1430–4.
102. Beverly-Burton M. Population genetics of *Anisakis simplex* (Nematoda: Ascaridoidea) in Atlantic salmon (*Salmo salar*) and their use as biological indicators of host stocks. Environ Biol Fish. 1978;3:369–77.
103. Mattiucci S, Nascetti G. Genetic diversity and infection levels of anisakid nematodes parasitic in fish and marine mammals from Boreal and Austral hemispheres. Vet Parasitol. 2007;148:43–57.
104. Lyons ET, Spraker TR, de Long RL, Ionita M, Melin SR, Nadler SA, Tolliver SC. Review of research on hookworms (*Uncinaria lucasi* Stiles, 1901) in northern fur seals (*Callorhinus ursinus* Linnaeus, 1758). Parasitol Res. 2011;109:257–65.
105. Campbell RA, Gales NJ, Lento GM, Baker CS. Islands in the sea: extreme female natal site fidelity in the Australian sea lion, *Neophoca cinerea*. Biol Lett. 2008;4:139–42.
106. Haynes BT, Marcus AD, Higgins DP, Gongora J, Gray R, Šlapeta J. Unexpected absence of genetic separation of a highly diverse population of hookworms from geographically isolated hosts. Infect Genet Evol. 2014;28: 192–200.
107. Nadler SA, Adams BJ, Lyons ET, De Long RL, Melin SR. Molecular and morphometric evidence for separate species of *Uncinaria* (Nematoda: Ancylostomatidae) in California sea lions and northern fur seals: hypothesis testing supplants verification. J Parasitol. 2000;86:1099–106.
108. Martín-Sánchez J, Paniagua I, Valero A. Contribution to the knowledge of *Hysterothylacium aduncum* through electrophoresis of the enzymes glucose phosphate isomerase and phosphoglucomutase. Parasitol Res. 1998;84:160–3.
109. Klimpel S, Kleinertz S, Hanel R, Rükert S. Genetic variability in *Hysterothylacium aduncum*, a raphidascarid nematode isolated from sprat (*Sprattus sprattus*) of different geographical areas of the northeastern Atlantic. Parasitol Res. 2007;101:1425–30.
110. Limborg MT, Pedersen JS, Hemmer-Hansen J, Tomkeiwicz J, Bekkevold D. Genetic population structure of European sprat *Sprattus sprattus*: differentiation across a steep environmental gradient in a small pelagic fish. Mar Ecol. 2009;379:213–24.
111. Martín-Sánchez J, Díaz M, Artacho ME, Valero A. Molecular arguments for considering *Hysterothylacium fabri* (Nematoda: Anisakidae) a complex of sibling species. Parasitol Res. 2003;89:214–20.
112. Mejía-Madrid HH, Vázquez-Domínguez E, Pérez-Ponce de León G. Phylogeography and freshwater basins in central Mexico: recent history as revealed by the fish parasite *Rhabdochona lichtenfelsi* (Nematoda). 2007;34: 787–801.
113. Li WX, Wang GT, Nie P. Genetic variation of fish parasite populations in historically connected habitats: undetected habitat fragmentation effect on populations of the nematode *Procamallanus fulvidraconis* in the catfish *Pelteobagrus fulvidraco*. J Parasitol. 2008;94:643–7.
114. Ma R, Yang G, Duan H, Jiang J, Wang S, Feng X. China's lakes at present: number, area and spatial distribution. Sci China Earth Sci. 2011;54:283–9.
115. Wu SG, Wang GT, Xi BW, Xiong F, Liu T, Nie P. Population genetic structure of the parasitic nematode *Camallanus cotti* inferred from DNA sequences of ITS1 rDNA and the mitochondrial COI gene. Vet Parasitol. 2009;164:248–56.
116. Blouin MS, Liu J, Berry RE. Life cycle variation and the genetic structure of nematode populations. Heredity. 1999;83:253–9.
117. Johnigk S-A, Ehlers R-U. Juvenile development and life cycle of *Heterorhabditis bacteriophora* and *H. indica* (Nematoda: Heterorhabditidae). Nematology. 1999;1:251–60.
118. Belaich MN, Buldain D, Ghiringhelli PD, Hyman B, Micieli MV, Achinelly MF. Nucleotide sequence differentiation of Argentine isolates of the mosquito parasitic nematode *Strelkovimermis spiculatus* (Nematoda: Mermithidae). 2015;40:415–8.
119. Crainey JL, Wilson MD, Post RJ. An 18S ribosomal DNA barcode for the study of *Isomermis lairdi*, a parasite of the blackfly *Simulium damnosum s.l.* Met Vet Entomol. 2009;23:238–44.
120. Tobias ZJ, Jorge F, Poulin R. Life at the beach: comparative phylogeography of a sandhopper and its nematode parasite reveals extreme lack of parasite mtDNA variation. Biol J Linn Soc. 2017;122:113–32.
121. Tang S, Hyman BC. Mitochondrial genome haplotype hypervariation within the isopod parasitic nematode *Thaumamermis cosgrovei*. Genetics. 2007;176: 1139–50.
122. Jobet E, Durand P, Langand J, Müller-Graf CDM, Hugot J-P, Bounnoux M-E, et al. Comparative genetic diversity of parasites and their hosts: population structure of an urban cockroach and its haplo-diploid parasite (oxyuroid nematode). Mol Ecol. 2000;9:481–6.
123. Morand S, Rivault C. Infestation dynamics of *Blatticola blattae* Graeffe (Nematoda: Thelastomatidae), a parasite of *Blattella germanica* (Dictyoptera: Blattellidae). Int J Parasitol. 1992;22:983–9.
124. Lin Q, Li HM, Gao M, Wang XY, Ren WX, Cong MM, et al. Characterization of *Baylisascaris schroederi* from Qinling subspecies of giant panda in China by the first internal transcribed spacer (ITS-1) of nuclear ribosomal DNA. Parasitol Res. 2012;110:1297–303.
125. Zhao GH, Li HM, Ryan UM, Cong MM, Hu B, Gao M, et al. Phylogenetic study of *Baylisascaris schroederi* isolated from Qinling subspecies of giant panda in China based on combined nuclear 5.8S and the second internal transcribed spacer (ITS-2) ribosomal DNA sequences. Parasitol Int. 2012;61: 497–500.
126. Zhou X, Xie Y, Zhang Z-H, Wang C-D, Sun Y, Gu X-B, et al. Analysis of the genetic diversity of the nematode parasite *Baylisascaris schroederi* from wild giant pandas in different mountain ranges in China. Parasit Vectors. 2013;6:233.
127. Xie Y, Zhou X, Zhang Z, Wang C, Sun Y, Liu T, et al. Absence of genetic structure in *Baylisascaris schroederi* populations, a giant panda parasite, determined by mitochondrial sequencing. Parasit Vectors. 2014;7:606.
128. Lu Z, Johnson WE, Menotti-Raymong M, Yuhki N, Martenson JS, Mainka S, et al. Patterns of genetic diversity in remaining giant panda populations. Conserv Biol. 2002;15:1596–607.
129. Peng Z, Zhang C, Shen M, Bao H, Hou Z, He S, et al. *Baylisascaris schroederi* infection in giant pandas (*Ailuropoda melanoleuca*) in Foping National Nature Reserve, China. J Wildlife Dis. 2017;53:854–8.
130. Wei F, Hu Y, Zhu L, Bruford MW, Zhan X, Zhang L. Black and white and read all over: the past, present and future of giant panda genetics. Mol Ecol. 2012;21:5660–74.
131. Solórzano-García B, Ellis EA, Rodríguez-Luna E. Deforestation and primate habitat availability in Los Tuxtlas Biosphere Reserve Mexico. Int J Ecosystem. 2012;2:61–6.
132. Solórzano-García B, Gasca-Pineda J, Poulin R, Pérez-Ponce de León G. Lack of genetic structure in pinworm populations from New World primates in forest fragments. Int J Parasitol. 2017;47:941–50.
133. Gasser RB, Woods WG, Blotkamp C, Verweij JJ, Storey PA, Polderman AM. Screening for nucleotide variations in ribosomal DNA arrays of *Oesophagostomum bifurcum* by polymerase chain reaction-coupled single-strand conformation polymorphism. Electrophoresis. 1999;20:1486–91.
134. De Gruijter JM, Ziem J, Verweij JJ, Polderman AM, Gasser RB. Genetic substructuring within *Oesophagostomum bifurcum* (Nematoda) from human and non-human primates from Ghana based on random amplified polymorphic DNA analysis. Am J Trop Med Hyg. 2004;71:227–33.
135. Gasser RB, de Gruijter JM, Polderman AM. Insights into the epidemiology and genetic make-up of *Oesophagostomum bifurcum* from human and non-human primates using molecular tools. Parasitology. 2006;132:453–60.
136. De Gruijter JM, Gasser RB, Polderman AM, Asigri V, Dijkshoorn L. High resolution DNA fingerprinting by AFLP to study the genetic variation

among *Oesophagostomum bifurcum* (Nematoda) from human and non-human primates from Ghana. Parasitology. 2005;130:229–37.
137. Labes EM, Wijayanti N, Deplazes P, Mathis A. Genetic characterization of *Strongyloides* spp. from captive, semi-captive and wild Bornean orangutans (*Pongo pygmaeus*) in Central and East Kalimantan, Borneo, Indonesia. Parasitology. 2011;138:1417–22.
138. Ravasi DF, O'Riain MJ, Davids F, Illing N. Phylogenetic evidence that two distinct *Trichuris* genotypes infect both humans and non-human primates. PLoS One. 2012;7:e44187.
139. Makouloutou P, Mbehang Nguema PP, Fujita S, Takenoshita Y, Hasegawa H, Yanagida T, Sato H. Prevalence and genetic diversity of *Oesophagostomum stephanostomum* in wild lowland gorillas at Moukalaba-Doudou National Park, Gabon. Helminthologia. 2014;51:83–93.
140. Blizzard EL, David CD, Henke S, Long DB, Hall CA, Yabsley MJ. Distribution, prevalence, and genetic characterization of *Baylisascaris procyonis* in selected areas of Georgia. J Parasitol. 2010;96:1128–33.
141. Sarkissian CA, Campbell SK, Dharmarajan G, Jacquot J, Page LK, Graham DH. Microgeographic population genetic structure of *Baylisascaris procyonis* (Nematoda: Ascaroidae) in western Michigan indicates the Grand River is a barrier to gene flow. J Parasitol. 2015;101:671–6.
142. Osten-Sacken N, Heddegrott M, Schleimer A, Anheyer-Behmenburg HE, Runge M, Horsburgh GJ, et al. Similar yet different: co-analysis of the genetic diversity and structure of an invasive nematode parasite and its invasive mammalian host. Int J Parasitol. 2018;48:233–43.
143. Dubey S, Shine R. Origin of the parasites of an invading species, the Australian cane toad (*Bufo marinus*): are the lungworms Australian or American? Mol Ecol. 2008;17:4418–24.
144. Sheng L, Cui P, Fang S-F, Lin R-Q, Zou F-C, Zhu X-Q. Sequence variability in four mitochondrial genes among rabbit pinworm (*Passalurus ambiguus*) isolates from different localities in China. Mitochondr DNA. 2015;26:501–4.
145. Mayr E. Animal Species and Evolution. Cambridge: Harvard University Press; 1963.
146. Gaither MR, Abey G, Vignon M, Meguro Y-I, Rigby M, Runyon C, et al. An invasive fish and the time-lagged spread of Its parasite across the Hawaiian Archipelago. PLoS One. 2013;8:e56940.
147. Gagne RB, Sprehn CG, Alda F, McIntyre PB, Gilliam JF, Blum MJ. Invasion of the Hawaiian Islands by a parasite infecting imperiled stream fishes. Ecography. 2018;41:528–39.
148. Knopf K, Mahnke M. Differences in susceptibility of the European eel (*Anguilla anguilla*) and the Japanese eel (*Anguilla japonica*) to the swim-bladder nematode *Anguillicola crassus*. Parasitology. 2004;129:491–6.
149. Rahhou I, Morand S, Lecomte-Finiger R, Sasal P. Biogeographical relationships of the eel parasite *Anguillicola crassus* revealed by random amplified polymorphic DNA markers (RAPDS). B Fr Pêch Piscic. 2005;378-379:87–98.
150. Wielgoss S, Tarachewski H, Meyer A, Wirth T. Population structure of the parasitic nematode *Anguillicola crassus*, an invader of declining North Atlantic eel stocks. Mol Ecol. 2008;17:3478–95.
151. Wielgoss S, Holland F, Wirth T, Meyer A. Genetic signatures in an invasive parasite of *Anguilla anguilla* correlate with differential stock management. J Fish Biol. 2010;77:191–210.
152. Wit J, Gilleard JS. Resequencing helminth genomes for population and genetic studies. Trends Parasitol. 2017;33:388–99.
153. Korhonen PK, Young ND, Gasser RB. Making sense of genomes of parasitic worms: tackling bioinformatic challenges. Biotechnol Adv. 2016;34:663–86.
154. Baird NA, Etter PD, Atwood TS, Currey MS, Shiver AL, Lewis ZA, et al. Rapid SNP discovery and genetic mapping using sequenced RAD markers. PLoS One. 2008;3e:3376.
155. Peterson BK, Webster JN, Kay EH, Fisher HS, Hoekstra HE. Double digest RADseq: an inexpensive method for de novo SNP discovery and genotyping in model and non-model species. PLoS One. 2012;7:e37135.
156. Da Fonseca RR, Albrechtsen A, Espregueira Themudo G, Ramos-Madrigal J, Andreas Sibbesen J, Maretty L, et al. Next-generation biology: sequencing and data analysis approaches for non-model organisms. Mar Genom. 2016; 30:3–13.
157. Puckett EE, Park J, Combs M, Blum MJ, Bryant JE, Caccone A, et al. Global population divergence and admixture of the brown rat (*Rattus norvegicus*). Proc R Soc B Biol Sci. 2016;283:20161762.
158. Anderson EC, Gerke JP, Shapiro JA, Crissman JR, Ghosh R, Bloom JS, et al. Chromosome-scale selective sweeps shape *Caenorhabditis elegans* genomic diversity. Nat Genet. 2012;44:285–90.
159. Li H, Durbin R. Inference of human population history from individual whole-genome sequences. Nature. 2011;475:493–6.
160. Jones FC, Grabherr MG, Chan YF, Russel P, Mauceli E, Johnson J, et al. The genomic basis of adaptive evolution in threespine sticklebacks. Nature. 2012;484:55–61.
161. Ott J, Wang J, Leal SM. Genetic linkage analysis in the age of whole-genome sequencing. Nat Rev Genet. 2015;16:275–84.
162. Fumagalli M. Assessing the effect of sequencing depth and sample size in population genetics inferences. PLoS One. 2013;8:e79667.
163. Hosono S, Faruqi AF, Dean FB, Du Y, Sun Z, Wu X, et al. Unbiased whole-genome amplification directly from clinical samples. Genome Res. 2003;13: 954–64.
164. Sabina J, Leamon JH. Bias in whole genome amplification: causes and considerations. Methods Mol Biol. 2015;1347:15–41.
165. Mobegi VA, Duffy CW, Amambua-Ngwa A, Loua KM, Laman E, Nwakanma DS, et al. Genome-wide analysis of selection on the malaria parasite *Plasmodium falciparum* in West African populations of differing infection endemicity. Mol Biol Evol. 2014;31:4190–9.
166. Coles GC, Jackson F, Pomroy WE, Prichard RK, von Samson-Himmelstjerna G, Silvestre A, et al. The detection of anthelmintic resistance in nematodes of veterinary importance. Vet Parasitol. 2006;136:167–85.
167. Choi Y-J, Bisset SA, Doyle SR, Hallsworth-Pepin K, Martin J, Grant WN, Mitreva M. Genomic introgression mapping of field-derived multiple-anthelmintic resistance in *Teladorsagia circumcincta*. PLoS Genet. 2017;13: e1006857.
168. Small ST, Reimer LJ, Tisch DJ, King CL, Christensen BM, Siba PM, et al. Population genomics of the filarial nematode parasite *Wuchereria bancrofti* from mosquitoes. Mol Ecol. 2016;25:1465–77.
169. Kikuchi T, Hino A, Tanaka T, Aung MPPTHH, Afrin T, Nagayasu E, et al. Genome-wide analyses of individual *Strongyloides stercoralis* (Nematoda: Rhabditoidea) provide insights into population structure and reproductive life cycles. PLoS Negl Trop Dis. 2016;10:e0005253.
170. Gendron St-Marseille A-F, Lord E, Véronneau P-Y, Brodeur J, Mimee B. Genome scans reveal homogenization and local adaptations in populations of the soybean cyst nematode. Front Plant Sci. 2018;9:987.
171. Lu F, Lipka AE, Glaubitz J, Elshire R, Cherney JH, Casler MD, et al. Switchgrass genomic diversity, ploidy, and evolution: novel insights from a network-based SNP discovery protocol. PLoS Genet. 2013;9:e1003215.
172. Chartier C, Reche B. Gastrointestinal helminths and lungworms of French dairy goats: prevalence and geographical distribution in Poitou-Charentes. Vet Res Commun. 1992;16:327–35.
173. Kataman KK, Thamsborg SM, Dalsgaard A, Kyvsgaard NC, Mejer H. Environmental contamination and transmission of *Ascaris suum* in Danish organic pig farms. Parasit Vectors. 2016;9:80.
174. Shokralla S, Spall JL, Gibson JF, Hadibabaei M. Next-generation sequencing technologies for environmental DNA research. Mol Ecol. 2012;21:1794–805.
175. Peham T, Steiner FM, Schlick-Steiner BC, Arthofer W. Are we ready to detect nematode diversity by next generation sequencing? Ecol Evol. 2017;7:4147–51.
176. Wimmer B, Craig BH, Pilkington JG, Pemberton JM. Non-invasive assessment of parasitic nematode species diversity in wild Soay sheep using molecular markers. Int J Parasitol. 2004;34:625–31.
177. Blouin MS, Dame JB, Tarrant CA, Courtney CH. Unusual population genetics of a parasitic nematode: mtDNA variation within and among populations. Evolution. 1992;46:470–6.
178. Höglund J, Engström A, Morrison DA, Mattsson JC. Genetic diversity assessed by amplified fragment length polymorphism analysis of the parasitic nematode *Dictyocaulus viviparus* the lungworm of cattle. Int J Parasitol. 2004;34:475–84.
179. Banks DJD, Singh R, Barger IA, Pratap B, le Jambre LF. Development and survival of infective larvae of *Haemonchus contortus* and *Trichostrongylus colubriformis* on pasture in a tropical environment. Int J Parasitol. 1990;20: 155–60.
180. Wright S. Evolution in Mendelian populations. Genetics. 1931;16:97–159.
181. Slatkin M. Gene flow in natural populations. Ann Rev Ecol Syst. 1985;16:393–430.
182. Stern C. The Hardy-Weinberg law. Science. 1943;97:137–8.
183. Andrews RH, Chilton NB. Multilocus enzyme electrophoresis: a valuable technique for providing answers to problems in parasite systematics. Int J Parasitol. 1999;29:213–53.
184. Slatkin M. Linkage disequilibrium - understanding the evolutionary past and mapping the medical future. Nat Genet. 2008;9:477–85.

185. Avise JC. Phylogeography: The History and Formation of Species. Cambridge: Harvard University Press; 2000.
186. Hartl DL. A primer of population genetics. Massachussets: Sinauer; 1988.
187. Lynch M, Mulligan BG. Analysis of population genetic structure with RAPD markers. Mol Ecol. 1994;3:91–9.
188. Powers TO, Todd TC, Burnell AM, Murray PCB, Fleming CC, Szalanski AL, et al. The rDNA internal transcribed spacer region as a taxonomic marker for nematodes. J Nematol. 1997;29:441–50.
189. McVean G. The structure of linkage disequilibrium around a selective sweep. Genetics. 2007:1395–406.
190. Obendorf DL, Beveridge I, Andrews RH. Cryptic species in populations of *Globocephaloides trifidospicularis* Kung (Nematoda: Trichostrongyloidea), parasitic in macropodid marsupials. Trans Roy Soc South Aus. 1991;115:213–6.
191. Jabbar A, Beveridge I, Mohandas N, Chilton NB, Littlewood DTJ, Jex AR, Gasser RB. Analyses of mitochondrial amino acid sequence datasets support the proposal that specimens of *Hypodontus macropi* from three species of macropodid hosts represent distinct species. BMC Evol Biol. 2013;13:259.
192. Chilton NB, Beveridge I, Andrews RH. Electrophoretic comparison of *Rugopharynx longibursaris* Kung and *R. omega* Beveridge (Nematoda: Strongyloidea), with the description of *R. sigma* n. sp. from pademelons, *Thylogale* spp. (Marsupialia: Macropodidae). Syst Parasitol. 1992;26:159–169.
193. Chilton NB, Beveridge I, Hoste H, Gasser RB. Evidence for hybridisation between *Paramacropostrongylus iugalis* and *P. typicus* (Nematoda: Strongyloidea) in grey kangaroos, *Macropus fuliginosus* and *M. giganteus*, in a zone of sympatry in eastern Australia. Int J Parasitol. 1997;27:475–82.
194. Chilton NB, Beveridge I, Andrews RH. Electrophoretic and morphological analysis of *Paramacropostrongylus typicus* (Nematoda: Strongyloidea), with the description of a new species, *Paramacropostrongylus iugalis*, from the eastern grey kangaroo *Macropus giganteus*. Syst Parasitol. 1993;24:35–44.
195. Beveridge I, Chilton NB, Andrews RH. Sibling species within *Macropostrongyloides baylisi* (Nematoda: Strongyloidea) from macropodid marsupials. Int J Parasitol. 1993;23:21–33.
196. Beveridge I, Chilton NB, Andrews RH. A morphological and electrophoretic study of *Rugopharynx zeta* (Johnston & Mawson, 1939) (Nematoda: Strongyloidea), with the description of a new species, *R. mawsonae*, from the black-striped wallaby *Macropus dorsalis* (Marsupialia: Macropodidae). Syst Parasitol. 1994;27:159–71.
197. Chilton NB, Smales LR. An electrophoretic and morphological analysis of *Labiostrongylus* (*Labiomultiplex*) *uncinatus* (Nematoda: Cloacinidae), with the description of a new species, *L. contiguus*, from *Macropus parryi* (Marsupialia: Macropodidae). Syst Parasitol. 1996;35:49–57.
198. Smales LR, Chilton NB. An electrophoretic and morphological analysis of *Labiostrongylus* (*Labiosimplex*) *bancrofti* (Johnston & Mawson, 1939) (Nematoda: Cloacinidae), from macropodid marsupials, with the description of two new species. Syst Parasitol. 1997;36:193–201.
199. Huby-Chilton F, Beveridge I, Gasser RB, Chilton NB. Redescription of *Zoniolaimus mawsonae* Beveridge, 1983 (Nematoda: Strongyloidea) and the description of *Z. latebrosus* n. sp. from the red kangaroo *Macropus rufus* (Marsupialia: Macropodidae) based on morphological and molecular data. Syst Parasitol. 2002;51:135–47.
200. Chilton NB, Huby-Chilton F, Gasser RB, Beveridge I. Review of *Papillostrongylus* Johnston & Mawson, 1939 (Nematoda: Strongyloidea) from wallabies and kangaroos (Marsupialia: Macropodidae) using morphological and molecular techniques, with the description of *P. barbatus* n. sp. Syst Parasitol. 2002;51:81–93.
201. Nascetti G, Paggi L, Orecchia P, Smith JW, Mattiucci S, Bullini L. Electrophoretic studies on the *Anisakis simplex* complex (Ascaridida: Anisakidae) from the Mediterranean and North-East Atlantic. Int J Parasitol. 1986;16:633–40.
202. Mattiucci S, Paggi L, Nascetti D, Portes Santos C, Costa G, di Beneditto AP, et al. Genetic markers in the study of *Anisakis typica* (Diesing, 1860): larval identification and genetic relationships with other species of *Anisakis* Dujardin, 1845 (Nematoda: Anisakidae). Syst Parasitol. 2002;51:159–70.
203. Abollo E, Paggi L, Pascual S, D'Amelio S. Occurrence of recombinant genotypes of *Anisakis simplex s.s.* and *Anisakis pegreffii* (Nematoda: Anisakidae) in an area of sympatry. Infect Genet Evol. 2003;3:175–81.
204. Martín-Sánchez J, Artacho-Reinoso ME, Díaz-Gavilán M, Valero-López A. Structure of *Anisakis simplex s.l.* populations in a region sympatric for *A. pegreffii* and *A. simplex s.s.*: absence of reproductive isolation between both species. Mol Biochem Parasitol. 2005;141:155–62.
205. Klimpel S, Busch MW, Kuhn T, Rhode A, Palm FW. The *Anisakis simplex* complex off the South Shetland Islands (Antarctica): endemic populations *versus* introduction through migratory hosts. Mar Ecol Prog Ser. 2010;403:1–11.
206. Baldwin RE, Rew MB, Johansson ML, Banks MA, Jacobson KC. Population structure of three species of *Anisakis* nematodes recovered from Pacific sardines (*Sardinops sagax*) distributed throughout the California current system. J Parasitol. 2011;97:545–54.
207. Cross MA, Collins C, Campbell N, Watts PC, Chubb JC, Cunningham CO, et al. Levels of intra-host and temporal sequence variation in a large CO1 sub-units from *Anisakis simplex sensu stricto* (Rudolphi, 1809) (Nematoda: Anisakisdae): implications for fisheries management. Mar Biol. 2007;151:695–702.
208. Ceballos-Mendiola G, Valero A, Polo-Vico R, Tejada M, Abattouy N, Karl H, et al. Genetic variability of *Anisakis simplex s.s.* parasitizing European hake (*Merluccius merluccius*) in the Little Sole Bank area in the Northeast Atlantic. Parasitol Res. 2010;107:1399–404.
209. Mladineo I, Poljak V. Ecology and genetic structure of zoonotic *Anisakis* spp. from Adriatic commercial fish species. Appl Environ Microbiol. 2014;80:1281–90.
210. Mattiucci S, Paggi L, Nascetti G, Abollo E, Webb SC, Pascual S, et al. Genetic divergence and reproductive isolation between *Anisakis brevispiculata* and *Anisakis physeteris* (Nematoda: Anisakidae). Int J Parasitol. 2001;31:9–14.
211. Mattiucci S, Nascetti G, Bullini L, Orecchia P, Paggi L. Genetic structure of *Anisakis physeteris*, and its differentiation from the *Anisakis simplex* complex (Ascaridida: Anisakidae). Parasitology. 1986;93:383–7.
212. Paggi L, Nascetti G, Webb SC, Mattiucci S, Cianchi R, Bullini L. A new species of *Anisakis* Dujardin, 1845 (Nematoda, Anisakidae) from beaked whales (Ziphiidae): allozyme and morphological evidence. Syst Parastitol. 1998;40: 161–74.
213. Valentini A, Mattiucci S, Bondanelli P, Webb SC, Mignucci-Giannone AA, Colom-Llavina MM, Nascetti G. Genetic relationships among *Anisakis* species (Nematoda: Anisakidae) inferred from mitochondrial *cox2* sequences, and comparison with allozyme data. J Parasitol. 2006;92:156–66.
214. Iglesias R, D'Amelio S, Ingrosso S, Farjallah S, Martínez-Cedeira JA, García-Estévez JM. Molecular and morphological evidence for the occurrence of *Anisakis* sp. A (Nematoda, Anisakidae) in the Blainville's beaked whale *Mesoplodon densirostris*. J Helminthol. 2008;82:305–8.
215. Mattiucci S, Paoletti M, Webb SC. *Anisakis nascettii* n. sp. (Nematoda: Anisakidae) from beaked whales of the southern hemisphere: morphological description, genetic relationships between congeners and ecological data. Syst Parasitol. 2009;74:199–217.
216. Paggi L, Nascetti G, Cianchi R, Orecchia P, Mattiucci S, D'Amelio S, et al. Genetic evidence for three species within *Pseudoterranova decipiens* (Nematoda, Ascaridida, Ascaridoidea) in the north Atlantic and Norwegian and Barents seas. Int J Parasitol. 1991;21:195–212.
217. Vrijenhoek RC. Genetic differentiation among larval nematodes infecting fishes. J Parasitol. 1978;64:790–8.
218. Nascetti G, Cianchi R, Mattiucci S, D'Amelio S, Orecchia P, Paggi L, et al. Three sibling species within *Contracaecum osculatum* (Nematoda, Ascaridida, Ascaridoidea) from the Atlantic arctic-boreal region: reproductive isolation and host preferences. Int J Parasitol. 1993;23:105–20.
219. Orecchia P, Mattiucci S, D'Amelio S, Paggi L, Plötz J, Cianchi R, et al. Two new members in the *Contracaecum osculatum* complex (Nematoda, Ascaridoidea) from the Antarctic. Int J Parasitol. 1994;24:367–77.
220. Mattiucci S, Cipriani P, Paoletti M, Nardi V, Santoro M, Bellisario B, Nascetti G. Temporal stability of parasite distribution and genetic variability values of *Contracaecum osculatum* sp. D and *C. osculatum* sp. E (Nematoda: Anisakidae) from fish of the Ross Sea (Antarctica). Int J Parasitol Parasites Wildl. 2015;4:356–67.
221. Arduino P, Nascetti G, Cianchi R, Plötz J, Mattiucci S, D'Amelio S, et al. Isozyme variation and taxonomic rank of *Contracaecum radiatum* (v. Linstow, 1907) from the Antarctic Ocean (Nematoda, Ascaridoidea). Syst Parasitol. 1995;30:1–9.
222. Zhu X, D'Amelio S, Hu M, Paggi L, Gasser RB. Electrophoretic detection of population variation within *Contracaecum ogmorhini* (Nematoda: Ascaridoidea: Anisakidae). Electrophoresis. 2001;22:1930–4.
223. Mattiucci S, Cianchi R, Nascetti G, Paggi L, Sardella N, Timi J, et al. Genetic evidence for two sibling species within *Contracaecum ogmorhini* Johnston & Mawson, 1941 (Nematoda: Anisakidae) from otariid seals of Boreal and Austral regions. Syst Parasitol. 2003;54:13–23.

224. Li A-X, D'Amelio S, Paggi L, He F, Gasser RB, Lun Z-R, et al. Genetic evidence for the existence of sibling species within *Contracaecum rudolphii* (Hartwich, 1964) and the validity of *Contracaecum septentrionale* (Kreis, 1955) (Nematoda: Anisakidae). Parasitol Res. 2005; 96:361–6.
225. Mattiucci S, Paoletti M, Olivero-Verbel J, Baldris R, Arroyo-Salgado B, Garbin L, et al. *Contracaecum bioccai* n. sp. from the brown pelican *Pelecanus occidentalis* (L.) in Colombia (Nematoda: Anisakidae): morphology, molecular evidence and its genetic relationship with congeners from fish-eating birds. Syst Parasitol. 2008;69:101–21.

14

Influence of confluent marine currents in an ecotonal region of the South-West Atlantic on the distribution of larval anisakids (Nematoda: Anisakidae)

Ana L Lanfranchi[1*], Paola E Braicovich[1], Delfina M P Cantatore[1], Manuel M Irigoitia[1], Marisa D Farber[2], Verónica Taglioretti[1] and Juan T Timi[1]

Abstract

Background: In the marine environment, transitional zones between major water masses harbour high biodiversity, mostly due to their productivity and by containing representatives of species characteristic of adjacent communities. With the aim of assessing the value of larval *Anisakis* as zoogeographical indicators in a transitional zone between subtropical and sub-Antarctic marine currents, larvae obtained from *Zenopsis conchifer* were genetically identified. Larvae from *Pagrus pagrus* and *Merluccius hubbsi* from two adjacent zoogeographical provinces were also sequenced.

Results: Four species were genetically identified in the whole sample, including *Anisakis typica, A. pegreffii, A. berlandi* and a probably new species related to *A. paggiae. Anisakis typica* and *A. pegreffii* were identified as indicators of tropical/subtropical and sub-Antarctic waters, respectively, and their presence evidenced the transitional conditions of the region. Multivariate analyses on prevalence and mean abundance of *Anisakis* spp. of 18 samples represented by 9 fish species caught south of 35°S determined that host trophic level and locality of capture were the main drivers of the distribution of parasites across zoogeographical units in the South-West Atlantic.

Conclusions: Most samples followed a clear zoogeographical pattern, but the sample of *Z. conchifer*, composed mostly of *A. typica*, was an exception. This finding suggests that population parameters of *A. typica* and *A. pegreffii* could differ enough to be considered as a surrogates of the identity of larvae parasitizing a given host population and, therefore, a step forward the validation of the use of larval *Anisakis* as biological indicators for studies on host zoogeography.

Keywords: *Anisakis pegreffii, Anisakis berlandi, Anisakis typica, Zenopsis conchifer*, Zoogeographical indicators

Background

Members of the genus *Anisakis* are known worldwide because of their implication in human health as the causative agents of anisakiosis, resulting from the ingestion of infective third-stage larvae in raw or undercooked marine fish products [1–4] and considered as one of the most significant emerging food-borne zoonoses [5]. Nevertheless, the biological relevance of anisakids in general goes beyond their epidemiological transcendence. Indeed, larval anisakids have been identified among the most suitable biological tags for stock discrimination because they have a lifespan or remain in an identifiable form in the host long enough to cover the timescale of such investigations [6–9]. However, a limitation to their effectiveness as markers is imposed by difficulties in their identification, since third-stage larvae of several species cannot be identified to species based on

* Correspondence: lanfra@mdp.edu.ar
[1]Laboratorio de Ictioparasitología, Instituto de Investigaciones Marinas y Costeras (IIMyC), Facultad de Ciencias Exactas y Naturales, Universidad Nacional de Mar del Plata - Consejo Nacional de Investigaciones Científicas y Técnicas (CONICET), (7600) Mar del Plata, 3350 Funes, Argentina
Full list of author information is available at the end of the article

traditional morphological analyses, except to the level of the morphotypes of Berland [10], *Anisakis* Type I and Type II [11]. Some of these cryptic species often occur in sympatry and syntopy in fish hosts and the lack of taxonomic resolution can affect comparative studies. This limitation in specific reconnaissance for larval stages of *Anisakis* can, however, be solved with the application of molecular tools, which have recently proved to be of value when parasites are used as biological tags, especially for studies carried out at large geographical scales [12–15].

The success of larval *Anisakis* as tags to discriminate host populations at large spatial scales relies on the fact that members of this genus display species-specific distribution patterns within different climate zones and oceans which, in turn, are congruent with those of their respective final hosts [16]. For this reason, the species composition of these parasites in fish can reveal the transitional nature of ecotonal zones between zoogeographical marine regions or interface areas between masses of water, such that observed for hake and blue whiting between the cold Atlantic and the warm Mediterranean waters [12, 17].

In the Argentine Sea, larvae of *Anisakis* are commonly reported in fish hosts (see [9] and references therein) as *Anisakis* sp. or *A. simplex* (*s.l.*). The only published reports of genetically identified species of *Anisakis* are that of *Anisakis pegreffii* in *Merluccius hubbsi* [4] and the skates *Sympterygia bonapartii* and *Zearaja chilensis* [18], and that of a single specimen of *Anisakis berlandi* in *S. bonapartii* [18], highlighting the considerable uncertainty existing in the species composition of this genus in this region. Adult *Anisakis* have been also reported in several species of cetaceans in the Argentine Sea [19], all of them based on morphological identifications, and most reported as *Anisakis* sp. or *A. simplex* (*s.l.*), although Berón-Vera et al. [20] also reported *A. physeteris*. A similar situation occurs in Brazilian waters, where some species have been morphologically identified in several species of marine cetaceans [21]. However, recent papers, based on genetic identification of larvae and adults, have recorded a higher diversity, *A. typica* being the most abundant and widely reported species of the genus, occurring in both cetaceans and fish hosts along Brazilian coasts [22, 23].

A promissory couple of species to evaluate the relative influence of confluent marine currents in the South-West Atlantic is represented by *A. typica* and *A. pegreffii*. According to data based on genetic identification, the former occurs in warmer temperate and tropical waters between 35°N and 30°S, whereas the distribution range of the later in the Southern Hemisphere extends in temperate to colder regions from 30°S to 60°S [4, 24]. However, in the South-West Atlantic, the border between the distributions of both species could be displaced to higher latitudes due to the influence of the Brazil Current, which flows southwards carrying subtropical waters to collide with the northward flowing Malvinas Current, composed of sub-Antarctic waters, on the continental slope around 38°S in the Argentine-Uruguayan Common Fishing Zone [25]. In the South-West Atlantic, cetacean species distribute differentially along a latitudinal-temperature gradient [26–28], and a contribution of different *Anisakis* species typical for warmer and colder regions should be expected in the confluence region. In a recent paper, Lanfranchi et al. [29] evaluated the utility of parasites as indicators of marine ecotones by analyzing data on the assemblages of long-lived larval parasites of *Zenopsis conchifer* inhabiting deep waters in the region of convergence between the Brazil and Malvinas currents, the southernmost limit of its distribution in the South American Atlantic. The ecology of *Z. conchifer* is little known; however, there is no evidence of migratory movements in the South-West Atlantic, except a shift towards deeper waters as fish grow [30]. Indeed, this fish is considered as a poor swimmer with restricted mobility [31, 32] and consequently constitutes a suitable model to evaluate the presence of infective stages of anisakids in their habitat, by acting as a passive sampler of the available larvae in their prey.

Lanfranchi et al. [29] included data on other host species recognized as harbouring parasite assemblages representative of neighbouring zoogeographical regions, characterized by these masses of water [9, 33, 34]. These waters, with subtropical and sub-Antarctic origins, affected the structure of parasite communities in the ecotone by acting as sources of infective stages of helminth species (acanthocephalans, nematodes, cestodes) typical of adjacent zoogeographical units, which were considered as reliable indicators to define such transitional regions. Among suitable markers, Lanfranchi et al. [29] reported larval *Anisakis* in *Z. conchifer*, identifying most of them as *A. simplex* (*s.l.*) based on morphology. These parasites were found at a prevalence of 77.3%, unexpectedly higher than the prevalences reported in more coastal fishes at similar latitudes. In the present paper, a genetic identification of a subsample of larval *Anisakis* from the same samples of *Z. conchifer* were carried out to assess the relative influence of sub-Antarctic and subtropical waters on the specific composition of this genus. Indeed, this region contained the distributional range of *A. pegreffii*; their occurrence in sympatry with *A. typica* should confirm the influence of the Brazil Current, as postulated by Lanfranchi et al. [29]. In fact, the only *Anisakis* larva found in a sample of ten *Z. conchifer* from Rio de Janeiro, Brazil was genetically identified as *A. typica* [35].

Prevalence and mean abundance of larval *Anisakis* in the Argentine Sea, presumed to be mostly *A. pegreffii*, follow a latitudinal pattern increasing southwards irrespective of the host species harbouring them [9, 18]. The locality of capture of *Z. conchifer* in the ecotonal region also provided the opportunity for evaluating whether population attributes of larval anisakids follow a general distribution pattern across fish species with a similar trophic level in the region, or if they depart from it. Such a departure could be considered not only as evidence of the presence of different species of *Anisakis* with their own distribution patterns, but also indicative of the influence of warmer waters on the distribution of *Anisakis* spp. in the subtropical-sub-Antarctic convergence region.

The aim of this paper is, therefore, threefold: (i) to unequivocally identify larval *Anisakis* in the Argentine Sea based on molecular techniques; (ii) to assess their value as zoogeographical indicators in an ecotonal zone; and (iii) to determine the possible drivers of the distribution of *Anisakis* spp. across fish species of similar trophic levels in the Argentine Sea. Our results will also contribute to the knowledge and inventory of this genus in the World Ocean, filling a gap on the extant knowledge on the distribution and global diversity of *Anisakis*.

Methods

Fish sampling and parasite inventories

A total of 46 specimens of *Z. conchifer* were examined for larval *Anisakis*. Fish were caught by trawl during a research cruise at the Argentine-Uruguayan Common Fishing Zone (35°32'–35°35'S, 53°06'–53°25'W) at depths between 94 and 117 m, in October 2011 (Fig. 1). Data of most of these fish correspond to a previously published paper [29]. Fish were either kept fresh or deep-frozen in plastic bags at -18 °C until examination. Females (n = 31) measured on average 28.4 cm (range 16.5–46.5 cm), males (n = 15) measured on average 24.5 cm (range 17.0–35.0 cm). After defrosting, larval *Anisakis* were recovered from the mesenteries, body cavity and liver after examination under a stereoscopic microscope. Prevalence and mean abundance were calculated following Bush et al. [36].

Genetic identification

The identification at the species level was obtained by direct sequences analysis of mitochondrial (mtDNA *cox*2) and nuclear (nDNA EF1 α-1) genes.

A subsample of 19 Type I larvae of *Anisakis* spp. (equivalent to 18.6% of the total collected) and a unique Type II larva, both from *Z. conchifer*, along with 16 preserved Type I larvae from another two fish hosts caught during previous studies (Fig. 1), all from the Magellanic zoogeographical province (9 worms from *Merluccius hubbsi*; 44°4'S, 63°29'W; January 2009), and Argentine zoogeographical province (7 worms from *Pagrus pagrus*; 36°S, 55°W; March 2016), were identified to the species level by genetic analyses.

DNA extraction was carried out using whole specimens with the DNeasy Blood and Tissue® Kit (Qiagen, Hilden, Germany) according to the manufacturer's instructions. The mtDNA *cox*2 gene was amplified using the primers 210R (5'-CAC CAA CTC TTA AAA TTA TC-3') and 211F (5'-TTT TCT AGT TAT ATA GAT TGR TTY AT-3') [37]. Additionally, to confirm their identity, the nDNA EF1 α-1 was amplified in larvae of *A. pegreffii* selected among those identified by the mtDNA *cox*2 gene using the primers EF-F (5'-TCC TCA AGC GTT GTT ATC TGT T-3') and EF-R (5'-AGT TTT GCC ACT AGC GGT TCC-3') [38]. All PCR reactions were set up in a 25 μl reaction volume using 12.5 μl of HotStarTaq Master Mix (Qiagen), 0.5 μM of each primer and 5 μl of DNA (≥ 10 ng) as a template. The PCR was carried out using the following conditions: 94 °C for 15 min (initial heat activation) followed by 35 cycles at 94 °C for 30 s (denaturation), 50 °C for 100 s (annealing) and 72 °C for 1 min (extension), followed by a final extension step at 72 °C for 10 min. Each PCR product was purified using QIAquick spin columns (QIAquick Gel Extraction Kit, Qiagen). The fragments were sequenced for both DNA strands using the PCR primers. Sequencing was performed using Big Dye Terminator v.3.1 and 3130xl Genetic analyzer (Applied Biosystems, Foster City, CA, USA) at the Genomic Unit, IB-INTA.

Sequences were edited manually in Proseq v.3.5 [39] and deposited in the GenBank database. Generated sequences at the mtDNA *cox*2 were compared against the NCBI database using the BLAST algorithm [40]. The same sequences were aligned by ClustalW [41] implemented in the MEGA 7.0 software package [42] and compared with subsets of ten sequences available in GenBank of each known species of *Anisakis*, except for *A. physeteris* and *A.* cf. *paggiae*, of which only four and one sequences, respectively, were available for comparison. In the case of *A. paggiae*, those sequences deposited by Quiazon et al. [43, 44], considered as *A. paggiae*-related by the authors, were excluded due to specific uncertainty. The interspecific and intraspecific genetic distance between currently described *Anisakis* species and sequences obtained in the present study were calculated using a Kimura-2-Parameters (K2P) model in MEGA. The sequences obtained at the EF1 α-1 gene (409 bp fragment) of the nDNA for the specimens of *A. pegreffii* were compared at the diagnostic positions 186 and 286 as previously detailed in [38].

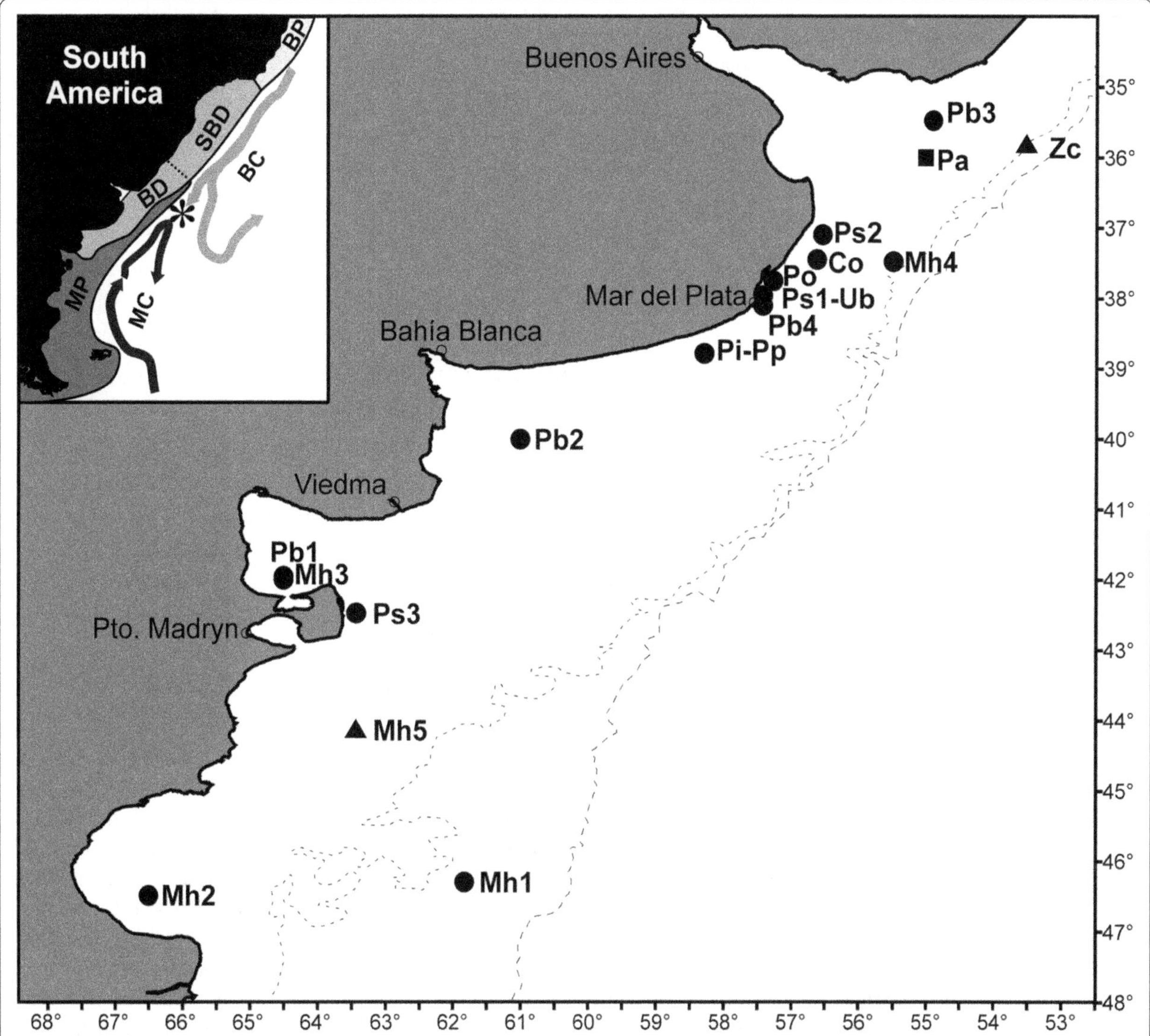

Fig. 1 Map showing the sampling localities, the zoogeographical regions and the main marine currents. Circles, samples of fish species included in quantitative analyses (sample codes as in Table 1); square, sample of *Pagrus pagrus* (Pa) included in genetic analyses; triangles, samples of *Zenopsis conchifer* (Zc) and *Merluccius hubbsi* (Mh5) included in both genetic and quantitative analyses. *Abbreviations*: BP, Brazilian Province; SBD, South Brazilian district of Argentine Province; BD, Bonaerensean district of Argentine Province; MP, Magellanic Province; BC, Brazil Current; MC, Malvinas Current. Asterisk (*), ecotone region (convergence zone)

Distribution of *Anisakis* spp. across fish species in the Argentine Sea

Data on prevalence and mean abundance of larval *Anisakis* in other fish species of the region were obtained from previous publications by the research team during the last 20 years (Table 1). Since host trophic level has been recognized as an important determinant of the abundance of long-lived parasites [45], and because the interest of the analyses relies on the geographical distribution of *Anisakis* spp., only those fish species with a high trophic level (> 3.5, obtained from Froese & Pauly [46]) and ichthyophagous diet [47] were retained (Table 1). In this sense, by having similar diets and due to the non-specificity of larval *Anisakis* in previous paratenic fish hosts, all host species are expected to be exposed to the same pool of infective stages, diminishing the effect of their trophic level, and therefore allowing other variables to arise as determinants of parasite burdens.

Including data for *Z. conchifer*, a total of 18 samples corresponding to 9 fish species were analyzed. Each sample was assigned to a region following pre-established zoogeographical schemes ([48] and references therein); these regions were the Bonaerensean District of the Argentine Province and the Magellanic Province, both displaying characteristic parasite faunas [9]. Samples caught at transitional areas between these two regions [48], namely San

Table 1 Composition of samples used for comparative analyses on the distribution of larval *Anisakis* in the Argentine Sea, including number of examined hosts (*n*), latitude S (Lat) and longitude W (Long) of capture, trophic level (TL) and mean total length (MTL) of hosts, and prevalence (P in %) and mean abundance (MA) of parasites

Host species (sample code)	*n*	Lat S[a]	Long W[a]	Region	Year	TL	MTL (cm)	P (%)	MA	Reference
Zenopsis conchifer (Zc)	46	35.55	53.25	Ecotone	2011	4.17	27.45	78.3	2.17	Present study
Conger orbignianus (Co)	50	37.50	56.65	Bonaerensean	2010	3.72	80.69	8.0	0.12	[50]
Merluccius hubbsi (Mh1)	115	46.33	61.83	Magellanic	1999	4.23	39.91	89.6	52.60	[79]
Merluccius hubbsi (Mh2)	80	46.50	66.50	Magellanic	1998	4.23	40.36	97.5	16.60	[79]
Merluccius hubbsi (Mh3)	83	42.00	64.50	Ecotone	1999	4.23	38.68	100	17.00	[79]
Merluccius hubbsi (Mh4)	42	37.50	55.50	Ecotone	2009	4.23	44.50	52.4	1.36	[29]
Merluccius hubbsi (Mh5)	50	44.07	63.48	Magellanic	2009	4.23	41.80	98.2	46.96	[29]
Paralichthys isosceles (Pi)	51	38.87	58.17	Bonaerensean	2009	4	27.95	0	0	[80]
Paralichthys patagonicus (Pp)	51	38.87	58.17	Bonaerensean	2010	3.9	35.20	9.8	0.18	[80]
Paralichthys orbignyanus (Po)	44	37.74	57.42	Bonaerensean	2004-2008	3.8	51.00	3.8	0.03	[81]
Percophis brasiliensis (Pb1)	32	42.00	64.51	Ecotone	2006	4.3	52.90	53.1	8.70	[78]
Percophis brasiliensis (Pb2)	51	40.00	61.00	Bonaerensean	2006	4.3	50.00	98.0	16.50	[78]
Percophis brasiliensis (Pb3)	35	35.50	54.83	Bonaerensean	2006	4.3	49.40	11.4	0.20	[78]
Percophis brasiliensis (Pb4)	59	38.13	57.53	Bonaerensean	2006	4.3	52.20	33.9	0.60	[78]
Pseudopercis semifasciata (Ps1)	30	38.03	57.30	Bonaerensean	2007	3.9	71.20	30.0	0.67	[82]
Pseudopercis semifasciata (Ps2)	20	37.25	56.38	Bonaerensean	2007	3.9	67.50	0	0	[78]
Pseudopercis semifasciata (Ps3)	50	42.37	63.50	Magellanic	2007	3.9	67.20	72.00	4.48	[78]
Urophycis brasiliensis (Ub)	62	38.00	57.50	Bonaerensean	2012	3.8	36.60	0	0	[33]

[a]Central point of distribution when two or more trawls were made

Matías Gulf and the outer shelf of the Bonaerensean region, influenced by sub-Antarctic waters which at these latitudes flow northwards along the slope bordering shelf waters, were assigned to a third region, defined as ecotone.

To analyze the relative contribution of host/abiotic variables on parasite distribution, Euclidean distance matrices of both prevalence and mean abundance were analyzed by distance-based multiple linear regressions (DistLM) [49] with significance testing based on 9999 permutations. As host-related predictor variables, the host species and their trophic level and mean total length were included in the models due to their known influence on parasite burdens [45, 50, 51]. Abiotic predictor variables were latitude, longitude and year of capture. The central year of the study period (2006) was adopted as the date of the sample Po. Draftsman plots and correlation matrices were used to check for multicollinearity in the predictor variables. Latitude and longitude were highly correlated each other ($R = 0.93$), due to the northeast to southwest orientation of the Argentine continental shelf, but were combined in a single predictor (locality).

Models including all possible combinations of predictor variables were generated using the Best procedure within the DistLM routine. An information theoretic approach based on modified Akaike's information criterion (AICc) was used to identify the best model; models with the lowest AICc were considered the most parsimonious [52]. The AICc was devised to handle situations where the number of samples (n) is small relative to the number (v) of predictor variables ($n/\text{v} < 40$) [49]. The difference (Δ_i) between the AICc value of the best model and the AICc value for each of the other models was calculated; models with Δ_i between 0 and 2 are considered as having a substantial level of empirical support of the model being therefore as good as the best model [53]; however, as suggested by Richards [54], models with Δi up to 6 should not be discounted, thus all models with $\Delta_i \leq 6$ were retained. For each selected model, the Akaike weights (w_i) were calculated following Burnham & Anderson [53] to identify and quantify the uncertainty in model selection and further used to estimate the relative importance of each predictor variable (predictor weight). For each predictor, the Akaike weights of all the models (with $\Delta_i < 6$) that contained that predictor were summed and these values were interpreted as the relative importance of that predictor. Indeed, those predictors occurring consistently in the most likely models have a w_i close to 1, whereas variables that are absent from or are only present in poorly fitting models (high AICc values) have a w_i close to 0 [52]. Additionally, the relative strength of each candidate model was assessed by calculating the evidence ratio (ER), which provides a measure of how much more likely the best model is than alternative models [52].

To visualize possible geographical patterns in the prevalence of larval *Anisakis* across the 18 samples, non-metric multidimensional scaling (nMDS) was carried out using Euclidean distances. A hierarchical agglomerative clustering was applied to the component communities using complete linkage, and resemblance levels were overlaid on the nMDS plot [55].

All multivariate analyses were implemented in PERMANOVA+ for the PRIMER7 package [49, 55].

Results

General results

A total of 103 larval *Anisakis* were found parasitizing *Z. conchifer*. All of them were identified as Type I larva (prevalence: 78.3%; mean abundance: 2.2; range: 0–13), except for one specimen classified as Type II.

Genetic identification

The identification through BLAST showed that sequences from the mtDNA *cox2* gene of larvae *Anisakis* Type I exhibited a similarity of 99–100% with sequences for *A. typica* available on GenBank (n = 20; 16 from *Z. conchifer*, accession numbers MH443102-MH443117 and 4 from *P. pagrus*, accession numbers MH443118-MH443121); of 99% with those for *A. berlandi* (n = 3; 2 from *Z. conchifer*, accession numbers MH443122-MH443123 and 1 from *P. pagrus*, accession number MH443124); and of 99–100% with sequences for *A. pegreffii* (n = 12, 1 from *Z. conchifer*, accession number MH443127; 2 from *P. pagrus*, accession numbers MH443126-MH443123; and 9 from *M. hubbsi*, accession numbers MH443128-MH443136). The only larva *Anisakis* Type II from *Z. conchifer* (accession number MH443137) showed a similarity of 95% with the sequences for *A. paggiae* available on GenBank and of 99% with an undetermined species sequence, *A.* cf. *paggiae*.

Interspecific genetic distances (Table 2) ranged between 0.10–0.20, except for those corresponding to the *A. simplex* complex and the pair *Anisakis* sp.-*A.* cf. *paggiae*, which ranged between 0.05–0.06. The distances between the sequences from the present study and those from GenBank to which they showed the maximum similarity were all 0.01–0.02, the range of most of the observed intraspecific distance, thereby confirming their specific status.

In addition, the presence of a T at the position 186 and of a C at the position 286 of the partial sequences of

Table 2 Averaged genetic distance calculated with the Kimura-2-parameter model at interspecific (below the diagonal) and intraspecific (diagonal, in italics) levels between specimens from the present study (denoted with *) and sequences deposited in GenBank

	A. sim	A. peg	A. peg*	A. ber	A. ber*	A. typ	A. typ*	A. zip	A. nas	A. phy	A. pag	A. cf. pag	A. sp.*	A. bre
A. sim	*0.02*	0.01	0.01	0.01	0.01	0.02	0.02	0.02	0.02	0.02	0.02	0.05	0.02	0.02
A. peg	0.05	*0.01*	0.003	0.01	0.01	0.02	0.02	0.01	0.02	0.02	0.02	0.04	0.02	0.02
A. peg*	0.05	**0.02**	*0.02*	0.01	0.01	0.02	0.02	0.01	0.02	0.02	0.02	0.04	0.02	0.02
A. ber	0.06	0.06	0.07	*0.01*	0.005	0.02	0.02	0.01	0.02	0.02	0.02	0.05	0.02	0.02
A. ber*	0.05	0.06	0.06	**0.02**	*0.02*	0.02	0.02	0.01	0.02	0.02	0.02	0.05	0.02	0.02
A. typ	0.14	0.14	0.14	0.14	0.14	*0.02*	0.003	0.02	0.02	0.02	0.02	0.06	0.02	0.02
A. typ*	0.14	0.14	0.13	0.14	0.14	**0.02**	*0.01*	0.02	0.02	0.02	0.02	0.06	0.02	0.02
A. zip	0.11	0.12	0.12	0.13	0.12	0.15	0.15	*0.02*	0.10	0.01	0.01	0.03	0.02	0.02
A. nas	0.14	0.13	0.13	0.14	0.13	0.13	0.13	0.10	*0.01*	0.02	0.02	0.04	0.02	0.02
A. phy	0.13	0.13	0.13	0.13	0.13	0.16	0.16	0.13	0.16	*0.01*	0.02	0.04	0.02	0.02
A. pag	0.13	0.12	0.12	0.14	0.14	0.17	0.17	0.12	0.14	0.13	*0.03*	0.02	0.01	0.01
A. cf. pag	0.16	0.15	0.15	0.17	0.17	0.20	0.21	0.12	0.16	0.16	0.06	–	0.01	0.04
A. sp.*	0.15	0.14	0.14	0.15	0.15	0.19	0.19	0.12	0.15	0.14	**0.06**	**0.01**	–	0.01
A. bre	0.16	0.16	0.16	0.17	0.17	0.20	0.20	0.14	0.18	0.11	0.13	0.13	0.12	*0.02*

Abbreviations: A. ber, *A. berlandi* (GenBank: KC809999-KC810001, JF423292-JF423297, MF353876); A. bre, *A. brevispiculata* (GenBank: KY421194, KP992462, EU560909, DQ116433, KJ786284, KJ786285, KC342900, KC342901, AB592803, AB592805); A. nas, *A. nascettii* (GenBank: FJ685642, GQ118164-GQ118169, GQ118171, GQ118173, JQ010980); A. phy, *A. physeteris* (GenBank: DQ116432, KU752202, KC479947, KC479948); A. sim, *A. simplex* (*s.l.*) (GenBank: KC810004, KC810003, KX158869, GQ338432, KT852475, KC479861, AB517570, JF423230, EU413959, MF358545); A. zip, *A. ziphidarum* (GenBank: KP992461, KT822146, DQ116430, KU752204, KU752205, KC821735, KC821737, KC821738; KF214804, KF214805), A. pag, *A. paggiae* (GenBank: KF693769, DQ116434, DQ116434, KJ786280, KJ786277, KJ786276, AB592809, AB592808, AB592810); A. cf. pag, *A. paggiae* related (see Di Azevedo et al. [56]) (GenBank: KF693770); A. sp., *Anisakis* sp.; A. peg, *A. pegreffii* (GenBank: EU933995, JQ341912, KR149283, KC480025, KC479888, KC479890, KC479993, KC809996, MF353877, MF353878); A. typ, *A. typica* (GenBank: KC821729, JQ859931, KP992467-KP992469, DQ116427, KF356646, KF032065, KF032063, KF701409)

Within group standard errors are given above the diagonal. Genetic distances between sequences of the present study and those from GenBank for the same species are in bold

the EF1 α-1 region of the nDNA obtained in 8 specimens, confirmed the identification of *A. pegreffii* (GenBank: numbers MH443138-MH443136).

Distribution of larval *Anisakis* across fish species in the Argentine Sea

The results of the DistLM on the prevalence data showed that the best model included host trophic level and locality as predictor variables (explaining 69.8% of the total variation of the data) (Table 3). The w_i indicated that it has 69.0% chance of being the best model and ER showed that it was nearly five times more likely to be the best approximating model than the subsequent one. Indeed, trophic level and locality were included in all and most models with Δ_i < 6, reaching a predictor weight of 1 and 0.9, respectively, indicating that both variables had the highest probabilities of being a component of the best model (Fig. 2). Regarding mean abundance, a higher number (10) of alternative models were obtained, the best one composed only by locality as a predictor variable (explaining 38% of the total variation of the data) (Table 3). The w_i indicated that the first model has a 22.8% chance of being the best one, a value very similar to that of the subsequent (composed by locality and trophic level). Evidence ratios showed that the first two models had similar chances of being the best one, but both were more than one and a half times more likely to be the best approximating models than the subsequent one. The predictor weights indicated that locality had the highest relative importance, followed by trophic level and year with considerably lower importance, whereas the mean host length had quite negligible relevance (Fig. 2). None of the models with Δ_i < 6 included host species as explanatory variable for the prevalence or mean abundance.

nMDS and cluster analyses on the prevalence data revealed apparent patterns of separation between samples following a zoogeographical pattern, which was substantially different from random as shown by it low stress level (0.01). Indeed, two main groups were evident (Fig. 3), one composed by most Bonaerensean samples and including samples Pb1 and Mh4 from the ecotone between Argentine and Magellanic Provinces and being more heterogeneous (branching at higher distances) than the second, which included the remaining Magellanic samples, but also the southernmost Bonaerensean Pb2 and *Z. conchifer.* A better picture of samples distribution is obtained by a three-dimensional nMDS (stress level = 0.01) (Additional file 1: Video S1).

Discussion

Molecular analyses identified four *Anisakis* species in the whole sample, including *A. typica*, *A. pegreffii*, *A. berlandi* and an unidentified species, *Anisakis* sp., which seems to be conspecific with *A.* cf. *paggiae* from *Kogia sima* from off north-east Brazil [56], indicating the possible presence of a new species of *Anisakis* in the

Table 3 Summary table of the results of the DISTLM analysis on prevalence and mean abundance of larval *Anisakis* in 18 samples corresponding to 9 fish species from the South-West Atlantic coasts. Results are ordered by the modified Akaike information criterion and only those models with Δ_i < 6 are included

Response variable	Model	AICc	R^2	Predictors[a]	Δ_i	Wi	ER
Prevalence	P1	121.28	0.70	1, 4	0	0.6903	–
	P2	124.65	0.71	1, 4, 5	3.37	0.1280	5.39
	P3	125.15	0.70	1, 2, 4	3.87	0.0997	6.92
	P4	126.78	0.42	1	5.50	0.0441	15.64
	P5	127.09	0.5	1, 5	5.81	0.0378	18.26
Mean abundance	MA1	97.83	0.38	4	0	0.2278	–
	MA2	98.01	0.48	1, 4	0.18	0.2080	1.09
	MA3	98.57	0.24	5	0.74	0.1573	1.45
	MA4	99.56	0.20	1	1.73	0.0959	2.37
	MA5	99.98	0.30	1, 5	2.15	0.0778	2.93
	MA6	100.39	0.29	2, 5	2.56	0.0633	3.60
	MA7	100.42	0.41	2, 4	2.59	0.0624	3.65
	MA8	101.02	0.39	4, 5	3.19	0.0462	4.93
	MA9	101.83	0.48	1, 4, 5	4.00	0.0308	7.39
	MA10	101.84	0.48	1, 2, 4	4.01	0.0307	7.43

Abbreviations: *AICc* modified Akaike information criterion, R^2 proportion of explained variation for the model, Δ_i difference between the AICc of the best model and the AICc for each of the other models, *Wi* Akaike weight, *ER* evidence ratio

[a]Predictor variables: 1, trophic level; 2, mean host length; 3, host species; 4, locality; 5, year

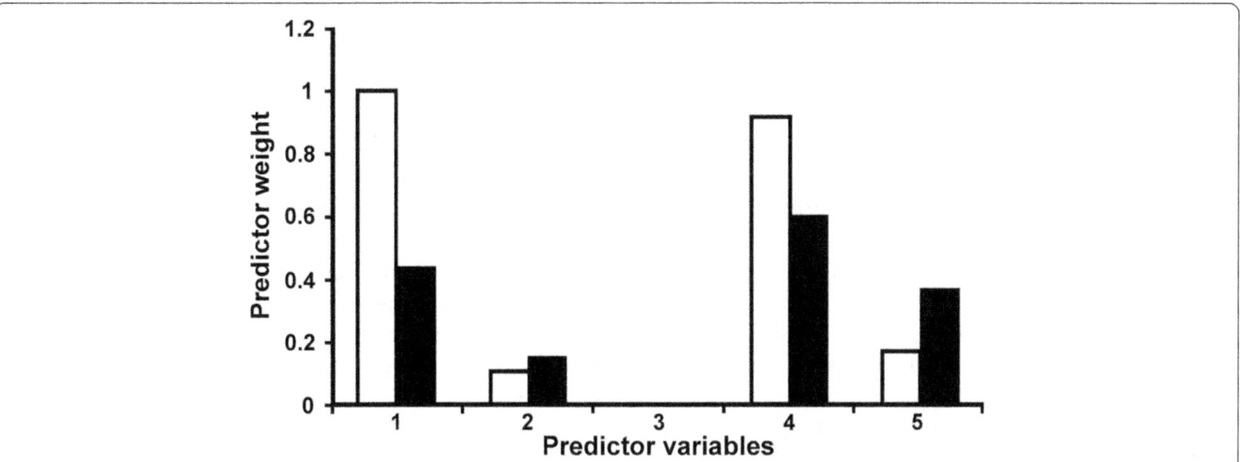

Fig. 2 Predictor weights of variables included in models with $\Delta_i < 6$ resulting of the DISTLM analyses on prevalence and mean abundance of *Anisakis simplex* (*s.l.*) in 18 samples corresponding to 9 fish species from the southern South-West Atlantic coasts. White bars, prevalence; black bars, mean abundance. Predictor variables: 1, trophic level; 2, mean host length; 3, host species; 4, locality; 5, year

South-West Atlantic. Indeed, the K2P distance between *A. paggiae* and *Anisakis* sp. was similar to those between the sibling species of the *A. simplex* complex. Similar distances have been reported for *A. paggiae*-related species in Japanese [43], Philippine [44] and Brazilian [56] waters. Our data support the existence of an *A. paggiae* species complex as suggested by these authors. It is noteworthy that this specimen of *Anisakis* sp. is the only larva Type II so far recorded by the authors in the region, not only in the present samples, but in many other fish species previously surveyed (personal observation).

Knowledge of geographical distribution patterns of *Anisakis* spp. is scarce for many species in the genus [16]. Indeed, most species have been reported from

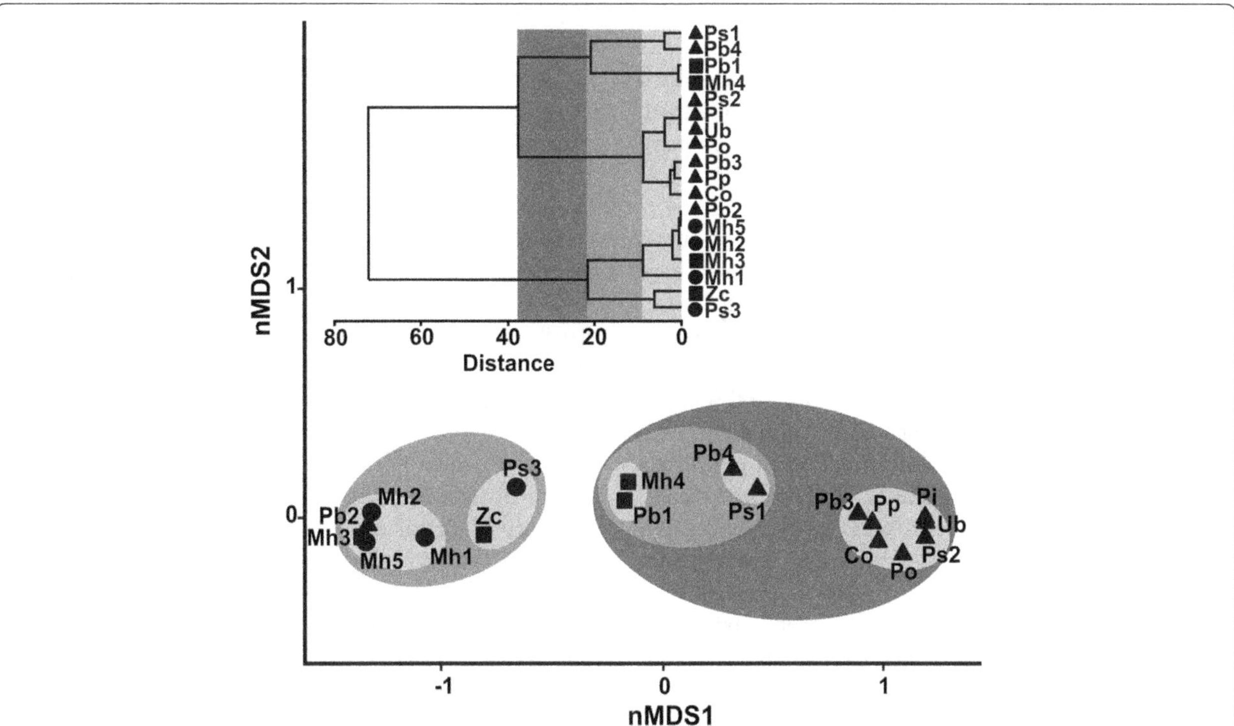

Fig. 3 Non-metric multi-dimensional scaling plot (nMDS) and cluster analyses based on the prevalence of larval *Anisakis* in 18 samples (Euclidean distance) corresponding to 9 fish species in the southern South-West Atlantic. Results of a hierarchical agglomerative clustering are overlaid on the nMDS plot with similarity levels represented by a grey scale. Sample codes as in Table 1. Circles, Magellanic Province; triangles, Argentine Province; squares, ecotone zones

temperate, subtropical and tropical waters between the equator and 35° north and south, being apparently more common in the boreal region [57]. The present findings increase the list of *Anisakis* species in marine fish from the West Atlantic, south to 35°S, by reporting for the first time *A. typica* and *Anisakis* sp. Together with the previously reported *A. pegreffii* and *A. berlandi*, this results in a regional richness of four species, a richness smaller than that recorded in Brazilian marine waters, where six of the nine known species of the genus [i.e. excepting *A. simplex* (*s.s.*), *A. pegreffii* and *A. berlandi*] have been recorded [56]. The record of larvae of *A. pegreffii* in a specimen of *Thunnus thynnus* from the region of Rio de Janeiro by Mattiucci et al. [58] is clearly a typing mistake (Table 3 of Mattiucci et al. [58]), which was subsequently replicated [56].

The composition of species observed in the study region reflects, furthermore, the transitional nature of its oceanographic conditions. *Anisakis typica* is known to be restricted to subtropical and tropical waters, and is the most common species in Brazilian waters [56], whereas *A. pegreffii* displays a discontinuous distribution, being known from the Mediterranean Sea, the Central East Atlantic and waters of China and Japan in the Northern Hemisphere and displaying a circumpolar distribution in the Southern Hemisphere [4, 24, 59]. *Anisakis pegreffii* is also the most reported species in the southern Argentine Sea, dominated by sub-Antarctic waters where 121 of 122 previously genetically identified worms were assigned to this species and only one to *A. berlandi* [18, 60, 61]. Therefore, *A. typica* and *A. pegreffii* can be considered as representatives of northern and southern regions of the South-West Atlantic, respectively. Despite being little represented in the examined samples, *A. berlandi* and *Anisakis* sp. also seem to have opposite geographical origins in the study region. *Anisakis berlandi* is typical from southern waters in the Southern Hemisphere [59, 61], although is also present in Pacific Canadian and Californian waters [62]. On the other hand, *Anisakis* sp. is apparently conspecific with *A.* cf. *paggiae* from *Kogia sima* from off north-east Brazil [56], a cetacean mainly distributed in deep-water habitats of tropical and temperate zones in the Central Atlantic Ocean [16]. In the marine environment, transitional zones between major water masses harbour high biodiversity, mostly due to their productivity [63], but also to an "edge effect", as defined by Odum [64]. Indeed, ecotones contain representatives of species characteristic of adjacent communities [65], which seems to explain the specific composition of *Anisakis* in the convergence regions where masses of water supply "northern" and "southern" species. The thermal gradient produced by these marine currents in the South-West Atlantic [66] explains the dominance of *A. pegreffii* in *M. hubbsi* off Patagonia (southern waters) and of *A. typica* in *Z. conchifer*. The presence of *A. typica* in *P. pagrus* caught at similar latitudes, but in coastal waters, evidences that the influence of the Brazil Current extends to shallower areas surrounding the convergence. This sparid is associated to hard substrates and exhibits considerable site fidelity, remaining in the same patch after recruitment [67], being therefore only exposed to infective stages present in its habitat.

In addition to the environmental conditions as determinants of distribution on *Anisakis* species, their distribution patterns at large spatial scales are congruent with those of their respective final hosts [16]. *Anisakis typica* has been recorded in subtropical and tropical waters from several species of dolphins (Delphinidae), but also in the harbour porpoise, *Phocoena phocoena* (Phocoenidae) and the franciscana dolphin, *Pontoporia blainvillei* (Pontoporidae) [4, 56, 58, 68]. Most of these cetaceans are typical of warmer temperate and tropical seas [58] and consequently the distribution of the parasite can be largely determined by that of their definitive hosts. However, some of these dolphins, namely *Tursiops truncatus* and *Delphinus delphis* are also distributed in higher latitudes, reaching the colder Patagonian waters, where larvae of *A. typica* have not been recorded yet in fishes, and where the adults paraizing them have been morphologically identified as *A. simplex* (*sensu lato*) [19, 69, 70]. Similarly, *P. blainvillei* is infested by *A. typica* in Uruguayan waters, but harbours *A. simplex* (*s.l.*) in central Argentine waters [71]. On the other hand, *A. pegreffii* has been never reported in Brazilian waters. Therefore, the presence of suitable definitive hosts is a necessary but not sufficient condition to explain the geographical patterns of *Anisakis* spp., evidencing that environmental conditions play a major role in such a distribution. In agreement with most records in fish and cetacean hosts from lower latitudes [56], *A. typica* dominated the anisakid community parasitizing *Z. conchifer* in waters on the continental slope at depths between 94 and 117 m and 5° south of its known distribution limit, evidencing a higher effect of the warmer Brazil current relative to other masses of water on the local distribution of larval *Anisakis*. The influence of subtropical waters could, therefore, occur through the transport of infective stages in previous intermediate hosts or be related to the migratory behaviour of the definitive hosts or infested fish from lower latitudes. However, the possibility of *A. typica* arriving to the study zone with migratory *Z. conchifer* from northern regions seems unlikely. Although this species seems to perform ontogenetic movements to deeper waters where large fish concentrate for reproduction [72] the occurrence of latitudinal migrations has not been reported. Furthermore, the size-at-maturity of females is 311 mm (that of males is unknown) [72], which indicates that most of the examined specimens were juvenile and consequently, based on the available information, they are most probably non-migratory individuals. The presence of *A. typica* in *P. pagrus*, as mentioned above, supports the transport of infective stages by the Brazil Current as the main cause of the southern extension in the range of this parasite.

Regarding the distribution of larval *Anisakis* across fish species south of 35°S, the explanatory variables mean host length and host species had little value as drivers of the prevalence and mean abundance of parasites. The lack of relationship between host species and parasite burdens is relevant since it indicates that, given the extremely low specificity of larval *Anisakis*, fish hosts act as passive samplers of infective stages through their diets. The identity and load of larvae in fish, therefore, depend on the trophic behaviour of fish hosts, as well as on the availability of larvae in the food web, modelled by environmental conditions, in each region. Indeed, despite only fish species with a high trophic level were considered, this variable was, together with locality, the main determinant of prevalence, being also highly relevant in explaining the mean abundance of larval *Anisakis*.

Larval anisakids are long-lived in fish hosts, and can be transmitted from one paratenic host to other, persisting in the food web and being potentially available for any host, independent of its trophic level. However, trophic level determines the range of preys a predator can consume, having a direct influence on the abundance and composition of parasite communities [73, 74]. In fact, ichthyophagous fish tend to accumulate higher numbers of larval parasites because they acquire packets of helminth species that travel together in paratenic hosts along food chains [73]. Therefore, the higher their trophic level, the higher the likelihood of becoming infected and the larger the number of infective stages acquired with each individual prey [45], determining the prevalence and the mean abundance of *Anisakis* spp. regardless of the locality of capture. The year of capture also had certain relevance in determining mean abundance, indicating that some changes could have occurred in the region during recent decades; however, a reliable explanation to these variations would require additional studies, beyond the scope of the present work. Finally, and as observed for larval *Anisakis* in skates of the Argentine Sea [18], the geographical origin of the samples was the main determinant of prevalence and mean abundance of parasites. The environmental conditions in the study region are determined by the subtropical and sub-Antarctic currents flowing along the continental slope [75]. The Malvinas Current dominates adjacent shelf waters, producing a latitudinal cline of temperature which decreases southwards, whereas the effect of the warm Brazil Current is marked at the northern limit of the Argentine sea [76]. This temperature gradient, characteristic of the study area [64], provides a series of environments in which *Anisakis* larvae are differentially distributed in terms of prevalence and abundance.

DistLM analyses were carried out irrespective of the *Anisakis* species comprising the assemblages of each sample. However, nMDS analyses showed that *Z. conchifer* departed from the general zoogeographical pattern displayed by the other samples, which in turn, agreed with biogeographical schemes recognized in the South-West Atlantic [48]. Indeed, the apparent separation of samples in two groups corresponding to the Bonaerensean District of the Argentine Province and to the Magellanic Province, characterized by low and high values of prevalence, respectively, confirms the value of larval *Anisakis* as zoogeographical indicators [9, 34]. On the other hand, the two ecotonal hake samples between these two zoogeographical units (Mh3 and Mh4) clustered with Magellanic and Bonaerensean samples, respectively, indicating a higher influence of each mass of water on the populations of *Anisakis* in fish at these transitional zones.

The exception to this pattern was the assignation of the southernmost Bonaerensean sample of *P. brasiliensis* (Pb2) to the Magellanic group of samples. This sample, together with that from the ecotonal Pb1 assigned to the Bonaerensean group, displayed the higher prevalence of larval *Anisakis* for this host. Although they were considered as different stocks based on their parasite assemblages [77], Avigliano et al. [78] determined, based on otholith microchemistry, that *P. brasilisensis* from these two localities represent a single stock. In the light of the present results, migratory movements of these *P. brasiliensis* between these latitudes could not be disregarded. Finally, *Z. conchifer* from deep waters at the convergence between subtropical and sub-Antarctic currents grouped with the distant Magellanic samples as a consequence of the unexpectedly high prevalence regarding other northern samples, even some very close ones, but caught on shelf waters. Taking into account that *A. typica* was the dominant species in *Z. conchifer*, and assuming that other samples are mostly composed of *A. pegreffii*, these results could indicate that interspecific differences of populations distribution exist between these congeners. This hypothesis requires further research because no other host species with a high trophic level from a similar latitude and depth have yet been analysed. In case these differences are confirmed in other fish samples, they may be useful tools as surrogates of the identity of larvae parasitizing a given host population.

The specific identification of larval *Anisakis* in a region where they are considered among the best biological indicators for studies on zoogeography and population distribution of their hosts is undoubtedly a step forward towards the validation of the use of this methodology. Furthermore, considering the diversity of species found, new perspectives for future studies also arise, since members of *Anisakis* have proven to be excellent tools for studying host-parasite cophylogeny, as indicators of trophic web stability and indicators of habitat disturbance of marine ecosystems [4, 24].

Knowledge on the distribution of *Anisakis* spp. in the World Ocean is indispensable for future studies on the epidemiology and pathogenicity of anisakiosis, as well as on the possibility of a changing risk of this zoonosis in the time of climate change [59].

Conclusions

The genetic identification of four species of larval *Anisakis* in fishes from the southern South-West Atlantic (three known and a probably new species related to *A. paggiae*) fill a gap in the knowledge of the global distribution of these zoonotic parasites. It was confirmed that, in the study region, larval *Anisakis* follow a clear zoogeographical pattern, being suitable indicators of tropical/subtropical and sub-Antarctic waters; the main drivers of that pattern were the host trophic level and locality of capture. This information is relevant for both human health and fishery industry, since the species in the genus exhibit differential levels of pathogenicity. The higher taxonomic resolution reached by molecular techniques represents a step forward the validation of the use of larval *Anisakis* as biological indicators for studies on host zoogeography.

Abbreviations

AICc: Modified Akaike's information criterion; *cox2*: Cytochrome *c* oxidase subunit 2; DistLM: Distance-based linear model; EF1 α-1: Elongation factor α-1; ER: Evidence ratio; K2P: Kimura 2-parameter model; nMDS: Non-metric multidimensional scaling; wi: Akaike weight

Acknowledgements

We thank the Instituto Nacional de Investigación y Desarrollo Pesquero (INIDEP), Mar del Plata, Argentina, for providing fish samples.

Funding

Financial support was provided by grants from CONICET (PIP # 112-201501-009763), ANPCYT (PICT 2015 # 2013) and UNMdP (Exa 915/18).

Authors' contributions

ALL, DMPC and VT were responsible for the fish sampling, dissection, microscopic examination and morphological data documentation. PEB, MMI and MDF performed DNA extraction, PCR screening, sequence alignments and bioinformatics analyses. JTT performed statistical analyses. All authors read and approved the final manuscript.

Competing interests

The authors declare that they have no competing interests.

Author details

[1]Laboratorio de Ictioparasitología, Instituto de Investigaciones Marinas y Costeras (IIMyC), Facultad de Ciencias Exactas y Naturales, Universidad Nacional de Mar del Plata - Consejo Nacional de Investigaciones Científicas y Técnicas (CONICET), (7600) Mar del Plata, 3350 Funes, Argentina. [2]Instituto de Biotecnología, Instituto Nacional de Tecnología Agropecuaria (INTA), Hurlingham, Buenos Aires, Argentina.

References

1. Smith JW, Wootten R. *Anisakis* and anisakiasis. Adv Parasitol. 1978;16:93–163.
2. Audicana MT, Ansotegui IJ, de Corres LF, Kennedy MW. *Anisakis* simplex: Dangerous-dead and alive? Trends Parasitol. 2002;18:20–5.
3. Audicana MT, Kennedy MW. *Anisakis simplex*: from obscure infectious worm to inducer of immune hypersensitivity. Clin Microbiol Rev. 2008;21:360–79.
4. Mattiucci S, Nascetti G. Advances and trends in the molecular systematics of anisakid nematodes, with implications for their evolutionary ecology and host-parasite co-evolutionary processes. Adv Parasitol. 2008;66:47–148.
5. McCarthy J, Moore TA. Emerging helminth zoonoses. Int J Parasitol. 2000;30:1351–60.
6. Timi JT. Parasites as biological tags for stock discrimination in marine fish from South American Atlantic waters. J Helminthol. 2007;81:107–11.
7. Lester RJG, MacKenzie K. The use and abuse of parasites as stock markers for fish. Fish Res. 2009;97:1–2.
8. Catalano SR, Whittington ID, Donnellan SC, Gillanders BM. Parasites as biological tags to assess host population structure: guidelines, recent genetic advances and comments on a holistic approach. Int J Parasitol Parasites Wildl. 2013;3:220–6.
9. Cantatore DMP, Timi JT. Marine parasites as biological tags in South American Atlantic waters, current status and perspectives. Parasitology. 2015;142:5–24.
10. Berland B. Nematodes from some Norwegian marine fishes. Sarsia. 1961; 2:1–50.
11. Cipriani P, Smaldone G, Acerra V, D'Angelo L, Anastasio A, Bellisario B, et al. Genetic identification and distribution of the parasitic larvae of *Anisakis pegreffii* and *Anisakis simplex* (*s.s.*) in European hake *Merluccius merluccius* from the Tyrrhenian Sea and Spanish Atlantic coast: implications for food safety. Int J Food Microbiol. 2015;198:1–8.
12. Mattiucci S, Abaunza P, Ramadori L, Nascetti G. Genetic identification of *Anisakis* larvae in European hake from Atlantic and Mediterranean waters for stock recognition. J Fish Biol. 2004;65:495–510.

13. Mattiucci S, Garcia A, Cipriani P, Santos MN, Nascetti G, Cimmaruta R. Metazoan parasite infection in the swordfish, *Xiphias gladius*, from the Mediterranean Sea and comparison with Atlantic populations: implications for its stock characterization. Parasite. 2014;21:35.
14. Mattiucci S, Cimmaruta R, Cipriani P, Abaunza P, Bellisario B, Nascetti G. Integrating *Anisakis* spp. parasites data and host genetic structure in the frame of a holistic approach for stock identification of selected Mediterranean Sea fish species. Parasitology. 2015;142:90–108.
15. Abaunza P, Murta AG, Campbell N, Cimmaruta R, Comesana AS, Dahle G, et al. Stock identity of horse mackerel (*Trachurus trachurus*) in the Northeast Atlantic and Mediterranean Sea: integrating the results from different stock identification approaches. Fish Res. 2008;89:196–209.
16. Kuhn T, García-Márquez J, Klimpel S. Adaptive radiation within marine anisakid nematodes: a zoogeographical modelling of cosmopolitan, zoonotic parasites. PLoS One. 2011;6:e28642.
17. Gómez-Mateos M, Valero A, Morales-Yuste M, Martín-Sánchez J. Molecular epidemiology and risk factors for *Anisakis simplex s.l.* infection in blue whiting (*Micromesistius poutassou*) in a confluence zone of the Atlantic and Mediterranean: differences between *A. simplex s.s.* and *A. pegreffii*. Int J Food Microbiol. 2016;232:111–6.
18. Irigoitia MM, Braicovich PE, Lanfranchi AL, Farber MD, Timi JT. Distribution of anisakid nematodes parasitizing rajiform skates under commercial exploitation in the Southwestern Atlantic. Int J Food Microbiol. 2018;267:20–8.
19. Hernández-Orts JS, Paso Viola MN, García NA, Crespo EA, González R, García-Varela M, Kuchta R. A checklist of the helminth parasites of marine mammals from Argentina. Zootaxa. 2015;3936:301–34.
20. Berón-Vera B, Crespo EA, Raga JA. Parasites in stranded cetaceans of Patagonia. J Parasitol. 2008;94:946–8.
21. Luque JL, Muniz-Pereira LC, Siciliano S, Siqueira LR, Oliveira MS, Vieira FM. Checklist of helminth parasites of cetaceans from Brazil. Zootaxa. 2010;2548:57–68.
22. Fonseca MCG, Knoff M, Felizardo NN, Di Azevedo MIN, Torres EJL, Gomes DC, et al. Integrative taxonomy of Anisakidae and Raphidascarididae (Nematoda) in *Paralichthys patagonicus* and *Xystreurys rasile* (Pisces: Teleostei) from Brazil. Int J Food Microbiol. 2016;235:113–24.
23. Di Azevedo MIN, Iñiguez AM. Nematode parasites of commercially important fish from the southeast coast of Brazil: morphological and genetic insight. Int J Food Microbiol. 2018;267:29–41.
24. Mattiucci S, Paoletti M, Cipriani P, Webb SC, Timi JT, Nascetti G. Inventorying biodiversity of anisakid nematodes from the Austral Region: a hotspot of genetic diversity? In: Klimpel S, Kuhn T, Mehlhorn H, editors. Biodiversity and Evolution of Parasitic Life in the Southern Ocean. Parasitology Research Monographs, vol. 9. Cham: Springer; 2017. p. 109–40.
25. Piola AR, Martínez Avellaneda N, Guerrero RA, Jardón FP, Palma ED, Romero SI. Malvinas-slope water intrusions on the northern Patagonia continental shelf. Ocean Sci. 2010;6:345–59.
26. Moreno IB, Zerbini AN, Danilewicz D, de Oliveira Santos MC, Simões-Lopes PC, Lailson-Brito J Jr, Azevedo AF. Distribution and habitat characteristics of dolphins of the genus *Stenella* (Cetacea: Delphinidae) in the southwest Atlantic Ocean. Mar Ecol Prog Ser. 2005;300:229–40.
27. Mandiola MA, Giardino GV, Bastida J, Rodríguez DH, Bastida RO. Marine mammal occurrence in deep waters of the Brazil-Malvinas Confluence off Argentina during summer. Mastozool Neotrop. 2015;22:397–402.
28. Di Tullio JC, Gandra TBR, Zerbini AN, Secchi ER. Diversity and distribution patterns of cetaceans in the subtropical southwestern Atlantic outer continental shelf and slope. PLoS One. 2016;11:e0155841.
29. Lanfranchi AL, Braicovich PE, Cantatore DMP, Alarcos AJ, Luque JL, Timi JT. Ecotonal marine regions - ecotonal parasite communities: helminth assemblages in the convergence of masses of water in the southwestern Atlantic. Int J Parasitol. 2016;46:809–18.
30. Haimovici M, Martins AS, Figueiredo JL, Vieira PC. Demersal bony fish of the outer shelf and upper slope of the southern Brazil Subtropical Convergence ecosystem. Mar Ecol Prog Ser. 1994;108:59–77.
31. Quéro JC, Du Buit MH, Vayne JJ. Les observations de poisons tropicaux et le réchauffement des eaux dans l'Atlantique européen. Oceanol Acta. 1998;21:345–51.
32. Ragonese S, Giusto GB. *Zenopsis conchifera* (Lowe, 1852) (Pisces, Actinopterygii, Zeidae): a new alien fish in the Mediterranean Sea. J Fish Biol. 2007;21:345–51.
33. Pereira AN, Pantoja C, Luque JL, Timi JT. Parasites of *Urophycis brasiliensis* (Gadiformes: Phycidae) as indicators of marine ecoregions in coastal areas of the South American Atlantic with the assessment of their stocks. Parasitol Res. 2014;113:4281–92.
34. Braicovich PE, Pantoja C, Pereira AN, Luque JL, Timi JT. Parasites of the Brazilian flathead *Percophis brasiliensis* reflect West Atlantic biogeograhic regions. Parasitology. 2017;144:169–78.
35. dos Reis Sardella CJ, Luque JL. Diagnóstico morfológico e molecular de larvas de *Anisakis typica* e *Anisakis brevispiculata* em peixes do litoral do Rio de Janeiro. Braz J Vet Med. 2016;38(Supl. 3):124–30.
36. Bush AO, Lafferty KD, Lotz JM, Shostak AW. Parasitology meets ecology on its own terms: Margolis et al. revisited. J Parasitol. 1997;83:575–83.
37. Nadler SA, Hudspeth DSS. Phylogeny of the Ascaridoidea (Nematoda: Ascaridida) based on three genes and morphology: hypothesis of structural and sequence evolution. J Parasitol. 2000;86:380–93.
38. Mattiucci S, Acerra V, Paoletti M, Cipriani P, Levsen A, Webb SC, et al. No more time to stay 'single' in the detection of *Anisakis pegreffii*, *A. simplex* (*s.s.*) and hybridization events between them: a multi-marker nuclear genotyping approach. Parasitology. 2016;143:998–1011.
39. Filatov DA. ProSeq: a software for preparation and evolutionary analysis of DNA sequence data sets. Mol Ecol Notes. 2002;2:621–4.
40. Altschul FS, Gish W, Miller W, Myers EW, Lipman DJ. Basic local alignment search tool. J Mol Biol. 1990;215:403–10.
41. Thompson JD, Higgins DG, Gibson TJ. CLUSTAL W: improving the sensitivity of progressive multiple sequence alignment through sequence weighting, position-specific gap penalties and weight matrix choice. Nucleic Acids Res. 1994;22:4673–80.
42. Kumar S, Stecher G, Tamura K. MEGA7: Molecular Evolutionary Genetics Analysis version 7.0 for bigger datasets. Mol Biol Evol. 2016;33:1870–4.
43. Quiazon K, Yoshinaga T, Santos M, Ogawa K. Identification of larval *Anisakis* spp. (Nematoda: Anisakidae) in Alaska pollock (*Theragra chalcogramma*) in northern Japan using morphological and molecular markers. J Parasitol. 2009;95:1227–32.
44. Quiazon K, Santos M, Yoshinaga T. *Anisakis* species (Nematoda: Anisakidae) of dwarf sperm whale *Kogia sima* (Owen, 1866) stranded off the Pacific coast of southern Philippine archipelago. Vet Parasitol. 2013;197:221–30.
45. Timi JT, Rossin MA, Alarcos AJ, Braicovich PE, Cantatore DMP, Lanfranchi AL. Fish trophic level and the similarity of larval parasite assemblages. Int J Parasitol. 2011;41:309–16.
46. Froese R, Pauly D. Fish Base. In: World Wide Web Electronic Publication; 2018. www.fishbase.org. Accessed 28 Feb 2018.
47. Cousseau MB, Perrotta RG. Peces Marinos de Argentina: Biología, Distribución, Pesca. 4th ed. Mar del Plata: Instituto Nacional de Investigación y Desarrollo Pesquero; 2013.
48. Menni RC, Jaureguizar AJ, Stehmann MFW, Lucifora LO. Marine biodiversity at the community level: zoogeography of sharks, skates, rays and chimaeras in the southwestern Atlantic. Biodivers Conserv. 2010;19:775–96.
49. Anderson MJ, Gorley RN, Clarke KR. PERMANOVA+ for PRIMER: Guide to Software and Statistical Methods. Plymouth: PRIMER-E; 2008.
50. Timi JT, Lanfranchi AL. Ontogenetic changes in heterogeneity of parasite communities of fish: disentangling the relative role of compositional *versus* abundance variability. Parasitology. 2013;140:309–17.
51. Braicovich PE, Ieno EN, Sáez M, Despos J, Timi JT. Assessing the role of host traits as drivers of the abundance of long-lived parasites in fish stock assessment studies. J Fish Biol. 2016;89:2419–33.
52. Symonds MRE, Moussalli A. A brief guide to model selection, multimodel inference and model averaging in behavioural ecology using Akaike's information criterion. Behav Ecol Sociobiol. 2011;65:13–21.
53. Burnham KP, Anderson DR. Model Selection and Multimodel Inference. 2nd ed. New York: Springer; 2002.
54. Richards SA. Testing ecological theory using the information theoretic approach: examples and cautionary results. Ecology. 2005;86:2805–14.
55. Clarke KR, Gorley RN. PRIMER v7: User Manual/Tutorial. Plymouth: PRIMER-E; 2015.
56. Di Azevedo MIN, Carvalho VL, Iñiguez AM. Integrative taxonomy of anisakid nematodes in stranded cetaceans from Brazilian waters: an update on parasite's hosts and geographical records. Parasitol Res. 2017;116:3105–16.
57. Klimpel S, Kuhn T, Busch MW, Horst K, Palm HW. Deep water life-cycle of *Anisakis paggiae* (Nematoda: Anisakidae) in the Irminger Sea indicates kogiid whale distribution in North Atlantic waters. Polar Biol. 2011;34:899–906.

58. Mattiucci S, Paggi L, Nascetti G, Santos CP, Costa G, Di Beneditto AP, et al. Genetic markers in the study of *Anisakis typica* (Diesing, 1860): larval identification and genetic relationships with other species of *Anisakis* Dujardin, 1845 (Nematoda: Anisakidae). Syst Parasitol. 2002;51:159–70.
59. Klimpel S, Palm HW. Anisakid nematode (Ascaridoidea) life cycles and distribution: increasing zoonotic potential in the time of climate change? In: Mehlhorn H, editor. Progress in Parasitology. Parasitology Research Monographs. Heidelberg: Springer Verlag; 2011;2:201–22.
60. Mattiucci S, Nascetti G, Cianchi R, Paggi L, Arduino P, Margolis L, et al. Genetic and ecological data on the *Anisakis simplex* complex with evidence for a new species (Nematoda, Ascaridoidea, Anisakidae). J Parasitol. 1997;83:401–16.
61. Mattiucci S, Nascetti G. Genetic diversity and infection levels of anisakid nematodes parasitic in fish and marine mammals from Boreal and Austral hemispheres. Vet Parasitol. 2007;66:47–148.
62. Klimpel S, Busch M, Khun T, Rohde A, Palm HW. The *Anisakis simplex* complex off the South Shetland Islands (Antarctica): endemic populations *versus* introduction through migratory hosts. Mar Ecol Prog Ser. 2010;34: 899–906.
63. Scales KL, Miller PI, Hawkes LA, Ingram SN, Sims DW, Votier SC. On the front line: frontal zones as priority at-sea conservation areas for mobile marine vertebrates. J Appl Ecol. 2014;51:1575–83.
64. Odum EP. Fundamentals of Ecology. 2nd ed. Philadelphia: Saunders; 1959.
65. Baker J, French K, Whelan RJ. The edge effect and ecotonal species: bird communities across a natural edge in southeastern Australia. Ecology. 2002; 83:3048–59.
66. Hoffmann J, Núñez M, Piccolo M. Características climáticas del océano Atlántico sudoccidental. In: Boschi EE, editor. El Mar Argentino y sus Recursos Pesqueros Tomo I. Antecedentes históricos de las exploraciones en el mar y las características ambientales. Mar del Plata: Instituto Nacional de Investigación y Desarrollo Pesquero; 1997. p. 163–93.
67. De Vries AD. The life history, reproductive ecology and demography of the red porgy, Pagrus pagrus, in the northeastern Gulf of Mexico. PhD Dissertation. Tallahassee: Florida State University; 2006.
68. Iñiguez AM, Carvalho VL, Motta MR, Pinheiro DC, Vicente AC. Genetic analysis of *Anisakis typica* (Nematoda: Anisakidae) from cetaceans of the northeast coast of Brazil: new data on its definitive hosts. Vet Parasitol. 2011; 178:293–9.
69. Berón-Vera B, Crespo EA, Raga JA, Fernández M. Parasites communities of common dolphins (*Delphinus delphis*) from Patagonia: the relation with host distribution and diet and comparison with sympatric host. J Parasitol. 2007; 93:1056–60.
70. Romero MA, Fernández M, Dans SL, García NA, González R, Crespo EA. Gastrointestinal parasites of bottlenose dolphins *Tursiops truncatus* from the extreme south western Atlantic, with notes on diet composition. Dis Aquat Org. 2014;108:61–70.
71. Aznar FJ, Raga JA, Corcuera J, Monzón F. Helminths as biological tags for franciscana (*Pontoporia blainvillei*) (Cetacea, Pontoporiidae) in Argentinian and Uruguayan waters. Mammalia. 1995;59:427–36.
72. Martins RS, Schwingel PR. Biological aspects of the sailfin dory *Zenopsis conchifer* (Lowe, 1852) caught by deep-sea trawling fishery off southern Brazil. Braz J Oceanogr. 2012;60:171–9.
73. Marcogliese DJ. Food webs and the transmission of parasites to marine fish. Parasitology. 2002;124:83–99.
74. Chen H-W, Liu W-C, Davis AJ, Jordan F, Hwang MJ, Shao K-T. Network position of hosts in food webs and their parasite diversity. Oikos. 2008;117: 1847–55.
75. Piola AR, Rivas AL. Corrientes en la plataforma continental. In: Boschi EE, editor. El Mar Argentino y Sus Recursos Pesqueros Tomo I. Antecedentes históricos de las exploraciones en el mar y las características ambientales. Mar del Plata: Instituto Nacional de Investigación y Desarrollo Pesquero; 1997. p. 119–32.
76. Guerrero RA, Piola AR. Masas de agua en la plataforma continental. In: Boschi EE, editor. El Mar Argentino y sus Recursos Pesqueros Tomo I. Antecedentes históricos de las exploraciones en el mar y las características ambientales. Mar del Plata: Instituto Nacional de Investigación y Desarrollo Pesquero; 1997. p. 107–18.
77. Braicovich PE, Timi JT. Parasites as biological tags for stock discrimination of the Brazilian flathead *Percophis brasiliensis* in the south-west Atlantic. J Fish Biol. 2008;73:557–71.
78. Avigliano E, Saez MB, Rico R, Volpedo AV. Use of otolith strontium: calcium and zinc: calcium ratios as an indicator of the habitat of *Percophis brasiliensis* Quoy & Gaimard, 1825 in the southwestern Atlantic Ocean. Neotrop Ichthyol. 2015;13:187–94.
79. Sardella NH, Timi JT. Parasites of Argentine hake in the Argentine Sea: population and infracommunity structure as evidence for host stock discrimination. J Fish Biol. 2004;65:1472–88.
80. Alarcos AJ, Timi JT. Parasite communities in three sympatric flounder species (Pleuronectiformes: Paralichthyidae). Similar ecological filters driving toward repeatable assemblages. Parasitol Res. 2012;110:2155–66.
81. Alarcos AJ, Etchegoin JA. Parasite assemblages of estuarine-dependent marine fishes from Mar Chiquita coastal lagoon (Buenos Aires Province, Argentina). Parasitol Res. 2010;107:1083–91.
82. Timi JT, Lanfranchi AL. The metazoan parasite communities of the Argentinean sandperch *Pseudopercis semifasciata* (Pisces: Perciformes) and their use to elucidate the stock structure of the host. Parasitology. 2009;136: 1083–91.

15

Fasciola hepatica-Pseudosuccinea columella interaction: effect of increasing parasite doses, successive exposures and geographical origin on the infection outcome of susceptible and naturally-resistant snails from Cuba

Annia Alba[1,2], Antonio A. Vázquez[1,4], Jorge Sánchez[1], David Duval[2], Hilda M. Hernández[1], Emeline Sabourin[3,4], Marion Vittecoq[3], Sylvie Hurtrez-Boussés[4] and Benjamin Gourbal[2*]

Abstract

Background: *Pseudosuccinea columella* is one of the most widespread vectors of *Fasciola hepatica*, a globally distributed trematode that affects humans, livestock and wildlife. The exclusive occurrence in Cuba of susceptible and naturally-resistant populations to *F. hepatica* within this snail species, offers a fascinating model for evolutionary biology, health sciences and vector control strategies. In particular, resistance in *P. columella* is characterized by the encapsulation of the parasite by host's immune cells and has been experimentally tested using different Cuban *F. hepatica* isolates with no records of successful infection. Here, we aimed to explore for the first time, the effect of different parasite doses, successive exposures and different parasite origins on the infection outcomes of the two phenotypes of *P. columella* occurring in Cuba.

Methods: To increase the chances for *F. hepatica* to establish, we challenged Cuban *P. columella* with increasing single parasite doses of 5, 15 or 30 miracidia and serial exposures (three-times) of 5 miracidia using a sympatric *F. hepatica* isolate from Cuba, previously characterized by microsatellite markers. Additionally, we exposed the snails to *F. hepatica* from different geographical origins (i.e. Dominican Republic and France). Parasite prevalence, redial burden and survival of snails were recorded at 25 days post-exposure.

Results: No parasite development was noted in snails from the resistant populations independent of the experimental approach. Contrastingly, an overall increase in prevalence and redial burden was observed in susceptible snails when infected with high miracidia doses and after serial exposures. Significant differences in redial burden between single 15 miracidia and serial 3 × 5 miracidia infected snails suggest that immune priming potentially occurs in susceptible *P. columella*. Compatibility differences of allopatric (Caribbean *vs* European) *F. hepatica* with susceptible snails were related to the geographical scale of the combinations.

(Continued on next page)

* Correspondence: benjamin.gourbal@univ-perp.fr
[2]University of Perpignan Via Domitia, Interactions Hosts Pathogens Environments UMR 5244, CNRS, IFREMER, Univ. Montpellier, F-66860 Perpignan, France
Full list of author information is available at the end of the article

(Continued from previous page)
Conclusions: Here, the effectiveness of *P. columella* resistance to *F. hepatica* does not decline with increasing parasite doses, successive infection or different geographical origins of parasite isolates, while presenting new evidence for specificity for infection in susceptible *P. columella* snails. Understanding the peculiarities of the *P. columella-F. hepatica* interaction and the extent of the resistant phenotype is crucial for an effective parasite control and for developing alternatives to tackle fasciolosis transmission.

Keywords: Snail-trematode interaction, Lymnaeidae, Liver fluke, Experimental infection, Immune priming, Compatibility, Allopatric parasites

Background

The liver fluke *Fasciola hepatica* Linnaeus, 1758 is the main causative agent of fasciolosis, a snail-borne parasitic disease that affects humans, livestock and wildlife [1]. The occurrence of this trematode in all continents except in Antarctica has been largely explained by the introduction of infected livestock and susceptible snails into new areas, with *F. hepatica* being able to parasitize a wide range of host species [1, 2]. The arrival of the liver fluke to the Americas presumably occurred during the early events of colonization of the New World by Europeans, with several native freshwater lymnaeid snails transmitting the parasite today [1].

Pseudosuccinea columella (Say, 1817), considered native from North America [3], can be also cited among the intermediate host species of *F. hepatica* in South America and the Caribbean [4–6]. In addition, it is a globally invasive freshwater snail that has been largely introduced out of its native range [3] with reports of established populations from Europe [7], Africa [8], Australia [9] and the Pacific islands [10, 11]. The global spread of some invasive genotypes of *P. columella* might complicate the epidemiological scenario of fasciolosis transmission [3].

Interestingly, in Cuba, *P. columella* displays two different phenotypes regarding *F. hepatica* infection with natural populations being either susceptible [5] or resistant to the liver fluke [12]. Notably, the resistant phenotype in field-occurring *P. columella* is characterized by the encapsulation of the parasite by the host's immune cells [12]. These populations have been extensively tested for infection using different Cuban isolates of *F. hepatica* but no successful parasite development has ever been recorded (see [12–14] for details). From a genetic perspective, studies exploring the existence of polymorphism in *P. columella* have shown that resistant snails cluster separately from susceptible populations in Cuba [13] and other regions of the world [3].

The challenging of resistant individuals of *P. columella* has been always carried out using a constant standard dose of five miracidia (infective larva for the snails). Therefore, we wanted to explore the effect of higher infective doses of the parasite, either by single or serial exposure trials on both susceptible and resistant *P. columella* using a known polymorphic *F. hepatica* isolate from Cuba (La Palma; [15]). With these approaches we aimed at tipping the scales in favour of the infection success by (i) increasing the probability of encounter of compatible host-parasite genotypes, and (ii) by circumventing or hijacking the effectiveness of host immune defences with large miracidia numbers and/or enhanced genetic diversity of the parasite at which each snail is confronted [16, 17].

In another experiment, given that resistant individuals had always been challenged with Cuban isolates of *F. hepatica*, we exposed for the first time, susceptible and resistant *P. columella* from Cuba to two allopatric liver fluke isolates from the Caribbean (short distance) and Europe (large distance), and compared their infection outcomes with those of the sympatric Cuban isolate. The theory of local adaptation predicts that parasites perform better on their local (sympatric) hosts rather than foreign (allopatric) hosts [18]. However, exceptions exist (e.g. [14, 19]), thus a differential exposure of a host population to an "unknown" entity (i.e. allopatric parasites) might result in differential outcomes and can test for different patterns of susceptibility or even resistance. Given the geographical isolation between the parasite isolates used, genetic differences are expected and should account for variations in compatibility with the snail host, particularly between the Cuban and the European isolates. With this experimental approach, it is likely that a higher infection success from exposing susceptible *P. columella* to sympatric *F. hepatica* would be observed, while the resulting outcome with resistant populations could give clues concerning the specificity of their resistance. If no infection occurs in resistant *P. columella* then we might hypothesize that this phenotypic response is not restricted only to local (Cuban) parasites but it has a broader or even global scale.

Here, we gain new insights on the susceptible *P. columella-F. hepatica* interaction, presenting evidence related to differences in compatibility and immune priming as factors affecting the infection outcomes (e.g. prevalence, redial burden, host survival) in this model. Moreover, we demonstrate that resistant populations described from

Cuba remain resistant to a high *F. hepatica* miracidial dose, after serial exposures or challenged with allopatric *F. hepatica* isolates. This highly resistant phenotype opened new perspectives of applications for fasciolosis control.

Methods

Fasciola hepatica isolates and laboratory-reared susceptible and resistant *P. columella*

We collected adults of *F. hepatica* in local abattoirs from eastern Cuba (sympatric isolate: La Palma, Pinar del Río Province), north-western Dominican Republic (allopatric isolate, narrow scale: Dajabón Province) and southern France (allopatric isolate, large scale: Camargue region). The genetic structure of eight *F. hepatica* isolates from Cuba (including parasites from La Palma and other regions within its vicinity) had been previously characterized [15]; this study demonstrated the existence of high polymorphism and genetic diversity within Cuban *F. hepatica* with no clear genetic differentiation among isolates due to a high genetic flow within the island and a preferential out-crossing as reproduction strategy. In particular, the La Palma isolate (local isolate used in the present study) showed over 75% prevalence in sacrificed bovines and a mean of five alleles per analysed microsatellite locus with an observed heterozygosity of 0.511 [15]. Unfortunately, no previous data on genetic diversity is available for the Dominican and French isolates used, but we can expect differences with Cuban flukes given the geographical isolation.

Flukes were collected from the liver of infected cattle and kept alive for 6 h in a solution of 0.85% NaCl (saline solution) and 5% glucose (Sigma-Aldrich, St. Quentin Fallavier, France) for egg laying. Eggs were preserved at 4 °C in the dark and in saline solution supplemented with gentamicin (Sigma-Aldrich, 40 mg/ml) until use.

We used two susceptible *P. columella* populations, Negrines (Havana Province) and Aurora (Mayabeque Province), and two resistant populations, La Coca (Havana Province) and La Palma (Pinar del Río Province). Snails were reared in the Laboratory of Malacology of the Institute of Tropical Medicine "Pedro Kourí", Cuba, for two to three generations and derived from field-collected populations of *P. columella*. Snails were cultured in Petri dishes with growing algae, in 26 °C de-chlorinated water complemented with crushed shells as a carbonate supplement as previously described [20]. The snails were fed on the algae *ad libitum* and routinely changed to other Petri dishes with growing algae to avoid starvation.

Experimental exposure of *P. columella* snails to *F. hepatica*

Experimental exposure of 2-weeks-old laboratory-reared *P. columella* from the four populations (two resistant and two susceptible) were carried out using freshly hatched miracidia, according to the methodology described by Vázquez et al. [14]. Briefly, eggs of *F. hepatica* were incubated in distilled water in total darkness at 28 °C for 15 days to complete maturation. Miracidia hatching was induced by direct exposure of eggs to light. For each assay, we always used 30 individuals of *P. columella* at varying conditions (see Fig. 1) as described below.

A. Exposure to different doses of F. hepatica miracidia

We exposed each *P. columella* population separately to single doses of 5, 15 and 30 miracidia (M) from the sympatric isolate of La Palma (Cuba) to increase the probability of exposing host populations to different parasite genotypes.

B. Serial exposure to F. hepatica miracidia

We explored the effect of serial infections with *F. hepatica* by exposing each *P. columella* population three times to the standard dose of 5 M [14] of the sympatric *F. hepatica* isolate of La Palma (Cuba; 3 × 5 M). Each exposure was performed at a three-day interval, after which each snail received a serially-delivered 15 M dose. The selection of the re-infection interval was based on the timing at which the immune response occurs (0 to 3–4 days post-exposure with patent parasite encapsulation as early as 24 h post-exposure; see Gutiérrez et al. [12]), which is also accompanied by possible "consumption" of defence related resources in the snail.

C. Exposure to sympatric and allopatric F. hepatica

We exposed each *P. columella* population separately to the standard dose of 5 M [14] of each allopatric *F. hepatica* isolate (Camargue, France and Dajabón, Dominican Republic). In order to save biological material, we used the results of the 5 M dose (see A above), for comparison against sympatric interactions.

In all trials and control groups, snails were individually allocated in 96-well plates and individually exposed overnight to *F. hepatica* miracidia. Each well was checked to record the penetration of all miracidia into the snails used for each experiment. Snails were maintained at 28 °C and monitored daily. Day-to-day mortality was recorded and exposed snails found dead were carefully dissected [21] to assess infection. Between days 7–10 post-exposure, infection was clearly patent by the presence of rediae in dissected individuals. The number of rediae per infected snail was counted to estimate the intensity of *F. hepatica* infection (redial burden) [14] per experimental group, always 25 days post-exposure or post-first-exposure in the case of serial exposure trials. Non-exposed snails from the same breeding batch were reared in the laboratory and subjected to the same conditions to serve as control of survival for the infection assays.

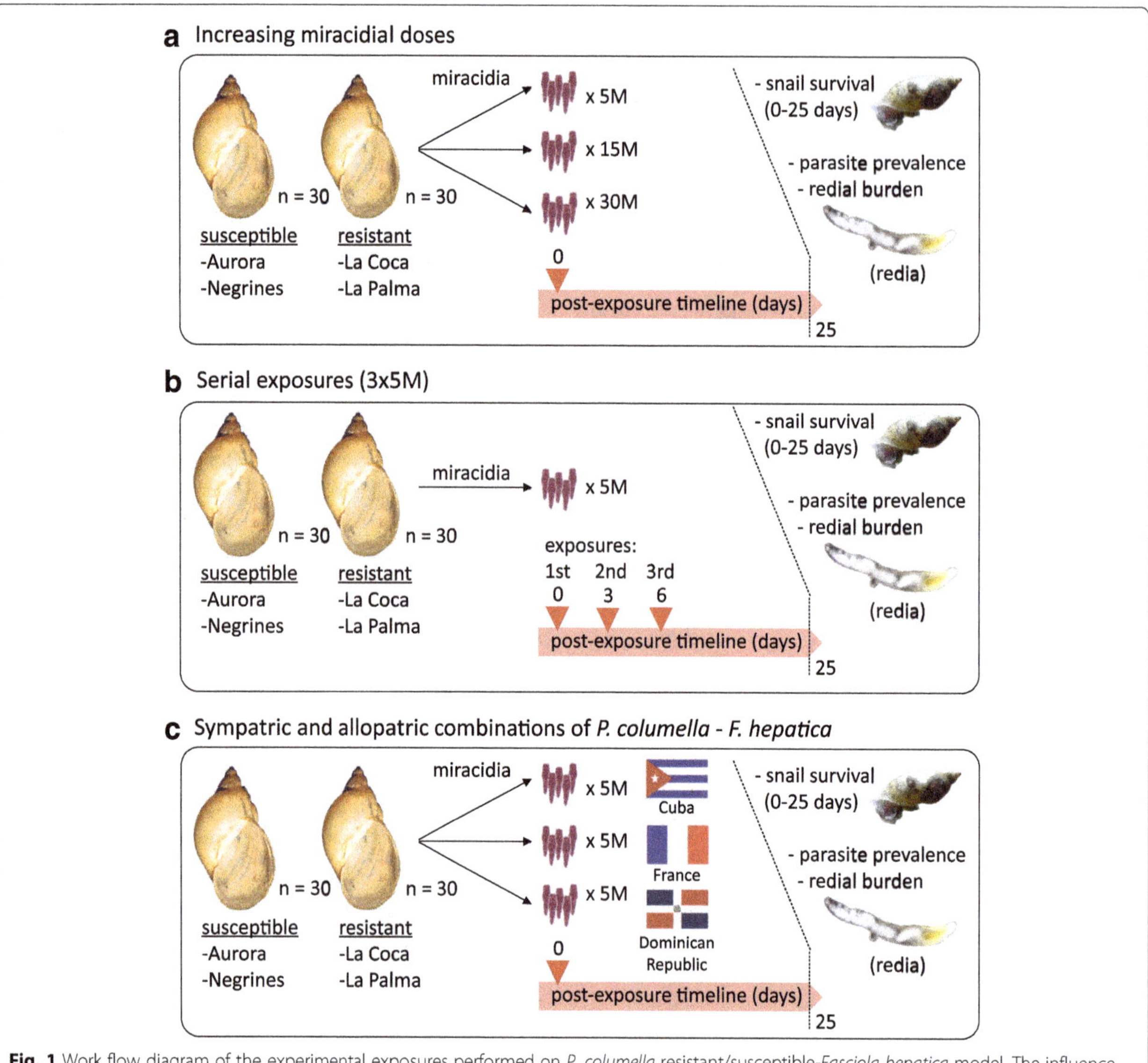

Fig. 1 Work flow diagram of the experimental exposures performed on *P. columella* resistant/susceptible-*Fasciola hepatica* model. The influence of different parasite doses (**a**) and serial parasite exposures (**b**) on *P. columella* phenotypes were assayed using sympatric (Cuban) *F. hepatica*. **c** Allopatric *F. hepatica* exposures

Data analysis

The prevalence of *F. hepatica* in each experimental group was expressed as the percentage of infected snails of all those initially exposed ($n = 30$); confidence limits were calculated at the 95% confidence level by the Wilson score interval. Differences in prevalence between groups were checked by Fisher's exact test. Survival curves of exposed snails [from 0–25 days post-(first-)exposure] were constructed based on the number of live snails at each time point divided by the number of exposed individuals and expressed as a percentage. We performed log-rank tests of Kaplan-Meier curves to assess the statistical differences on survivorship data. Data of *F. hepatica* redial counting per experimental group was checked for normality and variance homogeneity using Shapiro-Wilk and Levene tests, respectively. Factorial ANOVAs followed by a *post-hoc* multiple comparison Tukey test were carried out to assess statistical significance of the effect of (i) different miracidial doses and serial exposures within host populations, and (ii) allopatric and sympatric (data of experimental infection with Cuban *F. hepatica* at a 5 M dose) in redial burden. All calculations were performed in Statistica v.12 (StatSoft. Inc., Tulsa, OK, USA) and differences were always considered significant at values of $P < 0.05$.

Results

Results of host survival in the exposed groups are shown in Fig. 2. Overall, we observed a mortality peak on exposed snails occurring at 24–48 h post-exposure and a

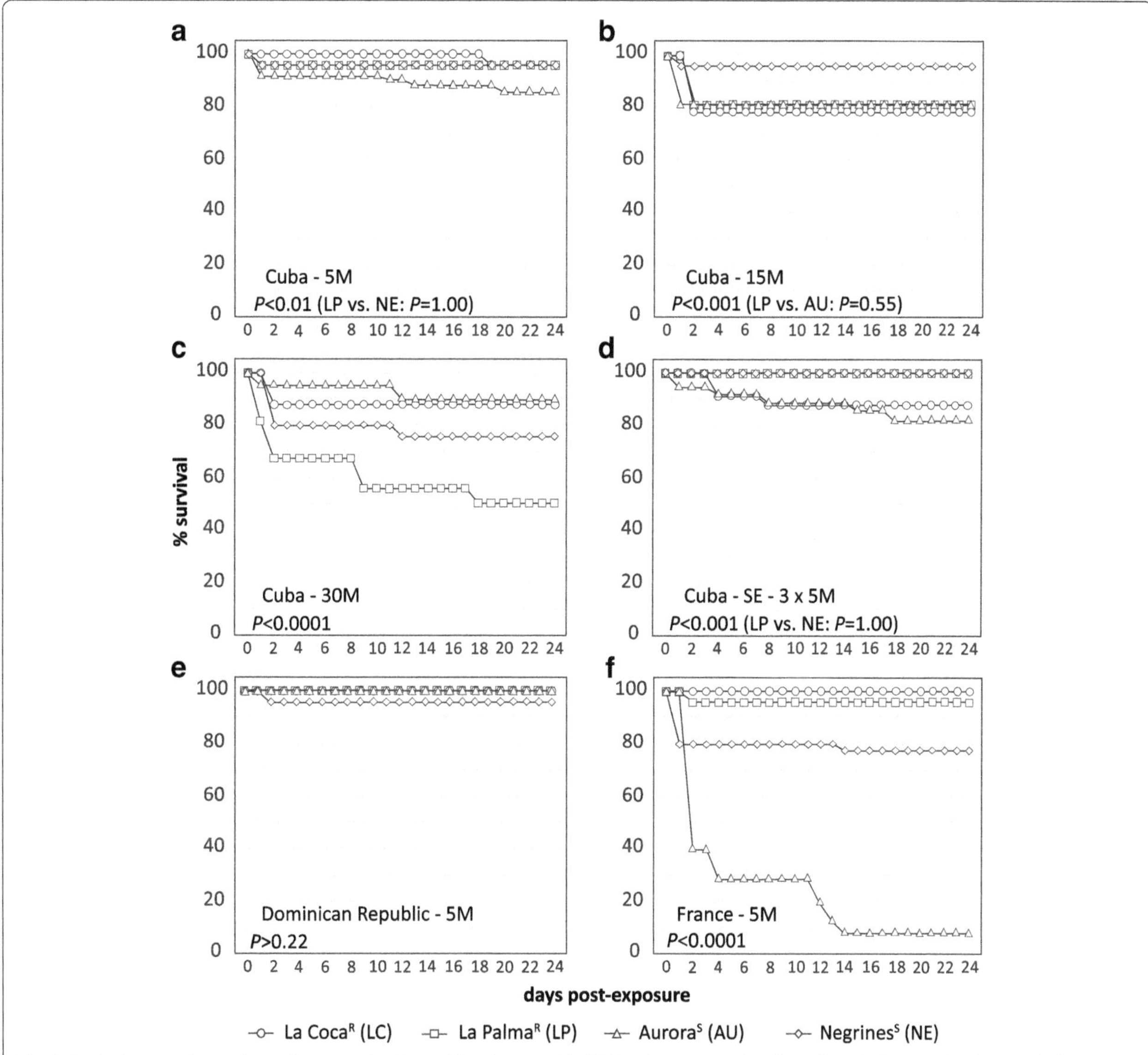

Fig. 2 Survival curves of experimentally-exposed resistant (R) and susceptible (S) *Pseudosuccinea columella* to *Fasciola hepatica*. Snails were challenged following different approaches: **a-c** increasing miracidial doses, **d** serial exposures (SE) and **e-f** exposure to allopatric *F. hepatica* isolates. Pairwise comparisons of snail survival between populations at each experimental trial were performed by log-rank tests and are shown. *Abbreviation*: M, miracidia

significant decrease of snail survival with increasing miracidia dose (Fig. 2a-d; log-rank tests: $P < 0.05$; Aurora, 5 M *vs* 30 M, $P = 0.24$; Negrines, 5 M *vs* 15 M, $P = 1$). No mortality was observed within the studied time frame in the control group (non-exposed snails; data not shown).

Infection outcome in resistant *P. columella*

As expected, while susceptible *P. columella* became infected after exposure to *F. hepatica*, resistant snails from La Palma and La Coca failed to develop larval stages and no sign of infection was observed following each of the experimental approaches tested (Table 1). Notably, resistant populations showed higher overall survival than susceptible *P. columella* (Fig. 2).

Infection outcome in susceptible *P. columella*, increasing miracidial dose and serial exposures

An overall increase of both prevalence (Fisher's exact test: Aurora, 5 M *vs* 30 M, $P = 0.021$; Negrines, 5 M *vs* 15 M / 3 × 5 M, $P < 0.03$; Table 1) and redial burden (Fig. 3a) was noted in susceptible individuals with the increase of the miracidial dose, either by single or serial exposure events. However, no significant differences in prevalence and redial burden were observed when snails were infected with 15 M or 30 M (Fisher's exact test: Aurora, 15 M *vs* 30 M, $P = 0.423$; Negrines, 15 M *vs* 30, $P = 0.472$; Fig. 3a).

An interesting result regarding redial burden was observed when comparing infection outcomes after

Table 1 Prevalence (95% confidence interval) of *Fasciola hepatica* in resistant and susceptible *Pseudosuccinea columella* using different experimental exposure approaches

Experimental infections	Experimental groups	*Pseudosuccinea columella* populations (%)			
		La Coca (n = 30)[a]	La Palma (n = 30)[a]	Aurora (n = 30)[b]	Negrines (n = 30)[b]
Increasing infective dose: sympatric *F. hepatica*	5 M	0	0	66.7 (48.1–85.2)	63.3 (44.4–82.2)
	15 M	0	0	83.0 (66.4–92.6)	90.0 (74.4–96.5)
	30 M	0	0	93.3 (78.7–98.2)	80.0 (62.7–90.5)
Serial exposure: sympatric *F. hepatica*	3 × 5 M	0	0	90.0 (74.4–96.5)	100 (88.7–100)
Exposure to allopatric *F. hepatica*	Dominican Republic 5 M	0	0	50.0 (33.1–66.9)	66.7 (48.8–80.8)
	France 5 M	0	0	13.3 (4.2–29.9)	60.0 (40.7–76.6)

Abbreviation: *M* miracidia
[a]Resistant populations
[b]Susceptible populations

exposures to 15 miracidia, either singly (15 M) or serially-delivered (3 × 5 M; Fig. 3a): it was significantly lower in serially-exposed susceptible snails (Aurora, P = 0.0145; Negrines, P = 0.0326; Fig. 3a). Contrastingly, a similar parasite prevalence was attained with both conditions (Fisher's exact test: Aurora, P = 0.7065; Negrines, P = 0.2372).

Infection outcome in susceptible *P. columella*, comparing exposure to sympatric and allopatric *F. hepatica* isolates

Infection with a 5 M dose of either Cuban and Dominican isolates produced similar prevalence and redial burden in the two susceptible *P. columella* populations (Table 1, Fig. 3b). However, compared to the Dominican isolate, a significant decrease on snail survivorship was observed with the Cuban parasite (Fig. 2a, e; log-rank tests: $P < 0.01$).

On the other hand, we found significant differences in compatibility between susceptible *P. columella* and the French *F. hepatica* isolate and this variability depended upon the snail-parasite combination (Table 1, Fig. 3b). A poor performance of French *F. hepatica*, in terms of prevalence and redial burden, was recorded when infecting Aurora snails but it appears as compatible as the Cuban isolate with Negrines (Table 1, Fig. 3b). It is noteworthy that an overall impairment of snail survival on susceptible populations was observed with the French parasite isolate when compared with the sympatric *F. hepatica* (Fig. 2f; log-rank tests: $P < 0.001$).

Discussion

P. columella resistance to *F. hepatica* remains after high parasite doses, serial exposures and parasites from different geographical origins

Fasciola hepatica infection of its snail host is a dynamic and complex process in which several stages (i.e. snail-finding, penetration, migration, establishment and larval development) and requirements (e.g. biochemical, physiological and immunological), accounting for host-parasite compatibility, must be met to ensure

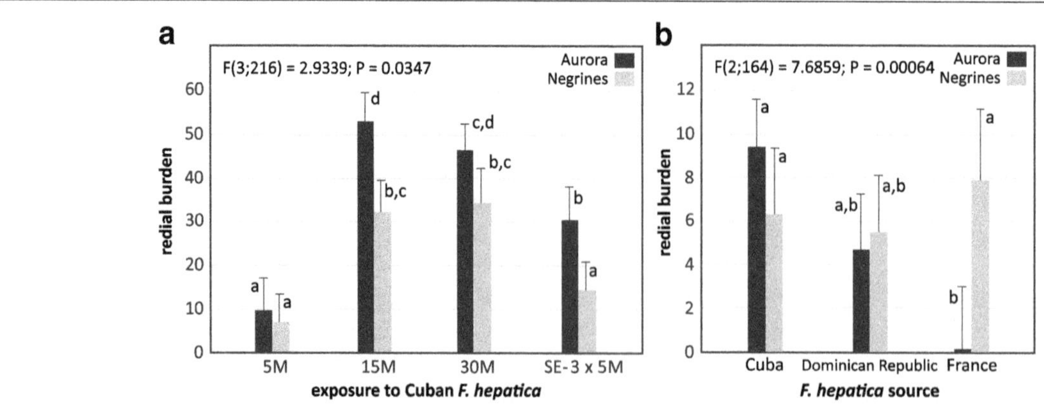

Fig. 3 Redial burden of *Fasciola hepatica* in two susceptible *Pseudosuccinea columella* populations using different experimental exposures (factorial ANOVA results). **a** Exposure to different doses of 5, 15 and 30 miracidia (M) and a serial (three times) exposure to 5 miracidia of Cuban *F. hepatica* (SE: 3 × 5 M) **b** Exposure to a dose of five miracidia of sympatric (Cuban) and allopatric *F. hepatica* isolates. Vertical bars denote 95% confidence interval and different letters show differences between means after a *post-hoc* Tukey test

parasite success [22]. In the present study, the experimental exposure of *P. columella* snails to *F. hepatica* was followed by the successful penetration of all miracidia into the snails in every trial. After this initial interaction, the first 24–48 h are crucial to the final outcome of the infection. In this time frame, a serial of fundamental events occurs inside the host: (i) complete transformation of miracidia into sporocysts [22]; (ii) migration within the digestive tract and first colonization attempts [23]; and (iii) orchestration of snail defence response, whether protective or not [12]. Either compatible *F. hepatica* larva survive and become established (the host becomes infected), or no further parasite development occurs and exposed snails are free from infection. Given the complexity of the initial interaction, it is not surprising that a peak of mortality in *P. columella* occurred during the first 24–48 h post-exposure, even in individuals from resistant populations (see Fig. 2).

As mentioned before, exposure to a large number of miracidia and/or to serial infections could differentially modify the parasite/host possibilities to infect or to be infected, most likely in favour of the parasite [17]. Our results on susceptible *P. columella* coincide with other investigations that have also rendered higher infection rates, mainly in sympatric snail-trematode combinations, after experimental infections with large numbers of parasite or serial miracidial exposures [17, 24, 25]. This strongly points at the pertinence of the first two experimental schemes used for tipping the scales in favour of parasite success. However, in this sense, the effectiveness of the resistant phenotype was not affected even after being challenged with a large number of miracidia and an enhanced genetic diversity of the parasite (either singly or serially delivered) with which each snail was confronted (*F. hepatica* isolate from La Palma isolate is known to be polymorphic [15]). Thus, host involvement in defence contributing to parasite elimination in resistant *P. columella* appears to be enough to protect the snails even from high infective doses without reversion of the resistant phenotype.

In addition, we investigated if resistant *P. columella* snails could resist other parasite isolates beyond the local (Cuban) isolates, challenging them with geographically distant *F. hepatica*, in an attempt to increase the chances of exposing the snails to parasites with different genetic diversity. Although there are no data on the genetic population structure of the allopatric *F. hepatica* isolates used, this species is known to be highly polymorphic with a preferential out-crossing reproduction [26]. Moreover, we should expect genetic differences among the isolates used given the geographical isolation, particularly between the Cuban and the European flukes. In this sense, the differences in *F. hepatica* performance between allopatric and sympatric isolates when infecting susceptible *P. columella* suggest significant differences in compatibility depending on host-parasite combination (as seen elsewhere [14]). These differences, most likely related with the assumed genetic differences, were highly marked between *F. hepatica* from Cuba and France. However, no infection developed in resistant snails exposed to either allopatric *F. hepatica* used, suggesting that the defence mechanisms involved in the resistant phenotype (protective immune response towards the parasite) might not be tightly restricted to a local genotype-genotype type interaction.

The underlying mechanism mediating the encapsulation of *F. hepatica* observed in resistant *P. columella* 24 h post-exposure [12] remains to be fully elucidated. However, mounting an efficient immune response against *F. hepatica*, or any other parasites, is expected to be costly [27] and would certainly results in trade-off against significant energy and resources of the host. However, host investment in defence might result all-too-costly for some individuals, particularly when parasites are highly pathogenic or virulent (as seen for the French *F. hepatica*-Aurora snails interaction), if the infective dose is high, or even if the regulatory mechanisms of the host response are not entirely effective. This may explain the decreased survival of resistant snails when exposed to a high miracidia dose, an effect that was also observed by Gutierrez et al. [12]. In any case, and considering both the individual and population levels, resistant *P. columella* populations failed to develop the infection.

Redial production in relation to high miracidial doses and successive exposure approaches

As for parasite prevalence, redial burden had an overall increase in susceptible snails when infected with doses higher than 5 M. However, the method of delivering the infective parasite dose influenced the parasite count (more rediae in a single 15 M dose compared to serially-exposed snails). This result could be linked to an increased ability to control parasite development on serially-exposed snails driven by boosting defences with the first exposure, a phenomenon commonly known as immune priming. Immune priming is acknowledged to occur in invertebrates and has been previously reported in the system *Biomphalaria glabrata-Schistosoma mansoni*, where enhanced protection of the host (ranging from decreased prevalence and parasite intensity to complete protection) may appear after subsequent parasite encounters [28–30]. According to these authors, the extent of such acquired protection increases towards genetically similar challenges and when re-exposure occurs 10 days after the primary infection. The demonstration of an immunological memory process in susceptible *P. columella-F. hepatica* deserves further investigations.

On the other hand, no significant variation was observed in infected snails exposed to 15 or 30 M which could be related to intraspecific competition of parasite larvae for host resources. Rondelaud et al. [31] referred that multiple miracidial infections could impact *F. hepatica* productivity in its intermediate host by limiting redial numbers on second and third generations.

Performance of allopatric *F. hepatica* with susceptible *P. columella* snails

In a previous study involving experimental infections with several Cuban *F. hepatica*-lymnaeid snail combination, Vázquez et al. [14] proposed the existence of a polymorphism of compatibility in this interaction when presented with a variety of outcomes in terms of snail survival and the parasite's prevalence and redial burden in susceptible snails. From our results, we also observed differences in compatibility between the local and allopatric *F. hepatica-P. columella* systems that varied depending on the host-parasite combinations.

In this sense, the significantly lower performance of French *F. hepatica* in susceptible *P. columella* from Cuba contrasted with what was observed with the Dominican allopatric isolate. The latter displayed a similar prevalence and redial burden to the local Cuban isolate. These results could be related with the peculiarities of the epidemiological scenario from each geographical area (Caribbean and Europe), especially concerning the differences on intermediate host species and environmental conditions. In fact, lymnaeid vectors of fasciolosis in Cuba (*Galba cubensis* and *P. columella*) are the same occurring in the Dominican Republic and in most of the Caribbean region [32, 33]. Thus, even when local adaptation of Dominican parasites to Cuban snail populations is improbable due to geographical isolation (both are separated islands), lower differences can be expected between allopatric parasites evolving under similar conditions (e.g. the same host species) and could explain the similar performances recorded between Cuban and Dominican *F. hepatica*. Conversely, *F. hepatica* transmission in France is mainly related to other snails (e.g. *Galba truncatula* and *Omphiscola glabra*) [34] which could lead to a divergent evolution of the European parasite and may explain its lower compatibility with Cuban *P. columella*. Rondelaud et al. [35] also observed differential redial development and cercarial production when parasites from Argentina and France were tested against a European *G. truncatula*. Thus, different vector species from different geographical regions could be particularly important when analysing compatibility of allopatric and sympatric *F. hepatica* isolates and might bring a deeper understanding on parasite evolution.

Conclusions

We found that resistance in *P. columella* to *F. hepatica* infection remains independent of the parasite dose, serial parasite exposures or the geographical origin of the parasite. Conversely, the *F. hepatica*-susceptible *P. columella* interaction seems specific for infection and is favoured by high parasite doses. Finally, our results endorse the potential use of resistant *P. columella* snails as an alternative for the control of parasite transmission.

Abbreviations

M: Miracidia; R: Resistant; S: Susceptible

Acknowledgements

The authors would like to thank Mercedes Vargas for kindly donating the *F. hepatica* isolate from the Dominican Republic. We would also like to thank two anonymous reviewers for making insightful comments and useful suggestions which greatly helped in improving the manuscript.

Funding

Partial financial support for this investigation was provided by the subventions granted to AA by the French Embassy in Cuba. BG was supported by ANR JCJC INVIMORY (number ANR 13-JSV7-0009) from the French National Research Agency (ANR). ES has been supported by the Tour du Valat and Labex CeMeb.

Authors' contributions

AA designed, performed and analysed the experiments and drafted the manuscript. AV, DD, SH and BG participated in design of the experiments, analysis and the reviewing process. JS, ML and ES participated in the experiments and reviewing process. HH participated in the reviewing process. All authors read and approved the final manuscript.

Competing interests

The authors declare that they have no competing interests.

Author details

[1]Centro de Investigaciones, Diagnóstico y Referencia, Instituto de Medicina Tropical "Pedro Kourí", La Habana, Cuba. [2]University of Perpignan Via Domitia, Interactions Hosts Pathogens Environments UMR 5244, CNRS, IFREMER, Univ. Montpellier, F-66860 Perpignan, France. [3]Centre de recherche de la Tour du Valat, Arles, France. [4]MIVEGEC, IRD, CNRS, Univ. Montpellier, Montpellier, France.

References

1. Mas-Coma S, Bargues MD, Valero MA. *Fasciola*, lymnaeids and human fascioliasis, with a global overview on disease transmission, epidemiology, evolutionary genetics, molecular epidemiology and control. Adv Parasitol. 2009;69:41–146.
2. Mas-Coma S. Epidemiology of fascioliasis in human endemic areas. J Helminthol. 2005;79:207–16.
3. Lounnas M, Correa AC, Vázquez AA, Dia A, Escobar JS, Nicot A, et al. Self-fertilization, long-distance flash invasion and biogeography shape the population structure of *Pseudosuccinea columella* at the worldwide scale. Mol Ecol. 2017;26:887–903.
4. Cruz-Reyes A, Malek E. Suitability of six limneaid snails for infection with *Fasciola hepatica*. Vet Parasitol. 1987;24:203–10.
5. Gutiérrez A, Vázquez AA, Hevia Y, Sánchez J, Correa AC, Hurtrez-Bouseès S, et al. First report of larval stages of *Fasciola hepatica* in a wild population of *Pseudosuccinea columella* from Cuba and the Caribbean. J Helminthol. 2011; 85:109–11.
6. Cucher M, Carnevale S, Prepelitchi L, Labbé J, Wisnivesky-Colli C. PCR diagnosis of *Fasciola hepatica* in field-collected *Lymnaea columella* and *Lymnaea viatrix* snails. Vet Parasitol. 2006;137:74–82.
7. Pointier JP, Coustau C, Rondelaud D, Theron A. *Pseudosuccinea columella* (Say 1817) (Gastropoda, Lymnaeidae), snail host of *Fasciola hepatica*: first record for France in the wild. Parasitol Res. 2007;101:1389–92.
8. Dar Y, Vignoles P, Rondelaud D, Dreyfuss G. Role of the lymnaeid snail *Pseudosuccinea columella* in the transmission of the liver fluke *Fasciola hepatica* in Egypt. J Helminthol. 2015;89:699–706.
9. Molloy JB, Anderson GR. The distribution of *Fasciola hepatica* in Queensland, Australia, and the potential impact of introduced snail intermediate hosts. Vet Parasitol. 2006;137:62–6.
10. Cowie R. Invertebrate invasions on Pacific Islands and the replacement of unique native faunas: a synthesis of the land and freshwater snails. Biol Invasions. 2001;3:119–36.
11. Pointier JP, Marquet G. Taxonomy and distribution of freshwater mollusks of French Polynesia. Jap J Malacol. 1990;48:147–60.
12. Gutiérrez A, Pointier JP, Yong M, Sánchez J, Théron A. Evidence of phenotypic differences between resistant and susceptible isolates of *Pseudosuccinea columella* (Gastropoda: Lymnaeidae) to *Fasciola hepatica* (Trematoda: Digenea) in Cuba. Parasitol Res. 2003;90:129–34.
13. Calienes AF, Fraga J, Pointier JP, Yong M, Sánchez J, Coustau C, et al. Detection and genetic distance of resistant populations of *Pseudosuccinea columella* (Mollusca: Lymnaeidae) to *Fasciola hepatica* (Trematoda: Digenea) using RAPD markers. Acta Trop. 2004;92:83–7.
14. Vázquez AA, Sánchez J, Pointier JP, Théron A, Hurtrez-Boussès S. *Fasciola hepatica* in Cuba: compatibility of different isolates with two intermediate intermediate hosts, *Galba cubensis* and *Pseudosuccinea columella*. J Helminthol. 2014;88:434–40.
15. Vázquez AA, Lounnas M, Sánchez J, Alba A, Milesi A, Hurtrez-Boussés S. Genetic and infective diversity of the common liver fluke *Fasciola hepatica* (Trematoda: Digenea) from Cuba. J Helminthol. 2016;90:719–25.
16. Jokela J, Schmid-Hempel P, Rigby MC. Dr. Pangloss restrained by the Red Queen - steps towards a unified defence theory. Oikos. 2000;89:267–74.
17. Osnas EE, Lively CM. Immune response to sympatric and allopatric parasites in a snail-trematode interaction. Front Zool. 2005;2:8.
18. Kawecki T, Ebert D. Conceptual issues in local adaptation. Ecol Lett. 2004;7: 1225–41.
19. Gasnier N, Rondelaud D, Abrous M, Carreras F, Boulard C, Diez-Baños P, et al. Allopatric combination of *Fasciola hepatica* and *Lymnaea truncatula* is more efficient than sympatric ones. Int J Parasitol. 2000;30:573–8.
20. Sánchez R, Perera G, Sánchez J. Cultivo de *Fossaria cubensis* (Pfeiffer) (Pulmonata: Lymnaeidae) hospedero intermediario de *Fasciola hepatica* (Linnaeus) en Cuba. Rev Cubana Med Trop. 1995;47:71–3.
21. Caron Y, Rondelaud D, Rosson B. The detection and quantification of a digenean infection in the snail host with emphasis in *Fasciola* sp. Parasitol Res. 2008;103:735–44.
22. Andrews SJ. The life cycle of *Fasciola hepatica*. In: Dalton JP, editor. Fasciolosis. Wallingford, UK: CAB International; 1999. p. 1–30.
23. Magalhães KC, Jannotti-Passos LK, Caldeira RL, Aires ME, Muller G, Carvalho OS, et al. Isolation and detection of *Fasciola hepatica* DNA in *Lymnaea viatrix* from formalin-fixed and paraffin-embedded tissues through multiplex-PCR. Vet Parasitol. 2008;152:333–8.
24. Théron A, Rognon A, Gourbal B, Mitta G. Multi-parasite host susceptibility and multi-host parasite infectivity: a new approach of the *Biomphalaria glabrata/Schistosoma mansoni* compatibility polymorphism. Infect Genet Evol. 2014;26:80–8.
25. Dar Y, Lounnas M, Djuikwo F, Teukeng FF, Mouzet R, Courtioux B, et al. Variations in local adaptation of allopatric *Fasciola hepatica* to French *Galba truncatula* in relation to parasite origin. Parasitol Res. 2013;112:2543–9.
26. Cwiklinsky K, Dalton JP, Dufresne PJ, La Course J, Williams DJL, Hodgkinson J, et al. The *Fasciola hepatica* genome: gene duplication and polymorphism reveals adaptation to the host environment and the capacity for rapid evolution. Genome Biol. 2015;16:71.
27. Carton Y, Nappi AJ, Poirie M. Genetics of anti-parasite resistance in invertebrates. Dev Comp Immunol. 2005;29:9–32.
28. Sire C, Rognon A, Theron A. Failure of *Schistosoma mansoni* to reinfect *Biomphalaria glabrata* snails: acquired humoral resistance or intra-specific larval antagonism? Parasitology. 1998;117:117–22.
29. Portela J, Duval D, Rognon A, Galinier R, Boissier J, Coustau C, et al. Evidence for specific genotype-dependent immune priming in the lophotrochozoan *Biomphalaria glabrata* snail. J Innate Immunol. 2013;5:261–76.
30. Pinaud S, Portela J, Duval D, Nowacki FC, Olive MA, Allienne JF, et al. A shift from cellular to humoral responses contributes to innate immune memory in the vector snail *Biomphalaria glabrata*. PLoS Pathog. 2016;12:e1005361.
31. Rondelaud D, Belfaiza M, Vignoles P, Moncef M, Dreyfuss G. Redial generations of *Fasciola hepatica*: a review. J Helminthol. 2009;83:245–54.
32. Gomez JD, Vargas M, Malek EA. Freshwater mollusks of the Dominican Republic. Nautilus. 1986;100:130–4.
33. Vázquez AA, Hevia Y, Sánchez J. Distribución y preferencia de hábitats de moluscos hospederos intermediarios de *Fasciola hepatica* en Cuba. Rev Cubana Med Trop. 2009;61:248–53.
34. Correa AC, De Meeûs T, Dreyfuss G, Rondelaud D, Hurtrez-Boussès S. *Galba truncatula* and *Fasciola hepatica*: Genetic costructures and interactions with intermediate host dispersal. Infect Genet Evol. 2017;55:186–94.
35. Rondelaud D, Sanabria R, Vignoles P, Dreyfuss G, Romero J. *Fasciola hepatica*: variations in redial development and cercarial production in relation to the geographic origin of the parasite. Parasite. 2013;20:33.

16

Seasonal dynamics of canine antibody response to *Phlebotomus perniciosus* saliva in an endemic area of *Leishmania infantum*

Rita Velez[1,2*], Tatiana Spitzova[3], Ester Domenech[4], Laura Willen[3], Jordi Cairó[4], Petr Volf[3] and Montserrat Gállego[1,2*]

Abstract

Background: Canine leishmaniosis (CanL) is an important zoonotic parasitic disease, endemic in the Mediterranean basin. In this region, transmission of *Leishmania infantum*, the etiological agent of CanL, is through the bite of phlebotomine sand flies. Therefore, monitoring host-vector contact represents an important epidemiological tool, and could be used to assess the effectiveness of vector-control programmes in endemic areas. Previous studies have shown that canine antibodies against the saliva of phlebotomine sand flies are specific markers of exposure to *Leishmania* vectors. However, this method needs to be further validated in natural heterogeneous dog populations living in CanL endemic areas.

Methods: In this study, 176 dogs living in 12 different locations of an *L. infantum* endemic area in north-east Spain were followed for 14 months. Blood samples were taken at 5 pre-determined time points (February, August and October 2016; January and April 2017) to assess the canine humoral immune response to whole salivary gland homogenate (SGH) and to the single salivary 43 kDa yellow-related recombinant protein (rSP03B) of *Phlebotomus perniciosus*, a proven vector of *L. infantum* naturally present in this region. Simultaneously, in all dogs, *L. infantum* infection status was assessed by serology. The relationship between anti-SGH and anti-rSP03B antibodies with the sampling month, *L. infantum* infection and the location was tested by fitting multilevel linear regression models.

Results: The dynamics of canine anti-saliva IgG for both SGH and rSP03B followed the expected trends of *P. perniciosus* activity in the region. Statistically significant associations were detected for both salivary antigens between vector exposure and sampling month or dog seropositivity to *L. infantum*. The correlation between canine antibodies against SGH and rSP03B was moderate.

Conclusions: Our results confirm the frequent presence of CanL vectors in the study area in Spain and support the applicability of SGH- and rSP03B-based ELISA tests to study canine exposure to *P. perniciosus* in *L. infantum* endemic areas.

Keywords: Canine leishmaniosis, *Phlebotomus perniciosus*, Saliva proteins, Markers of exposure, Longitudinal study, North-east Spain

Background

Leishmania infantum (Kinetoplastida: Trypanosomatidae) is the causative agent of canine leishmaniosis (CanL), a zoonotic vector-transmitted disease widespread in the Mediterranean region, as well as in other parts of the world [1–3]. Prevalence of *L. infantum* infection in canine populations from endemic areas is highly heterogeneous [4], and not all infected dogs will ever develop clinical signs of the disease [5]. However, infected asymptomatic dogs could act as a reservoir of the parasite and are capable of transmitting *L. infantum* to other dogs, as well as to humans [6, 7].

The transmission of the parasite is mainly vectorial, through the bite of phlebotomine sand flies. In the Mediterranean basin, eight species of the genus *Phlebotomus* have been implicated as vectors of *L. infantum*, according to conventional criteria. From these, all except one belong to the subgenus *Larroussius* [8]. In Spain, CanL transmission is mainly shared by *P.* (*L.*) *perniciosus* and *P.* (*L.*)

* Correspondence: rita.velez@isglobal.org; mgallego@ub.edu
[1]ISGlobal, Hospital Clínic - Universitat de Barcelona, Barcelona, Spain
Full list of author information is available at the end of the article

ariasi [9, 10], with the second species having a narrower distribution but being responsible for maintaining the infection at higher altitudes [11, 12]. Recently, *L. infantum* DNA was also found in another *Larroussius* species, *P. langeroni*, in the south of the country [13].

The detection of anti-sand fly salivary antibodies in the blood of vertebrate hosts has proven to be highly specific [14] and was successfully used as a marker of exposure to *L. infantum* vectors [15, 16]. In CanL endemic areas, monitoring the canine IgG response to sand fly saliva can be a useful epidemiological tool [15, 17], complementing studies of vector population dynamics and host-vector interactions, as well as enabling the assessment of risk of *Leishmania* infection [14, 18, 19]. Furthermore, it can be used to measure the effectiveness of vector-control programmes and to assist in the design of better control strategies for the disease [20, 21].

Originally, sand fly whole salivary gland homogenates (SGH) were used to investigate the presence of anti-sand fly saliva antibodies in vertebrate hosts [20–22]. However, its use in large-scale studies is impaired by technical limitations [23]. Additionally, the use of SGH in vector exposure tests may reduce the specificity of detection due to a possible cross-reactivity with saliva of sympatric and closely related sand fly species [24].

An alternative to the use of SGH is the identification of species-specific salivary proteins that can be expressed in recombinant forms and produced in large quantities for use in large-scale epidemiological studies [25, 26]. Recent studies identified *P. perniciosus* yellow-related protein rSP03B as the most promising candidate to replace SGH in the detection of host markers of exposure to this vector species [16, 17, 26]. This recombinant protein has been tested and validated in dogs and other animals in cross-sectional studies [16, 26], as well as in a canine longitudinal study [17], but no information exists on the seasonal dynamics of either SGH or rSP03B in natural heterogeneous dog populations from endemic areas.

Therefore, the objectives of this study were (i) to investigate the dynamics of *P. perniciosus* and their relative density in a previously uncharacterized CanL endemic area through the detection of anti-saliva IgG in dogs; and (ii) to evaluate the performance of both SGH and rSP03B antigens as markers of exposure to *P. perniciosus* in natural canine populations.

Results

Seasonal dynamics of IgG response against salivary proteins from *P. perniciosus*

Median values of normalized ELISA OD values for SGH ranged from 9.04 (range: 3.94–66.23) in January 2017 to 18.51 (7.93–100.58) in August 2016 (Table 1). For rSP03B, median OD values varied between 12.21 (6.75–53.71) and 19.53 (10.64–124.01) in January 2017 and August 2016, respectively. With both antigens, median OD readings raised from basal values in February 2016 (10.11 and 14.67 for SGH and rSP03B, respectively) to peak in August (18.51 and 19.53 for SGH and rSP03B, respectively), sustained higher readings in October (11.15 and 15.31 for SGH and rSP03B, respectively), and descended again to basal levels in January (9.04 and 12.21 for SGH and rSP03B, respectively) and April 2017 (9.54 and 13.44 for SGH and rSP03B, respectively). Median normalized ELISA OD results obtained per month for both SGH and rSP03B are described in Table 1 and plotted in Fig. 1.

Table 1 Median values of normalized OD readings for SGH and rSP03B obtained per sampling month in all locations

Variable	*N*	SGH Median (Range)	rSP03B Median (Range)
February 2016	174	10.11 (5.49–49.62)	14.67 (7.36–41.24)
August 2016	33	18.51 (7.93–100.58)	19.53 (10.64–124.01)
October 2016	164	11.15 (5.56–86.44)	15.31 (6.15–112.54)
January 2017	154	9.04 (3.94–66.23)	12.21 (6.75–53.71)
April 2017	148	9.54 (5.25–62.59)	13.44 (6.27–36.22)

Abbreviation: *N* number of dogs sampled per sampling month

Cut-off values were set at 13 for SGH and 22 for rSP03B. When these were applied to the OD readings obtained in August 2016, 75.76% (25/33) of the dogs were positive to anti-SGH IgG, and 36.36% (12/33) to anti-rSP03B antibodies. In October, these values dropped to 35.98% (59/164) for SGH and 18.9% (31/164) for rSP03B. During the non-transmission season (considered to extend from

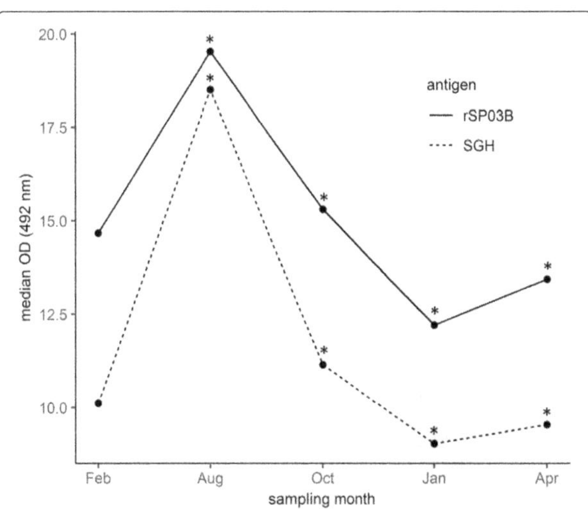

Fig. 1 Dynamics of anti-*P. perniciosus* salivary proteins IgG response in dogs from an endemic area during a sand fly activity season. Values presented refer to the normalized OD medians obtained at each sampling month for all dogs and locations. Statistically significant differences in median OD between two consecutive months are marked with an asterisk ($P < 0.05$)

November to May), the percentage of seropositive dogs ranged from 14.29% (25/175) in February 2016 to 17.57% (26/148) in April 2017 for SGH and 8.44% (13/154) in January 2017 to 12.16% (18/148) in April 2017 for rSP03B.

Correlation results for IgG response between SGH and rSP03B were r_S = 0.54 (95% CI: 0.48–0.60, P < 0.001) (Fig. 2).

Dogs' exposure to *P. perniciosus* in the study area

Exposure of dogs to phlebotomine vectors showed some variation according to the location. Median OD readings varied from 9.11 (range: 5.25–20.57) to 14.14 (7.44–55.45) for SGH ELISA and from 12.71 (7.53–64.44) to 17.87 (8.39–112.54) for rSP03B. Minimum median values of response to both SGH and rSP03B corresponded to the same location (Aiguaviva), but maximum median values were registered in different sites for each antigen (Sant Feliu de Guíxols for SGH and Montagut for rSP03B) (Table 2). Figure 3 presents the dynamics of dogs' IgG response to SGH (Fig. 3a) and rSP03B (Fig. 3b) in each locality.

The percentage of anti-sand fly saliva seropositive dogs per location, defined as the number of dogs that showed a positive IgG titre at least once during the study period, ranged from 13.33% (1/8) in Ordis to 100% in Canet d'Adri (8/8) and Sant Feliu de Guíxols (4/4) for SGH, and from 8.16% (1/12) in Hostalnou de Bianya to 100% (4/4) in Sant Feliu de Guíxols for rSP03B. Total anti-sand fly saliva seropositivity calculated for the study area was 49.43% (87/176) for anti-SGH IgG and 28.98% (51/176) for anti-rSP03B antibodies.

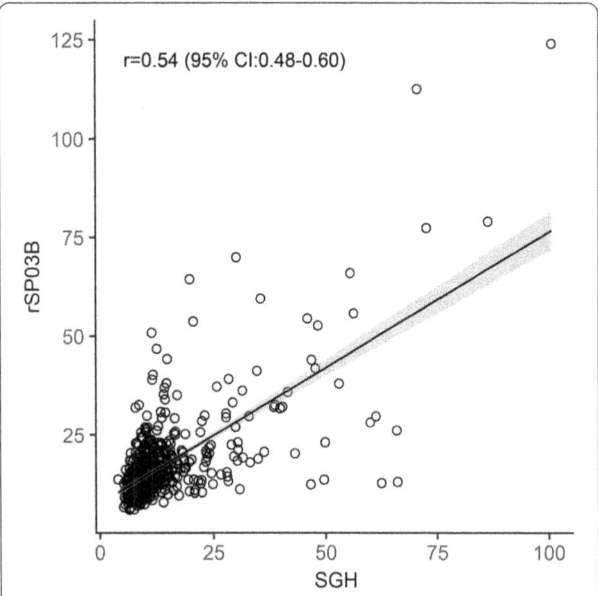

Fig. 2 Correlation between IgG recognizing SGH and rSP03B protein in dogs naturally exposed to *P. perniciosus*. Results from both SGH and rSP03B are presented in normalized OD (r_S = 0.54; 95% CI: 0.48–0.60, P < 0.001)

Dogs' exposure to *P. perniciosus* and *L. infantum* infection

Correlation results between antibody response to *P. perniciosus* saliva and *L. infantum* were low both for SGH (r_S = 0.27, 95% CI: 0.19–0.35, P < 0.001) and rSP03B protein (r_S = 0.25, 95% CI: 0.18–0.32, P < 0.001).

Multilevel analysis of the relationship between anti-*P. perniciosus* salivary proteins, month and location and *L. infantum* seropositivity

The multilevel model results confirmed the annual dynamics of anti-salivary proteins IgG responses. When compared to the first sampling month (February 2016), IgG responses to SGH significantly rose in August (t = 8.55, df = 491, P < 0.001) and October (t = 6.49, df = 491, P < 0.001) and dropped in January (t = -2.49, df = 491, P = 0.013) and April 2017 (no significant difference when compared to February 2016). As expected, the highest log OD estimate was observed in August 2016 and the lowest in January 2017 (Table 3). The same trend was observed in the model run for the rSP03B protein, with comparable levels of significance (Table 4). There were no significant differences in IgG responses for both antigens between each sampling location and the one set as reference, except for Montagut, where significantly higher OD levels were observed for SGH (t = 2.28, df = 166, P = 0.024) and rSP03B (t = 2.13, df = 164, P = 0.035). According to the multilevel model, seropositivity to *L. infantum* proved to be associated with a rise in anti-salivary proteins OD values for both SGH (t = 2.5, df = 491, P = 0.013) and rSP03B (t = 2.15, df = 493, P = 0.032).

Discussion

The quantification of anti-sand fly saliva antibodies in vertebrate hosts of *L. infantum* has been previously shown to be an effective way of measuring exposure to the parasite vectors [16]. In the case of dogs, the most frequent host and reservoir of *L. infantum*, this has been proven for *P. perniciosus* [15, 26], as well as for other sand fly species [27–29]. These markers of exposure can then be applied in host-vector epidemiological studies, in *L. infantum* infection risk assessment, and to assist in the design of control strategies for the disease. Therefore, it is important to validate these techniques in natural, heterogeneous populations from endemic areas, in which a higher individual variability is expected.

Phlebotomus perniciosus activity period in Spain shows two main peaks, the first in June-July and the second in September-October. These peaks also correspond to the periods of highest *L. infantum* transmission [30–32]. This trend was identified in our study and corresponds to the rise in anti-saliva antibody levels observed between

Table 2 Median values of normalized OD readings for SGH and rSP03B obtained per sampling location at all time points

Variable	*n* (Range)	Geographical coordinates	SGH Median (Range)	rSP03B Median (Range)
Ordis	8 (7–9)	42°13'37.7"N, 2°54'24.1E	9.14 (6.45–45.95)	15.16 (8.35–54.50)
Madremanya	14 (12–15)	41°58'47.0"N, 2°58'7.2"E	11.22 (6.79–49.84)	14.49 (8.95–43.99)
Vidreres	8 (7–9)	41°47'27.4"N, 2°45'0.4"E	10.59 (7.80–16.86)	13.46 (8.58–40.23)
Massanes	21 (20–23)	41°45'15.3"N, 2°38'44.0"E	9.31 (5.67–62.59)	16.35 (7.82–55.81)
Hostalnou de Bianya	12 (11–14)	42°13'26.0"N, 2°26'9.7"E	8.75 (5.35–33.16)	13.19 (6.27–46.82)
Montagut	13 (7–15)	42°14'7.7"N, 2°35'57.6"E	12.01 (3.94–72.61)	17.87 (8.39–112.54)
St. Esteve de Llémena	9 (9–10)	42°3'35.1"N, 2°37'1.4"E	9.49 (6.23–22.40)	14.18 (9.12–22.46)
Canet d'Adri	8 (4–10)	42°1'53.7"N, 2°44'15.3"E	10.61 (6.52–100.58)	14.03 (7.36–124.01)
Aiguaviva	19 (16–22)	41°54'27.2"N, 2°46'19.0"E	9.11 (5.25–20.57)	12.71 (7.53–64.44)
St. Feliu de Guíxols	4	41°47'2.3"N, 2°59'58.7"E	14.14 (7.44–55.45)	16.73 (8.57–65.97)
Riells i Viabrea	20 (18–21)	41°43'59"N, 2°33'39.3"E	10.02 (6.07–66.23)	13.43 (8.59–35.31)
Vilobí d'Onyar	23 (22–23)	41°53'3.2"N, 2°43'38.6"E	9.13 (5.17–16.49)	13.05 (6.15–38.07)

Abbreviation: *n* mean number of dogs sampled in each location

August and October. Humoral immune response to *P. perniciosus* saliva elicited in experimentally bitten dogs showed that antibody levels significantly rose after 2–4 weeks of continued exposure, peaking in week 5 [15]. In our field study, the highest IgG levels were in August, which clearly corresponded to the June-July *P. perniciosus* expected activity peak. Similarly, the high IgG readings obtained in October are likely to correspond to *P. perniciosus* second peak of activity. The lower rise in antibody levels observed at this time point can be explained by an earlier sampling at the beginning of October, which may have hindered the display of a complete seroconversion. The high overall levels of seropositivity to anti-sand fly saliva antigens, especially for SGH (49.43%), strongly support the CanL endemicity status for the region [33]. These results also validate both SGH and rSP03B as suitable antigens to assess exposure to *P. perniciosus* in natural canine populations from endemic areas.

An important remark when analysing the longitudinal dynamics of anti-sand fly saliva IgG in the study dog

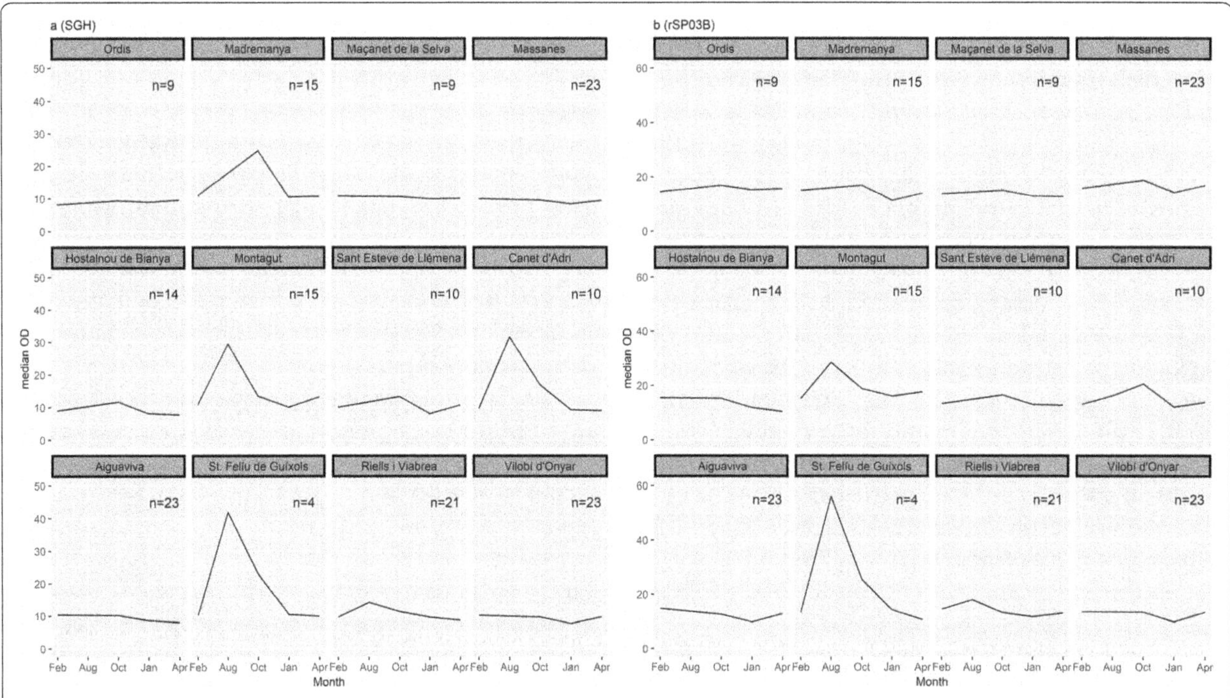

Fig. 3 Dynamics of dogs' IgG recognizing SGH (**a**) and rSP03B protein (**b**) in the different sampling locations during a sand fly activity season. Values presented refer to the normalized OD medians obtained at each sampling month

Table 3 Estimates of the multilevel linear regression model of the relationship between log transformed normalized SGH OD values and sampling time, location and dog seropositivity to *L. infantum*. "Dog" was included as a random effects variable

Variable	Levels	Estimate	SE	*P*-value[a]
Intercept		2.40	0.06	<0.001
Sampling month	February 2016	Ref	–	–
	August 2016	0.54	0.06	<0.001
	October 2016	0.20	0.03	<0.001
	January 2017	-0.06	0.03	0.013
	April 2017	-0.01	0.03	0.666
Location	Aiguaviva	Ref	–	–
	Ordis	0.07	0.11	0.562
	Madremanya	0.08	0.10	0.427
	Vidreres	0.10	0.11	0.393
	Massanes	0.07	0.09	0.441
	Hostalnou de Bianya	-0.08	0.10	0.404
	Montagut	0.22	0.10	0.024
	St. Esteve de Llémena	-0.03	0.11	0.786
	Canet d'Adri	-0.02	0.11	0.891
	St. Feliu de Guíxols	0.16	0.15	0.308
	Riells i Viabrea	0.03	0.09	0.703
	Vilobí d'Onyar	-0.02	0.09	0.791
L. infantum seropositivity	Seronegative	Ref	–	–
	Seropositive	0.10	0.04	0.013

Abbreviation: *SE* standard error
[a]Level of significance of *P*-value < 0.05 was used

Table 4 Estimates of the multilevel linear regression model of the relationship between log transformed normalized rSP03B OD values and sampling time, location and dog seropositivity to *L. infantum*. "Dog" was included as a random effects variable

Variable	Levels	Estimate	SE	*P*-value[a]
Intercept		2.79	0.06	<0.001
Sampling month	February 2016	Ref	–	–
	August 2016	0.39	0.06	<0.001
	October 2016	0.09	0.03	0.003
	January 2017	-0.13	0.03	<0.001
	April 2017	-0.06	0.03	0.016
Location	Aiguaviva	Ref	–	–
	Ordis	0.06	0.10	0.563
	Madremanya	-0.04	0.09	0.652
	Vidreres	-0.03	0.10	0.783
	Massanes	0.05	0.08	0.533
	Hostalnou de Bianya	-0.16	0.09	0.074
	Montagut	0.18	0.09	0.035
	St. Esteve de Llémena	-0.10	0.10	0.287
	Canet d'Adri	-0.05	0.10	0.641
	St. Feliu de Guíxols	-0.19	0.14	0.173
	Riells i Viabrea	-0.08	0.08	0.302
	Vilobí d'Onyar	-0.06	0.08	0.399
L. infantum seropositivity	Seronegative	Ref	–	–
	Seropositive	0.07	0.03	0.032

Abbreviation: *SE* standard error
[a]Level of significance of *P*-value < 0.05 was used

population is that there was a clear basal antibody level before the transmission season. After the expected rise in humoral response during summer months, IgG levels returned again to basal levels. These results show that, though exposed to repetitive bites during several months, dogs from endemic areas do not sustain high anti-saliva IgG levels throughout the year, allowing the detection of recent exposure to sand flies in natural populations. Similar results were recently reported in a longitudinal field study in Brazil, where canine IgG against *Lutzomyia longipalpis* saliva were evaluated [34]. Our study identified the same trends for both SGH and rSP03B, which reinforces the suitability of recombinant antigens in detecting recent exposure to phlebotomine vectors in endemic settings, particularly when considering the use of these tests in large-scale studies for vector control interventions [35, 36].

Antibodies recognizing both SGH and rSP03B followed similar dynamics throughout the field study. However, the correlation between the two antigens was only moderate ($r_S = 0.54$; 95% CI: 0.48–0.60, $P < 0.001$). Even so, available studies show that rSP03B is the most promising surrogate for SGH as a marker of exposure to *P. perniciosus* in the canine host. It has presented high levels of correlation with SGH in both experimentally [25] and naturally bitten dogs [16, 17, 26]. Two apyrase proteins (rSP01B and rSP01) have also shown a good correlation with SGH [25]. However, in a study where these three recombinant proteins presented similarly high correlations with SGH, rSP03B presented the lowest data dispersion and was considered a better option [16]. These results were confirmed in a field trial, where single rSP03B demonstrated a higher correlation coefficient with SGH than the combination of rSP03B with rSP01 [17].

A similar correlation between SGH and rSP03B to the one obtained in the present study has been observed before in Umbria region (central Italy) ($r_S = 0.56$; 95% CI: 0.38–0.71, $P < 0.001$; $n = 96$), in a screening study of dog exposure to *P. perniciosus* across European CanL endemic foci [26]. A possible reason for these discordant results may be the presence of other closely related phlebotomine species which could induce cross-reactivity with the SGH [22]. In some parts of Catalonia, *P. perniciosus* is sympatric with *P. ariasi*, also a proven vector of *L. infantum* [10]. Due to the close relationship between *P. perniciosus* and *P. ariasi*, both belonging to the subgenus *Larroussius*, it is expected that they share similar salivary antigens [37]. When comparing the percentage of seropositive dogs detected by both methods during the study, results for SGH are higher (49.43%) than for rSP03B (28.98%). Also, median results per sampling location show differences between SGH and rSP03B: in some cases, the trend between antigens is very similar (e.g. sera from Sant Feliu de Guíxols); in other cases, there is a recognizable peak in anti-SGH IgG, while anti-rSP03B IgG shows no change (e.g. sera from Madremanya). These differences can also be observed over time in the same location, with humoral responses to SGH and rSP03B peaking in different months along the transmission season (e.g. Canet d'Adri). We may hypothesize that SGH, because it contains more proteins than the single-antigen rSP03B, will more likely cross-react with antibodies against *P. ariasi*, inducing a stronger unspecific reaction to this vector species. It would also mean that the prevalence of sand fly species responsible for *L. infantum* transmission in the province varies according to the location, and possibly in the same location throughout the transmission season, for which it would be interesting to perform further entomological studies in the region.

Correlation indexes between levels of antibodies against both salivary antigens and *L. infantum* infection were low [SGH: $r_S = 0.27$ (95% CI: 0.19–0.35, $P < 0.001$); rSP03B: $r_S = 0.25$ (95% CI: 0.18–0.32, $P < 0.001$)]. Similar low correlations have been described before between sand fly bites and human visceral leishmaniasis (VL), while stronger correlations are reported between human cutaneous leishmaniasis (CL) and recent vector exposure (reviewed in [23]). This can be explained by VL's longer incubation period and/or the differences in host immune responses to cutaneous and visceral infection [38]. Results from some studies in human populations also suggest that the repeated contact with non-infected sand flies could be correlated with markers of protection for VL [39]. Partial protection against *L. major*, an agent of CL, has also been achieved in immunized mice by the bites of uninfected sand flies [40]. However, another study with BALB/c mice demonstrated that this type of immunity is limited to short-term exposure and questioned the efficacy of sand fly saliva-induced protection against *Leishmania* infection in CL endemic areas [41]. CanL follows a pattern which is more similar to VL than to CL, therefore a low correlation between humoral responses to sand fly saliva and *Leishmania* would be expected [15]. However, results of the multilevel linear regression model show a positive and statistically significant relationship between *P. perniciosus* bites and a seropositive status for *L. infantum*, both for SGH and rSP03B. Similar results have been described in other longitudinal field studies on both canine anti-*P. perniciosus* and anti-*L. longipalpis* IgG dynamics [17, 34]. Unlike cross-sectional surveys, longitudinal studies are able to detect the relationship between a higher number of sand fly bites at a given time point and a subsequent *L. infantum* infection. Therefore, this type of study is likely to better explain the relationship between these two events, which can take place several months apart.

Conclusions

The results of this study confirmed the applicability of both anti-*P. perniciosus* SGH and rSP03B IgG as markers of exposure to *L. infantum* vectors in natural dog populations from an endemic area. Canine humoral response to both antigens is compatible with the annual sand fly activity dynamics expected for the region. Significantly lower IgG levels were observed during the non-transmission season; despite the repeated exposure to sand flies during the summer months, there is a return to basal IgG levels in these dog populations during the winter. The comparative performance of SGH and rSP03B showed a moderate correlation, which might be explained by the occurrence of cross-reactions of SGH with other closely related sympatric sand flies. Further longitudinal studies in natural canine populations from endemic areas, together with entomological studies, should be carried out in order to corroborate this hypothesis. Nevertheless, both antigens are expected to detect only vectors of *L. infantum*, confirming their suitability for host-vector-parasite studies. Finally, the overall results support the CanL endemicity status for the study region, which had already been suggested by previous studies [33].

Methods

Experimental design

The study included a heterogeneous population of 176 dogs distributed by 12 locations in Girona Province (Catalonia, northeast of Spain), an area endemic for CanL [33]. These dogs were enrolled in a canine leishmaniosis vaccine field trial, but no statistically significant differences in *L. infantum* infection between groups were observed either during or at the end of the trial. These were all owned dogs, used mainly for hunting, but some breeding and racing individuals were also included. All animals were kept in large packs in open-air facilities, mostly in rural and periurban areas. Furthermore, no specific anti-sand fly insecticide treatments were applied, providing conditions for dog exposure to the vector. Dog density per study location varied between 4–23. The dogs were followed from February 2016 to April 2017 and blood samples, obtained by venepuncture and placed in 5 ml EDTA tubes, were collected at 5 pre-determined time points (Table 1). Plasma was obtained and stored at -40 °C until processing.

Sand flies and salivary proteins

A colony of *P. perniciosus* was reared under standard conditions as described previously [42]. Salivary glands were dissected from 4–6 day-old females, pooled at a concentration of 1 salivary gland per 1 µl of 20 mM Tris buffer with 150 mM NaCl and stored at -80 °C. The *P. perniciosus* 43 kDa yellow-related recombinant protein (rSP03B, Genbank accn. DQ150622) was obtained from Apronex s.r.o. (Prague, Czech Republic) and quantified by the Lowry method (Bio-Rad, Hercules, California, USA) following the manufacturer's protocol.

Serological detection of dog exposure to sand flies

Anti-*P. perniciosus* IgG was measured by an in-house enzyme-linked immunosorbent assay (ELISA) as described previously [17]. All samples from a single dog were processed in the same plate. Briefly, microtiter plates were coated either with salivary gland homogenate (SGH) (40 ng per well, equivalent to 0.2 salivary gland) or with rSP03B (5 µg/ml) in 20 mM carbonate-bicarbonate buffer (pH 9.5) and incubated overnight at 4 °C. Plates were then blocked with 6% (w/v) low fat dry milk in PBS with 0.05% Tween 20 (PBS-Tw). Canine plasma were diluted 1:200 for SGH and 1:100 for rSP03B in 2% (w/v) low fat dry milk/PBS-Tw. Secondary antibodies (anti-dog IgG, Bethyl laboratories) were diluted 1:9000 in PBS-Tw. The reaction was stopped with 10% H_2SO_4 and absorbance was measured at 492 nm using a Tecan Infinite M200 microplate reader (Tecan, Männedorf, Switzerland). Each sample was tested in duplicate and positive and negative controls were included in each plate. To account for the variability between plates, sample OD readings were normalized by dividing them by the mean OD of positive controls run in the same plate [43]. The normalized OD values were multiplied by 100. Positivity cut-offs were calculated as the mean plus 3 standard deviations from 14 dog samples from a non-endemic area.

Serological detection of *L. infantum* infection

All samples were tested for the presence of IgG against *L. infantum* through an in-house enzyme-linked immunosorbent assay (ELISA), using a technique described previously [44, 45]. Again, serial samples from a single dog were tested in parallel on the same plate. Briefly, dog plasma samples diluted at 1:400 were incubated in titration plates (Costar® Corning®, New York, USA) previously coated with sonicated whole promastigotes at a protein concentration of 20 µg/ml in 0.05 M carbonate buffer at pH 9.6. Protein A peroxidase (1:30,000, Sigma-Aldrich®, St. Louis, Missouri, USA) was used as conjugate and reactions were stopped with H_2SO_4 3M when a pre-determined calibrator control serum reached an optical density of 450 at 450 nm. Sample optical densities were read at 492 nm. All samples were run in duplicate and the calibrator, positive and negative sera were included in all plates. Results were expressed in standard units (U) compared to a calibrator control sample set arbitrarily at 100U. The positivity cut-off was established at 24U.

Statistical analysis

Statistical analyses were performed using R software (http://cran.r-project.org/) and Stata 15 software (StataCorp LP, College Station, TX, USA).

Correlations between IgG responses to *P. perniciosus* SGH and rSP03B and between each one of the salivary antigens and anti-*L. infantum* IgG levels were tested by the Spearman rank correlation test. Median OD values between time points were compared using the Wilcoxon signed rank sum test.

The relationship between anti-SGH and anti-rSP03B antibodies and sampling month, *L. infantum* infection status and location was tested by fitting multilevel linear regression models, taking into account the correlation between repeated measures of the same dogs over time. In the models, log-transformed anti-saliva or rSP03B normalized OD values were considered as continuous dependent variables and sampling month, *L. infantum* infection and location as categorical predictor variables. In order to assess variations in OD between the first sampling month and those following, "February 2016" was set as reference level for this variable. Likewise, the locality with the lowest median OD ("Aiguaviva") was considered to be the reference for the variable location. Finally, "seronegative" was set as the reference level for the variable *L. infantum* infection. The random component included dog and time to allow for variation at the intercept (between dogs) and the slope (over time). The inclusion of "dog" as a random effects variable significantly improved both models, with a between dog variance of 48% for SGH and of 47% for the rSP03B model. A *P*-value of < 0.05 was considered to indicate statistical significance.

Abbreviations

CanL: Canine leishmaniosis; CL: Human cutaneous leishmaniasis; ELISA: Enzyme-linked immunosorbent assay; IgG: Immunoglobulin G; OD: Optical density; rSP03B: 43 kDa yellow-related recombinant protein; SGH: Salivary gland homogenate; VL: Human visceral leishmaniasis

Acknowledgements

We thank all dog owners, for providing us access to their dogs. We also thank the reviewers for their helpful suggestions and comments, and Trelawny Bond-Taylor for language revision and editing of the final manuscript.

Funding
This project received funding from the European Union's Horizon 2020 research and innovation programme under Marie Sklodowska-Curie grant agreement n° 642609. The study was also partially supported by ERD Funds, project CePaViP (CZ.02.1.01/0.0/0.0/16_019/0000759), Research Centre UNCE (project 204072), Departament d'Universitats, Recerca i Societat de la Informació de la Generalitat de Catalunya (grant 2014SGR026), Plan Nacional de I+D+i and Instituto de Salud Carlos III, Subdirección General de Redes y Centros de Investigación Cooperativa, Ministerio de Economía y Competividad, Spanish Network for Research in Infectious Diseases (grant REIPI RD12/0015); co-financed by European Development Regional Fund (ERDF) "A way to achieve Europe". MG belongs to RICET, a Tropical Disease Cooperative Research Network in Spain (grant RD12/0018/0010). ISGlobal is a member of the CERCA Programme, Generalitat de Catalunya. The supporters had no role in study design, data collection and analysis, decision to publish, or preparation of the manuscript.

Authors' contributions
RV, LW, JC, PV and MG designed the study; RV, ED and MG performed the fieldwork; RV, TS and LW performed the lab work; TS and RV analysed and interpreted the data; RV and MG wrote the manuscript. All authors read and approved the final manuscript.

Competing interests
The authors declare that they have no competing interests.

Author details
[1]ISGlobal, Hospital Clínic - Universitat de Barcelona, Barcelona, Spain. [2]Secció de Parasitologia, Departament de Biologia, Sanitat i Medi Ambient, Facultat de Farmàcia i Ciències de l'Alimentació, Universitat de Barcelona, Barcelona, Spain. [3]Department of Parasitology, Faculty of Science, Charles University, Prague, Czech Republic. [4]Hospital Veterinari Canis, Girona, Spain.

References
1. WHO Expert Committee on the Control of the Leishmaniases & World Health Organization. Control of the leishmaniases: report of a meeting of the WHO Expert Commitee on the Control of Leishmaniases, Geneva, 22-26 March 2010. Geneva: World Health Organization. http://www.who.int/iris/handle/10665/44412. Accessed 15 Mar 2018
2. Dantas-Torres F. Canine leishmaniosis in South America. Parasit Vectors. 2009;2(Suppl. 1):S1.
3. Gállego M. Zoonosis emergentes por patógenos parásitos: las leishmaniosis. Rev Sci Tech. (OIE). 2004;23:661–76.
4. Franco AO, Davies CR, Mylne A, Dedet J-P, Gállego M, Ballart C, et al. Predicting the distribution of canine leishmaniasis in western Europe based on environmental variables. Parasitology. 2011;138:1878–91.
5. Baneth G, Koutinas AF, Solano-Gallego L, Bourdeau P, Ferrer L. Canine leishmaniosis - new concepts and insights on an expanding zoonosis: Part one. Trends Parasitol. 2008;24:325–30.
6. Borja LS, de Sousa OMF, Solcà MDS, Bastos LA, Bordoni M, Magalhães JT, et al. Parasite load in the blood and skin of dogs naturally infected by *Leishmania infantum* is correlated with their capacity to infect sand fly vectors. Vet Parasitol. 2016;229:110–7.
7. Molina R, Amela C, Nieto J, San-Andrés M, González F, Castillo JA, et al. Infectivity of dogs naturally infected with *Leishmania infantum* to colonized *Phlebotomus perniciosus*. Trans R Soc Trop Med Hyg. 1994;88:491–3.
8. Alten B, Maia C, Afonso MO, Campino L, Jiménez M, González E, et al. Seasonal dynamics of phlebotomine sand fly species proven vectors of Mediterranean leishmaniasis caused by *Leishmania infantum*. PLoS Negl Trop Dis. 2016;10:e0004458.
9. Rioux JA, Guilvard E, Gállego J, Moreno G, Pratlong F, Portús M, et al. Intervention simultanée de *Phlebotomus ariasi* Tonnoir, 1921 et *P. perniciosus* Newstead, 1911 dans un même foyer. Infestations par deux zymodemes syntopiques. A propos d'une enquête en Catalogne (Espagne). In: Leishmania: Taxonomie et Phylogenèse Applications Éco-épidémiologiques. Montpellier: IMEEE; 1986. p. 439–44.
10. Guilvard E, Gállego M, Moreno G, Fisa R, Rispail P, Pratlong F, et al. Infestation naturelle de *Phlebotomus ariasi* et *Phlebotomus perniciosus* (Diptera - Psychodidae) par *Leishmania infantum* (Kinetoplastida-Trypanosomatidae) en Catalogne (Espagne). Parasite. 1996;3:191–2.
11. Ballart C, Guerrero I, Castells X, Barón S, Castillejo S, Alcover MM, et al. Importance of individual analysis of environmental and climatic factors affecting the density of *Leishmania* vectors living in the same geographical area: the example of *Phlebotomus ariasi* and *P. perniciosus* in northeast Spain. Geospat Health. 2014;8:389–403.
12. Aransay AM, Testa JM, Morillas-Marquez F, Lucientes J, Ready PD. Distribution of sandfly species in relation to canine leishmaniasis from the Ebro Valley to Valencia, northeastern Spain. Parasitol Res. 2004;94:416–20.
13. Sáez VD, Morillas-Márquez F, Merino-Espinosa G, Corpas-López V, Morales-Yuste M, Pesson B, et al. *Phlebotomus langeroni* Nitzulescu (Diptera, Psychodidae) a new vector for *Leishmania infantum* in Europe. Parasitol Res. 2018;117:1105–13.
14. Rohousova I, Ozensoy S, Ozbel Y, Volf P. Detection of species-specific antibody response of humans and mice bitten by sand flies. Parasitology. 2005;130:493–9.
15. Vlkova M, Rohousova I, Drahota J, Stanneck D, Kruedewagen EM, Mencke N, et al. Canine antibody response to *Phlebotomus perniciosus* bites negatively correlates with the risk of *Leishmania infantum* transmission. PLoS Negl Trop Dis. 2011;5:e1344.
16. Martín-Martín I, Molina R, Rohoušová I, Drahota J, Volf P, Jiménez M. High levels of anti-*Phlebotomus perniciosus* saliva antibodies in different vertebrate hosts from the re-emerging leishmaniosis focus in Madrid, Spain. Vet Parasitol. 2014;202:207–16.
17. Kostalova T, Lestinova T, Sumova P, Vlkova M, Rohousova I, Berriatua E, et al. Canine antibodies against salivary recombinant proteins of *Phlebotomus perniciosus*: a longitudinal study in an endemic focus of canine leishmaniasis. PLoS Negl Trop Dis. 2015;9:e0003855.
18. Marzouki S, Ben Ahmed M, Boussoffara T, Abdeladhim M, Ben Aleya-Bouafif N, Namane A, et al. Characterization of the antibody response to the saliva of *Phlebotomus papatasi* in people living in endemic areas of cutaneous leishmaniasis. Am J Trop Med Hyg. 2011;84:653–61.
19. Carvalho AM, Cristal JR, Muniz AC, Carvalho LP, Gomes R, Miranda JC, et al. Interleukin 10-dominant immune response and increased risk of cutaneous leishmaniasis after natural exposure to *Lutzomyia intermedia* sand flies. J Infect Dis. 2015;212:157–65.
20. Gidwani K, Picado A, Rijal S, Singh SP, Roy L, Volfova V, et al. Serological markers of sand fly exposure to evaluate insecticidal nets against visceral leishmaniasis in India and Nepal: a cluster-randomized trial. PLoS Negl Trop Dis. 2011;5:e1296.
21. Clements MF, Gidwani K, Kumar R, Hostomska J, Dinesh DS, Kumar V, et al. Measurement of recent exposure to *Phlebotomus argentipes*, the vector of Indian visceral leishmaniasis, by using human antibody responses to sand fly saliva. Am J Trop Med Hyg. 2010;82:801–7.
22. Volf P, Rohoušova I. Species-specific antigens in salivary glands of phlebotomine sandflies. Parasitology. 2001;122:37–41.
23. Lestinova T, Rohousova I, Sima M, de Oliveira CI, Volf P. Insights into the sand fly saliva: blood-feeding and immune interactions between sand flies, hosts, and *Leishmania*. PLoS Negl Trop Dis. 2017;11:e0005600.
24. Lestinova T, Vlkova M, Votypka J, Volf P, Rohousova I. *Phlebotomus papatasi* exposure cross-protects mice against *Leishmania major* co-inoculated with *Phlebotomus duboscqi* salivary gland homogenate. Acta Trop. 2015;144:9–18.
25. Drahota J, Martin-Martin I, Sumova P, Rohousova I, Jimenez M, Molina R, et al. Recombinant antigens from *Phlebotomus perniciosus* saliva as markers of canine exposure to visceral leishmaniases vector. PLoS Negl Trop Dis. 2014; 8:e2597.
26. Kostalova T, Lestinova T, Maia C, Sumova P, Vlkova M, Willen L, et al. The recombinant protein rSP03B is a valid antigen for screening dog exposure to *Phlebotomus perniciosus* across foci of canine leishmaniasis. Med Vet Entomol. 2016;31:88–93.
27. Hostomska J, Rohousova I, Volfova V, Stanneck D, Mencke N, Volf P. Kinetics of canine antibody response to saliva of the sand fly *Lutzomyia longipalpis*. Vector Borne Zoonotic Dis. 2008;8:443–50.
28. Sima M, Ferencova B, Warburg A, Rohousova I, Volf P. Recombinant salivary proteins of *Phlebotomus orientalis* are suitable antigens to measure exposure of domestic animals to sand fly bites. PLoS Negl Trop Dis. 2016;10: e0004553.

29. Rohousova I, Talmi-Frank D, Kostalova T, Polanska N, Lestinova T, Kassahun A, et al. Exposure to *Leishmania* spp. and sand flies in domestic animals in northwestern Ethiopia. Parasit Vectors. 2015;8:360.
30. Morillas Marquez F, Guevara Benitez DC, Ubeda Ontiveros JM, Gonzalez Castro J. Fluctuations annuelles des populations de Phlébotomes (Diptera, Phlebotomidae) dans la province de Grenade (Espagne). Ann Parasitol Hum Comp. 1983;58:625–32.
31. Gálvez R, Descalzo MA, Miró G, Jiménez MI, Martín O, Dos Santos-Brandao F, et al. Seasonal trends and spatial relations between environmental/ meteorological factors and leishmaniosis sand fly vector abundances in central Spain. Acta Trop. 2010;115:95–102.
32. González E, Jiménez M, Hernández S, Martín-Martín I, Molina R. Phlebotomine sand fly survey in the focus of leishmaniasis in Madrid, Spain (2012–2014): seasonal dynamics, *Leishmania infantum* infection rates and blood meal preferences. Parasit Vectors. 2017;10:368.
33. Lladró S, Picado A, Ballart C, Portús M, Gállego M. Management, prevention and treatment of canine leishmaniosis in north-eastern Spain: an online questionnaire-based survey in the province of Girona with special emphasis on new preventive methods (CaniLeish vaccine and domperidone). Vet Rec. 2017;180:47.
34. Quinnell RJ, Soremekun S, Bates PA, Rogers ME, Garcez LM, Courtenay O. Antibody response to sand fly saliva is a marker of transmission intensity but not disease progression in dogs naturally infected with *Leishmania infantum*. Parasit Vectors. 2018;11:7.
35. Marzouki S, Kammoun-Rebai W, Bettaieb J, Abdeladhim M, Hadj Kacem S, Abdelkader R. Validation of recombinant salivary protein PpSP32 as a suitable marker of human exposure to *Phlebotomus papatasi*, the vector of *Leishmania major* in Tunisia. PLoS Negl Trop Dis. 2015;9:e0003991.
36. Souza AP, Andrade BB, Aquino D, Entringer P, Miranda JC, Alcantara R, et al. Using recombinant proteins from *Lutzomyia longipalpis* saliva to estimate human vector exposure in visceral leishmaniasis endemic areas. PLoS Negl Trop Dis. 2010;4:e649.
37. Anderson JM, Oliveira F, Kamhawi S, Mans BJ, Reynoso D, Seitz AE, et al. Comparative salivary gland transcriptomics of sandfly vectors of visceral leishmaniasis. BMC Genomics. 2006;7:52.
38. Kedzierski L, Evans KJ. Immune responses during cutaneous and visceral leishmaniasis. Parasitology. 2014;141:1544–62.
39. Andrade BB, Teixeira CR. Biomarkers for exposure to sand flies bites as tools to aid control of leishmaniasis. Front Immunol. 2012;3:121.
40. Kamhawi S, Belkaid Y, Modi G, Rowton E, Sacks D. Protection against cutaneous leishmaniasis resulting from bites of uninfected sand flies. Science. 2000;290:1351–4.
41. Rohoušová I, Hostomská J, Vlková M, Kobets T, Lipoldová M, Volf P. The protective effect against *Leishmania* infection conferred by sand fly bites is limited to short-term exposure. Int J Parasitol. 2011;41:481–5.
42. Volf P, Volfova V. Establishment and maintenance of sand fly colonies. J Vector Ecol. 2011;36:S1–9.
43. Sanchez J, Dohoo IR, Markham F, Leslie K, Conboy G. Evaluation of the repeatability of a crude adult indirect *Ostertagia ostertagi* ELISA and methods of expressing test results. Vet Parasitol. 2002;109:75–90.
44. Ballart C, Alcover MM, Picado A, Nieto J, Castillejo S, Portús M, et al. First survey on canine leishmaniasis in a non classical area of the disease in Spain (Lleida, Catalonia) based on a veterinary questionnaire and a cross-sectional study. Prev Vet Med. 2013;109:116–27.
45. Riera C, Valladares JE, Gállego M, Aisa MJ, Castillejo S, Fisa R, et al. Serological and parasitological follow-up in dogs experimentally infected with *Leishmania infantum* and treated with meglumine antimoniate. Vet Parasitol. 1999;84:33–47.

Limited genetic diversity of N-terminal of merozoite surface protein-1 (MSP-1) in *Plasmodium ovale curtisi* and *P. ovale wallikeri* imported from Africa to China

Ruilin Chu[1†], Xinxin Zhang[1†], Sui Xu[2], Limei Chen[1], Jianxia Tang[2], Yuhong Li[1], Jing Chen[2], Yinghua Xuan[1], Guoding Zhu[2], Jun Cao[1,2*] and Yang Cheng[1*]

Abstract

Background: *Plasmodium* merozoite surface protein-1 (MSP-1) is released into the bloodstream during merozoite invasion, and thus represents a crucial malarial vaccine target. Although substantial research effort has been devoted to uncovering the genetic diversity of MSP-1 for *P. falciparum* and *P. vivax*, there is minimal information available regarding the genetic profiles and structure of *P. ovale*. Therefore, the aim of the present study was to determine the extent of genetic variation among two subspecies of *P. ovale* by characterizing the MSP-1 N-terminal sequence at the nucleotide and protein levels.

Methods: N-terminal of MSP-1 gene were amplified from 126 clinical samples collected from imported cases of malaria in migrant workers returning to Jiangsu Province from Africa using a conventional polymerase chain reaction (PCR) assay. The PCR products were then sequenced and analyzed using the GeneDoc, MegAlign, MEGA7 and DnaSP v.6 programs.

Results: The average pairwise nucleotide diversities (π) of *P. ovale curtisi* and *P. ovale wallikeri* MSP-1 genes (*pomsp1*) were 0.01043 and 0.01974, respectively, and the haplotype diversity (*Hd*) were 0.746 and 0.598, respectively. Most of the nucleotide substitutions detected were non-synonymous, indicating that the genetic variations of *pomsp1* were maintained by positive diversifying selection, thereby suggesting their role as a potential target of a protective immune response. Amino acid substitutions of *P. ovale curtisi* and *P. ovale wallikeri* MSP-1 could be categorized into five and three unique amino acid variants, respectively.

Conclusions: Low mutational diversity was observed in *pomsp1* from the Jiangsu Province imported malaria cases; further studies will be developed such as immunogenicity and functional analysis.

Keywords: *Plasmodium ovale*, MSP-1, Imported malaria cases

Background

Malaria is one of the most serious infectious diseases of humans worldwide. An estimated 216 million cases of malaria were reported in 2016 and the global tally of malaria-caused deaths reached 445,000 [1]. Five species in the genus *Plasmodium* (*P. falciparum*, *P. vivax*, *P. malariae*, *P. ovale* and *P. knowlesi*) are known to cause human malaria under natural transmission [2]. In China, the majority of malaria cases are caused by *P. vivax* and *P. falciparum*, most of which are imported from malaria-endemic areas. Jiangsu Province, located in eastern China, was an unstable malaria transmission area and there has been no local malaria infection report since 2012. However, the number of imported malaria cases in Jiangsu ranked in the top three provinces in China, with 1799 imported malaria cases reported from 2005 to 2014 [3, 4]. As a neglected human parasite causing infection, *P. ovale* was first reported and named by Stephens in 1922 as one of the major *Plasmodium* species infecting humans [5].

* Correspondence: caojuncn@hotmail.com; woerseng@126.com
†Ruilin Chu and Xinxin Zhang contributed equally to this work.
1 Laboratory of Pathogen Infection and Immunity, Department of Public Health and Preventive Medicine, Wuxi School of Medicine, Jiangnan University, Wuxi, Jiangsu, People's Republic of China
Full list of author information is available at the end of the article

Plasmodium ovale has a wide geographic distribution, including the Middle East, Indonesia, and Southeast Asia [6–8]. In Africa, only 0.7–10% of human malaria cases are caused by *P. ovale* infections; thus, the diagnosis of *P. ovale* is often overlooked due to the low levels of parasitemia and mixed-species malaria infections [7, 9]. Notably, approximately 300 malaria cases in China imported from Africa annually are caused by *P. ovale*. There are two subspecies of *P. ovale*, *P. ovale curtisi* (classical type) and *P. ovale wallikeri* (variant type) [10], which show dimorphism of multiple genetic loci [2].

Merozoites surface proteins (MSPs) are released into the bloodstream of the host in extracellular forms, and are thus promising vaccine targets since they play a critical role in erythrocyte invasion [11]. As the predominant member of MSPs, MSP-1 has been detected in all examined *Plasmodium* species to date, and plays an important role during erythrocyte attachment [12]. Thus, naturally acquired antibodies to MSP-1 inhibit erythrocyte invasion and are associated with protection from clinical malaria in field studies [13]. However, MSP-1-based vaccines show low protective efficacy against clinical malaria, which may be attributed to the genetic diversity of MSP-1, leading to failure of anti-malaria parasite control measures. Moreover, antigenic diversity allows the parasite to evade natural immune responses, which may cause vaccines to lose efficacy [14]. The N-terminal fragments of the MSP-1 genes of *P. falciparum* and *P. vivax* (*pfmsp1* and *pvmsp1*, respectively) show polymorphism due to selection pressure, which has hindered MSP-1-based vaccine development [15, 16]. Comparatively, the C-terminal of MSP-1 is a conserved sequence, which is carried into the infected erythrocytes during merozoite invasion [17]. A recent study demonstrated the low diversity of the *pocmsp1* and *powmsp1* gene in 10 *P. ovale* isolated from symptomatic malaria patients in Thailand, which may be related to a low transmission rate or repeated bottleneck effects [18]. However, there is limited evidence of the genetic diversity of *pomsp1*. Therefore, characterization of *pomsp1* is necessary toward understanding the population genetic structure and finding a suitable candidate for vaccine development. Accordingly, in the present study, the *pomsp1* N-terminal sequence was analyzed from the both subspecies of *P. ovale* obtained from infected migrant workers returning to China from Africa. We determined the levels of polymorphisms and nucleotide divergence of *msp1* sequences to validate the classification of *P. ovale curtisi* and *P. ovale wallikeri* as distinct species or subspecies, and trace signatures of selection.

Methods

Study areas and sample collection

The samples of *P. ovale curtisi* and *P. ovale wallikeri* were obtained from febrile patients at local hospitals of Jiangsu Province in China between 2012 and 2016, who had recently returned from working in tropical regions of sub-Saharan Africa endemic for malaria. A total of 126 *P. ovale*-infected blood samples were collected. Identification of the isolates was confirmed using polymerase chain reaction (PCR) of specific gene sequences. Parasite species were distinguished by PCR amplification using the real-time TaqMan PCR [3].

PCR amplification and sequencing of the *pomsp1* N-terminal

The N-terminal nucleotide sequences of MSP-1 from *P. ovale curtisi* and *P. ovale wallikeri* were amplified by PCR using the primers designed as *pocmsp1*-Forward (5'-GAA ACG CTC GAA AAT TAT A-3') and *pocmsp1*-Reverse (5'-ACA GGA TCA GTA AAC AGA CCT T-3'), and *powmsp1*-Forward (5'-GAA ACG CTC GAA AAT TAT A-3') and *powmsp1*-Reverse (5'-ATC GGT AAA CAG ACC TTC CAT-3'), respectively. The *pocmsp1* (GenBank: KC137343) and *powmsp1* (GenBank: KC137341) sequences from the GenBank database were used as reference gene sequences. The reactions were carried out in a volume of 20 μl including 1 μl genomic DNA, 7.4 μl double-distilled water, 0.8 μl of each primer, 0.5 units DNA polymerase, and 2 mM deoxynucleoside triphosphate within 10 μl premix (2× Phanta® Max Master Mix, Nanjing, China). The PCR amplification was performed in a Mastercycler (Eppendorf, Hamburg, Germany) under the following programme: denaturation at 95 °C for 3 min; followed by 35 cycles of 95 °C for 15 s, 51 °C for 15 s and 72 °C for 30 s; and a final extension at 72 °C for 5 min. The amplified products were analyzed by 1% agarose gel electrophoresis and visualized under an ultraviolet transilluminator (Bio-Rad ChemiDoc MP, Hercules, USA). The size of the PCR products was estimated based on the mobility relative to the standard DNA marker (TRANSGEN BIOTECH, Beijing, China). PCR products were cloned into pUC57 vector and the universal primers M13F (5'-TGT AAA ACG ACG GCC AGT-3') and M13R (5'-CAG GAA ACA GCT ATG AC-3') were used for sequencing, which was performed by GENEWIZ (Suzhou, China) on an ABI 3730xl DNA Analyzer (Thermo Fisher Scientific, Waltham, USA).

Sequence alignment and data analysis

The geographical distribution map of *P. ovale curtisi* and *P. ovale wallikeri* was constructed using Arcgis10.2 software [19]. The primary structure of the PoMSP-1 protein was predicted with a bioinformatics tool (http://smart.embl-heidelberg.de/). To evaluate the diversity of the two subspecies, the *pocmsp1* (KC137343) and *powmsp1* (KC137341) sequences were used as templates and aligned using GeneDoc2.7.0 [20]. The nucleotide sequences of *pomsp1* were translated to deduced amino acid (aa) sequences using MegAlign module of Lasergene 7 software package DNASTAR [21] and then aligned with reference aa sequences. The codon-based test of purifying selection was conducted using the MEGA7 program [22]. The rates of non-synonymous mutations (*dN*) and synonymous mutations sites (*dS*) were computed by *Z*-test using the Nei & Gojobori method [23] with the Jukes and Cantor correction and 100 bootstrap replications.

The average pairwise nucleotide diversity (π), haplotype diversity (*Hd*), and number of haplotypes (*H*) were calculated by DnaSP v6 [24]. The nucleotide diversity was analyzed with a window length of 50 base pairs (bp) and a step size of 3 bp using DnaSP v6. Tajima's *D*, Fu and Li's D^*, and Fu and Li's F^* tests were used to measure the degree of deviation from neutrality [25, 26]. Phylogenetic trees of the N-terminal of MSP-1 were constructed using the neighbor-joining method according to the nucleotide sequences. The MSP-1 sequences of other *Plasmodium* species included the MSP-1 haplotypes of malaria parasites from humans (*P. falciparum, P. malariae, P. ovale* and *P. vivax*), gorillas (*P. praefalciparum, P. alderi* and *P. billcollinsi*), chimpanzees (*P. reichenowi, P. blacklocki* and *P. gaboni*), macaques (*P. knowlesi* and *P. cynomolgi*), and murine infections (*P. yoelii, P. chabaudi* and *P. berghei*), which were collected from the NCBI and PlasmoDB databases. Evolutionary relationships of the aligned sequences were determined using neighbor-joining approaches in MEGA 7.0.

Results

Geographical origin of *P. ovale curtisi* and *P. ovale wallikeri*

The total of 126 *P. ovale* clinical isolates showed a geographical distribution across 15 countries of sub-Saharan Africa. The isolates were mainly derived from Equatorial Guinea (n = 37, 29.7%), Angola (n = 27, 21.4%), Nigeria (n = 19, 15.1%), and the Republic of Congo (n = 13, 10.3%) located on the west coast of Africa (Fig. 1). Comparatively, the *P. ovale curtisi* isolates spanned a wider range of countries (15 countries) than *P. ovale wallikeri* isolates (10 countries). Overall, 61 (48.4%) cases of *P. ovale curtisi* infection and 65 (51.6%) cases of *P. ovale wallikeri* infection were identified in this study (Table 1).

Characterization of PoMSP-1

The lengths of MSP-1 encoded by the full-length *P. ovale curtisi* (GenBank: KC137343) and *P. ovale wallikeri* (GenBank: KC137341) genes were 1727 and 1672 (aa), respectively, each beginning with a predicted 19 aa signal peptide sequence (aa 1–19). Similar to PvMSP-1 and PfMSP-1, some other specific regions were identified in the *P. ovale curtisi* predicted protein primary structure, such as a coiled-coil region (aa 288–368 and 450–495), Pfam region (aa 1011–1546), and EGF domains (aa 1624–1660 and 1667–1705) (Fig. 2a). Similarly, the PowMSP-1 predicted protein primary structure contained a signal peptide (aa 1–19), coiled-coil region (aa 458–496), Pfam region (aa 950–1491 aa), and two EGF domains (aa 1569–1605 and 1612–1650) (Fig. 2b).

Nucleotide polymorphism of *pomsp1*

The MSP-1 genes of the 126 *P. ovale* isolates were amplified corresponding to nucleotide positions 58–1125 (Fig. 2c). There were five genotypes of the *pocmsp1* N-terminal, and 52 isolates (85.2%) showed a non-synonymous mutation compared with the reference GH01 strain, with 44 nucleotides (67.7%) showing a non-synonymous mutation in the *powmsp1* N-terminal. Interestingly, 31 *P. ovale curtisi* isolates had 27 serine residues, while only 21 serine residues existed in the others. There were six more non-synonymous aa changes detected in *P. ovale wallikeri* isolates (Fig. 3).

Overall, 26 single nucleotide polymorphisms (SNPs) were found among 61 samples with an average π value of 0.01043 in *pocmsp1*, and 42 SNPs were detected among 65 samples with an average π value of 0.01974 in *powmsp1*. A sliding method plot with a window length of 50 bp and a step size of 3 bp using DnaSP v6 revealed a π value in the range of 0–0.09688 and 0–0.19221 for *pocmsp1* and *powmsp1*, respectively. The conserved region was observed from 0.2–0.7 kb length in *pocmsp1* and before 0.6 kb in *powmsp1* with approximate π values of 0 (Fig. 4). The haplotype (gene) diversity of *pocmsp1* could be categorized into five distinct haplotypes with an estimated *Hd* of 0.746 and three distinct haplotypes with an estimated *Hd* of 0.598 in *powmsp1* samples (Table 2). The average number of nucleotide differences (*k*) for *pocmsp1* and *powmsp1* was 11.139 and 21.081, respectively.

Genetic population structure based on the *pomsp1* N-terminal

The population genetic structure of the *P. ovale* isolates was analyzed based on the MSP-1 N-terminal gene polymorphisms applied to the codon-based test of purifying selection according to average *dS* and *dN* values within each isolate. There was clear evidence of positive selection or diversifying selection in *P. ovale* MSP-1 [Prob = 1.000, $dS - dN$ = -0.06 (*pocmsp1*), -0.478 (*powmsp1*)]. In addition, Tajima's *D*, Fu and Li's D^* and F^* tests rejected a neutral model of polymorphism occurrence with values for *pocmsp1* (Tajima's D = 3.22138, $P < 0.01$; Fu and Li's D^* = 1.88498, $P < 0.02$; Fu and Li's F^* = 2.77112, $P < 0.02$) and *powmsp1* (Tajima's D = 4.57287, $P < 0.001$; Fu and Li's D^* = 2.00379, $P < 0.02$; Fu and Li's F^* = 3.5575, $P < 0.02$), respectively (Table 2).

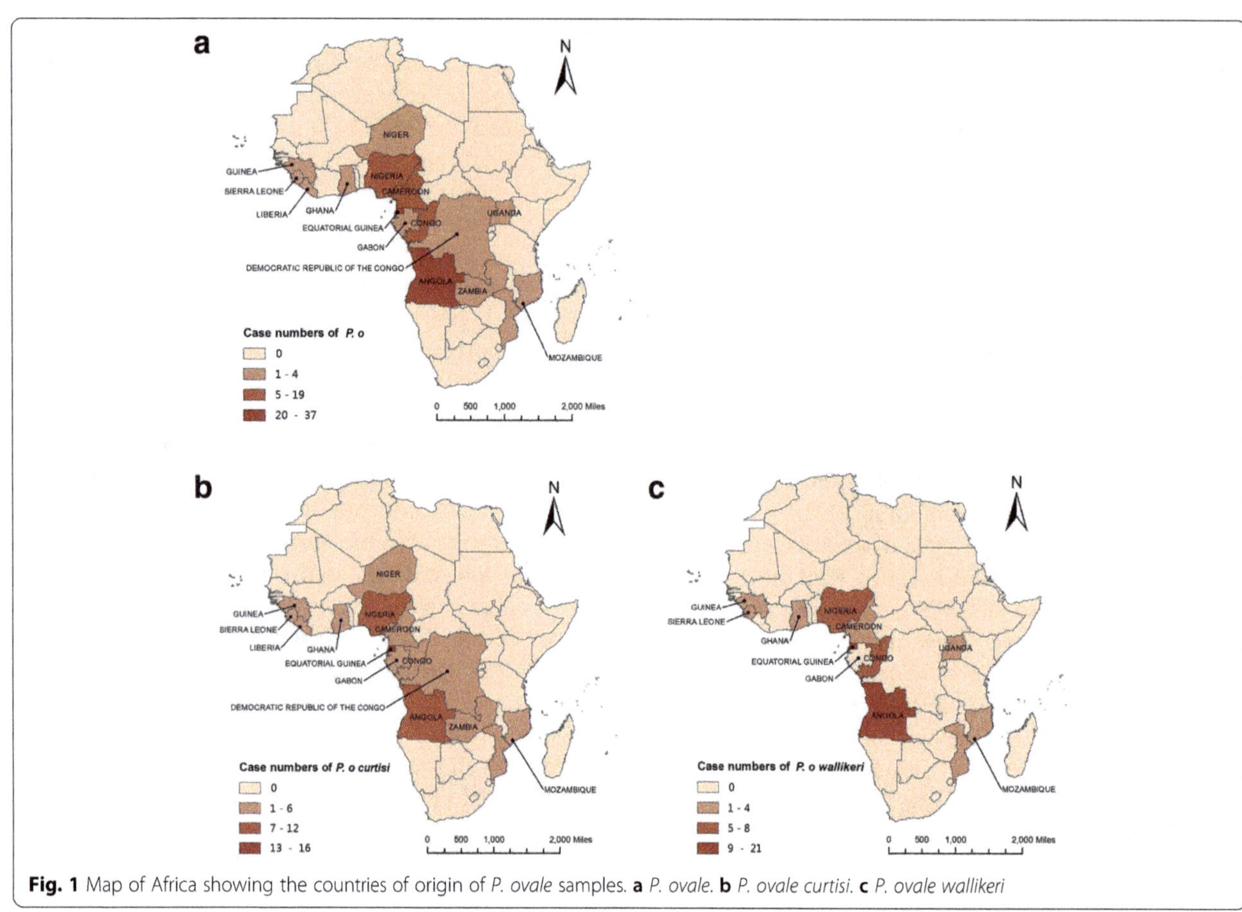

Fig. 1 Map of Africa showing the countries of origin of *P. ovale* samples. **a** *P. ovale*. **b** *P. ovale curtisi*. **c** *P. ovale wallikeri*

Table 1 Origin of imported *P. ovale curtisi* and *P. ovale wallikeri* in 2012–2016

Country	*P. ovale curtisi*		*P.ovale wallikeri*		Total
	Number	Percent	Number	Percent	Number
Angola	9	14.8	18	27.7	27
Equatorial Guinea	16	26.2	21	32.3	37
Republic of the Congo	5	8.2	8	12.3	13
Democratic Republic of the Congo	4	6.6	0	0	4
Guinea	1	1.6	2	3.1	3
Ghana	1	1.6	1	1.5	2
Gabon	1	1.6	0	0	1
Cameroon	6	9.8	4	6.2	10
Liberia	2	3.3	0	0	2
Mozambique	1	1.6	2	3.1	3
Niger	1	1.6	0	0	1
Nigeria	12	19.7	7	10.8	19
Sierra Leone	1	1.6	1	1.5	2
Zambia	1	1.6	0	0	1
Uganda	0	0	1	1.5	1
Total	61	100	65	100	126

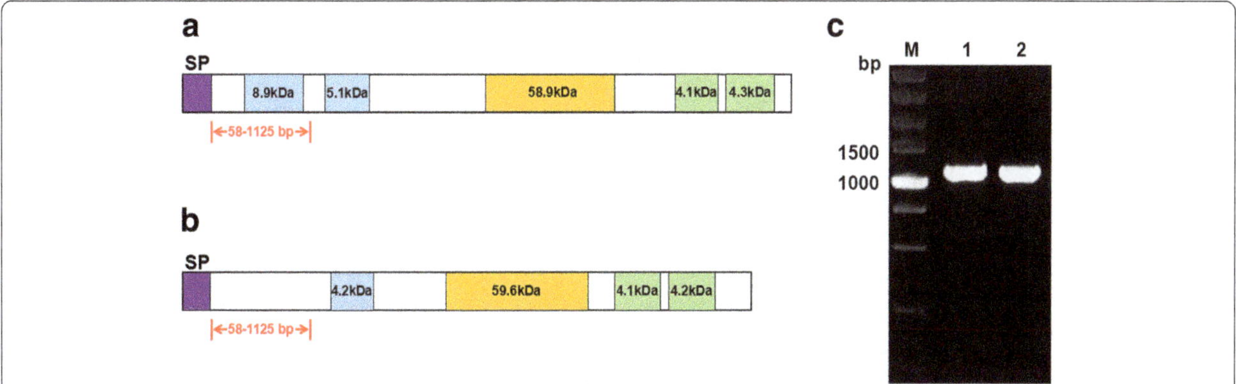

Fig. 2 Predicted *P. ovale* MSP-1 protein primary structure and MSP-1 N-terminal fragment size. **a** *P. ovale curtisi*. **b** *P. ovale wallikeri*. **c** *pomsp1* N-terminal fragment. *Abbreviations*: M, DNA marker; 1, *pocmsp1* N-terminal fragment; 2, *powmsp1* N-terminal fragment. Purple, blue, orange and green colors indicate signal peptide, coiled-coil, Pfam and EGF domains, respectively. Arrowheads indicate *pomsp1* N- terminal for sequencing

Phylogenetic analysis

As predicted based on the low level of genetic diversity and signature of positive selection described above, a close phylogenetic relationship was detected in *pomsp1* sequences between the subspecies based the branch lengths of *pocmsp1* and *powmsp1* with 100% bootstrap support (Fig. 5). Phylogenetic trees of 26 MSP-1 gene alleles from the 18 species of *Plasmodium* in human and non-human primates were constructed using the neighbor-joining method (Additional file 1: Figure S1).

Discussion

The life-cycle of the malaria parasite alternates between the human host and the mosquito vector, which is complex with extensive genetic and antigenic diversity across different stages of the parasite's life [14]. The genetic diversity of *P. ovale* might have impacted malaria transmission and the success of malaria control strategies. Gaining a deeper understanding of the mechanisms and patterns of genetic recombination and sequence variation may help in designing a vaccine that could represent the worldwide repertoire of polymorphic malaria surface antigens [27]. The sequences of *pocmsp1* and *powmsp1* showed a low level of diversity in a limited number of Asian isolates [18]. Hence, we analyzed the N-terminus of *pocmsp1* (61 isolates, 48.4%) and *powmsp1* (65, 51.6%), and found that *pocmsp1* was more conserved than *powmsp1* with 26 (14 synonymous, 12 non-synonymous) and 42 (26 synonymous, 16 non-synonymous) sites of nucleotide diversity, respectively.

Neutrality tests were further performed to determine the signatures of natural selection on the MSP-1 N-terminal fragment of *P. ovale*. Significantly positive values for these

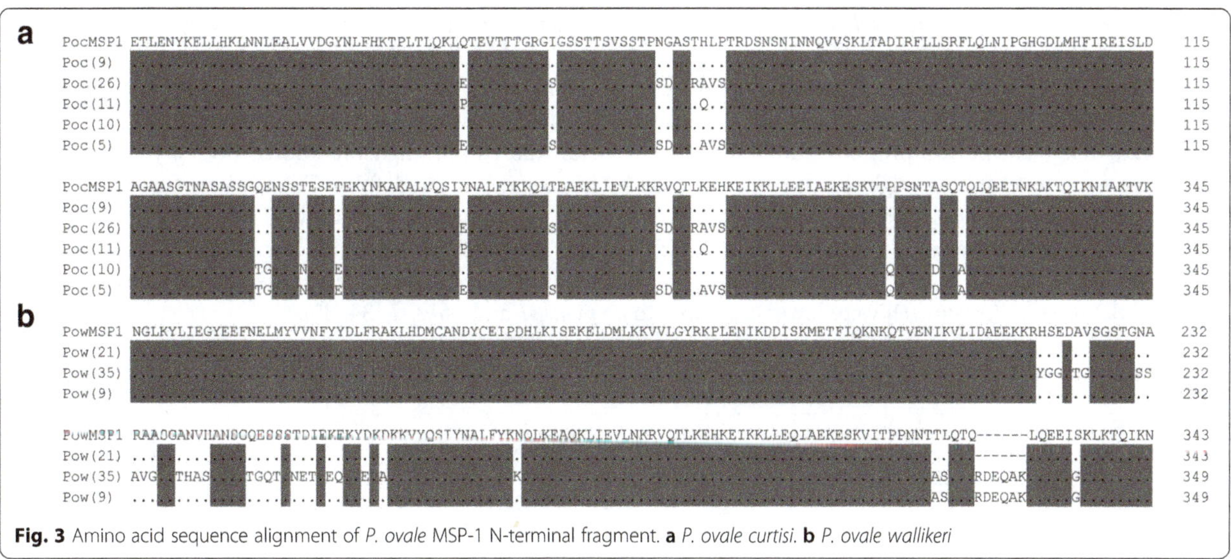

Fig. 3 Amino acid sequence alignment of *P. ovale* MSP-1 N-terminal fragment. **a** *P. ovale curtisi*. **b** *P. ovale wallikeri*

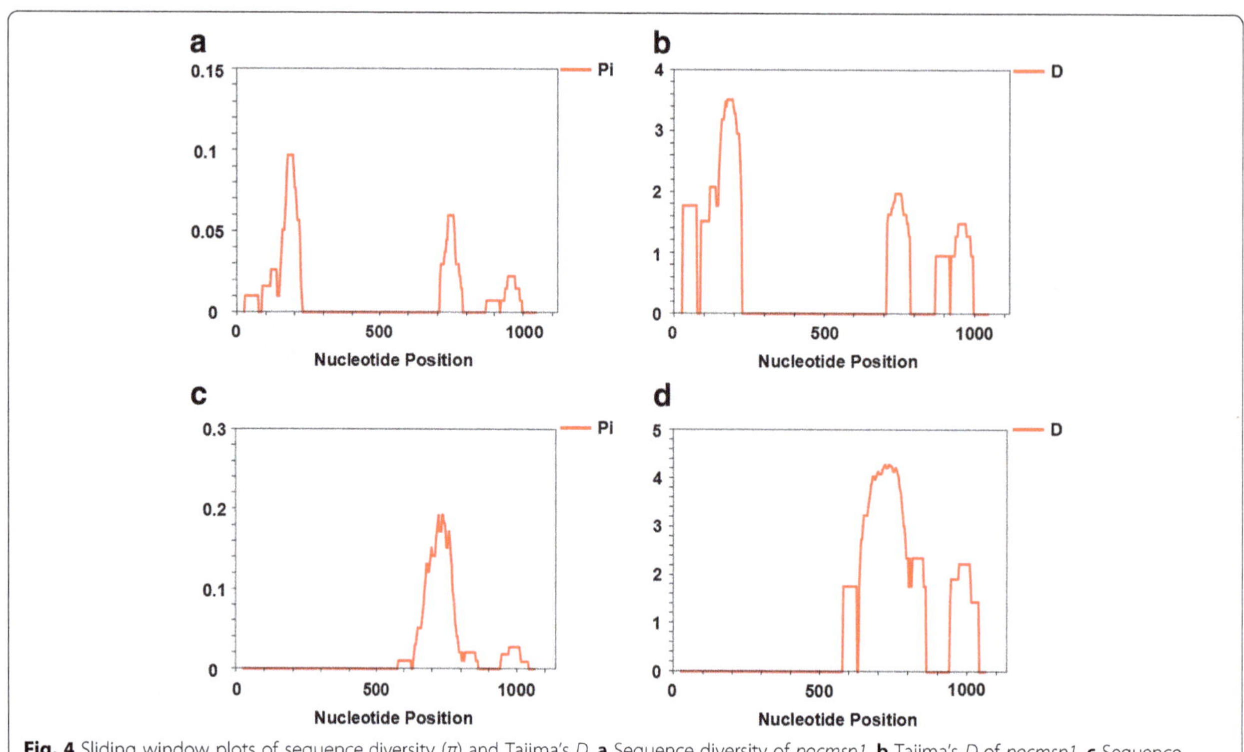

Fig. 4 Sliding window plots of sequence diversity (π) and Tajima's *D*. **a** Sequence diversity of *pocmsp1*. **b** Tajima's *D* of *pocmsp1*. **c** Sequence diversity of *powmsp1*. **d** Tajima's *D* of *powmsp1*

statistics reflect an excess of intermediate frequency alleles, which can result from population bottlenecks or balancing selection. The sequences for subspecies *P. ovale curtisi* and *P. ovale wallikeri* were further divided into five and three branches that were all within the same evolutionary branches. The MSP-1 N-terminal sequences placed the two subspecies in a distinct bifurcating branch, and the split of *pocmsp1* and *powmsp1* seems to be relatively more recent. Therefore, the MSP-1 N-terminal sequences of *P. ovale curtisi* and *P. ovale wallikeri* support the ancient divergence times of the malaria parasite lineage [28].

The *Z*-test ($dS - dN < 0$) indicated that strong positive or purifying selection within the parasite population. These results were in agreement with previous studies which suggested that such mechanisms might be in favour of parasites to evade targeted host immune responses [29]. In addition, the genetic diversities at the *P. ovale* MSP-1 N-terminal [π = 0.01043 ± SD 0.00061 (*pocmsp1*), π = 0.01974 ± SD 0.00055 (*powmsp1*)] were lower compared to that of *P. falciparum* and *P. vivax* [30], which may be related to the lower transmission rate of *P. ovale* from diverse geographical origins [8]. These findings were similar to previously published data demonstrating a low level of sequence diversity of the MSP-1 gene in *P. ovale* [18].

The intragenic recombination of MSP-1 gene is a major informative pattern at the level of population sequence diversity. The frequency of allelic recombination has important guiding significance for the population structure of parasites [31]. A previous study demonstrated that *P. falciparum* has a low level of genetic diversity in areas with low transmission rates and high level of sequence diversity in areas with high transmission rates [32]. High mutational diversity was observed in *pvmsp1* isolated from Thailand northwestern region [33]. The level of nucleotide diversity in both *pocmsp1* and *powmsp1* N-terminal sequences detected in this study showed lower magnitude than that reported for *pvmsp1* and *pfmsp1* [34, 35].

Table 2 Estimates of nucleotide diversity, natural selection, haplotype diversity and neutrality indices of *pomsp1* N-terminal fragment

Type	No. samples	G + C content (%)	No. haplotypes	*Hd*	Diversity ± SD		Tajima's *D*	Fu & Li's *D**	Fu & Li' s *F**
					Nucleotide	Haplotype			
P. ovale curtisi	61	34.1	5	0.746	0.01043 ± 0.00061	0.746 ± 0.035	3.22138	1.81498	2.77112
P. ovale wallikeri	65	35.2	3	0.598	0.01974 ± 0.00055	0.598 ± 0.036	4.57287	2.00379	3.5575

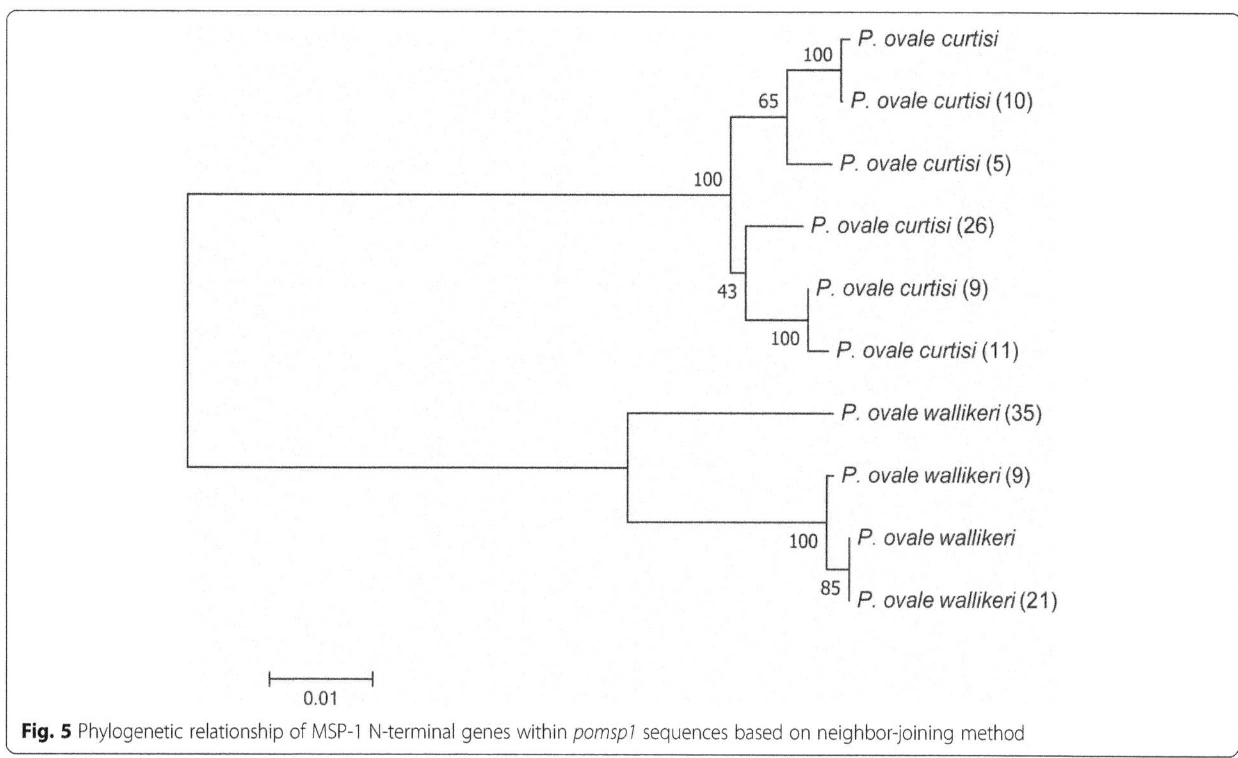

Fig. 5 Phylogenetic relationship of MSP-1 N-terminal genes within *pomsp1* sequences based on neighbor-joining method

Conclusions

This study provides valuable reference information on the genetic diversity of *P. ovale curtisi* and *P. ovale wallikeri* isolates imported from Africa to China based on analysis of the MSP-1 N-terminal sequence. To our knowledge, this is the first report of the genetic diversity, selection signature, and population structure of the N-terminal of *pomsp1* gene from an African population. The low level of genetic diversity indicated that these genes are under purifying selection. Therefore, these sequences have potential for vaccine development, which requires further investigation of the immunogenicity and antigenicity of *P. ovale* MSP-1.

Abbreviations

MSP-1: Merozoite surface protein-1; PCR: Polymerase chain reaction; aa: Amino acid; *Hd*: Haplotype diversity; SNP: Single nucleotide polymorphism; *dN*: Rates of non-synonymous substitutions; *dS*: Rates of synonymous substitutions; H: Haplotype; *Hd*: Haplotype diversity; *k*: Average number of pairwise nucleotide differences within the population; π: Nucleotide diversity

Acknowledgements

The authors thank all study participants, local health officials and doctors for their participation and support.

Funding

This study was funded by grants from National Natural Science Foundation of China (81601787), by Natural Science Foundation of Jiangsu Province (BK20160192, BK20150001), by the Jiangsu Provincial Key Research and Development Program (BE2016631), by the Fundamental Research Funds for the Central Universities funded by the Ministry of Education of China (JUSRP51710A), by Bill & Melinda Gates Foundation (OPP1161962), by National First-Class Discipline Program of Food Science and Technology (JUFSTR20180101), and by the Jiangsu Provincial Project of Invigorating Health Care through Science, Technology and Education.

Authors' contributions

YC and JC conceived and designed the study. SX, JXT, JC and GDZ collected the samples. RLC, XXZ and LMC performed the acquisition of data and data analysis. RLC, XXZ, YHL and YHX conducted the laboratory work, data handling and analysis and reviewed the manuscript. All authors read and approved the final version of the manuscript.

Competing interests

The authors declare that they have no competing interests.

Author details

[1]Laboratory of Pathogen Infection and Immunity, Department of Public Health and Preventive Medicine, Wuxi School of Medicine, Jiangnan University, Wuxi, Jiangsu, People's Republic of China. [2]Key Laboratory of National Health and Family Planning Commission on Parasitic Disease Control and Prevention, Jiangsu Provincial Key Laboratory on Parasite and Vector Control Technology, Jiangsu Institute of Parasite Diseases, Wuxi 214064, Jiangsu, People's Republic of China.

References

1. WHO. World Malaria Report (2008–2017). Geneva: World Health Organization; 2017. http://www.who.int/malaria/publications/world_malaria_report/en/
2. Sutherland CJ, Polley SD. Two nonrecombining sympatric forms of the human malaria parasite *Plasmodium ovale* occur globally. J Infect Dis. 2010;201:1544.
3. Cao Y, Wang W, Liu Y, Cotter C, Zhou H, Zhu G, et al. The increasing importance of *Plasmodium ovale* and *Plasmodium malariae* in a malaria elimination setting: an observational study of imported cases in Jiangsu Province, China, 2011–2014. Malar J. 2016;15:459.
4. Luo EP, Wang WM, Liu YB, Cao YY, Zhou HY, Xu T. Analysis of epidemic situation of malaria in Jiangsu Province from 2005 to 2014. Chin J Schisto Control. 2015;27:251–4 (In Chinese).
5. Stephens JWW. A new malaria parasite of man. Ann Trop Med Parasitol. 1922;16:383–8.
6. Collins WE, Jeffery GM. *Plasmodium ovale*: parasite and disease. Clin Microbiol Rev. 2005;18:570–81.
7. Win TT, Lin K, Mizuno S, Zhou M, Liu Q, Ferreira MU, et al. Wide distribution of *Plasmodium ovale* in Myanmar. Trop Med Int Health. 2010;7:231–9.
8. Kawamoto F, Liu Q, Ferreira MU, Tantular IS. How prevalent are *Plasmodium ovale* and *P. malariae* in East Asia? Parasitol Today. 1999;15:422–6.
9. Bichara C, Flahaut P, Costa D, Bienvenu AL, Picot S, Gargala G. Cryptic *Plasmodium ovale* concurrent with mixed *Plasmodium falciparum* and *Plasmodium malariae* infection in two children from Central African Republic. Malar J. 2017;16:339.
10. Win TT, Jalloh A, Tantular IS, Tsuboi T, Ferreira MU, Kimura M, et al. Molecular analysis of *Plasmodium ovale* variants. Emerg Infect Dis. 2004;10:1235–40.
11. Cowman AF, Crabb BS. Invasion of red blood cells by malaria parasites. Cell. 2006;124:755–6.
12. Holder AA, Blackman MJ, Burghaus PA, Chappel JA, Ling IT, Mccallumdeighton N, et al. A malaria merozoite surface protein (MSP1)-structure, processing and function. Mem Inst Oswaldo Cruz. 1992;87:37–42.
13. Egan AF, Morris J, Barnish G, Allen S, Greenwood BM, Kaslow DC, et al. Clinical immunity to *Plasmodium falciparum* malaria is associated with serum antibodies to the 19-kDa C-terminal fragment of the merozoite surface antigen, PfMSP-1. J Infect Dis. 1996;173:765–9.
14. Takala S, Branch O, Escalante AA, Kariuki S, Wootton J, Lal AA. Evidence for intragenic recombination in *Plasmodium falciparum*: identification of a novel allele family in block 2 of merozoite surface protein-1: asembo bay area cohort project XIV. Mol Biochem Parasitol. 2002;125:163–71.
15. Mayengue PI, Ndounga M, Malonga FV, Bitemo M, Ntoumi F. Genetic polymorphism of merozoite surface protein-1 and merozoite surface protein-2 in *Plasmodium falciparum* isolates from Brazzaville, Republic of Congo. Malar J. 2011;10:276.
16. Carmen FB, Sergi S, Marina B, Stanisic DI, Alves FP, Camargo EP, et al. Naturally-acquired humoral immune responses against the N- and C-termini of the *Plasmodium vivax*, MSP1 protein in endemic regions of Brazil and Papua New Guinea using a multiplex assay. Malar J. 2010;9:29.
17. Kaslow DC, Hui G, Kumar S. Expression and antigenicity of *Plasmodium falciparum* major merozoite surface protein (MSP119) variants secreted from *Saccharomyces cerevisiae*. Mol Biochem Parasitol. 1994;63:283.
18. Putaporntip C, Hughes AL, Jongwutiwes S. Low level of sequence diversity at *merozoite surface protein-1* locus of *Plasmodium ovale curtisi* and *P. ovale wallikeri* from Thai isolates. PLoS One. 2013;8:e58962.
19. ESRI. ArcGIS Desktop: Release 10. Redlands: Environmental Systems Research Institute. 2011.
20. Nicholas K, Nicholas H. GeneDoc: A tool for editing and annotating multiple sequence alignments. Ver. 2.7.000. 1996. Distributed by the author. 1997. http://iubio.bio.indiana.edu/soft/molbio/ibmpc/genedoc-readme.html.
21. Burland TG. Dnastar's lasergene sequence analysis software. Methods Mol Biol. 2000;132:71–91.
22. Kumar S, Stecher G, Tamura K. MEGA7: Molecular Evolutionary Genetics Analysis version 7.0 for bigger datasets. Mol Biol Evol. 2016;33:1870–4.
23. Nei M, Gojobori T. Simple methods for estimating the numbers of synonymous and nonsynonymous nucleotide substitutions. Mol Biol Evol. 1986;3:418–26.
24. Rozas J, Ferrermata A, Sánchezdelbarrio JC, Guiraorico S, Librado P, Ramosonsins SE, et al. DnaSP 6: DNA sequence polymorphism analysis of large datasets. Mol Biol Evol. 2017;34:3299–302.
25. Tajima F. Simple methods for testing the molecular evolutionary clock hypothesis. Genetics. 1993;135:599–607.
26. Fu YX, Li WH. Statistical tests of neutrality of mutations. Genetics. 1993;133: 693–709.
27. Bharti PK. Genetic diversity in the block 2 region of the merozoite surface protein-1 of *Plasmodium falciparum* in central India. Malar J. 2012;11:78.
28. Silva JC, Egan A, Friedman R, Munro JB, Carlton JM, Hughes AL. Genome sequences reveal divergence times of malaria parasite lineages. Parasitology. 2011;138:1737–49.
29. Chenet SM, Branch OH, Escalante AA, Lucas CM, Bacon DJ. Genetic diversity of vaccine candidate antigens in *Plasmodium falciparum* isolates from the Amazon basin of Peru. Malar J. 2008;7:93.
30. Atroosh WM, Almekhlafi HM, Mahdy MA, Saifali R, Almekhlafi AM, Surin J. Genetic diversity of *Plasmodium falciparum* isolates from Pahang, Malaysia based on MSP-1 and MSP-2 genes. Parasit Vectors. 2011;4:233.
31. Putaporntip C, Jongwutiwes S, Sakihama N, Ferreira MU, Kho WG, Kaneko A, et al. Mosaic organization and heterogeneity in frequency of allelic recombination of the *Plasmodium vivax* merozoite surface protein-1 locus. Proc Natl Acad Sci USA. 2002;99:16348–53.
32. Bannister LH, Hopkins JM, Fowler RE, Krishna S, Mitchell GH. Microsatellite markers reveal a spectrum of population structures in the malaria parasite *Plasmodium falciparum*. Mol Biol Evol. 2000;17:1467.
33. Putaporntip C, Hongsrimuang T, Seethamchai S, Kobasa T, Limkittikul K, Cui L, et al. Differential prevalence of *Plasmodium* infections and cryptic *Plasmodium knowlesi* malaria in humans in Thailand. J Infect Dis. 2009;199: 1143–50.
34. Versiani FG, Almeida ME, Mariuba LA, Orlandi PP, Nogueira PA. N-Terminal *Plasmodium vivax* merozoite surface protein-1, a potential subunit for malaria vivax vaccine. Clin Dev Immunol. 2013;2013:965841.
35. Tanabe K, Sakihama N, Rooth I, Björkman A, Färnert A. High frequency of recombination-driven allelic diversity and temporal variation of *Plasmodium falciparum* msp1 in Tanzania. Am J Trop Med Hyg. 2007;76:1037–45.

18

A chitinase-like protein from *Sarcoptes scabiei* as a candidate anti-mite vaccine that contributes to immune protection in rabbits

Nengxing Shen[1†], Haojie Zhang[1†], Yongjun Ren[2], Ran He[1], Jing Xu[1], Chunyan Li[1], Weimin Lai[1], Xiaobin Gu[1], Yue Xie[1], Xuerong Peng[3] and Guangyou Yang[1*]

Abstract

Background: Scabies is caused by *Sarcoptes scabiei* burrowing into the stratum corneum of the host's skin and is detrimental to the health of humans and animals. Vaccines are an attractive alternative to replace the acaricides currently used in their control.

Methods: In the present study, the *S. scabiei* chitinase-like protein 5 (SsCLP5) was characterized and recombinant SsCLP5 (rSsCLP5) was evaluated as a candidate vaccine protein for anti-mite protection in rabbits. The expression, characterization and immunolocalization of SsCLP5 were examined. Vaccination experiments were performed on three test groups (n = 12 per group) immunized with purified rSsCLP5. Control groups (n = 12 per group) were immunized with PBS, QuilA saponin or empty vector protein. After challenge, the inflammatory reaction and skin lesions were graded and rSsCLP5 indirect ELISA was used to detect antibody IgG levels in serum samples at the time of vaccination and post-challenge.

Results: The results showed that rSsCLP5 had high immunoreactivity and immunogenicity. In *S. scabiei*, SsCLP5 had a wide distribution in the chewing mouthpart, legs and exoskeleton, especially the outer layer of the exoskeleton. Vaccination with rSsCLP5 resulted in 74.3% (26/35) of rabbits showing no detectable lesions after challenge with *S. scabiei*.

Conclusions: Our data demonstrate that rSsCLP5 is a promising candidate for a recombinant protein-based vaccine against *S. scabiei*. This study also provides a method for studying scabies vaccine using rabbit as an animal model and a basis for screening more effective candidate proteins.

Keywords: *Sarcoptes scabiei*, Scabies, Chitinase-like protein 5, Recombinant protein, Vaccine

Background

Scabies is a highly contagious parasitic disease caused by the etiological agent *Sarcoptes scabiei*, which burrows into the stratum corneum of the host. Scabies or sarcoptic mange presents an enormous threat to the health of humans and animals worldwide [1, 2], occurring in more than 100 species of mammals [3] and causing clinical symptoms such as skin inflammation, itching and skin lesions [4]. Scabies occurs extensively in indigenous populations [5] and in the poorest areas of developing countries [6]. The uncontrolled spread of scabies or sarcoptic mange results in severe mortality, which has significant impacts in terms of welfare and economic loss [7–9]. Furthermore, in tropical climates, infection with *Streptococcus pyogenes* or *Staphylococcus aureus* often occurs, resulting in serious pyoderma of the skin lesions [10, 11].

At present, acaricides are used as a control measure for combating mite infestation; however, they can be toxic to humans and animals. For instance, neurotoxicity

* Correspondence: guangyou1963@aliyun.com
†Nengxing Shen and Haojie Zhang contributed equally to this work.
1Department of Parasitology, College of Veterinary Medicine, Sichuan Agricultural University, Chengdu 611130, China
Full list of author information is available at the end of the article

has been reported in children with widespread skin damage following treatment with benzyl benzoate [12] or lindane [13, 14]. Additionally, side effects have also been reported in dogs treated with moxidectin [15]. Furthermore, the risk of development of drug resistance in scabies mite due to intensive use of acaricides cannot be entirely ruled out and requires thorough consideration [16–18]. Moreover, acaricide residues have harmful effects on health and threaten the environment. An effective anti-mite vaccine, in contrast, has the potential to protect people and animals more efficiently in terms of safety, environmental friendliness and economic costs.

Sarcoptes scabiei infestation can induce both innate and adaptive immune responses in the host [19, 20]. Protective immune responses to mite infestation have been described [21–23], with findings suggesting that it is possible to develop a vaccine to control the scabies mite. To date, some vaccination studies have been published [22, 24]; however, no promising anti-mite vaccine candidate protein has been identified. The completed analysis of the genome [25], transcriptome [26] and proteome [27] of *S. scabiei* provides a basis for screening more effective candidate vaccine proteins.

Chitinase-like proteins (CLPs) and chitinases are a family of mediators increasingly associated with infection, T cell-mediated inflammation, wound healing, allergy and asthma [28]. CLPs are homologous to chitinases, both of which belong to the glycoside hydrolase family 18, but lack the ability to degrade chitin. Both play an important role in T-helper type 2 (Th2)-driven responses and possibly contribute to the repair process during inflammation [29–31]. In some parasitic infections [32–34], increased levels of chitinases and CLPs may contribute to the host's defense in mammals.

In this study, we describe the identification, characterization and immunolocalization of SsCLP5, a candidate protein for an anti-mite vaccine, and evaluate the potential of the rSsCLP5 protein in a vaccination trial for mite infestation in rabbits.

Methods

Animals and sources

Twenty New Zealand rabbits were purchased from Chengdu Tatsuo Biological Technology Co. Ltd. (Chengdu, China) and infested with *Sarcoptes scabiei* for a month. *Sarcoptes scabiei* was harvested by the Department of Parasitology, College of Veterinary Medicine, Sichuan Agricultural University. In brief, live mites including larvae, nymphs and adults were collected and isolated from severely affected rabbits by exposing the infested crust to 37 °C for 2 h. Partial mites were used for RNA and protein extraction and the remaining mites were used for a challenge test in a vaccination trial. RNA isolation from mites was performed using RNAprep pure Tissue Kit (TIANGEN, Beijing, China) and RNA was transcribed into cDNA using RevertAid First Strand cDNA Synthesis Kit (Thermo Fisher Scientific, Vilnius, Lithuania). Total crude protein was extracted from mites using Total Protein Extraction Kit (BestBio, Shanghai, China). cDNA and total crude protein were stored at -70 °C until assay.

Expression and purification of rSsCLP5

Based on genomic data (GenBank: JXLN01012673.1) and proteomics data (GenBank: KPM08736.1), we identified the *S. scabiei* chitinase-like protein 5 (SsCLP5) and amplified regions showing high sequence homology with other species according to the results of epitope analysis. Primers for amplification were designed using Primer 5.0 software and were as follows: forward (5'-CGG GAT CCA TGC AAG AGC TTC GTA A-3'), with a *Bam*HI restriction site (underlined), and reverse (5'-CCC TCG AGA TCA TAG AAG ATC ATA GAA AT-3'), with an *Xho*I restriction site (underlined; Invitrogen, Beijing, China). SsCLP5 was amplified using the following PCR cycling conditions: 94 °C for 5 min; 30 cycles of amplification at 94 °C for 45 s, 55 °C for 45 s, and 72 °C for 45 s; followed by a final extension at 72 °C for 10 min. The fragment was cloned into the pET-32a (+) expression vector (Invitrogen), which was transformed into *Escherichia coli* BL21 (DE3) cells. Protein expression was induced with 1 mM isopropyl-β-D-thiogalactoside (IPTG) at 37 °C for 6 h. Recombinant *S. scabiei* chitinase-like protein 5 (rSsCLP5) was purified using a Ni-NTA His-tag affinity chromatography kit (Bio-Rad Laboratories, California, USA), according to the manufacturer's instructions.

Sequence analysis

DNAMAN software was employed to compare sequence similarity between homologous genes. SsCLP5 was analysed using the online software SignalP 4.1 (http://www.cbs.dtu.dk/services/SignalP/), Transmembrane Prediction Server (http://www.sbc.su.se/~miklos/DAS/) and TargetP (http://www.cbs.dtu.dk/services/TargetP/) to assess potential signal peptides, transmembrane regions and subcellular localization, respectively. ExPasy (http://web.expasy.org/protparam/) was used to calculate predicted molecular weight and pI values. Homologous proteins were found in the NCBI database and comparative analysis was performed using the online software Clustal W2 (http://www.ebi.ac.uk/tools/msa/clustalw2/). Finally, we used MEGA 5.05 software for adjacent structure analysis of system evolution, and to build the evolutionary tree [35, 36].

Western blotting

Samples (40 μl of protein and 10 μl loading buffer) were boiled for 10 min. Protein samples were separated by

12% SDS-PAGE and transferred onto a nitrocellulose membrane for 35 min in an electrophoretic transfer cell (Bio-Rad Laboratories). Membranes were washed three times for 5 min in TBST (20 mM Tris-HCl, 150 mM NaCl, 0.05% [v/v] Tween 20, pH 7.4), blocked with 5% skim milk for 2 h, and then incubated overnight at room temperature with rabbit serum (diluted 1:100 with 0.01 M PBS). Next, the membranes were washed four times for 5 min each in TBST, then incubated with horseradish peroxidase (HRP)-conjugated goat anti-rabbit antibody (diluted 1:1000) for 2 h. The membranes were washed four times with PBS, and protein signals detected using diaminobenzidine reagent (TIANGEN, Beijing, China).

Immunolocalization

Adult mites were fixed in 1% molten agarose shortly after collection. The solid agarose containing the mites was then embedded in paraffin wax and cut into sections (5 μm) with a microtome. The sections were baked in a 60 °C oven for 2 h, dewaxed in xylene twice for 7 min each, in 100% ethanol twice for 3 min each, in 95% ethanol for 3 min, in 85% ethanol for 3 min and in 75% ethanol for 3 min, and were then rinsed with distilled water for 8 min. To inactivate endogenous peroxidase, the sections were incubated in blocking buffer (3% H_2O_2 in PBS) for 20 min at 37 °C. Next, heat-induced epitope retrieval was accomplished by immersing sections in 0.01 M sodium citrate buffer (pH 6.0) at 95 °C for 20 min. The sections were incubated in blocking buffer (5% bovine serum albumin in PBS) for 1 h at room temperature before incubation overnight at 4 °C with specific rabbit anti-rSsCLP5 antibodies (preparation of rSsCLP5 polyclonal antibody as described previously [37]) covering the sections (diluted 1:100 in PBS). After washing three times with PBS, the sections were incubated with fluorescein isothiocyanate (FITC) goat anti-rabbit IgG (H+L; diluted 1:100; EarthOx, LLC, San Francisco, CA, USA) in 0.1% Evans Blue for 1 h at 37 °C in the dark. Finally, sections were viewed with a microscope. In this experiment, the negative controls consisted of pre-immune rabbit serum antibody instead of specific antibodies.

Vaccination trial

A total of 72 three-month-old New Zealand rabbits (36 females and 36 males) were prepared for the vaccination trial by Chengdu Tatsuo Biological Technology Co. Ltd. Rabbits weighed 2.3 ± 0.2 kg at the beginning of the experiment and were immunized twice at a 14-day interval by subcutaneous injection of the neck. Rabbits were randomly divided into six groups of 12 rabbits each. Group one was inoculated with 1 ml 0.01 M PBS (137 mM NaCl, 2.7 mM KCl, 10 mM Na_2HPO_4, 2 mM KH_2PO_4, pH 7.4) as unvaccinated controls; group two was inoculated with 1 ml Quil-A saponin adjuvant (Sigma-Aldrich, St. Louis, MO, USA) at a concentration of 1 mg/ml (dissolved in PBS) as adjuvant controls; group three was inoculated with 100 μg (initial injection) and 200 μg (second injection) purified protein from the pET32a (+) empty vector with 1 ml Quil-A saponin at a concentration of 1 mg/ml (dissolved in PBS) as vector protein controls; and group four was immunized with 100 and 200 μg purified rSsCLP5 protein with 1 ml Quil-A saponin at a concentration of 1 mg/ml (dissolved in PBS) for the first and second immunizations, respectively. Group five and group six received the same immunization as group four and served as biological replicates. Two weeks after the second vaccination, each rabbit was challenged with approximately 2000 live mites on the two hind feet. In order to ensure proper and adequate infectivity, the live mites (larvae, nymphs and adults) were subjected to challenge test immediately after collection and counting under the microscope. The foot challenge area was chosen because mange lesions in naturally infested rabbits are most frequently initially observed in the hind limbs. Serum samples were obtained prior to vaccination and every week during vaccination and challenge until week 4 post-challenge. All sera samples were stored at -20 °C until use. Skin lesions of the hind legs were photographed weekly after the challenge. Mange lesion areas and the body weights were measured during the vaccination trial on a weekly basis.

Lesion score and mite burden

After the challenge, skin lesions caused by the mites were assessed at weekly intervals from weeks 1 to 4 post-infestation. The lesion areas were photographed and measured using a caliper. The inflammatory reaction and skin lesions were graded as follows: 0, no inflammatory reaction; 1, mild inflammatory reaction; 2, severe inflammatory reaction; 3, lesions first observed on the limbs (lesions ≤ 7.75 cm^2); 4, lesions of 7.75–15.5 cm^2 (including 15.5 cm^2) and 5, lesions of 15.5–31 cm^2 [22, 24]. Four weeks after the challenge, all tested rabbits were euthanized and the crusts from the hind limbs were collected and digested with 10% KOH. Then, the dead mites were concentrated by floating with saturated sucrose solution and counted under the light microscope [38].

Antibody responses

A checkerboard titration study was carried out to determine the optimal conditions for the rSsCLP5 and serum [39]. ELISA procedures were performed as previously described [37]. We used the rSsCLP5 indirect ELISA to detect antibody IgG levels in serum samples at the time of vaccination and post-challenge.

Data analysis

All analyses were performed with R Statistical Environment [40], with confidence intervals at 95% (α = 0.050).

All graphs were generated in GraphPad Prism version 5.0 (GraphPad Software). Statistical differences between groups were determined using IBM SPASS statistics 19.0 (SPASS Software). Analyses of variance for repeated measures for each dependent variable (IgG levels, lesion grades, lesion scores and weight) were performed using the *ez* package [41]. Data were analyzed using immunization group and time as fixed variables and the rabbit as a random variable to account for repeated measure variability.

Results

Identification and sequence analysis of SsCLP5

The SsCLP5 DNA complete sequence length is 1701 bp containing an open reading frame (ORF) of 1251 bp and encoding a putative protein with 416 amino acid residues. Based on the results of multiple species alignment and epitope prediction analysis, the highly similar region (nucleotides 457 to 1251 of the ORF) of SsCLP5 was amplified. The amplified region of SsCLP5 includes a 795 bp ORF encoding a putative protein of 264 amino acid residues (~30.9 kDa) with a pI of 8.92 that lacks signal peptide or transmembrane domains, and has strong hydrophilicity. The SsCLP5 protein sequence of *S. scabiei*, together with its 11 homologues, were subjected to phylogenetic analysis. The topological tree divided these 12 SsCLPs into five different clades. Specifically, SsCLP1, SsCLP4, SsCLP6, SsCLP8, SsCLP11 and SsCLP12 showed a close evolutionary relationship and formed the first branch, and SsCLP2, SsCLP3 and SsCLP9 formed the second branch (Fig. 1). However, others were presented separately in three branches. The SsCLP5 characterized here was classified into the fourth branch and shared 99% bootstrap values with the CLP from *Euroglyphus maynei* (Fig. 1).

Production and characterization of recombinant SsCLP5

The 795 bp ORF sequence was successfully cloned and then sub-cloned into the pet-32a (+) expression vector (Invitrogen) and expressed in *Escherichia coli* BL21 (DE3) cells. Protein expression level of SsCLP5 peaked at 6 h following induction with 1 mM IPTG. Recombinant SsCLP5 was expressed as soluble protein with a molecular mass of approximately 49 kDa (including vector-encoded amino acids; Fig. 2, Lane 2). The purification of the soluble protein was accomplished by immobilized metal affinity chromatography under denaturing conditions according to the manufacturer's instructions. After purification and concentration, the protein was assessed by 12% sodium dodecyl sulfate polyacrylamide gel electrophoresis (SDS-PAGE). Purified rSsCLP5 migrated as a single band at the predicted size of approximately 49 kDa (Fig. 2, Lane 3).

The immunoreactivity of rSsCLP5 was examined by immunoblot. Serum samples from rabbits naturally infested with *S. scabiei* (experimental group) and serum from rabbits vaccinated with rSsCLP5 both bound the ~49 kDa protein in the antigen preparation, signifying strong reactivity and good antigenicity of the SsCLP5 recombinant protein (Fig. 2, Lanes 5, 6). The serum from pre-immune rabbit (negative control) did not bind any protein component in the antigen preparation (Fig. 2, Lane 7). For the internal reference, ~45 kDa (416 amino acid residues) protein from the total mite extract was bound by the serum from the rabbits vaccinated with rSsCLP5 in experimental group (Fig. 2, Lane 8).

Localization of SsCLP5 in mites

Fluorescence immunohistochemistry was performed to examine SsCLP5 localization in mites. There was a wide distribution in the chewing mouthpart, legs and exoskeleton of *S. scabiei*, especially the outer layer of the exoskeleton (Fig. 3a). There was no fluorescence signal in the control group, which was treated with primary antibody from pre-immune rabbit serum (Fig. 3b). In addition, the hematoxylin-eosin (H & E) stained tissue sections of scabies mite including mouthparts, spicules and the integument of exoskeleton are depicted in Fig. 3c.

Vaccination trial, lesion areas and mite burden

The protective effects of the rSsCLP5-based vaccine were assessed by grading the inflammatory response and measurement of the lesion area after challenge. Five days post-challenge, inflammation in most of the infested hind feet and itching symptoms were observed in rabbits in all six groups. Ten days post-challenge, the clinical symptoms in 74.3% (26/35; one death) of the rabbits in the three test groups had resolved and showed no significant differences compared to the challenge-free rabbits. However, the three control groups showed more severe clinical symptoms than that of the test groups at 2 weeks post-challenge, including significant inflammation and itching. Meanwhile, some rabbits in the control groups began to produce crusts (Fig. 4b). With the progression of challenge infestation till 4 weeks, the differences in clinical symptoms between the control and test groups were more significant (Fig. 4c). As shown by the grades of the inflammatory reaction in Fig. 5a, each of the control groups had mean scores > 1 at 2 weeks post-challenge, and even the mean score of the PBS group was close to 2. Conversely, the test groups all had mean scores < 1. After 4 weeks post-challenge, the rabbits in the control groups presented severe scabies with mean scores > 4; however, only 9 rabbits had higher scores (≥ 3 points) in the test groups (Fig. 5b). The scores of the inflammatory reaction in the control groups (two deaths) were significantly higher compared to the test groups (one death) at 4 weeks post-challenge ($F_{(5,63)} = 23.38$, $P < 0.0001$), and the differences became more apparent over the course of the infestation.

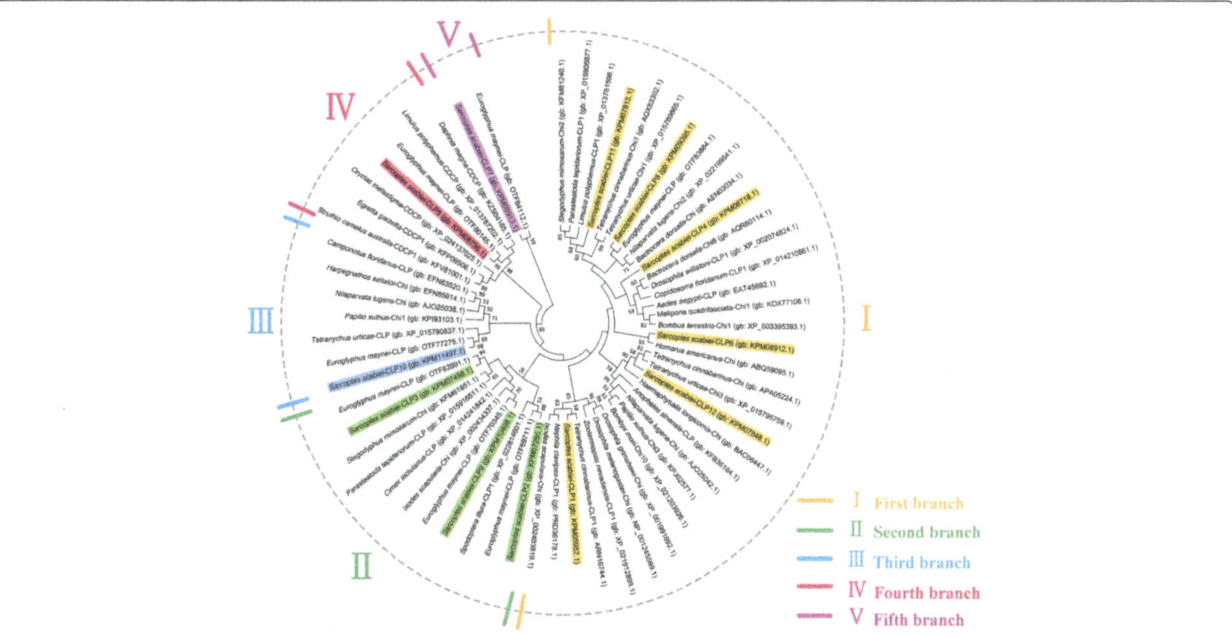

Fig. 1 Phylogenetic relationships between SsCLPs and CLPs and chitinases from other species. The unrooted phylogenetic tree was constructed using CLP and chitinase sequences from approximately 40 species by the maximum likelihood (ML) method in MEGA software. CLP sequences or chitinase sequences were used in the tree (with their GenBank or SwissProt accession numbers). The number behind the protein acronym (for example Chi1, CLP2, CLP3, etc.) is from the NCBI database which represents more than one kind of protein in the species. Accession numbers are as follows: *Stegodyphus mimosarum*-Chi2 (gb: KFM81240.1); *Parasteatoda tepidariorum*-CLP1 (gb: XP_015906877.1); *Limulus polyphemus*-CLP1 (gb: XP_013781598.1); *S. scabiei*-CLP11 (gb: KPM07813.1); *Tetranychus cinnabarinus*-Chi1 (gb: AQX83302.1); *Tetranychus urticae*-Chi1 (gb: XP_015789865.1); *S. scabiei*-CLP8 (gb: KPM09395.1); *E. maynei*-CLP (gb: OTF83884.1); *Nilaparvata lugens*-Chi2 (gb: XP_022199541.1); *Bactrocera dorsalis*-Chi (gb: AEN03034.1); *S. scabiei*-CLP4 (gb: KPM08718.1); *B. dorsalis*-Chi8 (gb: AQR60114.1); *Drosophila willistoni*-CLP1 (gb: XP_002074824.1); *Copidosoma floridanum*-CLP1 (gb: XP_014210861.1); *Aedes aegypti*-CLP (gb: EAT45692.1); *Melipona quadrifasciata*-Chi1 (gb: KOX77106.1); *Bombus terrestris*-Chi1 (gb: XP_003395393.1); *S. scabiei*-CLP6 (gb: KPM08912.1); *Homarus americanus*-Chi (gb: ABQ59095.1); *T. cinnabarinus*-Chi (gb: APA05224.1); *T. urticae*-Chi3 (gb: XP_015795759.1); *S. scabiei*-CLP12 (gb: KPM07848.1); *Haemaphysalis longicornis*-Chi (gb: BAC06447.1); *Anopheles sinensis*-CLP (gb: KFB36184.1); *N. lugens*-Chi (gb: AJO25042.1); *Papilio xuthus*-Chi3 (gb: KPJ02577.1); *Bombyx mori*-Chi10 (gb: XP_021203926.1); *Drosophila grimshawi*-Chi (gb: XP_001991892.1); *Drosophila melanogaster*-Chi (gb: NP_001245599.1); *Zootermopsis nevadensis*-CLP1 (gb: XP_021912899.1); *T. cinnabarinus*-CLP1 (gb: ARN16744.1); *S. scabiei*-CLP1 (gb: KPM05982.1); *Nephila clavipes*-CLP1 (gb: PRD36178.1); *Ixodes scapularis*-Chi (gb: XP_002403819.1); *S. scabiei*-CLP2 (gb: KPM07295.1); *E. maynei*-CLP (gb: OTF69711.1) ; *Spodoptera litura*-CLP1 (gb: XP_022814601.1); *S. scabiei*-CLP9 (gb: KPM10408.1); *E. maynei*-CLP (gb:OTF70345.1); *I. scapularis*-Chi (gb: XP_002434337.1); *Cimex lectularius*-CLP (gb: XP_014241842.1); *P. tepidariorum*-CLP (gb: XP_015916511.1); *S. mimosarum*-Chi (gb: KFM61851.1); *S. scabiei*-CLP3 (gb: KPM07498.1); *E. maynei*-CLP (gb: OTF83991.1); *S. scabiei*-CLP10 (gb: KPM11497.1); *E. maynei*-CLP (gb: OTF77275.1); *T. urticae*-CLP (gb: XP_015790837.1); *P. xuthus*-Chi1 (gb: KPI93103.1); *N. lugens*-Chi (gb: AJO25038.1); *Harpegnathos saltator*-Chi (gb: EFN85614.1); *Camponotus floridanus*-CLP (gb: EFN63520.1); *Struthio camelus australis*-CDCP1 (gb: KFV81001.1) CDCP1; *Egretta garzetta*-CDCP1 (gb: KFP09506.1); *Oryzias melastigma*-CDCP (gb: XP_024137025.1); *S. scabiei*-CLP5 (gb: KPM08736.1); *E. maynei*-CLP (gb: OTF80145.1); *L. polyphemus*-CDCP (gb: XP_013787202.1); *Daphnia magna*-CDCP (gb: KZS04185.1); *S. scabiei*-CLP7 (gb: KPM08913.1) and *E. maynei*-CLP (gb: OTF84112.1). *Abbreviations*: gb, GenBank or SwissProt accession numbers; Chi, chitinase; CLP, chitinase-like protein; CDCP, chitinase domain-containing protein

As for the lesion area at week 4 post-challenge, our results showed that the mean values of lesion areas in PBS, QuilA, and vector protein groups were 18.86 cm^2, 17.19 cm^2, and 14.74 cm^2, respectively. However, 74.3% of rabbits (26/35) immunized with rSsCLP5 had no detectable lesions or very sparse horny hyperplasia (Fig. 6). Moreover, the levels of skin lesions in control groups were significantly higher compared to the rSsCLP5 immunized groups ($F_{(5,63)}$ = 36.99, $P < 0.0001$). At the end of the trial, nearly 80% of the 69 rabbits showed different degrees of body weight gain from 0.1 to 0.35 kg at 4 weeks post-challenge compared to prior immunization weights (Fig. 7). Some of rabbits (13 rabbits, nearly 20%) from three control groups showed weight loss ranging from 0.05 to 0.25 kg; however, in the rSsCLP5 immunized group, weight loss (0.15 kg of body weight) was only observed in one rabbit (Fig. 7). Further observations revealed that the scabies did not spread to forelimbs at the end of the vaccination trial. We also analyzed the mite burden in the hind limbs, which serves as an indicator of the protective value of the rSsCLP5-based vaccine (Fig. 8). The mean number of mites was significantly higher ($F_{(5,63)}$ = 39.354, $P < 0.0001$) in the control groups (more than 4000 mites/rabbit) compared to rSsCLP5 vaccinated groups (nearly 1000 mites/rabbit).

Antibody responses

The optimal conditions for the rSsCLP5-based indirect ELISA were determined to be 4 μg/ml of rSsCLP5 protein,

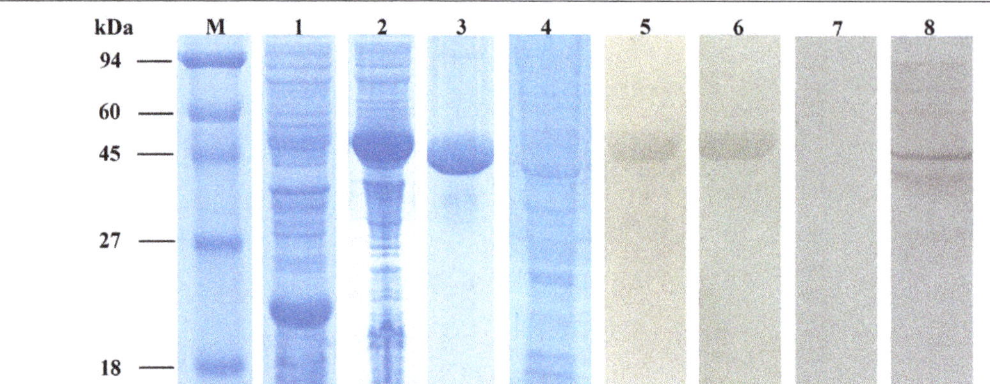

Fig. 2 SDS-PAGE and western blotting of SsCLP5. Lane M: protein molecular weight markers (in kDa); Lane 1: pet-32a (+) expression vector protein; Lane 2: non-purified rSsCLP5 [soluble protein expressed from *Escherichia* coli BL21 (DE3)]; Lane 3: purified rSsCLP5; Lane 4: total crude proteins from *S. scabiei*; Lane 5: purified rSsCLP5 detected by serum (diluted 1:120 with 0.01 M PBS) from a rabbit naturally infested with *S. scabiei* (experimental group); Lane 6: purified rSsCLP5 detected by serum (diluted 1:120 with 0.01 M PBS) from a rSsCLP5-vaccinated rabbit (positive control); Lane 7: purified rSsCLP5 detected by pre-immune rabbit serum (diluted 1:120 with 0.01 M PBS; negative control); Lane 8: total crude proteins detected with rabbit anti-rSsCLP5 serum (diluted 1:120 with 0.01 M PBS). Samples derived from the same experiment and gels/blots were processed in parallel

a 1:120 serum dilution, and a 1:3000 dilution of secondary antibody. Specific IgG antibody was detected by rSsCLP5-based indirect ELISA as previously described [37]. The results showed that the specific IgG antibodies increased at one week after the first vaccination in the rSsCLP5 vaccine groups, and levels were significantly higher than the antibody levels of three control groups ($F_{(5,63)}$ = 37.285, $P <$ 0.0001) (Fig. 9). At the same time, the IgG antibody levels observed in the vector protein group also increased, but at lower levels than in the rSsCLP5 vaccine groups. Two weeks after the second immunization, the specific IgG antibodies levels increased to the highest value (OD 450 nm ~1.4) and stabilized at high levels after the challenge in the three vaccinated groups. The IgG levels in the vaccinated groups were also significantly higher than in the controls at two weeks after the second immunization ($F_{(5,63)}$ = 614.491, $P < 0.0001$). In our pilot experiments, the high antibody levels increased to OD 450 nm ~1.8 and were stable for more than three months (data not shown). In the QuilA saponin and PBS control groups, the OD 450 nm values of specific IgG remained low throughout the experiment (Fig. 9). Additionally, the low levels antibody of the vector protein group rapidly decreased during the experimental period (Fig. 9).

Discussion

Chitinases and CLPs are a diverse group of proteins, as shown in the phylogenetic tree, with more than five categories of enzymes and proteins. It has been reported that these enzymes and proteins have a complex array of functions in mites and hosts, including roles in ecdysis, digestion, allergic reactions, immune response and resistance to infection, among others [42–44]. In western blotting experiments, the serum from rabbits infested with *S. scabiei* produced a strong signal on the blot, indicating that the SsCLP5 plays an important role in eliciting an immune response during natural infestation. When we used serum from rabbits inoculated with rSsCLP5 to probe the total body extracts of the mites, we detected the antigen signal at ~45 kDa, suggesting

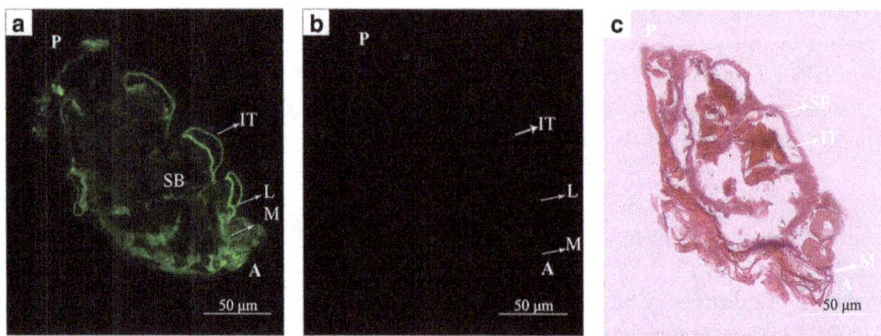

Fig. 3 Immunolocalization of SsCLP5 in *S. scabiei* tissue (**a**, **b**) and H & E sections of *S. scabiei*. **a** *S. scabiei* incubated with anti-rSsCLP5 antibody as the primary antibody. **b** Negative control (antibody of the pre-immune rabbit serum), **c** H & E sections of *S. scabiei*. *Abbreviations*: A, anterior end of mite; P, posterior end of mite; IT, integument of the exoskeleton; M, mouthparts; L, legs; SP, spicules; SB, stomach blocks

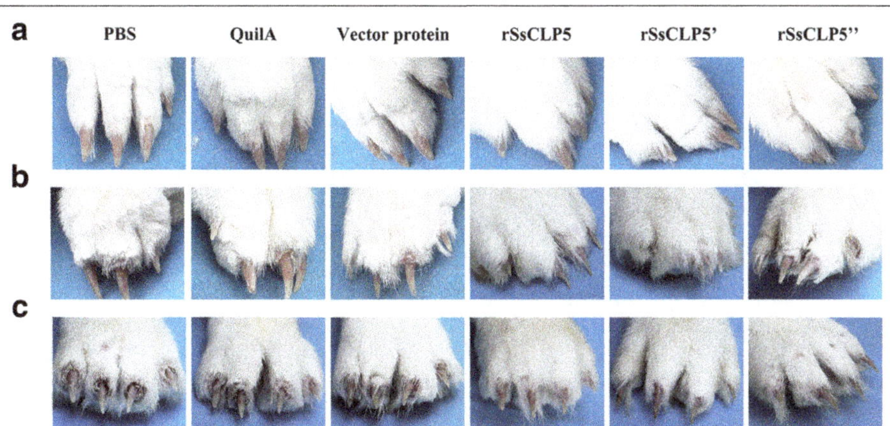

Fig. 4 Clinical symptoms in rabbits before, two and four weeks post-challenge. Series **a** shows normal hind limbs in rabbits before challenge, series **b** shows clinical symptoms of hind limbs in rabbits after challenge with scabies mites for two weeks, and series **c** shows clinical symptoms of hind limbs in rabbits after challenge with scabies mites for four weeks. *Key*: PBS, immunized with 1 ml 0.01 M PBS each time; Quil A, immunized with 1 ml QuilA saponin at concentration of 1 mg/ml (dissolved in PBS) each time; vector protein, immunized with 100 μg (first time) and 200 μg (second time) purified pET32a(+) vector protein with 1 ml QuilA saponin at concentration of 1 mg/ml (dissolved in PBS); rSsCLP5, rSsCLP5′, and rSsCLP5″ refer to the test groups immunized with 100 μg then 200 μg purified rSsCLP5 protein with 1 ml QuilA saponin at concentration of 1 mg/ml (dissolved in PBS) at the first and second immunizations

that the protein is high expression in mites as previously reported [26].

Fluorescence immunohistochemistry assays showed strong fluorescence signals of SsCLP5 present in the exoskeleton, chewing mouthpart and legs of *S. scabiei*. Signals were especially strong in the outer layer of the exoskeleton, suggesting that the SsCLP5 is highly expressed in the exoskeleton of scabies mites. Thus, it is possible that this protein presents in the epidermis of the rabbit after the death and lysis of mites, and the further recurrent immune responses in the host cannot be entirely ruled out. It has been reported that homologous proteins in other species are immune-related proteins that can cause different levels of immune responses in hosts [45–48]. The high expression of SsCLP5 supports its potential as a candidate vaccine protein against *S. scabiei*.

During the immunization trial, some rabbits in the mite control group examined at 4 weeks post-challenge showed severe scabies and weight loss, which is associated with scabies as a chronic wasting disease. Previous reports have similarly observed that severe scabies results in decreased body weight in rabbits and other animals, both in the wild and in laboratory animal models [49, 50]. In our study, the majority of rabbits vaccinated with rSsCLP5 and challenged with the scabies mite displayed weight gain due to the protective effects of rSsCLP5 and because the rabbits were in a growth and development stage. Interestingly, previous work has shown that re-infested animals show a reduced mite burden as compared to the initial mite infestation [20, 21, 51]. These reports demonstrate that mites or mite secretions induce immune protection in the host. Additionally, immunization of rabbits with whole body extracts of *S. scabiei* (var. *canis*) induced antibodies to more antigens than infestation with the mite [52]. Based on these and other recombinant protein studies [22, 24], we chose to immunize rabbits twice with an increasing dose of rSsCLP5 to obtain higher antibody levels. We created a grading scale to assess the severity of skin lesions caused by the mites. We observed that rabbits immunized with the rSsCLP5 acquired immune protection and the majority of the rabbits (74.3%) had no detectable lesions showing successful development of resistance against the scabies at four weeks post-challenge. We observed significant differences between the groups immunized with rSsCLP5 and control groups with respect to inflammation and lesion area at week 2 post-challenge ($F_{(5,63)}$ = 13.575, $P < 0.0001$) and at week 4 post-challenge ($F_{(5,63)}$ = 23.38, $P < 0.0001$). Approximately five days after the challenge, a comparison of all groups showed that the skin of the hind feet in all of the rabbits was severely inflamed. These symptoms gradually subsided by day 10 post-infestation. This could be associated with the release of substances that induce inflammatory and immune responses by the mites [53–55] and/or the inhibition of early immune responses by *S. scabiei* by downregulating the expression of pro-inflammatory mediators and cytokines [54, 56–58]. Studies of the life-cycle and infestation of *S. scabiei* found that most mites (*S. scabiei* var. *canis*) rapidly initiate penetration of the skin of the rabbit host [59] and develop from egg to adult in 10–13 days [60]. Immunomodulation by the mites, which appears to impact the development of the immune response during infestation in hosts, might explain why some animals fail to develop resistance to re-infestation by *S. scabiei* [61, 62]. In our study,

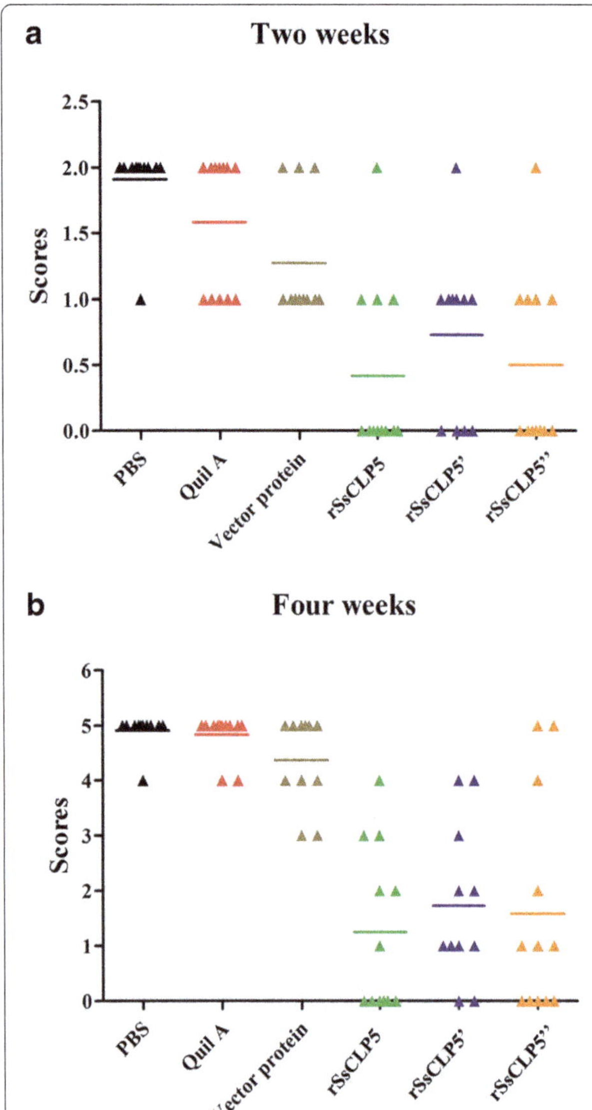

Fig. 5 Inflammatory reaction grades and skin lesions at two (**a**) and four weeks (**b**) post-challenge. The colored lines indicate the group average. *Key*: PBS, immunized with 1 ml 0.01 M PBS each time; Quil A, immunized with 1 ml QuilA saponin at concentration of 1 mg/ml (dissolved in PBS) each time; vector protein, immunized with 100 µg (first time) and 200 µg (second time) purified pET32a(+) vector protein with 1 ml QuilA saponin at concentration of 1 mg/ml (dissolved in PBS); rSsCLP5, rSsCLP5', and rSsCLP5" refer to the test groups immunized with 100 µg then 200 µg purified rSsCLP5 protein with 1 ml QuilA saponin at concentration of 1 mg/ml (dissolved in PBS) at the first and second immunizations. The grades of inflammatory reaction and skin lesions in the rSsCLP5 immunized groups (rSsCLP5, rSsCLP5', and rSsCLP5") were significantly lower compared to the control groups at week 2 post-challenge ($F_{(5,63)} = 13.575$, $P < 0.0001$) and at week 4 post-challenge ($F_{(5,63)} = 23.38$, $P < 0.0001$)

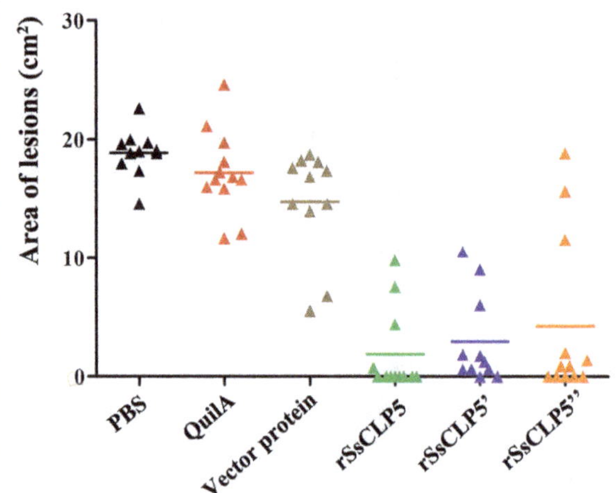

Fig. 6 Area of lesions on rabbit hind limbs at four weeks post-challenge. The colored lines indicate the group average. *Key*: PBS, immunized with 1 ml 0.01 M PBS each time; Quil A, immunized with 1 ml QuilA saponin at concentration of 1 mg/ml (dissolved in PBS) each time; vector protein, immunized with 100 µg (first time) and 200 µg (second time) purified pET32a(+) vector protein with 1 ml QuilA saponin at concentration of 1 mg/ml (dissolved in PBS); rSsCLP5, rSsCLP5', and rSsCLP5" refer to the test groups immunized with 100 µg then 200 µg purified rSsCLP5 protein with 1 ml QuilA saponin at concentration of 1 mg/ml (dissolved in PBS) at the first and second immunizations. The values of area of lesions in the rSsCLP5 immunized groups (rSsCLP5, rSsCLP5', and rSsCLP5") were significantly lower compared to PBS control, Quil A control and vector protein control at week 4 post-challenge ($F_{(5,63)} = 36.99$, $P < 0.0001$)

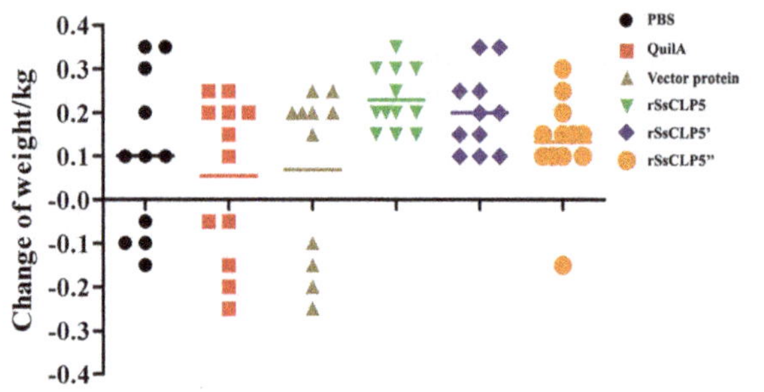

Fig. 7 Weight changes of the rabbits at week 4 post-challenge compared to prior immunization. The colored lines indicate the group average. *Key*: PBS, immunized with 1 ml 0.01 M PBS each time; Quil A, immunized with 1 ml QuilA saponin at concentration of 1 mg/ml (dissolved in PBS) each time; vector protein, immunized with 100 µg (first time) and 200 µg (second time) purified pET32a(+) vector protein with 1 ml QuilA saponin at concentration of 1 mg/ml (dissolved in PBS); rSsCLP5, rSsCLP5', and rSsCLP5" refer to the test groups immunized with 100 µg then 200 µg purified rSsCLP protein with 1 ml QuilA saponin at concentration of 1 mg/ml (dissolved in PBS) at the first and second immunizations. The weight changes of rabbits in the rSsCLP5 immunized groups (rSsCLP5 and rSsCLP5') were significantly higher compared to PBS control, Quil A control and vector protein control at week 4 post-challenge ($F_{(5,63)} = 2.689$, $P = 0.029$)

although we observed inflammation and lesions in some of the rabbits in the vaccinated group, the extent was lower than that observed in the infected control groups. On week 4 post-challenge, the mean values of the mite

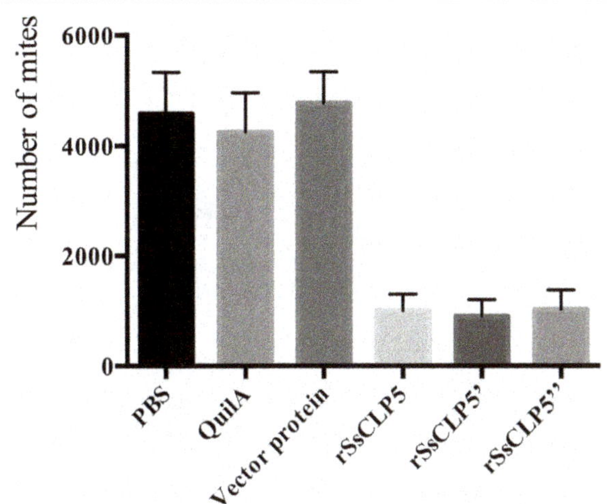

Fig. 8 Mite burden in rabbits at week 4 post-challenge. *Key*: PBS, immunized with 1 ml 0.01 M PBS each time; Quil A, immunized with 1 ml QuilA saponin at concentration of 1 mg/ml (dissolved in PBS) each time; vector protein, immunized with 100 μg (first time) and 200 μg (second time) purified pET32a(+) vector protein with 1 ml QuilA saponin at concentration of 1 mg/ml (dissolved in PBS); rSsCLP5, rSsCLP5', and rSsCLP5" refer to the test groups immunized with 100 μg then 200 μg purified rSsCLP protein with 1 ml QuilA saponin at concentration of 1 mg/ml (dissolved in PBS) at the first and second immunizations. Data columns correspond to the mean values; error bars represent the standard error. The mean values of mite burden in test groups immunized with rSsCLP5 were significantly lower compared to the control groups at week 4 post-challenge ($F_{(5,63)} = 39.354$, $P < 0.0001$)

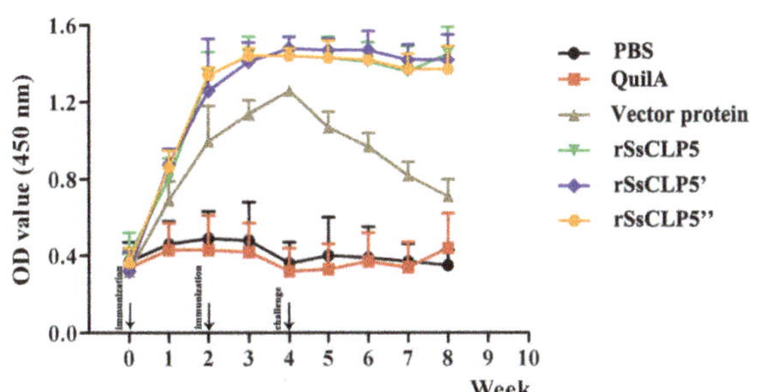

Fig. 9 Variation of specific IgG antibody levels in sera of immunized rabbits as detected by ELISA. Rabbits were immunized twice. *Key*: PBS, immunized with 1 ml 0.01 M PBS each time; Quil A, immunized with 1 ml QuilA saponin at concentration of 1 mg/ml (dissolved in PBS) each time; vector protein, immunized with 100 μg (first time) and 200 μg (second time) purified pET32a(+) vector protein with 1 ml QuilA saponin at concentration of 1 mg/ml (dissolved in PBS); rSsCLP5, rSsCLP5', and rSsCLP5" refer to the test groups immunized with 100 μg then 200 μg purified rSsCLP5 protein with 1 ml QuilA saponin at concentration of 1 mg/ml (dissolved in PBS) at the first and second immunizations. Data points correspond to the mean values; error bars represent the standard error. The groups immunized with the rSsCLP5 had significantly higher IgG levels compared to the control groups ($F_{(5,63)} = 37.285$, $P < 0.0001$) from week 1 after first immunization to the end of the experiment

burden in test groups were significantly lower compared to the control groups ($F_{(5,63)} = 39.354$, $P < 0.0001$). These differences in mite burden between the control and treated groups may be attributed to the immune protection induced by rSsCLP5 in the latter groups. Furthermore, immunization of rabbits with rSsCLP5 might have affected the ability of mites to infect, grow and reproduce.

A previous study found no protective effect when vaccinating goats with the extract of scabies mites [51]. Vaccination trials of rabbits with the recombinant antigens Ssag1 and Ssag2 (*S. scabiei* var. *hominis*) produced antibodies, but the rabbits displayed no protection or reduced mite burden [63]. In this study, we observed that the IgG levels in the adjuvant group and the PBS control group did not change significantly and maintained relatively stable levels after immunization. In the group immunized with the protein from the empty vector, antibody levels peaked 2 weeks after the second immunization. However, the antibody levels showed a very rapid decrease after a short time with no protective effects, indicating that the vector protein had little or no effect on the immunization effects of rSsCLP5 and production of the specific antibody. Additionally, both the inflammatory grades and lesion areas of animals in the vector protein group were higher than in the rSsCLP5 vaccinated groups. In the three test groups, the antibody levels reached the highest values (OD450 ~1.4) 2 weeks after the second immunization with rSsCLP5, with levels persisting for a longer period of time. Previous studies found that vaccinated rabbits exhibited high levels of IgG and increased total IgE levels when immunized with a mix of the recombinant antigens Ssλ20ΔB3 and GST-Ssλ15 (*S. scabiei* var. hominis); however, the rabbits had no protection against mite challenge [64]. In contrast, our study found high levels of antibodies to be produced and, importantly, our results showed that rSsCLP5 could induce immune protection. Three vaccinated groups showed different levels of protection against scabies mite infestation. The majority (74.3%) of rabbits did not show clinical symptoms of scabies after challenge with *S. scabiei*; however, some did show different degrees of infestation. The degree of infestation was not as serious as in the unvaccinated control groups and furthermore, rabbits will not develop scabies with an extremely small number of mites.

Taken together, our findings support the further testing of a rSsCLP5-based vaccine for *S. scabiei*. Future work focusing on optimizing parameters such as the protein concentrations required for an effective vaccine, the use of adjuvants, the number of immunizations, and the time interval between different injections will be of great value. In particular, investigations providing insights regarding the term protection of these candidate vaccine proteins are awaited.

Conclusions

In summary, SsCLP5 was identified and characterized in the present study. Furthermore, we evaluated rSsCLP5 as candidate vaccine protein for anti-mite protection in rabbits. Importantly, our data demonstrate that rSsCLP5 is a promising candidate for a recombinant protein-based vaccine against *S. scabiei*. This study also provides a method for studying scabies vaccine using rabbit as an animal model and a basis for screening more effective candidate proteins.

Abbreviations

CLPs: Chitinase-like proteins; ELISA: Enzyme-linked immunosorbent assay; HRP: Horseradish peroxidase; IPTG: Isopropyl-beta-D-thiogalactopyranoside; PBS: Phosphate-buffered saline; rSsCLP5: Recombinant *S. scabiei* chitinase-like protein 5; SsCLP5: *S. scabiei* chitinase-like protein 5; TBST: Tris-buffered saline and Tween 20

Acknowledgements

The authors thank Xibin Zhao and Yuchen Liu for their contributions. We are also extremely grateful to teachers and classmates at the Laboratory of Animal Infectious Disease and Microarray of Sichuan Province in Sichuan Agricultural University for kindly allowing us to conduct the protein purification experiments and use their fluorescence microscope in their laboratories. We would like to thank the native English speaking scientists of Elixigen Company (Huntington Beach, California) for editing our manuscript. We are also really appreciative of Christiana Angel from our department, whose native language is English, for correcting the English in the final version of the manuscript.

Funding

This work was supported by a grant from the Research Fund for the Chengdu Research of Giant Panda Breeding (project no. CPF2014-17). The funder had no role in study design, data collection and analysis, preparation or publication of the manuscript.

Authors' contributions

SNX participated in the design of the study, feeding experimental animals, the experiments, statistical analysis and manuscript writing. ZHJ fed experimental animals and performed the experiments. RYJ, HR, XJ and LCY contributed to sample collection and performed the experiments. YGY participated in the design of the study. LWM, GXB, XY and PXR helped in study design. All authors read and approved the final manuscript.

Competing interests

The authors declare that they have no competing interests.

Author details

[1]Department of Parasitology, College of Veterinary Medicine, Sichuan Agricultural University, Chengdu 611130, China. [2]Animal Breeding and Genetics Key Laboratory of Sichuan Province, Chengdu 610066, China. [3]Department of Chemistry, College of Life and Basic Science, Sichuan Agricultural University, Chengdu 611130, China.

References

1. Hengge UR, Currie BJ, Jäger G, Lupi O, Schwartz RA. Scabies: a ubiquitous neglected skin disease. Lancet Infect Dis. 2006;6:769–79.
2. Alasaad S, Rossi L, Heukelbach J, Pérez JM, Hamarsheh O, Otiende M, et al. The neglected navigating web of the incomprehensibly emerging and re-emerging *Sarcoptes* mite. Infect Genet Evol. 2013;17:253–9.
3. Bornstein S, Mörner T, Samuel WM. *Sarcoptes scabiei* and sarcoptic mange. Des Moines: Iowa State University Press; 2008. p. 107–19.
4. McCarthy J, Kemp DJ, Walton SF, Currie B. Scabies: more than just an irritation. Postgrad Med J. 2004;80:382–7.
5. Terry BC, Kanjah F, Sahr F, Kortequee S, Dukulay I, Gbakima AA. *Sarcoptes scabiei* infestation among children in a displacement camp in Sierra Leone. Public Health. 2001;115:208–11.
6. Heukelbach J, Scabies FH. Lancet. 2006;367:1767–74.
7. Walton SF, Holt DC, Currie BJ, Kemp DJ. Scabies: new future for a neglected disease. Adv Parasitol. 2004;57:309–76.
8. Rehbein S, Visser M, Winter R, Trommer B, Matthes HF, Maciel AE, et al. Productivity effects of bovine mange and control with ivermectin. Vet Parasitol. 2003;114:267–84.
9. Pence DB, Ueckermann E. Sarcoptic mange in wildlife. Rev Sci Et Tech. 2002;21:385–98.
10. Andrews RM, Mccarthy J, Carapetis JR, Currie BJ. Skin disorders, including pyoderma, scabies, and tinea infections. Pediatr Clin North Am. 2009;56: 1421–40.
11. WHO. The current evidence for the burden of group A streptococcal diseases. Sexual Health. Geneva: World Health Organization; 2004. p. 21.
12. Walker GJ, Johnstone PW. Interventions for treating scabies. Cochrane Database Syst Rev. 2000;3:CD000320.
13. Friedman SJ. Lindane neurotoxic reaction in nonbullous congenital ichthyosiform erythroderma. Arch Dermatol. 1987;123:1056–8.
14. Elgart ML. A risk-benefit assessment of agents used in the treatment of scabies. Drug Saf. 1996;14:386–93.
15. Wagner R, Wendlberger U. Field efficacy of moxidectin in dogs and rabbits naturally infested with *Sarcoptes* spp., *Demodex* spp. and *Psoroptes* spp. mites. Vet Parasitol. 2000;93:149–58.
16. Pasay C, Walton S, Fischer K, Holt D, Mccarthy J. PCR-based assay to survey for knockdown resistance to pyrethroid acaricides in human scabies mites (*Sarcoptes scabiei* var. *hominis*). Am J Trop Med Hyg. 2006;74:649–57.
17. Currie BJ, Harumal P, Mckinnon M, Walton SF. First documentation of *in vivo* and *in vitro* ivermectin resistance in *Sarcoptes scabiei*. Clin Infect Dis. 2004; 39:e8–e12.
18. Terada Y, Murayama N, Ikemura H, Morita T, Nagata M. *Sarcoptes scabiei* var. *canis* refractory to ivermectin treatment in two dogs. Vet Dermatol. 2010;21: 608–12.
19. Cote NM, Jaworski DC, Wasala NB, Morgan MS, Arlian LG. Identification and expression of macrophage migration inhibitory factor in *Sarcoptes scabiei*. Exp Parasitol. 2013;135:175–81.
20. Arlian LG, Morgan MS, Vyszenskimoher DL, Stemmer BL. *Sarcoptes scabiei*: the circulating antibody response and induced immunity to scabies. Exp Parasitol. 1994;78:37–50.
21. Mellanby K. The development of symptoms, parasitic infection and immunity in human scabies. Parasitology. 1944;35:197–206.
22. Casais R, Dalton KP, Millán J, Balseiro A, Oleaga Á, Solano P, et al. Primary and secondary experimental infestation of rabbits (*Oryctolagus cuniculus*) with *Sarcoptes scabiei* from a wild rabbit: factors determining resistance to reinfestation. Vet Parasitol. 2014;203:173–83.
23. Bhat SA, Mounsey KE, Liu X, Walton SF. Host immune responses to the itch mite, *Sarcoptes scabiei*. in humans. Parasit Vectors. 2017;10:385.
24. Zhang R, Jise Q, Zheng W, Ren Y, Nong X, Wu X, et al. Characterization and evaluation of a *Sarcoptes scabiei* allergen as a candidate vaccine. Parasit Vectors. 2012;5:176.
25. Rider SD Jr, Morgan MS, Arlian LG. Draft genome of the scabies mite. Parasit Vectors. 2015;8:585.
26. He R, Gu X, Lai W, Peng X, Yang G. Transcriptome-microRNA analysis of *Sarcoptes scabiei* and host immune response. PLoS One. 2017;12:e0177733.
27. Morgan MS, Arlian LG, Rider SD, Grunwald WC. Cool DR. A proteomic analysis of *Sarcoptes scabiei* (Acari: Sarcoptidae). J Med Entomol. 2016;53:553–61.
28. Sutherland TE, Maizels RM, Allen JE. Chitinases and chitinase-like proteins: potential therapeutic targets for the treatment of T-helper type 2 allergies. Clin Exp Allergy. 2009;39:943–55.

29. Bargagli E, Margollicci M, Luddi A, Nikiforakis N, Perari MG, Grosso S, et al. Chitotriosidase activity in patients with interstitial lung diseases. Respir Med. 2007;101:2176–81.
30. Zhu Z, Zheng T, Homer RJ, Kim Y, Chen NY, Cohn L, et al. Acidic mammalian chitinase in asthmatic Th2 inflammation and IL-13 pathway activation. Science. 2004;304:1678–82.
31. Nair MG, Gallagher IJ, Taylor MD, Loke P, Coulson PS, Wilson RA, et al. Chitinase and Fizz family members are a generalized feature of nematode infection with selective upregulation of Ym1 and Fizz1 by antigen-presenting cells. Infect Immun. 2005;73:385–94.
32. Chang NC, Hung SI, Hwa KY, Kato I, Chen JE, Liu CH, et al. A macrophage protein, Ym1, transiently expressed during inflammation is a novel mammalian lectin. J Biol Chem. 2001;276:17497–506.
33. Loke PN, Nair MG, Parkinson J, Guiliano D, Blaxter M, Allen JE. IL-4 dependent alternatively-activated macrophages have a distinctive in vivo gene expression phenotype. BMC Immunol. 2002;3:7.
34. Sandler NG, Mentinkkane MM, Cheever AW, Wynn TA. Global gene expression profiles during acute pathogen-induced pulmonary inflammation reveal divergent roles for Th1 and Th2 responses in tissue repair. J Immunol. 2003;171:3655–67.
35. Xie Y, Zhou X, Chen L, Zhang Z, Wang C, Gu X, et al. Cloning and characterization of a novel sigma-like glutathione S-transferase from the giant panda parasitic nematode, *Baylisascaris schroederi*. Parasit Vectors. 2015;8:1–13.
36. García-Varela M, Sereno-Uribe AL, Pinacho-Pinacho CD, Domínguez-Domínguez O. Pérez-Ponce de León G. Molecular and morphological characterization of *Austrodiplostomum ostrowskiae* Dronen, 2009 (Digenea: Diplostomatidae), a parasite of cormorants in the Americas. J Helminthol. 2016;90:174–85.
37. Shen N, He R, Liang Y, Xu J, He M, Ren Y, et al. Expression and characterisation of a *Sarcoptes scabiei* protein tyrosine kinase as a potential antigen for scabies diagnosis. Sci Rep. 2017;7:9639.
38. Rodríguezcadenas F, Carbajalgonzález MT, Fregenedagrandes JM, Allergancedo JM, Rojovázquez FA. Clinical evaluation and antibody responses in sheep after primary and secondary experimental challenges with the mange mite *Sarcoptes scabiei* var. *ovis*. Vet Immunol Immunopathol. 2010;133:109–16.
39. Crowther JR. The ELISA Guidebook. vol. 14. Nairobi: Springer Science & Business Media; 2000.
40. R Core Team. R: A language and environment for statistical computing. Vienna: R Foundation for Statistical Computing; 2013. p. 12–21.
41. Lawrence MA. ez: Easy analysis and visualization of factorial experiments. R package version. 2013;4:2-2 http://CRAN.R-project.org/package=ez. Accessed 26 Jul 2016.
42. de las Mercedes Dana M, Pintor-Toro JA, Cubero B. Transgenic tobacco plants overexpressing chitinases of fungal origin show enhanced resistance to biotic and abiotic stress agents. Plant Physiol. 2006;142:722–30.
43. Bussink AP, Speijer D, Aerts JM, Boot RG. Evolution of mammalian chitinase(-like) members of family 18 glycosyl hydrolases. Genetics. 2007;177:959–70.
44. Funkhouser JD, Aronson NN. Chitinase family GH18: evolutionary insights from the genomic history of a diverse protein family. BMC Evol Biol. 2007;7:96.
45. Jin HM, Copeland NG, Gilbert DJ, Jenkins NA, Kirkpatrick RB, Rosenberg M. Genetic characterization of the murine Ym1 gene and identification of a cluster of highly homologous genes. Genomics. 1998;54:316–22.
46. Welch JS, Escoubet-Lozach L, Sykes DB, Liddiard K, Greaves DR, Glass CK. TH2 cytokines and allergic challenge induce Ym1 expression in macrophages by a STAT6-dependent mechanism. J Biol Chem. 2002;277:42821–9.
47. Gordon S. Alternative activation of macrophages. Nat Rev Immunol. 2003;3:23–35.
48. Pesce J, Kaviratne M, Ramalingam TR, Thompson RW, Urban JF, Cheever AW, et al. The IL-21 receptor augments Th2 effector function and alternative macrophage activation. J Clin Invest. 2006;116:2044–55.
49. Baccouche K, Sellam J, Guegan S, Aractingi S, Berenbaum F. Crusted Norwegian scabies, an opportunistic infection, with tocilizumab in rheumatoid arthritis. Joint Bone Spine. 2011;78:402–4.
50. Lokuge B, Kopczynski A, Woltmann A, Alvoen F, Connors C, Guyula T, et al. Crusted scabies in remote Australia, a new way forward: lessons and outcomes from the East Arnhem Scabies Control Program. Med J Aust. 2014;200:644–8.
51. Tarigan S, Huntley JF. Failure to protect goats following vaccination with soluble proteins of *Sarcoptes scabiei*: evidence for a role for IgE antibody in protection. Vet Parasitol. 2005;133:101–9.
52. Morgan MS, Arlian LG. Serum antibody profiles of *Sarcoptes scabiei* infested or immunized rabbits. Folia Parasitol. 1994;41:223–7.
53. Walton SF, Meeusen EN, Engwerda CR. The immunology of susceptibility and resistance to scabies. Parasite Immunol. 2010;32:532–40.
54. Arlian LG, Morgan MS, Neal JS. Modulation of cytokine expression in human keratinocytes and fibroblasts by extracts of scabies mites. Am J Trop Med Hyg. 2003;69:652–6.
55. Mullins JS, Arlian LG, Morgan MS. Extracts of *Sarcoptes scabiei* De Geer downmodulate secretion of IL-8 by skin keratinocytes and fibroblasts and of GM-CSF by fibroblasts in the presence of proinflammatory cytokines. J Med Entomol. 2009;46:845–51.
56. Arlian LG, Morgan MS, Neal JS. Extracts of scabies mites (Sarcoptidae: *Sarcoptes scabiei*) modulate cytokine expression by human peripheral blood mononuclear cells and dendritic cells. J Med Entomol. 2004;41: 69–73.
57. Arlian LG, Fall N, Morgan MS. *In vivo* evidence that *Sarcoptes scabiei* (Acari: Sarcoptidae) is the source of molecules that modulate splenic gene expression. J Med Entomol. 2007;44:1054–63.
58. Elder BL, Arlian LG, Morgan MS. *Sarcoptes scabiei* (Acari: Sarcoptidae) mite extract modulates expression of cytokines and adhesion molecules by human dermal microvascular endothelial cells. J Med Entomol. 2006;43:910–5.
59. Arlian LG, Runyan RA, Achar S, Estes SA. Survival and infectivity of *Sarcoptes scabiei* var. *canis* and var. *hominis*. J Am Acad Dermatol. 1984;11:210–5.
60. Arlian LG, Vyszenskimoher DL. Life cycle of *Sarcoptes scabiei* var. *canis*. J Parasitol. 1988;74:427–30.
61. Little SE, Davidson WR, Rakich PM, Nixon TL, Bounous DI, Nettles VF. Responses of red foxes to first and second infection with *Sarcoptes scabiei*. J Wildl Dis. 1998;34:600–11.
62. Sarasa M, Rambozzi L, Rossi L, Meneguz PG, Serrano E, Granados JE, et al. *Sarcoptes scabiei*: specific immune response to sarcoptic mange in the Iberian ibex *Capra pyrenaica* depends on previous exposure and sex. Exp Parasitol. 2010;124:265–71.
63. Harumal P, Morgan M, Walton SF, Holt DC, Rode J, Arlian LG, et al. Identification of a homologue of a house dust mite allergen in a cDNA library from *Sarcoptes scabiei* var. *hominis* and evaluation of its vaccine potential in a rabbit/*S. scabiei* var. *canis* model. Am J Trop Med Hyg. 2003; 68:54–60.
64. Casais R, Granda V, Balseiro A, Del Cerro A, Dalton KP, Gonzalez R, et al. Vaccination of rabbits with immunodominant antigens from *Sarcoptes scabiei* induced high levels of humoral responses and pro-inflammatory cytokines but confers limited protection. Parasit Vectors. 2016;9:435.

19

Field effectiveness and safety of fluralaner plus moxidectin (Bravecto® Plus) against ticks and fleas: a European randomized, blinded, multicenter field study in naturally-infested client-owned cats

Nadja Rohdich[1*], Eva Zschiesche[1], Oliver Wolf[2], Wolfgang Loehlein[2], Thierry Pobel[3], Maria José Gil[3] and Rainer K. A. Roepke[1]

Abstract

Background: A spot-on formulation containing fluralaner (280 mg/ml) plus moxidectin (14 mg/ml) (Bravecto® Plus) has been developed to provide broad spectrum parasite protection for cats. The effectiveness and safety of this product against ticks and fleas was assessed in a randomized, controlled, 12-week study in client-owned cats in Germany and Spain.

Methods: Eligible households containing at least one cat with at least two fleas and/or two ticks were allocated randomly in a 2:1 ratio to a single treatment with fluralaner plus moxidectin on Day 0, or three 4-weekly treatments with fipronil (Frontline®). Veterinary staff, masked to treatment, completed tick and flea counts on each cat at 14 ± 2 (2 weeks), 28 ± 2 (4 weeks), 56 ± 2 (8 weeks) and 84 ± 2 days (12 weeks) after the initial treatment.

Results: In total, 707 cats (257 with ticks) from 332 households (236 with fleas) were included. *Ixodes ricinus* (78%) and *Rhipicephalus sanguineus* complex (18%) ticks were the most commonly identified. Tick and flea counts were lower in the fluralaner plus moxidectin group than in the fipronil group throughout the study and the efficacy of fluralaner plus moxidectin exceeded 97 and 98%, respectively. At 12 weeks, 94.1 and 93.3% of cats from the fluralaner plus moxidectin and 92.2 and 60.3% of cats from the fipronil group were free of ticks and fleas, respectively. Fluralaner plus moxidectin was non-inferior to fipronil ($P < 0.0001$) at all assessments and superior to fipronil at 2 and 8 weeks for the proportion of cats free of ticks ($P < 0.0001$). Fluralaner plus moxidectin was superior to fipronil for the proportion of both households and cats free of fleas ($P < 0.0001$). Both products were safe and well tolerated.

Conclusions: A single application of fluralaner plus moxidectin spot-on was well tolerated by cats and highly effective for 12 weeks against ticks and fleas. Fluralaner plus moxidectin was non-inferior to fipronil for the proportion of ectoparasite-free and consistently superior to fipronil in controlling fleas.

Keywords: Bravecto Plus, Ectoparasites, Feline, Fipronil, Fleas, Fluralaner, Isoxazoline, Moxidectin, *Rhipicephalus*, Ticks

* Correspondence: nadja.rohdich@msd.de
[1]MSD Animal Health Innovation GmbH, Zur Propstei, 55270 Schwabenheim, Germany
Full list of author information is available at the end of the article

Background

A key part of veterinary preventive healthcare in cats is the treatment and/or prevention of ecto- and endoparasite infestations. The prevalence of flea infestations in cats is generally higher than that of ticks [1]. However, there is a dearth of information on feline tick infestations. The most common genera of ticks that are found on cats are *Ixodes* spp. and *Rhipicephalus* spp. [2, 3], but the overall prevalence of tick infestations is likely underestimated since they may go unnoticed, unless attached to prominent sites on a cat's head, or be removed by grooming behaviour. A recent survey in Austria, Belgium, France, Hungary, Italy, Romania and Spain confirmed tick and/or flea infestation in 16.7% of 1519 client-owned cats [1]. Interestingly, co-infection with gastrointestinal nematodes (most commonly *Toxocara cati*) was found to be common (11.9%).

The modern era of ectoparasite control for cats began in the mid-1990s with the advent of low-volume, monthly-applied topical products. The earliest of these products, fipronil (effective against fleas, with some tick efficacy) and imidacloprid (fleas only), were more convenient in terms of formulation (spot-on, compared to sprays, dusts and bathing) and safer than earlier flea control products (e.g. organophosphates) [4]. The early 2000's saw the introduction of selamectin, a topically applied but systemically acting macrocyclic lactone. Despite lacking tick efficacy in cats, topically applied selamectin provided owners with improved convenience because of its extended spectrum of activity beyond fleas and ear mites (*Otodectes cynotis*) to include treatment of adult intestinal roundworms and intestinal hookworms and prevention of heartworm disease [5]. In 2009, a monthly spot-on combination product containing imidacloprid plus the systemically active macrocyclic lactone moxidectin was registered for use in cats with a similar spectrum of activity as selamectin [6, 7]. More recently, a monthly spot-on product introduced for cats combined fipronil with the insect growth regulator (*S*)-methoprene, the anticestodal agent praziquantel and the macrocyclic lactone eprinomectin to provide efficacy against fleas, ticks, gastrointestinal nematodes, lungworms and tapeworms, and prevention of heartworm disease [8]. In 2017, a combination of selamectin and the isoxazoline sarolaner, both with a systemic mode of action, was commercialized in Europe as a monthly spot-on for cats, extending the spectrum of the selamectin product to include ticks [9]. Thus there has been a substantial evolution in the convenience and spectrum of activity of topically applied products available for cat owners.

Nonetheless, despite these advances, a potential limitation of these products lies in the need for repeated monthly applications. This is important in light of a recent survey in Europe showing that cats treated less than four times per year with monthly products are at a significantly greater risk of flea infestation than those treated more frequently [1]. Similarly, the control of endoparasites is dependent on owner compliance, such as the minimum of four treatments per annum proposed by the European Scientific Council Companion Animal Parasites [10]. Despite this expert guidance, ensuring pet owner compliance with control measures for internal and external parasites in cats and dogs continues to present a substantial challenge for the veterinary profession [11–14]. Therefore there is an ongoing need for products with the potential to improve owner compliance with veterinary treatment recommendations.

A spot-on formulation of fluralaner, an extended-duration isoxazoline compound with potent insecticidal and acaracidal activity in these species, was introduced to help address that need. Clinical studies in client-owned dogs and cats have confirmed the safety and effectiveness of fluralaner in providing up to 12 weeks control of flea and tick infestations under field conditions [15–19]. While there are no reports of methods that would facilitate improved cat owner compliance with veterinary-recommended parasite control programs, a study of dog owners found that fluralaner's sustained activity could lead to improved compliance with such programs [14].

In order to provide a broader spectrum of activity in a low volume spot-on formulation, fluralaner was combined with moxidectin, a well-known safe and effective macrocylic lactone with potent nematocidal activity, long half-life and safety profile that have enabled its use in extended duration formulations in dogs [20]. Moxidectin has been used in cats for more than 15 years in a monthly spot-on product at a dose rate of 1 mg/kg. This novel spot-on solution containing fluralaner (minimum recommended dose rate of 40 mg/kg) plus moxidectin (minimum recommended dose rate of 2 mg/kg), is now approved for cats for the treatment and control of tick and flea infestations for 12 weeks, for the prevention of heartworm disease for 8 weeks, and the treatment of nematode infections. A European field study demonstrated the effectiveness and safety of this product in the treatment of natural infections with gastrointestinal parasites (roundworms and hookworms) and *Capillaria* spp. in client-owned cats [21]. The present study reports the effectiveness and safety of this combination product in the treatment and control of natural tick and flea infestations of client-owned cats.

Methods

Study design

This was a multicenter, positive-controlled, randomized, investigator-blinded study, conducted from March until October 2015, in 33 veterinary practices located in Germany and Spain. The study was conducted in consideration of Good Clinical Practice VICH guideline

GL9, EMEA, 2000, Guideline on Statistical Principles for Veterinary Clinical Trials (EMEA, 2010), Guideline for the testing and evaluation of the efficacy of antiparasitic substances for the treatment and prevention of tick and flea infestation in dogs and cats (EMEA/CVMP/EWP/005/2000-Rev.2) and the World Association for the Advancement of Veterinary Parasitology (WAAVP) guidelines for evaluating the efficacy of parasiticides for the treatment, prevention and control of tick and flea infestation on dogs and cats [22–25]. Cat owners completed an informed consent form for the inclusion of all cats in a household into the study prior to any enrollment and prior to initiation of treatment.

Animals and households

Healthy cats at least 10 weeks-old and weighing at least 1.2 kg were eligible for inclusion. Cats with chronic medical conditions could be included at the discretion of the investigator in each clinic. Households were eligible for enrollment if they contained at least one cat with at least two fleas and/or at least two ticks, and were excluded if they contained a pregnant or lactating cat, if more than five cats were present, or if they contained non-feline animals capable of hosting fleas or ticks. All cats in each enrolling household received the same treatment.

To be eligible for enrollment, cats could not have received ectoparasiticide treatment within the previous 7 to 30 days, depending on the expected duration of effect of the treatment. No household environmental flea treatment was allowed for two months before the start of the study. During the study, the use of any non-study products with insecticidal or insect growth regulator properties was not permitted on either pets or premises of participating households. Grooming and bathing were allowed during the study, but should not have been performed for three days before a scheduled visit or for three days after treatment.

In the European Union, the guideline for the demonstration of efficacy against ticks and fleas requires 50 treated cases per region in two geographical regions for each of ticks and fleas, meaning a total of 150 cats infested with ticks would be included in the study (100 cats in the fluralaner plus moxidectin group and 50 in the fipronil group) [24]. Assuming a drop-out rate of 15% and an average of two tick-infested cats per household, 90 households with 180 tick-infested cats were to be included. A similar calculation for households with flea-infested cats provided the same household enrollment requirement. It was assumed that 50% of enrolling households with a tick-infested cat would have at least one flea-infested cat, so that the total number of households to be enrolled was 225 (based on the resulting assumption of 45 households with ticks only, 45 households with ticks and fleas and 135 with fleas only).

Owners were instructed to record any between-visit observations related to tick or flea infestation and to ensure that ticks were collected and brought to the practice within one week of observation, or to immediately arrange for an additional visit. Collected ticks were shipped to a central laboratory in Germany (IDEXX laboratories, Ludwigsburg) for identification to the genus and species level. If lesions of flea allergy dermatitis were present, the size, type (erythema, papules, crusts, scales, alopecia, excoriation) and localization of the largest lesion were also documented. Clinic staff administering treatment were not blinded; all clinic staff involved in study assessments were masked to treatment.

Randomization and treatment

Using computer-generated randomization lists, households were randomly allocated to treatment groups stratified by site in blocks of three, in a 2:1 ratio for the fluralaner plus moxidectin spot-on to a commercially-available fipronil spot-on product. All treatments were administered within each clinic, by clinic staff.

The fluralaner (280 mg/ml) plus moxidectin (14 mg/ml) product (Bravecto® Plus spot-on for cats) was supplied in pipettes containing 0.4, 0.89 and 1.79 ml for cats of 1.2–2.8 kg, > 2.8–6.25 kg and > 6.25–12.5 kg body weight, respectively. Treatment was applied topically on a single occasion, Day 0, at a dose rate of 40–94 mg fluralaner plus 2.0–4.65 mg moxidectin/kg body weight. For application, the cat was required to be standing or lying in sternal recumbency with its back horizontal. Treatment was applied by placing the tip of the pipette on the skin at the base of the cat's skull and then gently squeezing to apply the entire contents directly onto the cat's skin. The potential for product run-off was minimized by limiting the amount applied to any one spot: if two spots were needed, the first was applied at the base of the skull and the second between the shoulder blades.

Fipronil (Frontline® spot-on cat 10% w/v solution, Boehringer Ingelheim, Ingelheim, Germany) was supplied in pipettes containing 0.5 ml for cats weighing at least 1 kg body weight. Treatment was applied topically on Days 0, 28 ± 2 and 56 ± 2, based on the minimum treatment interval for the product of 4 weeks, at a dose rate of approximately 7.5–15 mg/kg body weight. The product was applied as spots along the back: one at the base of the skull and a second, if needed, 2 to 3 cm distal to this, according to manufacturer's instructions. Care was taken to apply the product directly to the skin and to avoid excessive wetting of the hair at the treatment spot, as the manufacturer reports that it causes a sticky appearance for up to 24 h after application.

After treatment, each cat was inspected to determine if there had been any product run-off. Cats were observed for 10 min to determine if any skin irritation was present at the application site. Owners were instructed to observe their cats for any adverse events (i.e. unfavorable or unexpected events), and to contact the investigator to report any such events immediately after they were observed.

Assessments

On Day 0, each cat was thoroughly examined by the investigator to determine general health and suitability for inclusion in the study. At this and all scheduled subsequent visits after 14 ± 2 (2 weeks), 28 ± 2 (4 weeks), 56 ± 2 (8 weeks) and 84 ± 2 days (12 weeks), physical examinations were completed, ticks and fleas were counted, ticks were collected for identification and signs of flea allergy dermatitis assessed. Safety assessments were based on all observations of adverse events by owners or clinic staff in all cats enrolled and allocated to a treatment group [intention-to-treat (ITT) population].

Tick and flea counts were performed by trained clinic staff using the comb-counting method described in WAAVP guidelines for evaluating the efficacy of parasiticides for the treatment, prevention and control of tick and flea infestations on cats [25]. If required, cats could be sedated immediately prior to combing. Assessment of tick infestations involved pushing against the natural lay of the hair to expose any fleas or ticks, whether or not attached. All ticks were gently removed using forceps, counted and classified as live or dead. Assessments continued in this manner for at least 5 min. After this assessment was completed, cats were combed from front (including the whole head, ears and neck) to back (including the tail, flanks, legs, chest, axillae, groin, ventral thorax and abdomen) using overlapping strokes, for at least 5 min with a fine-toothed flea comb (approximately 11–13 teeth/cm). Special attention was paid to ectoparasite predilection sites (in hair whorls beneath the ears and hind legs, axillae and ventral abdomen, tail-base and back just cranial to the tail). If ticks and/or fleas were recovered during combing, the procedure was continued for a further 5 min until no ticks or fleas were recovered, making the total assessment time at least 10 min per cat. Between visits, owners were instructed to observe their cats for the presence of any live ticks and/or fleas and record the numbers. Any attached ticks that were observed between visits were to be removed with forceps and placed in clinic-supplied tubes labeled with the cat's name, and taken to the clinic within one week for classification and identification. In the event that tick removal by the owner was not possible, the cat was to be brought to the clinic for an unscheduled visit.

Statistical analysis

The primary endpoint of the study assessed all cats that were treated and examined according to the protocol [per protocol (PP) population]. The primary efficacy criterion was the percent reduction in tick and flea counts for each product at each follow-up visit, in comparison to the initial tick and flea burden. The statistical unit was the individual animal for tick efficacy and the household for flea efficacy. Efficacy analyses were also completed for the ITT population.

Study group means were determined for each visit (pre-treatment on Day 0 and follow-up visits at 14 ± 2, 28 ± 2, 56 ± 2 and 84 ± 2 days). The calculation was based on live ticks and fleas, in cats initially infested with ticks and in flea-infested households, respectively. The percent reduction in geometric and arithmetic mean counts was calculated for each study group and each follow-up visit according to the formula:

$$\text{Reduction }(\%) = \left(\bar{X}_{\text{pre}} - \bar{X}_{\text{post}}/\bar{X}_{\text{pre}}\right) \times 100$$

where $\bar{X}_{pre}$ represents the mean of live ticks or fleas on Day 0, and $\bar{X}_{post}$ is the mean at each post-Day 0 assessment. To allow the calculation in case of zero counts, the geometric mean was calculated as follows:

$$x_g = \left(\prod_{i=1}^{n}(x_i + 1)\right)^{\frac{1}{n}} - 1$$

To compensate for the skewed distribution of geometric means, the tick or flea counts were log-transformed prior to statistical analysis: $x_i' = \ln(x_i + 1)$. Tick and flea counts at follow-up visits were compared pairwise to the pre-treatment counts using a one-sided, two-sample t-test. The level of significance (α) was set at 0.025.

Secondary efficacy was based upon the percentage of cats free of live ticks and/or fleas and households free of fleas. For each post-treatment follow-up visit, non-inferiority and superiority of the percentage of tick or flea-free cats in the fluralaner plus moxidectin group were compared to the percentage of tick or flea-free cats in the fipronil group. A test of non-inferiority for the risk difference was used with an α of 0.025 and a tolerated difference (δ) of 0.15 [26]. The *P*-value and the lower 97.5% one-sided confidence limits were calculated. If the lower confidence limit was above -0.15, it was concluded that fluralaner plus moxidectin was no less effective (non-inferior) to fipronil. If the lower confidence limit was above 0, it was concluded that fluralaner plus moxidectin was superior to fipronil.

Frequency tables were used to compare the distribution of sex, breed, hair length, living conditions, number of cats in the household and presence of skin lesions possibly related to flea allergy dermatitis in both treatment groups. The presence of clinical signs of flea allergy dermatitis and improvement in those signs were evaluated descriptively.

Results

In total, 332 households with at least one cat qualified for enrollment. The targets for inclusion of tick-infested cats (*n* = 50) and flea-infested households (*n* = 50) were met in both Germany and Spain. For ticks, the PP population included 229 cats (136 in Germany, 93 in Spain) and the ITT population 257 cats (154 in Gemany, 103 in Spain). For fleas, the PP population included 208 households with at least one flea-infested cat (88 in Gemany, 120 in Spain) and the ITT population 236 households (103 in Gemany, 133 in Spain). There were 707 cats involved in the ITT population and 635 cats in the PP population. Initial homogeneity between study groups was demonstrated at inclusion (Day 0) for cats from all households. There was more than one cat in approximately 60% of households in each group, 14 and 16% of cats in the fluralaner plus moxidectin and fipronil groups, respectively, were reported as inside cats, and 79 and 73% of cats, respectively, were reported by owners to spend time both inside and outside. The breed distribution was similar between groups and included European (*n* = 380), mixed breed (*n* = 28), Persian (*n* = 22) and Siamese (*n* = 14) cats, with low numbers of British shorthair (*n* = 5), Maine Coone (*n* = 4), Birman (*n* = 3), Ragdoll (*n* = 2), Tonkinese (*n* = 1), Turkish Angora (*n* = 1), Havana (*n* = 1) and Chartreux (*n* = 1). For the ITT population the average age was 4.9 years in the fluralaner plus moxidectin group and 4.8 years in the fipronil group. The mean weights were 4.2 and 4.1 kg, respectively. Males comprised 57% of cats in the fluralaner plus moxidectin group and 52% of cats in the fipronil group, and 83% of cats in each group had been neutered.

At enrollment, six cats with concomitant disease (epilepsy, hyperthyroidism, hypertension, congestive heart failure, feline leukemia virus infection) requiring long-term treatment (phenobarbital, carbimazole or thiamazole, amlodipine, benazepril and interferon-alpha, respectively) were included in the fluralaner plus moxidectin group. A single cat in the fipronil group was stabilized at enrollment on benazepril and furosemide for congestive heart failure, and this was continued during the study.

During the study 72 cats were either withdrawn, lost to follow up, or excluded from a visit analysis: 35 cats were excluded from the efficacy analysis because of protocol violations, mainly due to being washed or groomed within the proscribed pre- or post-treatment interval, or for failure to adhere to the scheduled visits; data from 17 fluralaner plus moxidectin group cats were excluded from the efficacy analysis (but were included in the safety analysis) because the incorrect pipette was used, meaning that the applied dose rate exceeded the maximum recommended; 13 cats were lost to follow-up; 5 cats in the fluralaner plus moxidectin group died [two road traffic accidents, two with no further details were available (one accidentally, one found dead) and one was euthanized due to weight loss, lymphadenopathy and dyspnea (attributed to a malignant lymphoma)]. None of these deaths were attributable to treatment. One cat from the fluralaner plus moxidectin group was withdrawn by the owner due to a reported lack of efficacy, and one cat from the fipronil group cat was withdrawn because of a reported intolerance to the product.

A total of 873 ticks (ITT population) were collected at inclusion: the most frequent tick species found was *Ixodes ricinus* (*n* = 684, 78.4%, 1–57 per cat) in both Germany and Spain; *Rhipicephalus sanguineus* complex (*n* = 154, 17.6%, 1–4 per cat) mainly in Spain (two cats in Germany were infested); and *Dermacentor reticulatus* (*n* = 2, 0.2%, 1 per cat), *Dermacentor marginatus* (*n* = 2, 0.2%, 1 per cat), *Haemaphysalis concinna* (*n* = 2, 0.2%, 2 ticks per cat) and *Ixodes* spp. (*n* = 1, 0.1%) were also found, as well as *Ixodes* spp. larvae (*n* = 15, 1.7%, 1–4 per cat) and nymphs (*n* = 13, 1.5%, 1–2 per cat) in Spain.

At each follow-up assessment, mean tick and flea count reductions in both groups were significant relative to Day 0 (Tables 1, 2; Figs. 1, 2). The mean tick and flea count reductions from baseline in the fluralaner plus moxidectin group were greater than in the fipronil group at all post-Day 0 assessments. For the PP population at 2, 4, 8 and 12 weeks, the geometric mean live tick count reductions in the fluralaner plus moxidectin group were at least 97.2%, and in the fipronil group were at least 92.7%. For the PP population at 2, 4, 8 and 12 weeks, the geometric mean flea count reductions in the fluralaner plus moxidectin group were at least 98.9% (arithmetic means at least 96.6%) while in the fipronil group these reductions were at least 86.3% (arithmetic mean 74.9%), and exceeded 90% on only one occasion, two weeks following the first treatment (Table 2, Fig 2).

For secondary efficacy between-group comparisons, with the lower 97.5% one-sided confidence limit well above the non-inferiority limit of -0.15, fluralaner plus moxidectin non-inferiority to fipronil for tick and flea efficacy was shown ($P < 0.0001$) in the PP and ITT populations at each follow-up visit (Tables 3, 4). At all assessments following Day 0, the proportion of cats free of ticks was higher in the fluralaner plus moxidectin group than in the fipronil group. The fluralaner plus moxidectin treatment was superior to fipronil at 2 and 4 weeks for the number of cats free of ticks ($P < 0.0001$) and at 2, 4, 8 and 12 weeks for the proportion of households free of fleas and cats free of fleas ($P < 0.0001$). For the PP population at 2, 4, 8 and 12 weeks, at least 92.8 and 81.8% of tick-infested cats from the fluralaner plus moxidectin and

Table 1 Geometric (arithmetic) mean counts of live ticks and percent reduction from baseline in each group

Visit	Mean	Reduction (%)	*t*-statistic (t_{df})	*P*-value (Pr > t)	Mean	Reduction (%)	*t*-statistic (t_{df})	*P*-value (Pr > t)
Per protocol population								
	Fluralaner + moxidectin (*n* = 152)				Fipronil (*n* = 77)			
1	2.59 (3.67)	–			2.17 (2.61)	–		
2	0.05 (0.09)	98.3 (97.7)	$t_{(200.37)} = 26.6$	<0.0001	0.12 (0.21)	94.4 (92.0)	$t_{(152)} = 17.9$	<0.0001
3	0.07 (0.16)	97.2 (95.7)	$t_{(228.96)} = 24.9$	<0.0001	0.11 (0.23)	94.9 (91.0)	$t_{(152)} = 17.6$	<0.0001
4	0.07 (0.15)	97.3 (95.9)	$t_{(228.17)} = 25.0$	<0.0001	0.16 (0.23)	92.7 (91.0)	$t_{(144.27)} = 17.5$	<0.0001
5	0.05 (0.09)	97.9 (97.5)	$t_{(199.31)} = 26.5$	<0.0001	0.07 (0.10)	97.0 (96.0)	$t_{(119.53)} = 21.0$	<0.0001
Intent to treat population								
	Fluralaner + moxidectin (*n* = 171)				Fipronil (*n* = 86)			
1	2.54 (3.61)	–			2.22 (2.70)	–		
2	0.04 (0.08)	98.4 (97.9)	$t_{(219.73)} = 28.1$	<0.0001	0.17 (0.34)	92.2 (87.6)	$t_{(170)} = 16.0$	<0.0001
3	0.08 (0.15)	96.9 (95.6)	$t_{(255.62)} = 25.9$	<0.0001	0.15 (0.35)	93.2 (87.0)	$t_{(169)} = 16.1$	<0.0001
4	0.07 (0.14)	97.3 (96.0)	$t_{(252.87)} = 26.2$	<0.0001	0.15 (0.22)	93.4 (92.0)	$t_{(156.24)} = 18.6$	<0.0001
5	0.06 (0.10)	97.6 (97.1)	$t_{(230.92)} = 27.2$	<0.0001	0.07 (0.11)	96.9 (96.0)	$t_{(132.43)} = 21.6$	<0.0001

fipronil groups, respectively, were free of ticks. For the PP population at 2, 4, 8 and 12 weeks, at least 93.3 and 60.3% of cats from the fluralaner plus moxidectin and fipronil groups, respectively, were free of fleas.

In the PP population there were 30 fluralaner plus moxidectin-treated cats (7.1%) and 6 fipronil-treated cats (2.8%) with clinical signs of flea allergy dermatitis at inclusion. Of these cats, in the fluralaner plus moxidectin group 86.7% had improved or were graded as clinically cured, compared with 66.7% in the fipronil group. Clinical cures were recorded in 53.3% of the fluralaner plus moxidectin cats and 33.3% of fipronil cats.

There were no treatment-related serious adverse events in either group. Adverse event reports in the fluralaner plus moxidectin group included a single report of itching at the site of application on Day 0; another cat was reported to show dyspnoea and was suspected to have been licking the application site the day after treatment; small spots of hair loss were reported in one cat on Day 4 and mild alopecia in a further eight cats, on a single occasion for each, between Days 13 through 15. In the fipronil group, alopecia at the application site was reported in two cats on Day 28; in a third cat crusting at the application site was observed on Day 35. On Day 0,

Table 2 Geometric (arithmetic) mean household flea counts and percent reduction from baseline

Visit	Mean	Reduction (%)	*t*-statistic (t_{df})	*P*-value (Pr > t)	Mean	Reduction (%)	*t*-statistic (t_{df})	*P*-value (Pr > t)
Per protocol population								
	Fluralaner + moxidectin (*n* = 135)				Fipronil (*n* = 73)			
1	6.89 (14.93)	–			6.38 (9.23)	–		
2	0.06 (0.51)	99.1 (96.6)	$t_{(186.21)} = 24.9$	<0.0001	0.50 (1.34)	92.1 (85.5)	$t_{(144)} = 13.0$	<0.0001
3	0.06 (0.10)	99.1 (99.3)	$t_{(154.39)} = 26.4$	<0.0001	0.71 (2.44)	88.8 (73.6)	$t_{(131.94)} = 10.7$	<0.0001
4	0.04 (0.06)	99.5 (99.6)	$t_{(145)} = 27.2$	<0.0001	0.66 (1.60)	89.7 (82.6)	$t_{(144)} = 12.0$	<0.0001
5	0.08* (0.18)	98.9 (98.8)	$t_{(168.67)} = 25.6$	<0.0001	0.87 (2.32)	86.3 (74.9)	$t_{(134.98)} = 10.3$	<0.0001
Intent to treat population								
	Fluralaner + moxidectin (*n* = 152)				Fipronil (*n* = 84)			
1	6.82 (14.26)	–			6.44 (10.0)	–		
2	0.08 (0.50)	98.9 (96.5)	$t_{(214.76)} = 26.6$	<0.0001	0.52 (1.46)	91.9 (85.4)	$t_{(166)} = 13.4$	<0.0001
3	0.06 (0.11)	99.1 (99.3)	$t_{(174.87)} = 28.4$	<0.0001	0.71 (2.49)	88.9 (75.1)	$t_{(156.73)} = 11.2$	<0.0001
4	0.03 (0.05)	99.5 (99.6)	$t_{(1628.1)} = 29.4$	<0.0001	0.61 (1.48)	90.5 (85.2)	$t_{(164)} = 13.0$	<0.0001
5	0.07 (0.16)	99.0 (98.9)	$t_{(189.22)} = 27.7$	<0.0001	0.81 (2.15)	87.4 (78.5)	$t_{(163)} = 11.2$	<0.0001

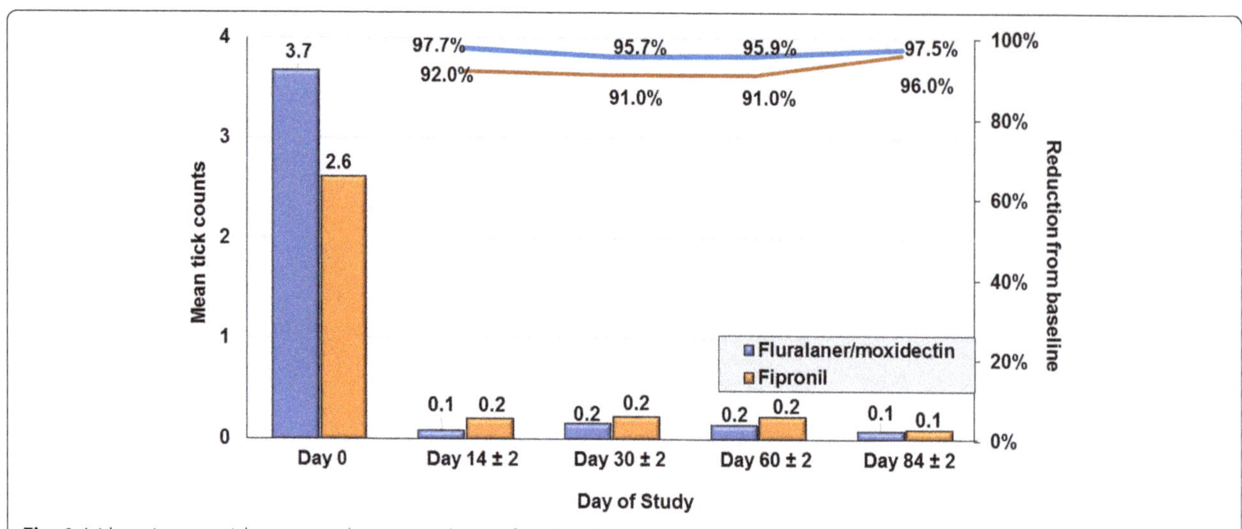

Fig. 1 Arithmetic mean tick counts and percent reduction from baseline at each subsequent visit for topical fluralaner plus moxidectin- or fipronil-treated cats (bars indicate arithmetic mean tick counts; lines indicate percent reductions from baseline)

salivation and lethargy in one cat from the fluralaner plus moxidectin group was considered to be possibly treatment-related. In the fipronil group, salivation and tremor observed in one cat on Day 0 was considered by the investigator to be probably treatment-related, as was itching, without further detail, observed in one cat on Day 29 and in two cats on Day 85. Isolated instances of mild, generally transient gastrointestinal signs considered unlikely to be treatment-related were reported to have occurred in both treatment groups at different times during the study.

Discussion

To the best of our knowledge, this is the first reported field study demonstrating the 12-week field efficacy and safety of fluralaner against ticks in cats, and the first European field study confirming the 12-week efficacy and safety of fluralaner against fleas in cats. The new spot-on formulation of fluralaner plus moxidectin for cats (Bravecto® Plus) administered topically at 12-week intervals was safe and highly effective gainst natural tick and flea infestations in cats. The efficacy of fluralaner plus moxidectin was non-inferior to fipronil ($P < 0.0001$) at all time-points and superior to fipronil at two weeks and two months post-treatment for the proportion of cats free of ticks ($P < 0.0001$), and at all time-points for the proportion of households free of fleas and the proportion of cats free of fleas ($P < 0.0001$).

The numbers of ticks on fluralaner plus moxidectin-treated cats were reduced by at least 97.2% at all time-points after a single treatment. This tick efficacy in cats is consistent with that shown in a European field

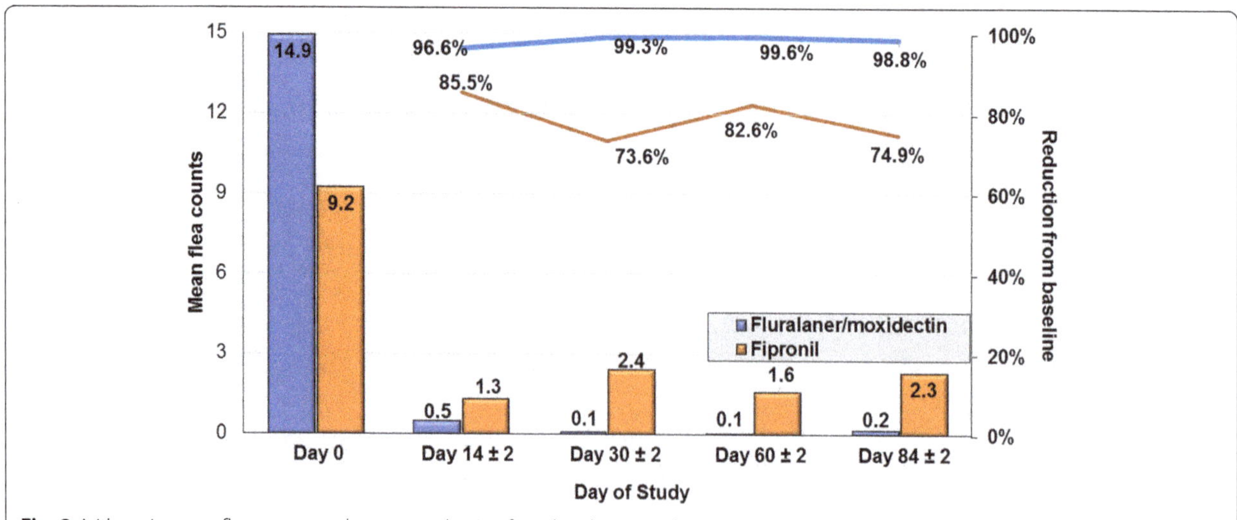

Fig. 2 Arithmetic mean flea counts and percent reduction from baseline at each subsequent visit for topical fluralaner plus moxidectin- or fipronil-treated cats (bars indicate arithmetic mean flea counts; lines indicate percent reductions from baseline)

Table 3 Percent of cats infested with ticks on Day 0 that were free of ticks at subsequent visits

Treatment group	Cats free of ticks (%)			
	Visit 2	Visit 3	Visit 4	Visit 5
Per protocol population				
Fluralaner + moxidectin	96.1	92.8	93.4	94.1
Fipronil	88.3	89.6	81.8	92.2
Lower 97.5% one-sided confidence limit[a]	0.0008	-0.0456	0.0294	-0.0534
P-value for non-inferiority[b]	<0.0001	<0.0001	<0.0001	<0.0001
Intent to treat population				
Fluralaner + moxidectin	96.5	91.8	93.4	93.3
Fipronil	86.1	88.2	83.1	91.6
Lower 97.5% one-sided confidence limit[a]	0.0293	-0.0403	0.0215	-0.0530
P-value for non-inferiority[b]	<0.0001	<0.0001	<0.0001	<0.0001

[a]Lower 97.5% one-sided confidence limit was well above the non-inferiority limit of -0.15. If the lower confidence limit was above 0, superiority was concluded
[b]Farrington-Manning method

study (Germany, France and Spain) of fluralaner in dogs where tick counts were reduced by at least 99% at 2, 4, 8 and 12 weeks following a single treatment [15]. The results of the present study also compare favorably to those of two separate reports of isoxazolines described in European 12-week field studies in tick-infested, client-owned cats. In one study the efficacy against ticks of three consecutive monthly applications of a topical formulation of sarolaner and selamectin (an isoxazoline and macrocyclic lactone, respectively) was ≥ 92.6%, while the efficacy of fipronil administered according to the same schedule ranged from 74.6 to 93.4% [27]. The sarolaner-selamectin combination was non-inferior to fipronil at all time-points and superior on Days 30 and 60. In the other study, the efficacy of orally administered lotilaner against ticks ranged from 98.3 to 100%, and for fipronil from 89.6 to 99.6% [28]. Lotilaner was superior to fipronil from Days 14 to 70 and non-inferior on the other assessment days. The accumulated findings therefore indicate that while fipronil continues to be generally effective against ticks, it may be inferior to those isoxazolines against which it has been tested.

The results of this study in flea-infested households, a 98.9–99.5% reduction from baseline in geometric mean flea counts, provide evidence to support the immediate and sustained reduction in flea burdens for 12 weeks following a single fluralaner plus moxidectin treatment of cats. The results provide further substantiation of the efficacy of fluralaner against *Ctenocephalides felis*, which has been shown to be the dominant flea species in Europe [29]. These findings reinforce those from a USA field study where there was a 98.6–99.1% reduction in flea counts in treated cats for 12 weeks following a single fluralaner treatment [16]. In other studies with

Table 4 Percent of households with at least one cat initially infested with at least two fleas that were free of fleas at subsequent visits

Treatment group	Households free of fleas (%)			
	Visit 2	Visit 3	Visit 4	Visit 5
Per protocol population				
Fluralaner + moxidectin	95.6	94.1	95.6	93.3
Fipronil	76.7	69.9	68.5	60.3
Lower 97.5% one-sided confidence limit[a]	0.0929	0.1388	0.1673	0.2190
P-value for non-inferiority[b]	<0.0001	<0.0001	<0.0001	<0.0001
Intent to treat population				
Fluralaner + moxidectin	94.7	93.4	96.0	93.9
Fipronil	75.0	70.2	69.5	61.7
Lower 97.5% one-sided confidence limit[a]	0.1046	0.1337	0.1682	0.2169
P-value for non-inferiority[b]	<0.0001	<0.0001	<0.0001	<0.0001

[a]Lower 97.5% one-sided confidence limit was well above the non-inferiority limit of -0.15. If the lower confidence limit was above -0.15, non-inferiority was concluded. If the lower confidence limit was above 0, superiority was concluded
[b]Farrington-Manning method

shorter-acting spot-on or oral products in cats, three consecutive monthly administrations have been required to reach 12 weeks of efficacy whereas fluralaner (with or without moxidectin) has been shown to achieve this efficacy duration following a single dose. The results of the present study compare favorably with those from two European (non-inferiority) field studies in cats, one investigating the flea control arising from three monthly applications of a combination of sarolaner and selamectin compared to three applications of a topical formulation of imidacloprid and moxidectin, the other comparing a single oral administration of lotilaner with a single application of fipronil/(S)-methoprene. In the former study, the three applications of sarolaner-selamectin resulted in mean flea count reductions from baseline of 97.3, 98.8 and 99.4% on Days 30, 60 and 90, respectively, and 83.6, 87.7 and 96.3% in the imidacloprid/moxidectin-treated group [27]. In the latter study, mean flea count reductions were 97.2 and 98.1% at two and four weeks post-treatment with lotilaner, respectively, while the corresponding efficacy for fipronil/(S)-methoprene was just 48.3 and 46.4% [30], respectively.

The low efficacy of fipronil in that study aligns with the findings in our study in which the fipronil group household mean flea count reductions were less than 90% on all but one occasion (2 weeks after the first treatment), and there was a low proportion of households (60.3%) that were free of fleas, despite the treatment being applied at the veterinary practice at 4-week intervals. While failures in the control of fleas on dogs and cats are common, they are frequently due to inappropriate control measures [30]. However, in the present study, fipronil treatment was applied every four weeks by the veterinary team. There is also considerable variation in the susceptibility of flea strains to insecticides [31, 32] and this may result in flea infestations that are difficult to control with certain agents under field conditions. It is clear from the results of our study and of other studies in Europe and the USA that fipronil, which in earlier papers had been shown to perform well under field conditions, often appears to perform poorly against fleas under the controlled conditions of a field study [16, 17, 30, 33–38].

While fleas are long established as important parasites of cats in Europe, concern about tick infestations in cats has received much less attention. Our finding of so many tick-infested cats, similar to that reported in 2017 by Geurden et al. [27], is an indicator that cats are at substantial risk from tick infestation, and therefore of the associated risk of infection with tick-borne pathogens. These recent findings suggest that more attention should be placed on the risks of tick infestations of cats, and of the potential such infestations have to result in vector-borne disease.

In the present study, in Germany and Spain, the predominant ticks prior to treatment were the sheep tick (*I. ricinus*, 78.4%) as well as other *Ixodes* spp. ticks (0.1%) including nymphs (1.5%) and larvae (1.7%) and the brown dog tick (*R. sanguineus* complex, 17.6%). Other *Ixodes* spp. found on cats, sometimes the predominate tick, can include the hedgehog tick (*I. hexagonus*) as reported in Belgium, France, Germany and Italy [2, 39, 40]. Both the sheep tick and brown dog tick also predominated in a study with sarolaner plus selamectin, although in that study *R. sanguineus* was found only on cats in France and Italy but not in Germany and Hungary. The same study reported low numbers of the ornate cow tick (*D. reticulatus*) on cats in Germany and Hungary and this was found in Spain in the present study along with low numbers of the ornate sheep tick (*D. marginatus*). The present study also found the relict tick (*H. concinna*), a common rodent tick, in low numbers on cats in Spain. This Eurasian hard tick has been previously reported in low numbers on dogs in Hungary [39, 40] but appears not to have been previously reported in cats. These findings underline that cats, through their behaviour can encounter questing ticks, meaning that a variety of ticks can be found.

Both immediate and persistent efficacy of ectoparasiticides are particularly important under field conditions where cats are exposed not only to re-infestation with ticks and fleas from the environment, but also to the risk of vector-borne pathogens that they carry. The extended-duration fluralaner plus moxidectin spot-on product tested in the present study was confirmed under field conditions to provide 12 weeks of activity following a single topical application. This will help to provide safe and effective extended duration ectoparasite control for cats in a form that reduces potential gaps in protection and is convenient to cat owners.

Conclusions

The topical formulation of fluralaner plus moxidectin spot-on solution for cats was highly effective for 12 weeks against ticks [*I. ricinus*, *Ixodes* spp. (including nymphs and larvae), *R. sanguineus* complex, *D. reticulatus*, *D. marginatus*, *H. concinna*] and fleas (*Ctenocephalides* spp.) on naturally infested cats. It was safe and the percentage of parasite-free cases in the fluralaner-moxidectin group was higher and always significantly non-inferior to the registered fipronil spot on for cats.

Abbreviations

EMEA: European Medicines Agency; FAD: Flea allergy dermatitis; ITT: Intent-to-treat; PP: Per protocol; VICH: International Cooperation on Harmonisation of Technical Requirements for Registration of Veterinary Medicinal Products; WAAVP: World Association for Veterinary Parasitology; $\overline{X}_{pre}$: Mean of live ticks or fleas on Day 0; $\overline{X}_{post}$: Mean at each post-Day 0 assessment

Acknowledgments
The authors would like to thank the veterinarians and their clients for participating in the study. Thanks also to Dr Bill Ryan of Ryan Mitchell Associates LLC and Dr Linda Horspool for guidance and support with preparation of the manuscript.

Funding
The study was funded by MSD Animal Health.

Authors' contributions
NR, EZ and RKAR authored the study design and protocol. The study was conducted by NR, OW, WL, TP and MJG. EZ completed the statistical calculations. All authors revised, read and approved the final manuscript.

Competing interests
NR, EZ and RKAR are employees of MSD Animal Health. OW, WL, TP and MJG declare that they have no competing interests.

Author details
[1]MSD Animal Health Innovation GmbH, Zur Propstei, 55270 Schwabenheim, Germany. [2]Loehlein & Wolf Vet Research, Maistrasse 69, 80337 Munich, Germany. [3]TPC Biomed, C/Los Betetas 12-4°D, 42002 Soria, Spain.

References

1. Beugnet F, Bourdeau P, Chalvet-Monfray K, Cozma V, Farkas R, Guillot J, et al. Parasites of domestic owned cats in Europe: co-infestations and risk factors. Parasit Vectors. 2014;7:291.
2. Claerebout E, Losson B, Cochez C, Casaert S, Dalemans AC, De Cat A, et al. Ticks and associated pathogens collected from dogs and cats in Belgium. Parasit Vectors. 2013;6:183.
3. Savary De Beauregard B. Contribution à l'étude épidémiologique des maladies vectorielles bactériennes observées chez le chat dans le sud de la France. Veterinary Thesis. Ecole Nationale Vétérinaire de Toulouse; 2003.
4. Taylor MA. Recent developments in ectoparasiticides. Vet J. 2001;16:253–68.
5. Bishop BF, Bruce CI, Evans NA, Goudie AC, Gration KAF, Gibson SP, et al. Selamectin: a novel broad-spectrum endectocide for dogs and cats. Vet Parasitol. 2000;91:163–76.
6. Arther RG, Charles S, Ciszewski DK, Davis WL, Settje TS. Imidacloprid/moxidectin topical solution for the prevention of heartworm disease and the treatment and control of flea and intestinal nematodes of cats. Vet Parasitol. 2005;133:219–25.
7. Venco L, Mortarino M, Carro C, Genchi M, Pampurini F, Genchi C. Field efficacy and safety of a combination of moxidectin and imidacloprid for the prevention of feline heartworm (*Dirofilaria immitis*) infection. Vet Parasitol. 2008;154:67–70.
8. European Medicines Agency. Summary of product characteristics. Broadline. 2017. https://www.ema.europa.eu/documents/product-information/broadline-epar-product-information_en.pdf. Accessed 1 Oct 2018.
9. Otranto D, Little S. Tradition and innovation: selamectin plus sarolaner. A new tool to control endo- and ectoparasites of cats - a European perspective. Vet Parasitol. 2017;238(Suppl. 1):S1–2.
10. European Scientific Counsel Companion Animal Parasites (ESCCAP). ESCCAP Guideline 1: Worm control in dogs and cats. 3rd edition. 2017. https://www.esccap.org/. Accessed 30 Mar 2018.
11. Cummings J, Vickers L, Marbaugh J. Evaluation of veterinary dispensing records to measure clinic compliance with recommended heartworm prevention programs. In: Soll MD, Knight DH, editors. Proceedings of the Heartworm Symposium '95. Batavia, IL: American Heartworm Society; 1995. p. 183–6.
12. Gates MC, Nolan TJ. Factors influencing heartworm, flea, and tick preventative use in patients presenting to a veterinary teaching hospital. Prev Vet Med. 2010;93:193–200.
13. Atkins CE, Murray MJ, Olavessen LJ, Burton KW, Marshall JW, Brooks CC. Heartworm 'lack of effectiveness' claims in the Mississippi delta: computerized analysis of owner compliance - 2004–2011. Vet Parasitol. 2014;206:106–13.
14. Lavan RP, Tunceli K, Zhang D, Normile D, Armstrong R. Assessment of dog owner adherence to veterinarians' flea and tick prevention recommendations in the United States using a cross-sectional survey. Parasit Vectors. 2017;10:284.
15. Rohdich N, Roepke RK, Zschiesche E. A randomized, blinded, controlled and multi-centered field study comparing the efficacy and safety of Bravecto (fluralaner) against Frontline (fipronil) in flea- and tick-infested dogs. Parasit Vectors. 2014;7:83.
16. Meadows C, Guerino F, Sun F. A randomized, blinded, controlled USA field study to assess the use of fluralaner topical solution in controlling feline flea infestations. Parasit Vectors. 2017;10:37.
17. Meadows C, Guerino F, Sun F. A randomized, blinded, controlled USA field study to assess the use of fluralaner topical solution in controlling canine flea infestations. Parasit Vectors. 2017;10:36.
18. Dryden MW, Canfield MS, Kalosy K, Smith A, Crevoiserat L, McGrady JC, et al. Evaluation of fluralaner and afoxolaner treatments to control flea populations, reduce pruritus and minimize dermatologic lesions in naturally infested dogs in private residences in west central Florida USA. Parasit Vectors. 2016;9:365.
19. Crosaz O, Chapelle E, Cochet-Faivre N, Ka D, Hubinois C, Guillot J. Open field study on the efficacy of oral fluralaner for long-term control of flea allergy dermatitis in client-owned dogs in Ile-de-France region. Parasit Vectors. 2016;9:174.
20. Prichard R, Ménez C, Lespine A. Moxidectin and the avermectins: consanguinity but not identity. Int J Parasitol Drugs Drug Resist. 2012;2:134–53.
21. Rohdich N, Zschiesche E, Wolf O, Loehlein W, Kirkova Z, Iliev P, et al. A randomized, blinded, controlled, multicentered field study assessing the treatment of nematode infections in cats with fluralaner plus moxidectin spot-on solution (Bravecto® Plus). Parasit Vectors. 2018 (In Press).
22. EMEA. Guideline on good clinical practices. VICH Topic GL9. GCP. 2000. http://www.ema.europa.eu/docs/en_GB/document_library/Scientific_guideline/2009/10/WC500004343.pdf. Accessed 17 May 2018.
23. EMEA. Guideline on statistical principles for veterinary clinical trials. http://www.ema.europa.eu/docs/en_GB/document_library/Scientific_guideline/2009/10/WC500004329.pdf. Accessed 4 Apr 2018.
24. EMEA. Guideline for the testing and evaluation of the efficacy of antiparasitic substances for the treatment and prevention of tick and flea infestation in dogs and cats (EMEA/CVMP/EWP/005/2000-Rev.2). http://www.ema.europa.eu/ema/pages/includes/document/open_document.jsp?webContentId=WC500004596. Accessed 01 Oct 2018.
25. Marchiondo AA, Holdsworth PA, Fourie LJ, Rugg D, Hellmann K, Snyder DE, et al. World Association for the Advancement of Veterinary Parasitology (W.A.A.V.P.) second edition: Guidelines for evaluating the efficacy of parasiticides for the treatment, prevention and control of flea and tick infestations on dogs and cats. Vet Parasitol. 2013;194:84–97.
26. Farrington CP, Manning G. Test statistics and sample size formulae for comparative binomial trials with null hypothesis of non-zero risk difference or non-unity relative risk. Stat Med. 1990;9:1447–54.
27. Geurden T, Becskei C, Farkas R, Lin D, Rugg D. Efficacy and safety of a new spot-on formulation of selamectin plus sarolaner in the treatment of naturally occurring flea and tick infestations in cats presented as veterinary patients in Europe. Vet Parasitol. 2017;238(Suppl. 1):S12–7.
28. Cavalleri D, Murphy M, Seewald W, Drake J, Nanchen S. A randomized, controlled study to assess the efficacy and safety of lotilaner (Credelio™) in controlling ticks in client-owned cats in Europe. Parasit Vectors. 2018;11:411.
29. Gálvez R, Musella V, Descalzo MA, Montoya A, Checa R, Marino V, et al. Modelling the current distribution and predicted spread of the flea species *Ctenocephalides felis* infesting outdoor dogs in Spain. Parasit Vectors. 2017;10:428.
30. Cavalleri D, Murphy M, Seewald W, Drake J, Nanchen S. A randomized, controlled study to assess the efficacy and safety of lotilaner (Credelio™) in controlling fleas in client-owned cats in Europe. Parasit Vectors. 2018;11:410.
31. Dryden MW, Rust MK. The cat flea: biology, ecology and control. Vet Parasitol. 1994;52:1–19.

32. Bossard RL, Hinkle NC, Rust MK. Review of insecticide resistance in cat fleas (Siphonaptera: Pulicidae). J Med Entomol. 1998;35:415–22.
33. Dryden MW, Ryan WG, Bell M, Rumschlag AJ, Young LM, Snyder DE. Assessment of owner-administered monthly treatments with oral spinosad or topical spot-on fipronil/(S)-methoprene in controlling fleas and associated pruritus in dogs. Vet Parasitol. 2013;191:340–6.
34. Dryden MW, Payne PA, Smith V, Chwala M, Jones E, Davenport J, et al. Evaluation of indoxacarb and fipronil (s)-methoprene topical spot-on formulations to control flea populations in naturally infested dogs and cats in private residences in Tampa FL, USA. Parasit Vectors. 2013;6:366.
35. Cavalleri D, Murphy M, Seewald W, Drake J, Nanchen S. A randomised, blinded, controlled field study to assess the efficacy and safety of lotilaner tablets (Credelio™) in controlling fleas in client-owned dogs in European countries. Parasit Vectors. 2017;10:526.
36. Beugnet F, Franc M. Results of a European multicentric field efficacy study of fipronil-(S) methoprene combination on flea infestation of dogs and cats during 2009 summer. Parasite. 2010;17:337–42.
37. Dryden MW, Denenberg TM, Bunch S. Control of fleas on naturally infested dogs and cats and in private residences with topical spot applications of fipronil or imidacloprid. Vet Parasitol. 2000;93:69–75.
38. Dryden MW, Payne PA, Vicki S, Riggs B, Davenport J, Kobuszewski D. Efficacy of dinotefuran-pyriproxyfen, dinotefuran-pyriproxyfen-permethrin and fipronil-(S)-methoprene topical spot-on formulations to control flea populations in naturally infested pets and private residences in Tampa, FL. Vet Parasitol. 2011;182:281–6.
39. Földvári G, Farkas R. Ixodid tick species attaching to dogs in Hungary. Vet Parasitol. 2005;129:125–31.
40. Cavalleri D, Murphy M, Seewald W, Drake J, Nanchen S. A randomized, controlled study to assess the efficacy and safety of lotilaner (Credelio™) in controlling ticks in client-owned dogs in Europe. Parasit Vectors. 2017;10:531.

20

Trichinella britovi muscle larvae and adult worms: stage-specific and common antigens detected by two-dimensional gel electrophoresis-based immunoblotting

Sylwia Grzelak, Bożena Moskwa and Justyna Bień*

Abstract

Background: *Trichinella britovi* is the second most common species of *Trichinella* that may affect human health. As an early diagnosis of trichinellosis is crucial for effective treatment, it is important to identify sensitive, specific and common antigens of adult *T. britovi* worms and muscle larvae. The present study was undertaken to uncover the stage-specific and common proteins of *T. britovi* that may be used in specific diagnostics.

Methods: Somatic extracts obtained from two developmental stages, muscle larvae (ML) and adult worms (Ad), were separated using two-dimensional gel electrophoresis (2-DE) coupled with immunoblot analysis. The positively-visualized protein spots specific for each stage were identified through liquid chromatography-tandem mass spectrometry (LC-LC/MS).

Results: A total of 272 spots were detected in the proteome of *T. britovi* adult worms (Ad) and 261 in the muscle larvae (ML). The somatic extracts from Ad and ML were specifically recognized by *T. britovi*-infected swine sera at 10 days post infection (dpi) and 60 dpi, with a total of 70 prominent protein spots. According to immunoblotting patterns and LC-MS/MS results, the immunogenic spots recognized by different pig *T. britovi*-infected sera were divided into three groups for the two developmental stages: adult stage-specific proteins, muscle larvae stage-specific proteins, and proteins common to both stages. Forty-five Ad proteins (29 Ad-specific and 16 common) and thirteen ML proteins (nine ML-specific and four common) cross-reacted with sera at 10 dpi. Many of the proteins identified in Ad (myosin-4, myosin light chain kinase, paramyosin, intermediate filament protein B, actin-depolymerizing factor 1 and calreticulin) are involved in structural and motor activity. Among the most abundant proteins identified in ML were 14-3-3 protein zeta, actin-5C, ATP synthase subunit d, deoxyribonuclease-2-alpha, poly-cysteine and histide-tailed protein, enolase, V-type proton ATPase catalytic and serine protease 30. Heat-shock protein, intermediate filament protein ifa-1 and intermediate filament protein B were identified in both proteomes.

Conclusions: To our knowledge, this study represents the first immunoproteomic identification of the antigenic proteins of adult worms and muscle larvae of *T. britovi*. Our results provide a valuable basis for the development of diagnostic methods. The identification of common components for the two developmental stages of *T. britovi* may be useful in the preparation of parasitic antigens in recombinant forms for diagnostic use.

Keywords: *Trichinella britovi*, Adult worm, Muscle larvae, 2-DE, Mass spectrometry, Immunoblotting

* Correspondence: jbien@twarda.pan.pl
Witold Stefański Institute of Parasitology, Polish Academy of Sciences, Twarda 51/55, 00-818 Warsaw, Poland

Background

Trichinellosis is an important food-borne parasitic worldwide zoonosis caused by nematodes belonging to the genus *Trichinella* and is known to have high socioeconomic and medical significance. Humans typically acquire trichinellosis through the consumption of raw or improperly-processed meat of either farmed or wild animals containing infective muscle larvae (ML) of *Trichinella* [1–3]. The entire life-cycle of the parasite takes place in a single host. *Trichinella* displays three major antigenic stages: muscle larvae (ML), adult worms (Ad), and newborn larvae (NBL). Muscle larvae ingested with animal-derived meat are released into the host stomach upon the activation of digestive enzymes; they then migrate to the epithelial cells of the small intestine where they molt and transform into adult worms (Ad) within 48 hours post-infection (pi). Newborn larvae (NBL) are released after five days post-infection (dpi) and move through the lymphatic vessels to reach the striated muscle, where they grow and develop into encapsulated and non-encapsulated forms [4, 5]. All developmental stages of *Trichinella* elicit a protective immune response, as well as antigens which can be used for serological detection of *Trichinella* spp. infection. Several reports note that the *Trichinella* antigens produced by adult worms, new-born larvae and muscle larvae are stage-specific [6–8]. Our previous study indicated that together with stage-specific proteins, *T. spiralis* produces species-specific and common proteins for each developmental stage [9–11]. Although a few *Trichinella* antigens have been fully characterized, the complex interactions between the parasite and the host's immune system are not yet fully understood [12–16]. Thus, there is still a need to find other parasite proteins which may play an important role during the establishment of infection, which influence immune evasion strategies or modulate the host response. Recent studies have shown that a serine protease inhibitor released by *T. spiralis* may allow it to escape immune attack, and is related to the survival and colonization of the parasite in the hosts [17]. Identification of these proteins is not only important for understanding parasite-host interrelations, but is also a key factor in the development of serological diagnostic methods for species-specific differentiation and for detecting early-stage infection.

The combination of two-dimensional gel electrophoresis (2-DE) and mass spectrometry has been widely used to characterize the protein profiles of various *Trichinella* species [9, 18–21]. When used together with immunoblotting, the techniques enable the identification of the proteins that induce immune response and which could be used for immunodiagnosis. This immunoproteomics tool has previously been used to determine both the characteristics of immunogenic proteins and the serological response directed against parasites, such as *Schistosoma japonicum* [22], *Toxoplasma gondii* [23], *Ascaris lumbricoides* [24] and *Taenia solium* [25]. As *T. spiralis* is considered the main etiological agent of most human infections and deaths, most studies have focused only on the identification of potentially immunogenic proteins expressed by *T. spiralis* stages [20, 26–29]. Although *T. spiralis* is commonly used as a representative species of the genus *Trichinella*, *T. pseudospiralis*, *T. nativa* and the T8 genotype, have also been described as being valuable sources of information regarding the parasite proteins needed for the development of immunological diagnostics [18, 19, 30].

Over the years, numerous cases with trichinellosis have been attributed to *T. britovi*, considered the second-most common species of *Trichinella and one* that may affect human health [31–36]. Although the clinical and biological features observed during human infection caused by *T. spiralis* and *T. britovi* are different, it is not possible to attribute these features to a single species because the number of infective larvae is unknown. *Trichinella spiralis* infections are typically more severe than those caused by *T. britovi*, and the main distinctions between the two types of infections were that patients infected with *T. spiralis* displayed a longer duration of parasite-specific IgG, increased CPK levels, and a more severe intestinal symptomatology than those infected with *T. britovi*. This could be due to the fact that the fecundity of *T. britovi* females is lower than those of *T. spiralis* [36]. Our previous proteomic study of the excretory-secretory proteins of *T. britovi* muscle larvae found that the 5'-nucleotidase and serine protease may be potential proteins for diagnosis [9]. Currently, little is known about the protein profile shared by all developmental stages of *T. britovi*. Therefore, there is a need for more information about common and stage-specific *T. britovi* proteins to aid the development of species-specific diagnostics, and to better understand the adaptation of *T. britovi* to a parasitic niche and its host-parasite relationship.

The aim of the present study was to identify the *T. britovi* proteins that may be used in specific diagnostics. Somatic antigen extracts obtained from two developmental stages of *T. britovi*, muscle larvae (ML) and adult worms (Ad), were separated by two-dimensional gel electrophoresis (2-DE) coupled with immunoblot analysis. In addition, any positively-visualized proteins specific for each stage were further identified by liquid chromatography-tandem mass spectrometry (LC-LC/MS).

Methods

Experimental animals and collection of *T. britovi* adult worms and muscle larvae

The *T. britovi* nematodes had been maintained by several passages in male C3H mice at the Institute of

Parasitology, PAS. To generate ML and Ad forms of *T. britovi*, the mice were orally infected with a dose of 700 ML *T. britovi*. ML were collected 42 days post-infection (dpi), and Ad were collected at 4 dpi. Muscle larvae of *T. britovi* were recovered by HCl-pepsin digestion from the previously-infected mice [37]. The recovered ML were subsequently purified several times with water through succeeding steps of sedimentation in cylinders. After the final sedimentation, the ML were collected into 1.5 ml tubes. The larval pellet was extensively washed three times in phosphate-buffered saline (PBS) supplemented with antibiotics (50 U/ml penicillin, 50 µg/ml streptomycin). The adult worms were collected from the small intestine of C3H mice (3–4 months-old). Briefly, after recovery, the intestines were washed with sterile water with the use of a syringe, cut longitudinally and crosswise into 1–2 cm pieces, placed on a mesh in a conical dish filled with RPMI 1640 medium (Sigma-Aldrich Chemie GmbH, Steinheim, Germany) supplemented with 25 mM HEPES, 2 mM L-glutamine, antibiotics (50 U/ml penicillin, 50 µg/ml streptomycin) and incubated for three hours at 37 °C. Any Ad worms located on the bottom of the dish were then collected into 15 ml tubes, and washed three times with PBS supplemented with antibiotics. The *T. britovi* stages were then stored at -70 °C before protein extraction and proteomic analysis.

Protein extraction

The same protein sample preparation procedure was used for both *T. britovi* stages. After thawing, the collected *T. britovi* ML and Ad were again extensively washed three times in PBS and then suspended in a lysis buffer (8 M Urea, 4% CHAPS, 40 mM Trizma base), supplemented with protease inhibitor cocktail (Roche, Berlin, Germany). The protein extract was then homogenized in glass Potter-homogenizer and disintegrated by sonication three times for 10 s. The lysis extract was clarified by centrifugation at 14,000× *g* at 4 °C for 15 min. The supernatant was collected, placed in new 1.5 ml tubes, and protein concentration was measured with the use of a NanoDrop-1000 Uv/Vis Spectrometer (NanoDrop Technologies, Wilmington, USA). The proteins were frozen at -70 °C for further analysis.

Two dimensional gel electrophoresis (2-DE)

Three replicates of *T. britovi* protein samples were run in parallel on three immobilized pH-gradient IPG strips (RioRad, Hercules, USA). The 100 µg samples of previously prepared protein extracts from *T. britovi* Ad and ML were purified with the 2-D Clean-Up Kit (GE Healthcare, New Jersay ,USA) in accordance with the manufacturer's protocol. After the final centrifugation step, the protein pellets were rehydrated overnight in 250 µl of 2-D Starter Kit Rehydration/Sample Buffer (BioRad, Hercules, USA) and loaded onto a 7 cm pH 3-10 IPG strips (BioRad, Hercules, USA) for first dimension separation. The protein samples were separated in accordance with their pI values through isoelectric focusing (IEF) using a Protean IEF Cell (BioRad) device at 20 °C as follows: first step 15 min at 250 V; second step rapid ramping to 4000 V for two hours; and third step for 15,500 Vhrs (current limit of 50 µA/IPG strip). After focusing, the strips were submitted for two steps of equilibration, the first for 25 min in ReadyPrep 2-D starter Kit Equilibration Buffer I, containing DTT (BioRad, USA), and the second for 25 min in ReadyPrep 2-D Starter Kit Equilibration Buffer II containing iodoacetamide (BioRad, USA) instead of DTT. The two-dimensional SDS-PAGE was run using 12% acrylamide separating gels and 4% polyacrylamide stacking gels in a Mini-PROTEAN Tetra Cell electrophoresis chamber (BioRad, USA) at 200 V for approximately 50 min. The PageRuler Unstained Protein Ladder (Thermo Fisher Scientific, Massachusetts, USA) was loaded onto each gel as a weight marker. All gels were separated in the same conditions.

Silver staining and 2-DE immunoblotting

After 2-DE electrophoresis gels were silver-stained using PlusOne Silver Staining Kit (GE Healthcare) in accordance with manufacturer's protocol, while those used for 2-DE immunoblotting were not stained. The obtained gels were scanned with ChemiDoc MP system (BioRad, USA) and analyzed in Image Lab 5.2.1. software (BioRad, USA).

In addition, proteins from unstained gels were transferred onto Immuno-Blot polyvinylidene fluoride (PVDF) membranes (BioRad) by a wet transfer system (BioRad, USA) at 95 V for one hour in cool conditions. The PVDF membranes with the Ad and ML proteins were blocked in Pierce Protein-Free T20 (TBS) Blocking Buffer (Thermo Fisher Scientific) for one hour at room temperature. Following this, the PVDF membranes were incubated overnight at 4 °C with *T. britovi*-infected pig sera (dose of 20,000 ML) diluted 1:100, at 10 dpi and 60 dpi. Adult worm proteins transferred onto the membrane were treated with antisera taken at 10 dpi while the ML proteins were treated with antisera from 10 dpi and 60 dpi. The secondary antibody HRP-conjugated goat anti-pig IgG were diluted 1:35 000 (Sigma-Aldrich, Louis, USA). The uninfected sera were used as parallel negative controls. The negative control experiment used the same method as mentioned above. The immunoreactive proteins were visualized on a film using a Super Signal West Pico Chemiluminescent Substrate (Thermo Fisher Scientific,

Walthman, USA) according to the provided instruction. Reproducibility of the immune recognition was verified by repeating the immunoblot at least three times.

LC-MS/MS

Spots of interest visible on the films were gently excised from compatible silver-stained gels and analyzed by liquid chromatography coupled to a mass spectrometer in the Laboratory of Mass Spectrometry, Institute of Biochemistry and Biophysics, Polish Academy of Sciences (Warsaw, Poland). Samples were concentrated and desalted on a RP-C18 pre-column (Waters), and further peptide separation was achieved on a nano-Ultra Performance Liquid Chromatography (UPLC) RP-C18 column (Waters, BEH130 C18 column, 75 μm i.d., 250 mm long) in a nanoACQUITY UPLC system, using a 45 minute linear acetonitrile gradient. The column outlet was directly coupled to an Electrospray ionization (ESI) ion source of a Orbitrap Velos type mass spectrometer (Thermo Scientific, Waltham, USA), operating in a regime of a data-dependent MS to MS/MS switch with HCD-type peptide fragmentation. An electrospray voltage of 1.5 kV was used.

Bioinformatics

Raw data files were pre-processed with Mascot Distiller software (version 2.4.2.0, MatrixScience). The obtained peptide masses and fragmentation spectra were matched to the National Center Biotechnology Information (NCBI) non-redundant database (115,488,495 sequences/ 42,334,050,411 residues), with a Nematoda filter (748,652 sequences) using the Mascot search engine (Mascot Daemon v. 2.4.0, Mascot Server v. 2.4.1, MatrixScience). The following search parameters were applied: enzyme specificity was set to trypsin, peptide mass tolerance to ± 30 ppm and fragment mass tolerance to ± 0.1 Da. The protein mass was left as unrestricted, and mass values as monoisotopic, with one missed cleavage being allowed. Alkylation of cysteine by carbamidomethylation as fixed, oxidation of methionine was set as a variable modification. Protein identification was performed using the Mascot search engine (MatrixScience), with a probability-based algorithm. The expected value threshold of 0.05 was used for the analysis, which means that all peptide identifications had less than a one-in-20 chance of being a random match. All proteins identified in the MASCOT search were subsequently assigned to the UniProtKB database (https://www.uniprot.org/) and QuickGO (http://www.ebi.ac.uk/QuickGO/) and classified in gene ontology (GO) in accordance with its molecular function, biological process and cellular component information.

Results

2-DE and immunoblot analysis of Ad and ML proteins of *T. britovi*

To identify species-specific parasite antigens, extracts of *T. britovi* Ad and ML were separated by IEF on 7 cm, pH 3–10 strips. Figures 1a and 2a represent one of the three replicated silver-stained proteome gels used for further analysis. The proteomes of Ad and ML presented 261 and 272 spots, respectively, with a pH range of 3–10 and molecular weight (MW) ranging from 10 kDa to 250 kDa (Figs. 1a, 2a). The results of the 2-DE immunoblot of the Ad and ML extracts are given in Figs. 1b and 2b, c. Approximately 31 Ad-immunoreactive protein spots and nine ML protein spots were positively recognized by *T. britovi*-infected swine sera at 10 dpi. Sera taken from pigs at 60 dpi recognized 30 ML protein spots. Potentially immunogenic proteins migrated with a MW between 10 and 150 kDa (Figs. 1b, 2b, c). These immunoreactive spots matched to the corresponding protein spots on silver stained gels, and were selected for further LC-MS/MS identification. No protein reacted to uninfected swine sera (Figs. 1c, 2d).

LC-MS/MS analysis of antigenic proteins of *T. britovi* specific for adult worms

The protein data obtained in the present study were compared against deposited protein sequences available for other *Trichinella* spp. The obtained MS/MS datasets were therefore searched against the NCBI database with the Mascot search engine, and the samples detected as *Trichinella* spp.-specific were selected based on score, matches and sequence coverage data. Thirty-one of the positive spots recognized by the *T. britovi*-infected serum samples taken at 10 dpi were matched and located on the silver-stained gels and then subjected to LC-MS/MS analysis (Table 1). The results revealed the presence of 45 proteins with potential antigenic character, among which 29 were specific only for the adult stage of *T. britovi*. Five of these antigenic proteins were present in more than one spot (Table 2), and most of the analyzed spots contained more than one protein. The highest number of proteins were identified from spot number 22, containing five proteins, spots 6, 7 and 19 containing four proteins, and spots 8, 23, 28, 30 and 31 containing three proteins (Table 1). Only one protein was present in nine spots (nos 2, 4, 11, 12, 13, 14, 24, 25 and 29). No protein set was found in spot no. 21. Several of the immunogenic proteins specific for adult worms were matched to myosin, actin-depolymerizing factor 1, isoforms a/b, heat-shock cognate 71 kDa protein, stress-70 protein, Rho GDP-dissociation inhibitor 1, paramyosin or serine/arginine-rich splicing factor 1 (Tables 1 and 2).

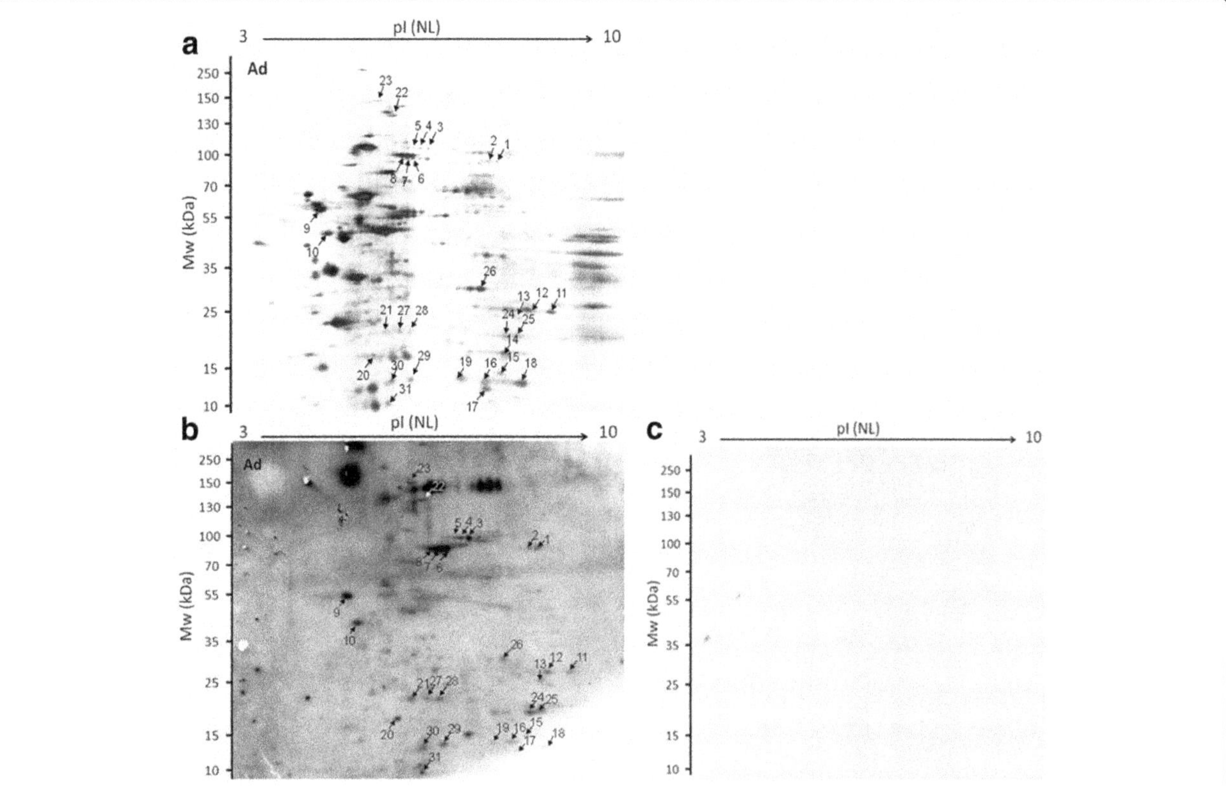

Fig. 1 An image of 2-DE separations and immunoblot analysis of somatic antigen extract of *T. britovi* adult worms (Ad). **a** 2-DE gels were stained with a silver stain. **b** 2D-immunoblot of Ad proteins were probed with infected pig sera at 10 dpi. **c** 2D-immunoblot of Ad proteins probed with uninfected swine sera. Matched spots selected for subsequent LC-MS/MS analysis are marked

LC-MS/MS analysis of antigenic proteins of *T. britovi* specific for muscle larvae

Nine ML protein spots cross-reacting with *T. britovi* infected swine sera were identified by MS analysis at 10 dpi, and 30 spots were found at 60 dpi (Tables 3 and 4).

LC-MS/MS analysis revealed the presence of 13 immunoreactive ML proteins recognized by sera at 10 dpi samples, nine of which were stage-specific (Table 5). In the samples at 60 dpi, 39 proteins were recognized by sera, with only 25 being stage-specific (Table 6). One protein recognized by sera at 10 dpi was present in two spots (nos 29, 30) (Table 5) and seven proteins recognized by sera at 60 dpi were present in more than one spot (Table 6). The highest number of proteins, i.e. seven, were observed in spot number 30, followed by four proteins in spots 17 and 29, and three proteins in spots 4, 6, 12, 20, 30 and 32 (Table 4). The remaining spots contained fewer than three proteins (Tables 3 and 4). Only spot no 34 contained no proteins recognized by sera at 10 dpi, while at 60 dpi, three spots contained no recognized proteins (7, 8 and 28) (Tables 3 and 4).

The following immunogenic proteins specific for the ML stage were identified in the 10 dpi serum samples: 26S protease regulatory subunit 7; actin-5C; enolase; protein disulfide-isomerase 2; V-type proton ATPase catalytic subunit A; and serine protease 30 (Table 5). The following were identified in the 60 dpi samples: 14-3-3 protein zeta; 40S ribosomal protein SA; calponin-like protein OV9M; propionyl-CoA carboxylase alpha chain; Rab GDP dissociation inhibitor alpha; secernin-3; serine protease 30; Toll-interacting protein (Table 6). Finally, the following proteins were identified in both the 10 and 60 dpi samples: actin 5C; serine protease; intermediate filament protein (IFA-1); and mitochondrial-processing peptides subunit beta (Tables 5 and 6).

LC-MS/MS analysis of antigenic proteins common for both stages of *T. britovi*

Although some proteins were found to be specific for both the Ad and ML stages of *T. britovi*, most were common to both stages (Table 7). The following proteins appeared in both proteomes, and were most frequently identified from multiple spots: heat-shock protein beta-1 (present in five spots - Ad 10 dpi, four spots - ML 60 dpi); intermediate filament protein IFA-1; partial (present in five spots - Ad 10 dpi, three spots - ML 60 dpi, four spots - ML 10 dpi); intermediate filament protein IFA-1 (present in five spots - Ad 10 dpi, three spots - 10 dpi and one spot - ML 60 dpi); peroxiredoxin-2/partial (present in three spots - Ad 10

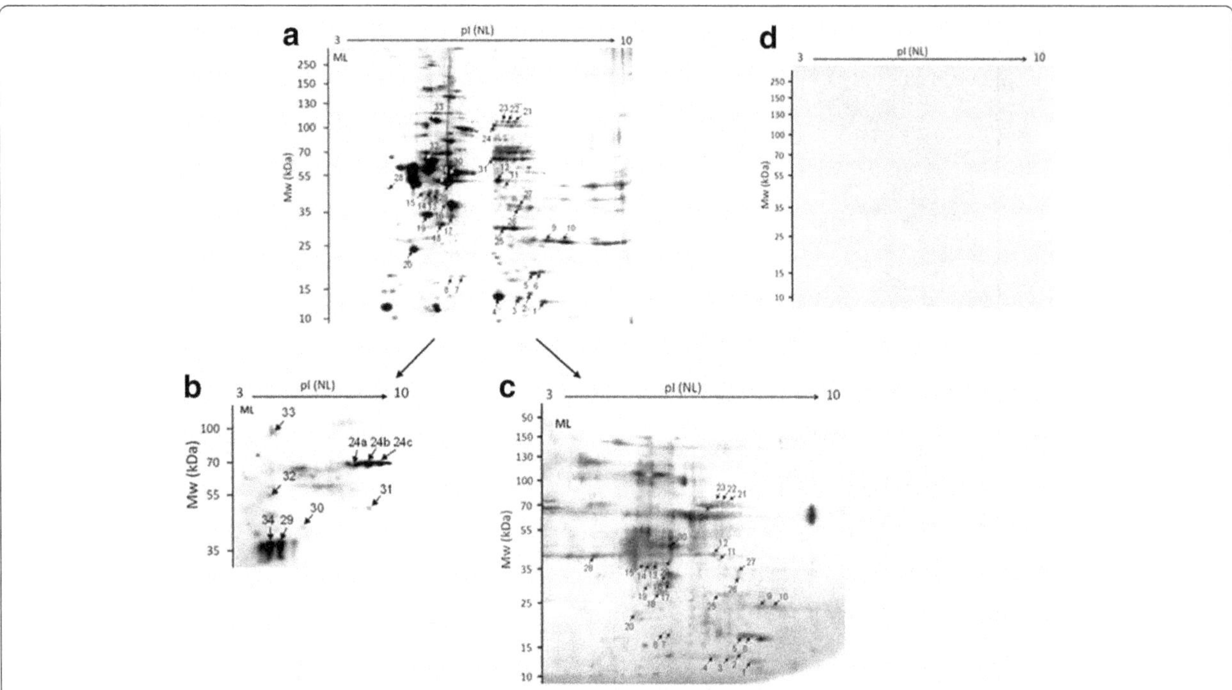

Fig. 2 An image of 2-DE separations and immunoblot analysis of somatic antigen extract of *T. britovi* muscle larvae (ML). **a** 2-DE gels were stained with a silver stain. 2D-immunoblot of ML proteins were probed with infected pig sera at 10 dpi (**b**) and at 60 dpi (**c**). **d** 2D- immunoblot of ML proteins probed with uninfected swine sera. Matched spots selected for subsequent LC-MS/MS analysis are marked

dpi, two spots - ML 60 dpi); tropomyosin (present in one spot - Ad 10 dpi, four spots - ML 60 dpi); and heat-shock 70 kDa protein (present in four spots - Ad 10 dpi, one spot - ML 60 dpi) (Tables 1, 3, 4 and 7). The presence of these different isoforms could be attributed to differences in amino acid sequence, alternative splicing or post-translational modifications. The dominant proteins for both stages were identified as heat-shock protein 70 kDa, heat-shock protein beta-1, intermediate filament B and IFA-1 (Table 7).

Gene ontology (GO) analysis

The gene ontology (GO) database was used to identify the antigenic proteins of the Ad and ML stages according to their molecular function, cellular component and biological process.

For the *T. britovi* adult stage, the proteins were classified according to molecular function (39), cellular components (21) and biological process (21). Seven subcategories of molecular function were determined, the most abundant of which were binding (24) and catalytic activity (18); however, structural molecule activity (6), molecular function regulation (3), transporter activity (2), signal transducer (1) or peroxiredoxin activity (1) subcategories were also observed. Eight subcategories for cellular component were determined, the most numerous being the cell part subcategory (18); however, intracellular organelle part (7), macromolecular complex (7), organelle (6), membrane part (5), intermediate filament (4), membrane (3) or cell (1) subcategories were also observed to a lesser extent. Seven subcategories of biological process were determined. The most abundant were assigned to the cellular process (16) and the metabolic process (11) subcategories, while the remainder were assigned to biological regulation (5), localization (3), transport (2), response to oxidative stress (1), cell adhesion (1) or cellular component organization (1) (Fig. 3a-c). Based on the gene ontology analysis, the potentially antigenic proteins of *T. britovi* muscle larvae which reacted with both 10 dpi and 60 dpi pig sera, were categorized according to molecular function (35), cellular component (24) or biological process (18). Six subcategories for molecular function were determined. The most abundant were binding (20), and catalytic activity (20), whereas structural molecule activity (6), transmembrane transporter activity (3), molecular function regulation (2) or peroxiredoxin activity (1) were visibly less numerous. Eight cellular component subcategories were determined, with the most numerous subcategory being cell part (18), followed by intracellular organelle part (9), macromolecular complex (7), polymeric cytoskeletal fiber (6), membrane part (5), membrane (3), organelle (3) and cell (1). Four subcategories for biological process were determined. The cellular process (15) subcategory was the most numerous, followed by metabolic process (11), biological regulation (5) and localization (5) (Fig. 3a-c).

Table 1 Results of LC-MS/MS analysis of *Trichinella britovi* adult worms (Ad) selected spots which reacted with pig sera collected at 10 dpi

Spot	NCBIprot accession no.	MS[a]	MP[b]	Seq[c]	SC (%)[d]	emPAI[e]	Mr(kDa)/pI[f]	Description
1	KRZ04300.1	746	11	10	15	0.82	71.823/6.58	Transketolase, partial
	KRY23714.1	363	5	5	8	0.33	75.949/8.54	Succinate dehydrogenase (ubiquinone) flavoprotein subunit, mitochondrial, partial
2	KRY10810.1	817	13	11	16	1.08	70.999/6.60	Transketolase
3	KRY09282.1	1067	18	17	25	1.86	73.168/6.07	Intermediate filament protein ifa-1
	KRY23083.1	1015	16	16	22	1.19	76.326/6.17	Stress-70 protein, mitochondrial, partial
4	KRY23083.1	405	6	6	10	0.32	76.326/6.17	Stress-70 protein, mitochondrial, partial
5	KRY23083.1	247	3	3	5	0.18	76.326/6.17	Stress-70 protein, mitochondrial, partial
	KRZ06996.1	99	2	2	2	0.12	74.844/5.78	Intermediate filament protein ifa-1, partial
6	KRY11608.1	1889	36	26	40	4.74	75.526/6.24	Intermediate filament protein B
	KRY09282.1	1883	31	27	38	4.10	73.168/6.07	Intermediate filament protein ifa-1
	KRY16427.1	1772	33	22	22	1.78	108.386/6.14	Heat-shock cognate 71 kDa protein, partial
	CAA73574.1	1612	30	21	31	3.15	71.860/5.77	Heat-shock protein 70
7	KRY58599.1	1946	38	26	23	1.54	131.529/6.88	Heat-shock cognate 71 kDa protein, partial
	KRY11608.1	1933	37	23	38	5.03	75.526/6.24	Intermediate filament protein B
	CAA73574.1	1773	32	25	36	3.87	71.860/5.77	Heat-shock protein 70
	KRY09282.1	1503	25	21	29	2.95	73.168/6.07	Intermediate filament protein ifa-1
8	CAA73574.1	1633	35	22	33	3.42	71.860/5.77	Heat-shock protein 70
	KRY11608.1	1094	18	17	25	1.62	75.526/6.24	Intermediate filament protein B
	KRZ06996.1	906	13	12	17	0.98	74.844/5.78	Intermediate filament protein ifa-1, partial
9	KRY21440.1	646	12	9	16	0.97	62.134/5.04	Calreticulin
	KRY19442.1	329	5	5	15	0.81	35.572/9.61	Y-box factor -like protein
10	KRY21426.1	507	8	7	27	1.80	29.821/4.64	Myosin light chain kinase, smooth muscle
	AET09716.1	215	3	3	15	0.78	22.620/4.54	Tropomyosin, partial
11	KRZ13803.1	412	6	5	17	1.07	35.565/8.61	32 kDa beta-galactoside-binding lectin lec-3 (Galectin)
12	KRY20423.1	465	8	6	21	1.48	33.995/7.69	32 kDa beta-galactoside-binding lectin (Galectin)
13	KRX13351.1	62	1	1	4	0.15	29.477/8.21	RNA-binding protein rnp-1
14	KRX46812.1	497	7	6	32	2.26	22.941/7.07	Peroxiredoxin-2, partial
15	KRZ77496.1	378	6	4	3	0.08	23.7876/6.48	Dedicator of cytokinesis protein 1
	KRY20040.1	140	3	2	10	0.97	18.977/6.97	Heat-shock protein beta-1
16	KRY20040.1	445	12	6	34	3.69	18.977/6.97	Heat-shock protein beta-1
	KRX20324.1	323	6	4	28	1.33	19.886/8.12	OV-16 antigen, partial
17	KRY20040.1	405	11	5	30	3.01	18.977/6.97	Heat-shock protein beta-1
	KRX20324.1	369	6	4	28	1.43	19.886/8.12	OV-16 antigen, partial
18	KRX47621.1	701	19	9	53	7.94	18.951/6.97	Heat-shock protein beta-1
	KRX19442.1	106	2	2	10	0.57	18.490/8.74	Transcription factor BTF3 -like protein 4
19	KRX16844.1	358	11	6	30	2.86	18.894/6.32	Alpha-crystallin B chain
	KRY20040.1	297	6	4	26	2.06	18.977/6.97	Heat-shock protein beta-1
	KRZ07637.1	278	3	3	14	0.75	23.026/6.12	Stromal cell-derived factor 2
	KRZ08373.1	75	2	2	9	0.47	22.324/7.60	Peroxiredoxin 2
20	KRX18074.1	398	8	6	9	0.74	54.209/4.92	BAG family molecular chaperone regulator 2, partial
	KRZ17076.1	165	3	2	10	0.75	22.920/5.45	Rho GDP-dissociation inhibitor 1

Table 1 Results of LC-MS/MS analysis of *Trichinella britovi* adult worms (Ad) selected spots which reacted with pig sera collected at 10 dpi *(Continued)*

Spot	NCBIprot accession no.	MS[a]	MP[b]	Seq[c]	SC (%)[d]	emPAI[e]	Mr(kDa)/pI[f]	Description
21	Unidentified	–	–	–	–	–	–	–
22	KRY31449.1	1224	26	15	20	1.11	91.608/5.31	Transitional endoplasmic reticulum ATPase - like protein 2
	KRZ08767.1	1011	13	13	7	0.27	234.755/5.91	Myosin-4, partial
	KRZ03705.1	287	3	3	4	0.13	101.672/5.38	Paramyosin
	KRY00202.1	206	4	3	5	0.20	92.727/5.26	Heat-shock 70 kDa protein 4L
	KRY14731.1	172	3	3	3	0.10	131.892/6.63	CAP-Gly domain-containing linker protein 1
23	KRY18882.1	994	15	12	14	0.79	108.605/5.51	LIM domain and actin-binding protein 1
	KRZ08767.1	345	6	6	3	0.12	234.755/5.91	Myosin-4, partial
	KRZ13693.1	302	5	5	4	0.20	125.148/6.31	Integrin alpha pat-2
24	KRZ06959.1	252	3	3	11	0.61	28.479/7.74	Triosephosphate isomerase, partial
25	KRZ12367.1	299	4	4	24	1.19	24.385/7.01	GTP-binding nuclear protein Ran
26	KRX15368.1	656	14	10	33	3.52	34.025/6.29	32 kDa beta-galactoside-binding lectin, partial
	KRY59871.1	115	2	2	12	0.32	30.478/9.08	Serine/arginine-rich splicing factor 1, partial
	KRX23478.1	101	2	2	4	0.27	35.530/6.82	Protein MEMO1, partial
27	KRX41818.1	376	5	5	21	1.13	29.431/5.58	Putative phosphomannomutase
	KRY00151.1	137	3	2	4	0.25	59.844/5.54	ATP synthase subunit beta, mitochondrial
	KRY00848.1	114	2	2	2	0.09	108.425/6.27	Heat-shock 70 kDa protein, partial
28	KRX20997.1	368	6	6	8	0.40	76.565/8.34	Guanine nucleotide-binding proteinalpha-12 subunit, partial
	KRX16428.1	294	6	5	23	1.65	26.141/5.80	V-type proton ATPase subunit E
	KRZ10894.1	177	3	3	9	0.58	27.709/7.55	GrpE -like protein 1, mitochondrial
29	KRY01036.1	394	8	5	27	2.16	22.274/6.88	Actin-depolymerizing factor 1, isoforms a/b, partial
30	KRY01036.1	440	8	5	27	2.12	22.274/6.88	Actin-depolymerizing factor 1, isoforms a/b, partial
	KRY17912.1	295	4	4	18	1.63	17.440/6.18	Uncharacterized protein T12_13420
	KRY00151.1	143	4	2	4	0.33	59.844/5.54	ATP synthase subunit beta, mitochondrial
31	KRY01216.1	278	5	5	21	1.85	19885/5.43	Ubiquitin-conjugating enzyme E2 G1, partial
	KRY21297.1	199	4	3	14	1.15	21.790/8.89	Peptide methionine sulfoxide reductase MsrB
	KRY15966.1	185	4	3	10	0.44	34.259/6.31	Hypothetical protein T12_8663

[a]Mascot score
[b]Matched peptide
[c]Sequence
[d]Sequence coverage (%)
[e]Exponentially modified protein abundance index
[f]Experimental nominal mass (kDa) and isoelectric point

Discussion

Recent reports indicate most cases of *Trichinella britovi* infection occur amongst patients unaware of eating improperly cooked meat products [32–34, 38]. Early diagnosis of trichinellosis is crucial, as anthelmintic drug treatment is much more effective if administered during the initial phases before muscle larvae become encapsulated [39].

In trichinellosis, the interaction between the parasite and the host is influenced by the *Trichinella* life-cycle, which includes a range of stage-specific antigens, immune evasion strategies and modulatory effects on host responses. The combination of immunoblot analysis and proteomic techniques, such as the two-dimensional gel electrophoresis and mass spectrometry used in the present study, is a comprehensive approach to identifying *Trichinella* proteins [40]. Although most proteomic studies have focused on the identification of proteins characteristic of *T. spiralis* life-cycle stages, same of them were dedicated to other *Trichinella* species/genotypes including *T. pseudospiralis*, *T. nativa*, *T. papuae* and T8 [18, 19, 21, 26, 41].

However, further effort is still needed to identify the *T. britovi* proteins that may play an important role in

Table 2 Alphabetical list of stage-specific antigenic proteins of adult worms of *T. britovi*, which reacted with pig sera collected at 10 dpi, together with spot number information. Identification by LC-MS/MS

Protein name	Spot number
Actin-depolymerizing factor 1, isoforms a/b, partial	29, 30
BAG family molecular chaperone regulator 2, partial	20
Calreticulin	9
CAP-Gly domain-containing linker protein 1	22
GrpE-like protein 1, mitochondrial	28
Guanine nucleotide-binding protein alpha-12 subunit, partial	28
Heat-shock 70 kDa protein 4L	22
Heat-shock cognate 71 kDa protein, partial	6, 7
Hypothetical protein T12_8663	31
Integrin alpha pat-2	23
LIM domain and actin-binding protein 1	23
Myosin-4, partial	22, 23
Myosin light chain kinase, smooth muscle	10
Paramyosin	22
Peptide methionine sulfoxide reductase MsrB	31
Putative phosphomannomutase	27
Rho GDP-dissociation inhibitor 1	20
RNA-binding protein rnp-1	13
Serine/arginine-rich splicing factor 1, partial	26
Stress-70 protein, mitochondrial	3, 4, 5
Stromal cell-derived factor 2	19
Succinate dehydrogenase (ubiquinone) flavoprotein subunit, mitochondrial, partial	1
Transitional endoplasmic reticulum ATPase -like protein 2	22
Transketolase /partial	1, 2
Triosephosphate isomerase, partial	24
Ubiquitin-conjugating enzyme E2 G1, partial	31
Uncharacterized protein T12_13420	30
Y-box factor -like protein	9
V-type proton ATPase subunit E	28

understanding host-parasite interactions, and to develop immunological diagnostic methods. Only two papers have addressed the identification of antigenic proteins from *T. britovi*, the second-most common species of *Trichinella* that may affect human health [9, 30]. Dea-Ayuela & Bolaz-Fernandez [30], using 2-DE immunoblot, identified the *T. britovi* proteins that likely belong to the *Trichinella* TSL-1 group of antigens: enolase; P49 antigen; and actins. These proteins play a part in parasite invasion and migration through the host cells. Other studies based on the immunoproteomics of the excretory-secretory systems of *T. britovi* muscle larvae identified a range of proteins, including various glycoproteins (gp43, p49), serine-protease and 5'-nucleotidase [9], that play a role in the development and migration of NBL in host tissue and in the regulation of the immune response by modulating nucleotide levels during infection [42].

The purpose of the present study, therefore, was to identify the *T. britovi*-specific immunodominant proteins present in adult worms and muscle larvae. The crude protein extracts of both stages were separated by 2-DE, subjected to immunoblot analysis with sera from animals infected with *T. britovi* (at 10 dpi and 60 dpi), and identified by LC-MS/MS. A previous immunoproteomic study performed on *T. spiralis* antigens showed that 64 proteins from adult worm crude extract were recognized by sera from pigs and mice infected with *T. spiralis* at 7 dpi, but only seven proteins in muscle larvae crude extract were detected using sera from *T. spiralis*-infected mice and pigs at 5 dpi and 45 dpi, respectively [11, 15, 27].

In the present study, the immunogenic spots recognized by the various pig *T. britovi*-infected sera were divided into three groups according to immunoblotting pattern and LC-MS/MS results: adult (Ad) stage-specific proteins; muscle larvae (ML) stage-specific proteins; and proteins common to both developmental stages. Forty-five proteins in the Ad samples (29 stage-specific for Ad and 16 common) and 13 proteins in the ML samples (9 stage-specific for ML and 4 common) cross-reacted with sera at 10 dpi, while 39 proteins in the ML samples (25 stage-specific for ML and 14 common) reacted with the sera taken at 60 dpi.

Additionally, to further understand the functions of the *T. britovi* proteins, these proteins were categorized according to the GO into biological processes, molecular function and cellular components. The results reveal the presence of a range of proteins known to be antigens involved in the mechanisms of invasion of host tissue and cells, larval migration or molting, immune modulation, metabolic processes in other helminths: actin; heat-shock proteins; paramyosin; 14-3-3-protein; myosin; serine protease; enolase; poly-cysteine and histidine-tailed protein; and deoxyribonuclease-2-alpha [21, 26, 27, 43–45]. Of these proteins, the following were common for both tested *T. britovi* stages: 32 kDa beta galactoside-binding lectin lec-3 (Galectin); heat-shock 70 kDa protein; heat-shock protein beta-1; intermediate filament protein IFA-1; intermediate filament protein B; GTP-binding nuclear protein Ran; OV-16 antigen; protein MEMO1; transcription factor BTF3-like protein 4; tropomyosin; and peroxiredoxin-2. These have previously been found to be present and active throughout the parasite development process; however, they were present in varying amounts, as indicated by the observed dissimilarities in spot intensities.

Table 3 Results of LC-MS/MS analysis of *Trichinella britovi* muscle larvae (ML) selected spots which reacted with pig sera collected at 10 dpi

Spot		NCBIprot accession No.	MS[a]	MP[b]	Seq[c]	SC (%)[d]	emPAI[e]	Mr(kDa)/pI[f]	Description
24	a	KRY11608.1	1765	36	26	36	4.01	75.526/6.24	Intermediate filament protein B
		KRY09282.1	1457	30	22	30	2.92	73.168/6.07	Intermediate filament protein ifa-1
	b	KRY11608.1	1903	40	29	39	5.11	75.526/6.24	Intermediate filament protein B
		KRY09282.1	1541	33	23	33	3.30	73.168/6.07	Intermediate filament protein ifa-1
	c	KRY11608.1	930	14	13	19	1.24	75.526/6.24	Intermediate filament protein B
		KRY09282.1	2328	66	34	47	7.99	73.168/6.07	Intermediate filament protein ifa-1
29		XP_003373575.1	1206	52	15	41	4.74	42.210/5.30	Actin-5C
30		XP_003373575.1	527	9	8	25	1.47	42.210/5.30	Actin-5C
		KRY50178.1	415	8	6	15	0.89	46.783/5.44	Hypothetical protein T03_17187
		KRZ06996.1	160	3	3	4	0.12	74.844/5.78	Intermediate filament protein ifa-1, partial
		KRZ09733.1	323	5	5	5	0.28	96.031/6.00	Mitochondrial-processing peptidase subunit beta, partial
		KRX47705.1	293	4	4	3	0.14	150.442/6.28	Serine protease 30
31		KRZ02603.1	1083	28	14	34	2.98	50.922/6.01	Enolase, partial
		KRY13126.1	544	10	9	20	1.47	48.623/5.41	26S protease regulatory subunit 7
32		KRY18793.1	883	19	14	30	3.45	54.997/5.00	Protein disulfide-isomerase 2
		OUC40875.1	749	17	10	26	2.73	48.387/4.87	Putative Tubulin/FtsZ family, GTPase domain protein
		KRY00151.1	655	14	8	17	1.31	59.844/5.54	ATP synthase subunit beta, mitochondrial
33		KRX41020.1	1127	27	16	27	1.92	72.856/5.09	Heat-shock 70 kDa protein C, partial
		KRY00702.1	364	6	5	9	0.46	68.894/5.08	V-type proton ATPase catalytic subunit A
34		Unidentified	–	–	–	–	–	–	–

[a]Mascot score
[b]Matched peptide
[c]Sequence
[d]Sequence coverage (%)
[e]Exponentially modified protein abundance index
[f]Experimental nominal mass (kDa) and isoelectric point

Adult *T. britovi* are frequently found to contain proteins involved in structural and motor activity, such as myosin-4, myosin light chain kinase, paramyosin, intermediate filament protein B, actin-depolymerizing factor 1 and calreticulin. These cytoskeleton proteins with an actin binding function, are responsible for cellular component organization and actin filament depolymerization, thus facilitating the parasite growth and development processes. Some of them, including actin-depolymerizing factor 1 and paramyosin, were identified in the ML stage but not the early stage of *Trichinella* development [11, 46]. One of these, carleticulin, belongs to the carleticulin family of proteins, which are involved in the protein folding process, and were recently reported to facilitate *T. spiralis* immune evasion by interacting with the first component of the human classical complement pathway, C1q [47]. In addition to its role in muscle length and stability determination, paramyosin also possess immunomodulatory functions. The surface-exposed paramyosin is thought to act as a protective agent during the host inflammatory processes by inhibiting the complement activation cascade and membrane attack complex (MAC) formation [48]. However, V-type proton ATPase subunit E, a member of the ATPase protein family, is activated at a wide pH range and possesses interesting properties under certain biochemical conditions. ATPases are involved in metabolite movements, purging of toxins and energy generation for metabolic processes; they also take part in the environmental response [49, 50] and hence are thought to be involved in the nematode immune response course. Most of the analyzed *T. britovi* antigens are derived from the muscle stage of the larvae. GO analysis of the obtained results showed that some of the proteins participate in various cellular and metabolic processes mostly associated with the synthesis and degradation of macromolecules (nucleotides, proteins) which play an important role in the invasion

Table 4 Results of LC-MS/MS analysis of *Trichinella britovi* muscle larvae (ML) selected spots which reacted with pig sera collected at 60 dpi

Spot	NCBIprot accession No.	MS[a]	MP[b]	Seq[c]	SC (%)[d]	emPAI[e]	Mr(kDa)/pI[f]	Description
1	KRX47621.1	732	22	10	53	13.42	18.951/6.97	Heat-shock protein beta-1
	KRX19442.1	133	2	2	10	0.64	18.490/8.74	Transcription factor BTF3 -like protein 4
2	KRX14469.1	241	3	3	2	0.06	247.333/6.85	Dedicator of cytokinesis protein 1
	KRZ13097.1	165	5	3	13	1.75	19.090/5.43	Heat-shock protein beta-1, partial
3	KRY20040.1	376	8	6	34	4.92	18.977/6.97	Heat-shock protein beta-1
	KRX20324.1	310	5	4	28	1.64	19.886/8.12	OV-16 antigen, partial
4	KRX16844.1	662	60	10	66	10.33	18.894/6.32	Alpha-crystallin B chain
	KRY20040.1	396	8	7	35	4.78	18.977/6.97	Heat-shock protein beta-1
	KRY18783.1	109	2	2	9	0.18	25.119/6.44	Stromal cell-derived factor 2
5	KRX46812.1	546	11	8	41	4.02	22.941/7.07	Peroxiredoxin-2, partial
6	KRX46812.1	409	8	6	28	2.07	22.941/7.07	Peroxiredoxin-2, partial
	KRZ12367.1	292	4	4	19	1.02	24.385/7.01	GTP-binding nuclear protein Ran
	KRX18658.1	226	3	3	15	0.73	23.516/6.92	ATP synthase subunit d, mitochondrial
7	Unidentified	–	–	–	–	–	–	–
8	Unidentified	–	–	–	–	–	–	–
9	KRZ13803.1	406	7	5	17	1.11	35.565/8.61	32 kDa beta-galactoside-binding lectin lec-3 (Galectin)
10	KRZ13803.1	584	9	7	24	1.58	35.565/8.61	32 kDa beta-galactoside-binding lectin lec-3 (Galectin)
	KRY30017.1	304	6	5	17	0.82	34.995/8.74	Putative 3-hydroxyacyl-CoA dehydrogenase
11	KRZ13161.1	105	2	2	6	0.23	42.112/7.12	Glutamine synthetase
12	KRY11984.1	432	7	7	15	0.90	49.560/6.59	Poly-cysteine and histidine-tailed protein
	KRX28313.1	364	7	6	14	1.01	45.667/6.09	Calponin -like protein OV9M, partial
	KRX47308.1	240	3	3	3	0.14	107.151/6.52	Deoxyribonuclease-2-alpha
13	KRY01407.1	324	4	4	10	0.46	51.099/5.91	Cuticlin-1, partial
14	KRY01407.1	319	4	4	10	0.48	51.099/5.91	Cuticlin-1, partial
	KRY00848.1	166	3	3	2	0.15	108.425/6.27	Heat-shock 70 kDa protein, partial
15	CBX25713.1	322	5	5	14	1.14	32.896/4.65	Tropomyosin, partial
16	KRY09099.1	476	8	8	22	1.47	38.218/5.20	Hypothetical protein T12_13379, partial
	KRX15676.1	174	3	3	7	0.43	35.904/5.46	40S ribosomal protein SA, partial
17	KRY09099.1	381	6	6	16	1.20	38.218/5.20	Hypothetical protein T12_13379, partial
	KRZ15717.1	217	4	3	9	0.46	39.852/5.63	Guanine nucleotide-binding protein subunit beta-1, partial
	KRY18502.1	203	4	3	3	0.26	65.700/4.95	Microtubule-associated protein RP/EB family member 3, partial
	KRX15059.1	126	3	2	5	0.52	36.189/5.00	Disorganized muscle protein 1
18	KRX21567.1	504	11	6	21	1.66	40.427/5.49	Pyruvate dehydrogenase E1 component subunit beta, mitochondrial
19	KRX15059.1	667	23	9	28	2.96	36.189/5.00	Disorganized muscle protein 1
	KRZ03570.1	403	6	6	18	1.20	34.457/4.75	Tropomyosin
20	XP_003378934.1	1001	20	12	46	6.93	28.294/4.83	14-3-3 protein zeta
	AET09716.1	248	4	4	19	1.09	22.620/4.54	Tropomyosin, partial
	KRX19348.1	159	3	3	13	0.56	28.034/4.82	Toll-interacting protein
21	KRZ50222.1	917	16	14	3	0.17	449.723/6.87	Propionyl-CoA carboxylase alpha chain, mitochondrial

Table 4 Results of LC-MS/MS analysis of *Trichinella britovi* muscle larvae (ML) selected spots which reacted with pig sera collected at 60 dpi *(Continued)*

Spot	NCBIprot accession No.	MS[a]	MP[b]	Seq[c]	SC (%)[d]	emPAI[e]	Mr(kDa)/pI[f]	Description
22	KRZ50222.1	1081	18	17	4	0.19	449.723/6.87	Propionyl-CoA carboxylase alpha chain, mitochondrial
23	KRY09873.1	557	9	9	2	0.09	441.173/6.76	Propionyl-CoA carboxylase alpha chain, mitochondrial
24	KRY45949.1	1999	45	29	42	6.80	73.429/6.07	Intermediate filament protein ifa-1
	KRY09282.1	1720	36	26	36	4.01	75.526/6524	Intermediate filament protein B
25	KRX15368.1	437	7	7	20	1.80	34.025/6.29	32 kDa beta-galactoside-binding lectin, partial
	KRZ10402.1	91	2	2	4	0.33	35.568/6.67	Protein MEMO1, partial
	KRZ78587.1	42	3	1	2	0.11	48.445/5.59	Secernin-3
26	KRY07641.1	341	6	5	18	1.14	38.033/6.38	1,5-anhydro-D-fructose reductase
27	KRY07641.1	239	4	4	12	0.63	38.033/6.38	1,5-anhydro-D-fructose reductase
28	Unidentified	–	–	–	–	–	–	–
29	XP_003373575.1	1255	39	15	41	4.48	42.210/5.30	Actin-5C
	AET09716.1	168	2	2	11	0.45	22.620/4.54	Tropomyosin, partial
	KRY38295.1	160	3	3	6	0.26	54.444/6.39	Secernin-3
	KRZ06996.1	232	3	3	4	0.19	74.844/5.78	Intermediate filament protein ifa-1, partial
30	KRY50178.1	993	18	15	40	4.11	46.783/5.44	Hypothetical protein T03_17187
	XP_003373575.1	527	9	8	25	1.47	42.210/5.30	Actin-5C
	KRZ06996.1	363	6	6	9	0.47	74.844/5.78	Intermediate filament protein ifa-1, partial
	KRX47705.1	293	4	4	3	0.14	150.442/6.28	Serine protease 30
	KRZ09733.1	323	5	5	5	0.28	96.031/6.00	Mitochondrial-processing peptidase subunit beta, partial
	KRZ17128.1	256	4	4	9	0.51	46.607/5.26	Putative histone-binding protein Caf1
	KRY13378.1	250	5	5	9	0.54	54.969/5.66	Rab GDP dissociation inhibitor alpha

[a]Mascot score
[b]Matched peptide
[c]Sequence
[d]Sequence coverage (%)
[e]Exponentially modified protein abundance index
[f]Experimental nominal mass (kDa) and isoelectric point

Table 5 Alphabetical list of stage-specific antigenic proteins of muscle larvae of *T. britovi*, which reacted with pig sera collected at 10 dpi, together with spot number information. Identification by LC-MS/MS

Protein name	Spot number
26S protease regulatory subunit 7	31
Actin-5C	29/30
Enolase, partial	30
Hypothetical protein T03_17187	30
Protein disulfide-isomerase 2	32
Putative Tubulin/FtsZ family, GTPase domain protein	32
V-type proton ATPase catalytic subunit A	33
Mitochondrial-processing peptidase subunit beta, partial	30
Serine protease 30	30

and development of *Trichinella* in the host [10, 26, 28, 51]. The most frequently identified immunodominant antigens of ML *T. britovi* recognized by infection sera include 14-3-3 protein zeta, actin-5C, ATP synthase subunit d, deoxyribonuclease-2-alpha, poly-cysteine and histide-tailed protein, enolase, V-type proton ATPase catalytic and serine protease 30. For example, the actin-5c protein (recognized by sera at 10 dpi/60 dpi), known to bind ATP molecules (GO), has previously been identified with the use of early and late infection sera [26, 52]. This protein is related to the invasion of a parasite into the intestinal epithelial cells and plays a critical role in larval development [53]. Serine protease 30, with peptidase and hydrolase activities, was recognized by sera at 10 dpi/60 dpi. The

Table 6 Alphabetical list stage-specific antigenic proteins of muscle larvae of *T. britovi*, which reacted with pig sera collected at 60 dpi, together with spot number information. Identification by LC-MS/MS

Protein name	Spot number
1,5-anhydro-D-fructose reductase	26, 27
14-3-3 protein zeta	20
40S ribosomal protein SA, partial	16
Actin-5C	29, 30
ATP synthase subunit d, mitochondrial	6
Calponin -like protein OV9M, partial	12
Cuticlin-1, partial	13, 14
Deoxyribonuclease-2-alpha	12
Disorganized muscle protein 1	17, 19
Glutamine synthetase	11
Guanine nucleotide-binding protein subunit beta-1, partial	17
Hypothetical protein T03_17187	30
Hypothetical protein T12_13379, partial	16, 17
Microtubule-associated protein RP/EB family member 3, partial	17
Mitochondrial-processing peptidase subunit beta, partial	30
Poly-cysteine and histidine-tailed protein	12
Propionyl-CoA carboxylase alpha chain, mitochondrial	21, 22, 23
Putative 3-hydroxyacyl-CoA dehydrogenase	10
Putative histone-binding protein Caf1	30
Pyruvate dehydrogenase E1 component subunit beta, mitochondrial	18
Rab GDP dissociation inhibitor alpha	30
Secernin-3	25, 29
Serine protease 30	30
Stromal cell-derived factor 2	4
Toll-interacting protein	20

protein belongs to serine protease family, along with enzymes that take part in digestion, blood coagulation and fibrinolysis processes. It is involved in host tissues and cell invasions, and plays a pivotal role in nematode molting [54]. Additionally, deoxyribonuclease 2-alpha of the deoxyribonuclease II family was identified, which plays an important role in *Trichinella* invasion, development and survival [55]. The 60 dpi sera also identified the 14-3-3 protein. This is a key regulator of multiple biological processes, including signal transduction, cell differentiation and cell survival, it is also known to induce humoral and cellular immune response and has been tested as a potential vaccine target [56, 57]. The GO analysis revealed that some of the isolated proteins possess catalytic, ligase, hydrolase and peptidase activities, and are responsible for ATP and glutamine synthesis processes; these include ATP-synthase subunit d, glutamine synthase and propionyl-CoA carboxylase alpha chain, all of which were recognized in the 60 dpi sera. GO analysis also showed mitochondrial-processing peptidase (MPP) subunit beta, secernin-3 protein and the previously mentioned serine protease 30 to demonstrate proteolytic and peptidase activity [58]. Microtubule-associated protein RP/EB family member 3 and cuticlin-1, classified as a cellular component belonging to the ML proteome and recognized by sera at 60 dpi, possesses a microtubule binding function. In *Caenorhabditis elegans*, cuticlin-1 contributes to the formation of extracellular envelopes, thereby protecting the organism from the environment [59].

It is important to note that in accordance with previous studies [11, 60, 61], the 10 dpi sera in the present study identified the protein enolase in crude ML extract. Bernal et al. [61] revealed that enolase plays a part in many processes, including fibrinolysis and degradation of the extracellular matrix, through the activation of plasminogen (a proenzyme of the serine protease plasmin). Moreover, this enzyme may contribute to tissue migration during all *T. spiralis* developmental stages [59]. Dea-Ayuela & Bolas-Fernandez [30] confirmed that enolase the immunoreactive property using a combination of 2D-immunoblot and MS. Our findings also confirm the presence of a common proteins for both *T. britovi* stages which was recognized by sera from pigs at 10 dpi and 60 dpi. One particularly well-studied group of proteins comprises the heat-shock proteins (Hsps), which are known to assist the parasite in tissue invasion and intracellular survival, as well as protect it against injury or stress conditions arising as a result of host immune response stimulation [62]. This is consistent with earlier results which identified Hsps as being a common to the adult and muscle larvae stages [10, 26, 51, 55, 63], and were recognized by sera at 15 dpi and 45 dpi [11]. The present GO analysis demonstrated that the identified Hsp proteins present oxidoreductase and structural molecule activity, and that they are located on ribosomes and take part in the translation processes, suggesting that they participate in host cellular stress and immune responses, as well as in the regulation of gene expression and parasite development [27, 64].

Our findings also indicate that the heat-shock protein beta identified in both the Ad and ML proteomes belongs to the small heat-shock proteins (sHsp), which are considered to be an important focus of research in the fight against parasitic diseases [65]. Wu et al. [66]

Table 7 Alphabetical list of antigenic proteins, common for both adult worms (Ad) and muscle larvae (ML) stages *T. britovi* recognized by sera at 60 dpi and 10 dpi, together with spot number information. Identification by LC-MS/MS

Protein name	Spot number Ad *T. britovi*	Spot number ML *T. britovi*	
	10 dpi	10 dpi	60 dpi
32 kDa beta-galactoside-binding lectin lec-3 (Galectin)	11	–	9, 10
32 kDa beta-galactoside-binding lectin, partial (Galectin)	12, 26	–	25
Alpha-crystallin B chain	19	–	4
ATP synthase subunit beta, mitochondrial	27, 30	32	–
Dedicator of cytokinesis protein 1	15	–	2
GTP-binding nuclear protein Ran	25	–	6
Heat-shock 70 kDa protein, partial	6, 7, 8, 27	–	14
Heat-shock protein beta-1	15, 16, 17, 18, 19	–	1, 2, 3, 4
Intermediate filament protein B	6, 7, 8	24 a,b,c	24
Intermediate filament protein ifa-1, partial	3, 5, 6, 7, 8	24a/b/c, 30	24, 29, 30
OV-16 antigen, partial	16, 17	–	3
Peroxiredoxin-2, partial	14, 19, 30	–	5, 6
Protein MEMO1, partial	26	–	25
Transcription factor BTF3 -like protein 4	18	–	1
Tropomyosin, partial	10	–	15, 19, 20, 29
V-type proton ATPase subunit E	28	33	–

reported that sHsp likely play a role in enhancing the survival of the *T. spiralis* muscle larvae under conditions of chemical and physical stress, as well as in the development of larvae. Wang et al. [64] suggested that recombinant Hsp70 is an immunogenic protein released by parasites and that it is exposed to the host immune system during infection.

Intermediate filament protein (IFA-1) and intermediate filament protein B were identified in both *T. britovi* proteomes. These are members of the diverse family of intermediate filaments; these are cytoskeletal components of animal cells which contribute to their mechanical strength and facilitate growth [67]. In nematodes, they allow epidermal elongation in the larvae, worm growth and muscle stability maintenance [68]. Peroxiredoxin-2 has antioxidant and oxidoreductase activity, participates in cellular oxidant detoxification processes and preserves cell redox homeostasis. It therefore plays a crucial role during the host immune response by protecting parasites from endogenous and host-derived ROS, and is possibly involved in cellular signaling [69].

The present study examined somatic extracts taken from adult worms (AW) and muscle larvae of *T. britovi*. Some of the proteins present in these somatic extracts might not be excretory-secretory (E-S) proteins, and they cannot be exposed to the host immune system and induce the specific antibody response. Hence, some of the identified proteins may have less serodiagnostic value, or perhaps no significance at all. Nevertheless, in the process of *Trichinella* infection, the E-S antigens produced by the AW and ML are directly exposed to the immune system and elicit the production of specific anti-*Trichinella* antibodies by the host. Immunoproteomics studies have identified the early diagnostic antigens associated with the E-S proteins of *T. spiralis* AW and ML in animal or patient sera during early infection, and the recombinant 31 kDa antigen from *T. spiralis* ML E-S proteins has been proved to be valuable for early diagnosis of trichinellosis [70, 71]. Hence, further diagnostic antigens for *T. britovi* infection may be identified by future studies on the E-S antigens of AD and ML with early infection sera.

Few proteomic studies examine *T. britovi* exclusively or compare the findings with those of different *Trichinella* spp. [9], and those that have been performed focus on the characterization of mitochondrial genomes [72]. This approach results in the acquisition of a narrow range of knowledge regarding the nuclear genomic or transcriptomic data associated with this parasite, and this narrow focus presents a serious obstacle in the identification of its proteins, and the understanding of their precise function during parasite invasion. Therefore, many proteins are not represented in existing studies, and their precise function can only be assumed on the basis of indirect resemblance analysis.

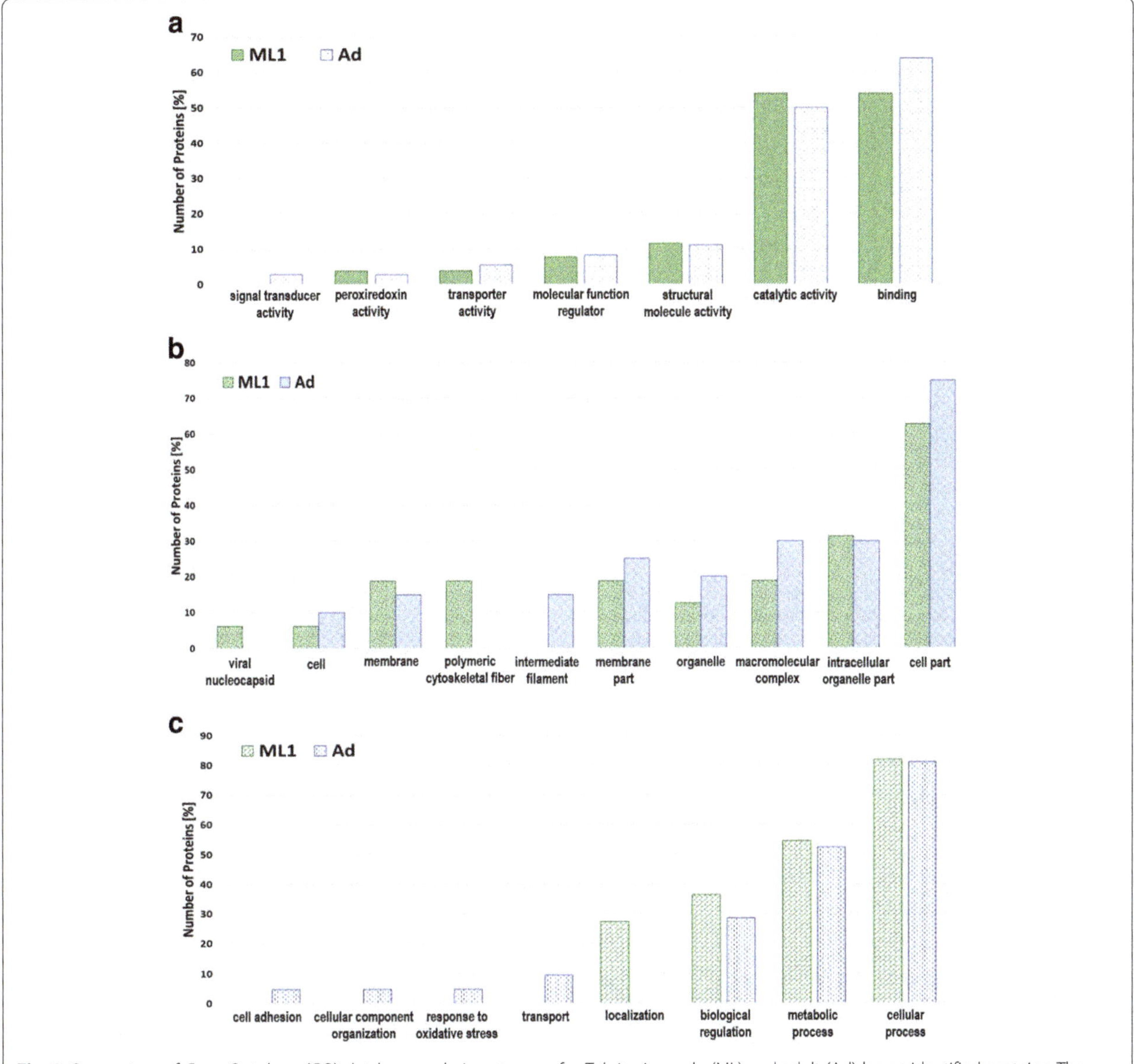

Fig. 3 Comparison of Gene Ontology (GO) database analysis outcomes for *T. britovi* muscle (ML) and adult (Ad) larvae identified proteins. The proteins were categorized according to molecular function (**a**), cellular component (**b**) and biological process (**c**)

Conclusions

To our knowledge, the present study describes the first immunoproteomic identification of the antigenic proteins of adult worm and muscle larvae of *T. britovi*. The somatic extracts from adult worms and muscle larvae of *T. britovi* were specifically recognized by *T. britovi*-infected pig sera at 10 dpi and 60 dpi; a total of 70 prominent protein spots were thus identified, and these were found to contain 45 adult worm and 52 muscle larvae proteins. Adult worms and muscle larvae of *T. britovi* produce proteins (both stage-specific and common proteins) with antigenic properties, some of which have been identified in other helminths as potential diagnostic targets and vaccine candidates. The presence of common and stage-specific proteins for both investigated *T. britovi* stages was confirmed; these included heat-shock proteins, intermediate filament protein IFA-1, 32 kDa beta-galactosidase-binding lectin, peroxiredoxin-2 or 14-3-3 protein, actin-5C, paramyosin, intermediate filament protein B, calreticulin, deoxyribonuclease-2-alpha, enolase, serine protease. These proteins were related to many significant molecular functions, cellular components and biological processes of the parasite, suggesting that the somatic proteins of these two developmental stages may induce a humoral immune response, making them potential antigens for the development of diagnostic methods for *T. britovi* infection.

Abbreviations

2-DE: Two-dimensional electrophoresis; Ad: Adult worms; dpi: Days post-infection; ELISA: Enzyme-linked immunosorbent assay; ES: Excretory-secretory; IEF: Isoelectric focusing; LC-MS/MS: Liquid chromatography-tandem mass spectrometry; ML: Muscle larvae; MW: Molecular weight; NBL: Newborn larvae; pI: Isoelectric point; PVDF: Polyvinylidene fluoride membrane

Acknowledgements

We are grateful to K. Nöckler (Federal Institute for Risk Assessment, Berlin, Germany) for providing experimentally *Trichinella*-infected sera.

Funding

Financial support for this study was provided by the National Science Centre Poland (grant UMO-2015/18/E/NZ6/00502).

Authors' contributions

JB designed and supervised the experiments. JB and SG performed the experiments, analyzed the data and drafted the manuscript. BM contributed in the data analysis and manuscript preparation. All authors read and approved the final manuscript.

Competing interests

The authors declare that they have no competing interests.

References

1. Pozio E. The opportunistic nature of *Trichinella* - exploitation of new geographies and habitats. Vet Parasitol. 2013;194:128–32.
2. Pozio E. World distribution of *Trichinella* spp. infections in animals and humans. Vet Parasitol. 2007;149:3–21.
3. Rostami A, Gamble HR, Dupouy-Camet J, Khazan H, Bruschi F. Meat sources of infection for outbreaks of human trichinellosis. Food Microbiol. 2017;64:65–71.
4. Gottstein B, Pozio E, Nöckler K. Epidemiology, diagnosis, treatment, and control of trichinellosis. Clin Microbiol Rev. 2009;22:127–45.
5. Ortega-Pierres G, Vaquero-Vera A, Fonseca-Liñán R, Bermúdez-Cruz RM, Argüello-García R. Induction of protection in murine experimental models against *Trichinella spiralis*: an up-to-date review. J Helminthol. 2015;89:526–39.
6. Philipp M, Parkhouse RM, Ogilvie BM. Changing proteins on the surface of a parasitic nematode. Nature. 1980;287:538–40.
7. Bioreau P, Vayssier M, Fabien JF, Perret C, Calamel M, Soulé C. Characterization of eleven antigenic groups in *Trichinella* genus and identification of stage and species markers. Parasitology. 1997;115:641–51.
8. Takahashi Y. Antigens of *Trichinella spiralis*. Parasitol Today. 1997;13:104–6.
9. Bień J, Nareaho A, Varmanen P, Goździk K, Moskwa B, Cabaj W, et al. Comparative analysis of excretory-secretory antigens of *Trichinella spiralis* and *Trichinella britovi* muscle larvae by two-dimensional difference gel electrophoresis and immunoblotting. Proteome Sci. 2012;10:10.
10. Bień J, Cabaj W, Moskwa B. Recognition of antigens of three different stages of the *Trichinella spiralis* by antibodies from pigs infected with *T. spiralis*. Exp Parasitol. 2013;134:129–37.
11. Bień J, Cabaj W, Moskwa B. Proteomic analysis of potential immunoreactive proteins from muscle larvae and adult worms of *Trichinella spiralis* in experimentally infected pigs. Folia Parasitol. 2015;62:022.
12. Tang B, Liu M, Wang L, Yu S, Shi H, Boirea P, et al. Characterisation of a high-frequency gene encoding a strongly antigenic cystatin-like protein from *Trichinella spiralis* at its early invasion stage. Parasit Vectors. 2015;8:78.
13. Sun GG, Song YY, Jiang P, Ren HN, Yan SW, Han Y, et al. Characterization of *Trichinella spiralis* putative serine protease. Study of its potential as sero-diagnostic tool. PLoS Negl Trop Dis. 2018;12:e0006485.
14. Zhang Y, Wang Z, Li L, Cui J. Molecular characterization of *Trichinella spiralis* aminopeptidase and its potential as a novel vaccine candidate antigen against trichinellosis in BALB/c mice. Parasit Vectors. 2013;6:246.
15. Yang W, Li LG, Liu RD, Sun GG, Liu CY, Zhang SB, et al. Molecular identification and characterization of *Trichinella spiralis* proteasome subunit beta type-7. Parasit Vectors. 2015;8:18.
16. Sun GG, Ren HN, Liu RD, Song YY, Qi X, Hu CX, et al. Molecular characterization of a putative serine protease from *Trichinella spiralis* and its elicitedimmune protection. Vet Res. 2018;49:59.
17. Song YY, Zhang Y, Yang D, Ren HN, Sun GG, Jiang P, et al. The immune protection induced by a serine protease inhibitor from the foodborne parasite *Tricinella spiralis*. Front Microbiol. 2018;9:1544.
18. Näreaho A, Ravanko K, Hölttä E, Sukura A. Comparative analysis of *Trichinella spiralis* and *Trichinella nativa* proteins by two-dimensional gel electrophoresis. Parasitol Res. 2006;98:349–54.
19. Robinson MW, Greig R, Beattie KA, Lamont DJ, Connolly B. Comparative analysis of the excretory-secretory proteome of the muscle larva of *Trichinella pseudospiralis* and *Trichinella spiralis*. Int J Parasitol. 2007;37:139–48.
20. Liu P, Wu XP, Bai X, Wang XL, Yu L, Rosenthal B, et al. Screening of early antigen genes of adult-stage *Trichinella spiralis* using pig serum from different stages of early infection. Vet Parasitol. 2013;194:222–5.
21. Somboonpatarakun C, Rodpai R, Intapan PM, Sanpool O, Sadaow L, Wongkham C, et al. Immuno-proteomic analysis of *Trichinella spiralis*, *T. pseudospiralis*, and *T. papuae* extracts recognized by human *T. spiralis*-infected sera. Parasitol Res. 2018;117:201–12.
22. Wang J, Zhao F, Yu CX, Xiao D, Song LJ, Yin XR, et al. Identification of proteins inducing short-lived antibody responses from excreted/secretory products of *Schistosoma japonicum* adult worms by immunoproteomic analysis. J Proteomics. 2013;87:53–67.
23. Sun XM, Ji YS, Elashram SA, Lu ZM, Liu XY, Suo X, et al. Identification of antigenic proteins of *Toxoplasma gondii* RH strain recognized by human immunoglobulin G using immunoproteomics. J Proteomics. 2012;77:423–32.
24. Acevedo N, Mohr J, Zakzuk J, Samonig M, Briza P, Erler A, et al. Proteomic and immunochemical characterization of glutathione transferase as a new allergen of the nematode *Ascaris lumbricoides*. PLoS One. 2013;8:e78353.
25. Santivanez SJ, Hernandez-Gonzalez A, Chile N, Oleaga A, Arana Y, Palma S, et al. Proteomic study of activated *Taenia solium* oncospheres. Mol Biochem Parasitol. 2010;171:32–9.
26. Yang J, Pan W, Sun X, Zhao X, Yuan G, Sun Q, et al. Immunoproteomic profile of *Trichinella spiralis* adult worm proteins recognized by early infection sera. Parasit Vectors. 2015;8:20.
27. Bermúdez-Cruz RM, Fonseca-Liñán R, Grijalva-Contreras LE, Mendoza-Hernández G, Ortega-Pierres MG. Proteomic analysis of antigens from early developmental stages of *Trichinella spiralis*. Vet Parasitol. 2016;231:22–31.
28. Cui J, Liu RD, Wang L, Zhang X, Jiang P, Liu MY, et al. Proteomic analysis of surface proteins of *Trichinella spiralis* muscle larvae by two-dimensional gel electrophoresis and mass spectrometry. Parasit Vectors. 2013;6:355.
29. Robinson MW, Connolly B. Proteomic analysis of the excretory-secretory proteins of the *Trichinella spiralis* L1 larva, a nematode parasite of skeletal muscle. Proteomics. 2005;5:4525–32.
30. Dea-Ayuela MA, Bolas-Fernandez F. Two-dimensional electrophoresis and mass spectrometry for the identification of species-specific *Trichinella* antigens. Vet Parasitol. 2005;132:43–9.
31. Pozio E, Cossu P, Marucci G, Amati M, Ludovisi A, Morales MA, et al. The birth of a *Trichinella britovi* focus on the Mediterranean island of Sardinia (Italy). Vet Parasitol. 2009;159:361–3.
32. Fichi G, Stefanelli S, Pagani A, Luchi S, De Gennaro M, Gómez-Morales MA, et al. Trichinellosis outbreak caused by meat from a wild boar hunted in an

Italian region considered to be at negligible risk for *Trichinella*. Zoonoses Public Health. 2015;62:285–91.
33. Akkoc N, Kuruuzum Z, Akar S, Yuce A, Onen F, Yapar N, et al. A large-scale outbreak of trichinellosis caused by *Trichinella britovi* in Turkey. Zoonoses Public Health. 2009;56:65–70.
34. Gomez-Garcia V, Hernandez-Quero J, Rodriguez-Osorio M. Short report: Human infection with *Trichinella britovi* in Granada. Spain. Am J Trop Med Hyg. 2003;68:463–4.
35. Messiaen P, Forier A, Vanderschueren S, Theunissen C, Nijs J, Van Esbroeck M, et al. Outbreak of trichinellosis related to eating imported wild boar meat, Belgium, 2014. Euro Surveill. 2016;21. https://doi.org/10.2807/1560-7917.ES.2016.21.37.30341.
36. Pozio E, Varese P, Morales MA, Croppo GP, Pelliccia D, Bruschi F. Comparison of human trichinellosis caused by *Trichinella spiralis* and by *Trichinella britovi*. Am J Trop Med Hyg. 1993;48:568–75.
37. Kapel CM, Gamble HR. Infectivity, persistence, and antibody response to domestic and sylvatic *Trichinella* spp. in experimentally infected pigs. Int J Parasitol. 2000;30:215–21.
38. Romano F, Motta A, Melino M, Negro M, Gavotto G, Decasteli L, et al. Investigation on a focus of human trichinellosis revealed by an atypical clinical case: after wild-boar (*Sus scrofa*) pork consumption in northern Italy. Parasite. 2011;18:85–7.
39. Nunez GG, Costantino SN, Venturiello SM. Detection of coproantibodies and faecal immune complexes in human trichinellosis. Parasitology. 2007;134:723–7.
40. Wang L, Cui J, Hu DD, Liu RD, Wang ZQ. Identyfication of early diagnostic antigens from major excretory-secretory proteins of *Trichinella spiralis* muscle larvae using immunoproteomics. Parasit Vectors. 2014;7:40.
41. Zocevic A, Mace P, Vallee I, Blaga R, Liu M, Lacour SA, et al. Identification of *Trichinella spiralis* early antigens at the pre-adult and adult stages. Parasitology. 2011;138:463–71.
42. Gounaris K. Nucleotidase cascades are catalyzed by secreted proteins of the parasitic nematode *Trichinella spiralis*. Infect Immun. 2002;70:4917–24.
43. Sulima A, Bień J, Savijoki K, Näreaho A, Sałamatin R, Conn DB, et al. Identification of immunogenic proteins of the cysticercoid of *Hymenolepis diminuta*. Parasit Vectors. 2017;10:577.
44. Sun R, Zhao X, Wang Z, Yang J, Zhao L, Zhan B, et al. *Trichinella spiralis* paramyosin binds human complement C1q and inhibits classical complement activation. PLoS Negl Trop Dis. 2015;9:e0004310.
45. Wang Y, Bai X, Zhu H, Wang X, Shi H, Tang B, et al. Immunoproteomic analysis of the excretory-secretory products of *Trichinella pseudospiralis* adult worms and newborn larvae. Parasit Vectors. 2017;10:579.
46. Gunning PW, Ghoshdastider U, Whitaker S, Popp D, Robinson RC. The evolution of compositionally and functionally distinct actin filaments. J Cell Sci. 2015;128:2009–19.
47. Zhao L, Shao S, Chen Y, Sun X, Sun R, Huang J, et al. *Trichinella spiralis* calreticulin binds human complement C1q as an immune evasion strategy. Front Immunol. 2017;8:636.
48. Zhang Z, Yang J, Wei J, Yang Y, Chen X, Zhao X, et al. *Trichinella spiralis* paramyosin binds to C8 and C9 and protects the tissue-dwelling nematode from being attacked by host complement. PLoS Negl Trop Dis. 2011;5:e1225.
49. Knight AJ, Behm CA. Minireview: the role of the vacuolar ATPase in nematodes. Exp Parasitol. 2012;132:47–55.
50. Rosa BA, Townsend R, Jasmer DP, Mitreva M. Functional and phylogenetic characterization of proteins detected in various nematode intestinal compartments. Mol Cell Proteomics. 2015;14:812–27.
51. Liu RD, Cui J, Liu XL, Jiang P, Sun GG, Zhang X, et al. Comparative proteomic analysis of surface proteins of *Trichinella spiralis* muscle larvae and intestinal infective larvae. Acta Trop. 2015;150:79–86.
52. Wang ZQ, Wang L, Cui J. Proteomic analysis of *Trichinella spiralis* proteins in intestinal epithelial cells after culture with their larvae by shotgun LC-MS/MS approach. J Proteom. 2012;75:2375–83.
53. MacQueen AJ, Baggett JJ, Perumov N, Bauer RA, Januszewski T, Schriefer L, et al. ACT-5 is an essential *Caenorhabditis elegans* actin required for intestinal microvilli formation. Mol Biol Cell. 2005;16:3247–59.
54. Dzik JM. Molecules released by helminth parasites involved in hosts colonization. Acta Biochim Pol. 2006;53:33–64.
55. Liao C, Liu M, Bai X, Liu P, Wang X, Li T, et al. Characterisation of a plancitoxin-1-like DNase II gene in *Trichinella spiralis*. PLoS Negl Trop Dis. 2014;8:e3097.
56. Luo QL, Qiao ZP, Zhou YD, Li XY, Zhong ZR, Yu YJ, et al. Application of signaling protein 14-3-3 and 26 kDa glutathione-S-transferase to serological diagnosis of *Schistosomiasis japonica*. Acta Trop. 2009;112:91–6.
57. Yang J, Zhu W, Huang J, Wang X, Sun X, Zhan B, et al. Partially protective immunity induced by the 14-3-3 protein from *Trichinella spiralis*. Vet Parasitol. 2016;231:63–8.
58. Nomura H, Athauda SB, Wada H, Maruyama Y, Takahashi K, Inoue H. Identification and reverse genetic analysis of mitochondrial processing peptidase and the core protein of the cytochrome bc1 complex of *Caenorhabditis elegans*, a model parasitic nematode. J Biochem. 2006; 139:967–79.
59. Sapio MR, Hilliard MA, Cermola M, Favre R, Bazzicalupo P. The Zona Pellucida domain containing proteins, CUT-1, CUT-3 and CUT-5, play essential roles in the development of the larval alae in *Caenorhabditis elegans*. Dev Biol. 2005;282:231–45.
60. Nakada T, Nagano I, Wu Z, Takahashi Y. Molecular cloning and functional expression of enolase from *Trichinella spiralis*. Parasitol Res. 2005;96:354–60.
61. Bernal D, de la Rubia JE, Carrasco-Abad AM, Toledo R, Mas-Coma S, Marcilla A. Identification of enolase as a plasminogen-binding protein in excretory-secretory products of *Fasciola hepatica*. FEBS Lett. 2004;563:203–6.
62. Nagano I, Wu Z, Takahashi Y. Functional genes and proteins of *Trichinella* spp. Parasitol Res. 2009;104:197–207.
63. Ko RC, Fan L. Heat shock response of *Trichinella spiralis* and *T. pseudospiralis*. Parasitology. 1996;96:89–95.
64. Wang S, Zhu X, Yang Y, Yang J, Gu Y, Wei J, et al. Molecular cloning and characterization of heat shock protein 70 from *Trichinella spiralis*. Acta Trop. 2009;110:46–51.
65. Pérez-Morales D, Espinoza B. The role of small heat shock proteins in parasites. Cell Stress Chaperones. 2015;20:767–80.
66. Wu Z, Nagano I, Boonmars T, Takahashi Y. Thermally induced and developmentally regulated expression of a small heat shock protein in *Trichinella spiralis*. Parasitol Res. 2007;101:201–12.
67. Wang N, Stamenović D. Contribution of intermediate filaments to cell stiffness, stiffening, and growth. Am J Physiol Cell Physiol. 2000;279:C188–94.
68. Woo WM, Goncharov A, Jin Y, Chisholm A. Intermediate filaments are required for *C. elegans* epidermal elongation. Dev Biol. 2004;267:216–29.
69. Gretes MC, Poole LB, Karplus PA. Peroxiredoxins in parasites. Antioxid Redox Signal. 2012;17:608–33.
70. Wang L, Wang ZQ, Hu DD, Cui J. Proteomic analysis of *Trichinella spiralis* muscle larvae excretory-secretory proteins recognized by early infection sera. Biomed Res Int. 2013;2013:139745.
71. Wang ZQ, Liu RD, Sun GG, Song YY, Jiang P, Zhang X, et al. Proteomic analysis of *Trichinella spiralis* adult worm excretory-secretory proteins recognized by sera of patients with early trichinellosis. Front Microbiol. 2017;8:986.
72. Mohandas N, Pozio E, La Rosa G, Korhonen PK, Young ND, Koehler AV, et al. Mitochondrial genomes of *Trichinella* species and genotypes - a basis for diagnosis, and systematic and epidemiological explorations. Int J Parasitol. 2014;44:1073–80.

21

Transcriptomic insights into the early host-pathogen interaction of cat intestine with *Toxoplasma gondii*

Meng Wang[1], Fu-Kai Zhang[1], Hany M. Elsheikha[2], Nian-Zhang Zhang[1], Jun-Jun He[1*], Jian-Xun Luo[1] and Xing-Quan Zhu[1,3*]

Abstract

Background: Although sexual reproduction of the parasite *Toxoplasma gondii* exclusively occurs in the cat intestine, knowledge about the alteration of gene expression in the intestine of cats infected with *T. gondii* is still limited. Here, we investigated the temporal transcriptional changes that occur in the cat intestine during *T. gondii* infection.

Methods: Cats were infected with 100 *T. gondii* cysts and their intestines were collected at 6, 12, 18, 24, 72 and 96 hours post-infection (hpi). RNA sequencing (RNA-Seq) Illumina technology was used to gain insight into the spectrum of genes that are differentially expressed due to infection. Quantitative RT-PCR (qRT-PCR) was also used to validate the level of expression of a set of differentially expressed genes (DEGs) obtained by sequencing.

Results: Our transcriptome analysis revealed 2363 DEGs that were clustered into six unique patterns of gene expression across all the time points after infection. Our analysis revealed 56, 184, 404, 508, 400 and 811 DEGs in infected intestines compared to uninfected controls at 6, 12, 18, 24, 72 and 96 hpi, respectively. RNA-Seq results were confirmed by qRT-PCR. DEGs were mainly enriched in catalytic activity and metabolic process based on gene ontology enrichment analysis. Kyoto Encyclopedia of Genes and Genomes pathway analysis showed that transcriptional changes in the intestine of infected cats evolve over the course of infection, and the largest difference in the enriched pathways was observed at 96 hpi. The anti-*T. gondii* defense response of the feline host was mediated by Major Histocompatibility Complex class I, proteasomes, heat-shock proteins and fatty acid binding proteins.

Conclusions: This study revealed novel host factors, which may be critical for the successful establishment of an intracellular niche during *T. gondii* infection in the definitive feline host.

Keywords: *Toxoplasma gondii*, Cat, RNA-Seq, Gene expression, Immune response, Xenobiotic metabolism

Background

Toxoplasmosis, caused by the intracellular parasite *Toxoplasma gondii*, is a disease of global importance. *Toxoplasma gondii* has been reported in nearly all warm-blooded animals [1]. However, its only definitive host is the cat, including members of the family Felidae, where the sexual cycle occurs in the enterocytes of the small intestine. Cat infection occurs *via* the ingestion of bradyzoite-containing tissue cysts, and following excystation of bradyzoites in the gut, the parasites infect the epithelium and progress from the asexual merozoite stage into sexual stages called gametes (micro- and macrogametocytes). Male and female gametes fuse to form microscopic zygotes/oocysts, which are excreted in cat feces into the environment where they mature into sporulated oocysts [2]. Infected cats can produce millions of oocysts through a single infection [3]. These environmentally resistant oocysts can remain infectious for long periods of time in the environment [4, 5]. When

* Correspondence: hejunjun617@163.com; xingquanzhu1@hotmail.com
[1]State Key Laboratory of Veterinary Etiological Biology, Key Laboratory of Veterinary Parasitology of Gansu Province, Lanzhou Veterinary Research Institute, Chinese Academy of Agricultural Sciences, Lanzhou, Gansu Province 730046, People's Republic of China
Full list of author information is available at the end of the article

ingested by intermediate hosts, infectious sporozoites are liberated from the oocysts and differentiate into tachyzoites in order to complete the life-cycle.

Humans (an intermediate host) can be infected not only *via* eating meat containing parasite cysts, but also *via* accidental ingestion of water contaminated with oocysts [6], ingestion of oocysts in contaminated food sources [7], or *via* gardening or cleaning cat litter. Although *T. gondii* does not seem to cause major illness in healthy people [8], patients with an immunocompromised status, such as with AIDS or cancer may develop fatal encephalitis, mainly because of the reactivated tissue cysts [9]. *Toxoplasma gondii* can also cause serious health complications in an unborn child if the primary infection occurred during pregnancy. Other intermediate hosts, such as herbivorous and omnivorous animals, are infected by eating oocysts in contaminated food sources or water supplies [1].

Despite the crucial epidemiological role played by *T. gondii* oocysts in the dissemination of infection to humans and animals [10], studies investigating the gene regulatory pathways that are involved in the early stages of feline intestinal infection and the formation of oocysts are still limited. The intestinal epithelium can function as a physical barrier to protect the host against microbial infection [11, 12], and also participates in host innate immunity through the production of cytokines, chemokines and antimicrobial peptides [13–15]. Thus, enhanced understanding of the host-pathogen interactions that permit *T. gondii* to develop into sexual stages in the cat intestine would help advance the development of improved preventative and therapeutic approaches to thwart the infection at the main source in the definitive host.

The lack of knowledge about the transcriptional changes that occur in cat intestine during early stage of *T. gondii* infection has prompted us to map the temporal changes that occur in the cat intestinal transcriptome during the first 96 hours after infection. In this study, we used RNA sequencing to illustrate the transcriptional changes that occur in the intestine of cats during early stages of *T. gondii* infection. Our findings provide new insight into defense strategies in the feline intestine and uncover host genes modulated during infection, including genes required for host defense and genes required for the growth of the parasite.

Methods

Animals

Female (2- to 3-month-old) domestic cats (*Felis catus*) of the Chinese Li Hua breed were purchased from a local breeder and housed in a controlled environment. Prior to the experiment, all cats were confirmed to be negative from *T. gondii* using the modified agglutination test (MAT) and free of major viral infections (e.g. feline immunodeficiency virus, feline parvovirus, feline calicivirus, feline coronavirus and feline leukemia virus) based on serological examination. Cats received commercial cat diets (Royal Canine Inc., St. Charles, USA) and water *ad libitum* during the two weeks prior to experimentation in order to minimize any potential dietary impact on the study results. After challenging with *T. gondii*, each cat was fed individually once per day based on their daily energy requirements and water was available *ad libitum*.

Parasite infection and sample collection

Toxoplasma gondii PRU strain belongs to the predominant genotype II reported in cats [16–18]. The capacity of the PRU strain to produce cysts in the brain of mice and oocysts in the gut of cats makes it a suitable candidate for experimental infections of cats [19]. *Toxoplasma gondii* PRU strain was maintained by passage through Kunming mice [20]. We used a low passage PRU strain to preserve the biological attributes and fidelity to the original strain. Brain cysts of *T. gondii* were examined microscopically and their number was adjusted to 100 cysts/ml in phosphate buffered saline (PBS, pH 7.4). Cats (n = 21) were randomly allocated to 7 groups (i.e. 3 cats per group). Six groups were subjected to infection, where each cat was infected by intragastric inoculation with 100 cysts in 1 ml sterile PBS. One group of cats (remained uninfected as a control group) received 1 ml of sterile PBS only. Cat intestinal tissue was collected at different time points [6, 12, 18, 24, 72 and 96 hours post-infection (hpi)] from cats infected with *T. gondii*. Intestinal tissue was also collected from three cats in the uninfected group. The collected tissues were rinsed trice in PBS and kept frozen in liquid nitrogen until further processing.

RNA isolation and quantification

Total RNA from each intestine was extracted by TRIzol Reagent (Invitrogen Co. Ltd, San Diego, USA). RNA degradation and contamination were examined by electrophoresis on 1% agarose gels. RNA purity was checked by a NanoPhotometer® spectrophotometer (Implen, Westlake Village, CA, USA). RNA concentration was measured using a Qubit® RNA Assay Kit in a Qubit® 2.0 Fluorometer (Life Technologies, Carlsbad, CA, USA). RNA integrity was assessed using an RNA Nano 6000 Assay Kit and an Agilent Bioanalyzer 2100 system (Agilent Technologies, Santa Clara, CA, USA), demonstrating an RNA integrity number > 8.

Confirmation of *T. gondii* infection in the intestines

RNA (1 μg) collected at each time point stated above were reverse-transcribed to a single strand cDNA using a PrimeScript™ RT reagent kit with gDNA Eraster (Takara, Dalian, China). Infection was detected in the intestinal tissues using quantitative real-time PCR (qRT-PCR), which targets surface antigen one (SAG1) of *T. gondii* using forward primer: 5'-CAC AGA GCC TCC CAC TCT TG-3' and reverse primer: 5'-AGA CTA GCA GAA TCC CCC GT-3'. qRT-PCR was performed using a 7500 system (ABI), employing SYBR® Premix *Ex Taq*™ II (Takara). The reaction was performed in a final volume of 20 μl containing 10.4 μl Premix *Ex Taq* II, 0.8 μl of each primer, 2 μl of cDNA template, and 6 μl of double-distilled water (ddH_2O). PCR conditions were as follows: initial denaturation step at 95 °C for 30 s, followed by 40 cycles of 95 °C for 5 s and 60 °C for 34 s. All templates were examined in triplicate and controls without template were also included. The results of qRT-PCR were calculated by determination of the $2^{-\Delta\Delta CT}$ (where CT is the threshold cycle) (relative expression) level.

Library preparation for sequencing

Three micrograms of RNA per intestinal sample were used as an input for the RNA sample preparations. Sequencing libraries were generated using an NEBNext® Ultra™ RNA Library Prep Kit for Illumina® (NEB, Ipswich, USA) following manufacturer's recommendations and index codes were added to correlate sequences to their respective samples. The mRNA was purified from total RNA using poly-T oligo-attached magnetic beads. Fragmentation was performed using divalent cations under elevated temperature in NEBNext First Strand Synthesis Reaction Buffer (5×). First strand cDNA was synthesized using random hexamer primer and M-MuLV Reverse Transcriptase (RNase H). Second strand cDNA synthesis was subsequently performed using DNA Polymerase I and RNase H. Remaining overhangs were converted into blunt ends *via* exonuclease/polymerase activities. After adenylation of the 3' ends of DNA fragments, NEBNext Adaptors with a hairpin loop structure were ligated to prepare for hybridization. In order to select cDNA fragments preferentially ~150–200 bp in length, the library fragments were purified with AMPure XP system (Beckman Coulter, Beverly, USA). Then, 3 μl of USER Enzyme (NEB) were used with size-selected, adaptor-ligated cDNA at 37 °C for 15 min followed by 5 min at 95 °C before PCR. The PCR was performed with Phusion High-Fidelity DNA polymerase, Universal PCR primers and Index (X) Primer. PCR products were purified (AMPure XP system) and the quality of the libraries was assessed using an Agilent Bioanalyzer 2100 system. The clustering of the index-coded samples was performed on a cBot Cluster Generation System using TruSeq PE Cluster Kit v3-cBot-HS (Illumina, San Diego, USA) according to the manufacturer's instructions.

Differential expression analysis

Raw reads of fastq format were processed using in-house Perl scripts. Clean reads were obtained by removing reads adapters, poly-N containing reads and low-quality reads from raw data. The Q20, Q30 and GC content of the clean data were determined. All downstream analyses were based on the clean data. The *Felis catus* genome was used as the reference genome and gene model annotation files were downloaded from the cat genome website (ftp://ftp.ensembl.org/pub/release-76/fasta/felis_catus/dna/). Index of the reference genome was built using Bowtie v.2.2.3 and paired-end clean reads were aligned to *F. catus* reference genome using TopHat v.2.0.12. TopHat was selected as the mapping tool since it can produce a database of splice junctions based on the gene model annotation file and provides a better mapping result than other mapping tools [21]. HTSeq v.0.6.1 was used to count the read numbers mapped to each gene. Fragments per kilobase of transcript sequence per million base pairs sequenced (FPKM) of each gene was calculated in order to determine the level of gene expression. Differential expression analysis of two groups (three replicates per group) was performed using the DESeq R package (1.18.0) [22]. The *P*-values were adjusted using the Benjamini-Hochberg correction for multiple testing. Genes were determined to be significantly differentially expressed if they had a |log2(fold change)| > 0.58 and false-discovery rate (FDR) < 0.05.

Pearson's correlation analysis of samples used for RNA sequencing was carried out to examine the correlation between gene expression levels among samples. The square of the Pearson's correlation coefficient (R^2) < 0.92 indicates optimal sampling selection and experimental conditions. The distribution of differentially expressed genes (DEGs) on the chromosomes of cat genomes was examined. Clustering analysis of the DEGs was performed to determine the co-expression pattern of genes at different time points after infection. The genes with the same or similar expression pattern were grouped together into a cluster. *K*-means cluster was achieved based on the relative expression level of DEGs $\log_2$(fold change).

Gene Ontology (GO) and Kyoto Encyclopedia of Genes and Genomes (KEGG) analysis

GO enrichment analysis of DEGs was carried out using the *GOseq* R package [23]. All DEGs were mapped to GO terms in the database (http://www.geneontology.org/), and then gene numbers were calculated for every GO term using the hypergeometric test in order to obtain the significantly enriched GO terms for the DEGs; these were compared to the genomic background. GO terms with a corrected *P*-value less than 0.05 were considered significantly enriched by DEGs. KOBAS software was used to perform pathway analysis and to test the statistical enrichment of the DEGs in KEGG (http://www.genome.jp/kegg/) [24, 25]. This analysis was used to identify significantly enriched genes involved in metabolic or signalling pathways.

Validation of the RNA-Seq data

The expression of 10 to 14 selected genes was investigated by qRT-PCR to confirm the RNA sequencing based transcriptional response of cat intestine to *T. gondii* infection. These genes were identified by sequencing analysis as differentially upregulated or downregulated following the infection. Total RNA was isolated from the intestinal tissues obtained from *T. gondii*-infected and uninfected (control) cats at different time points after infection using RNeasy Mini Kit (Qiagen, Hilden, Germany). DNase-digested total RNA (1 μg) was reverse-transcribed to single strand cDNA using the Primer Script™ RT Reagent Kit with gDNA Eraser (Takara). SYBR Premix *Ex Taq*™ II (Takara) was used to perform qRT-PCR on an ABI real-time PCR cycler (ABI 7500). Forward (F) and reverse (R) primers used to amplify the selected genes are listed in Table 1. The amplification reactions were performed using the following conditions: 95 °C for 10 min followed by 40 cycles of 95 °C for 15 s and 60 °C for 1 min. Melting curve analysis was performed using the following conditions: 1 min at 95 °C, 65 °C for 2 min and progressive increase from 65 to 95 °C to ensure that a single product was amplified in each reaction. The relative fold change in gene expression was calculated following actin normalization using the $2^{-\Delta\Delta CT}$ method. The mean values of the control cats were used to calculate the fold change for the infected cats.

Results

Confirmation of *T. gondii* infection

Detection and amplification of *T. gondii SAG1* gene was confirmed in all infected cats by qRT-PCR assay. The three cats in the control group were qRT-PCR-negative. The results also revealed that *SAG1* gene was amplified in intestinal samples of cats starting from 6 hpi and peaking at 96 hpi.

RNA-Seq data

We employed RNA-Seq to investigate the temporal gene expression patterns of cat intestine during early infection with *T. gondii* PRU strain. Over 25,000,000 raw reads were obtained from each intestinal sample and more than 24,000,000 clean reads were obtained after removing adaptors and low-quality reads. About 83% of the clean reads were mapped to the reference genome and more than 70% of the clean reads were located in the exon regions; the rest were in the introns or intergenic. Pearson's correlation coefficient of gene expression among different time points was close to 1, indicating the high similarity of the gene expression patterns between samples (Fig. 1). The distribution of DEGs on cat chromosomes is shown in Fig. 2. The chromosomal location of DEGs across the different time points after infection showed more upregulated gene expression on chromosomes D2, D3 and E2, and a skewed pattern of downregulated genes on the X chromosome (Additional file 1: Table S1).

Gene expression analysis

Differential gene expression analysis was performed by comparing the gene transcriptional level in response to *T. gondii* infection to that in the uninfected control samples at each time point after infection (FDR < 0.05 and |log2(fold change)| > 0.58). Transcriptome analysis revealed 2363 infection-specific DEGs, of which 56, 184, 404, 508, 400 and 811 genes were differentially expressed at 6, 12, 18, 24, 72 and 96 hpi, respectively (Fig. 3, Additional file 2: Table S2). qRT-PCR results of the examined set of genes at 6, 12, 18, 24, 72 and 96 hpi in cat intestine were consistent with the RNA-Seq results, confirming the validity of sequencing data (Fig. 4).

Cluster analysis

Hierarchical cluster analysis using k-means grouped all DEGs into six clusters according to their expression pattern across the six time points post-infection (Fig. 5). Cluster 1 (containing 433 genes) and cluster 3 (127 genes) showed a progressive increase in the expression with time after infection. Genes in cluster 2 (409 genes) and cluster 4 (214 genes) were downregulated as *T. gondii* infection proceeds. Cluster 5 (38 genes) and cluster 6 (15 genes) showed a bi-phasic upregulated expressional pattern, but at different time points after infection. Venn diagram analysis revealed 70 genes that were differentially co-expressed in infected samples at all time points (12, 18, 24, 72 and 96 hpi) compared with control samples (Fig. 6). The highest number of specific DEGs was detected at 96 hpi (347), which was significantly higher than that of any other time point. The number of DEGs from 72 and 96 hpi were less than that from 24 and 96 hpi. The mechanisms that underpin these temporal changes of gene expressions remain to be investigated. These aforementioned results indicate that most of the upregulated genes were grouped in clusters 1, 3 and 5, whereas clusters 2 and 4 contained most of the downregulated genes.

Gene ontology (GO) classifications

GO analysis showed that DEGs were overrepresented by GO terms involved in immune responses, such as chemokine receptor binding and cytokine activity. The top 30 differentially expressed GO terms of the DEGs in cat intestine are shown in Table 2. GO analysis of DEGs at various time points post-infection revealed the dynamic changes in biological processes, molecular function and cellular component during early stages of *T. gondii* infection in the cat intestine. The top 30 most enriched GO terms with the corresponding

Table 1 Primers used in the qRT-PCR in the present study

Gene	Sequence (5'-3')	Primer length (mer)	Tm (°C)	GC %	Product length (bp)
β-actin	ATTCCACGGCACAGTCAAGG	20	63.39	55	110
	CACCAGCATCACCCCATTT	19	61.75	52.63	
RSAD2	CACCAGCGTCAACTACCACT	20	59.97	55	140
	AATATTCACCGGCTTCCTGC	20	58.32	50	
SYCN	AAGACGCGCAAGTTCTCGAC	20	61.28	55	117
	AAGGCATCAGTAACACCTGCAA	22	60.49	45.45	
CELA1	ATGCTACGCTTCTTGGTGCT	20	60.04	50	239
	CGGAAGGTCATTTTGCGGTC	20	59.83	50	
GKN2	CTTGAAGGTGGTATGCCTGGT	21	60	52.38	214
	CCTGGATGCGATGTAGCGAT	20	60.04	55	
TFF2	ATGCGTCATGGAAGTCTCGG	22	62.14	50	198
	TGACAGTCGTCAACGGACATC	24	61.04	45.83	
LYPF	TTACACCCGACAAACCCTGA	20	59.24	52.38	132
	CAGGTCTCCGGCCTTTATTCT	21	60.67	55	
CYP1A1	TCGATACCTACCCAACCCTG	20	58.22	55	246
	ACTGTGTCAAATCCAGCTCCG	21	60.61	52.38	
CLPS	TGCTCTGCCAAGACACTCTAT	21	58.82	47.62	222
	5'CAATCAGACAAGGGAGGTGCT	21	60	52.38	
CPA2	TGCTCAGTCATCTACCAAGCC	21	59.79	52.38	100
	ATCGACCTGTGTCCCTCAGT	20	60.25	55	
PRSS2	TACTTCTGCCGCCATGACTC	20	59.82	55	227
	TCACTTGGATGCGAGACTTGT	21	59.66	47.62	
CPA1	AACGATTTACCAAGCCAGCGG	21	61.55	52.38	210
	GCCGAAGGACCAGTTCAGTA	20	59.39	55	
FLNC	AGTGGTGCCACCCTGTAACC	20	62.06	60	181
	CTCTCGCACTTTCACTGGCT	20	60.32	55	
FN1	GAACACTAATGTCAACTGCCCA	22	58.85	45.45	125
	TGGACCTTGGCAGAGAATCC	20	59.38	55	
DES	ATGTCCAAGCCAGACCTCAC	20	59.67	55	240
	GGAATCGTTGGTGCCCTTGA	20	60.61	55	
ACTG2	GTATACTCGGTGCTCAAGCC	20	58.15	55	243
	TAGGATCCCTCGCTTGCTCT	20	60.11	55	
FABP6	CCCACAGCTACCAACGCTAC	20	60.74	60	185
	ATTCTGCTGGAGAGCATCTTCAAT	24	60.39	41.67	
MYH11	GCATGCTGCAAGATCGAGAG	20	59.42	55	147
	CTTGCGTGATGCTTGTGTCC	20	60.11	55	
FGB	CCCAATCAACCTTCGTGTGC	20	59.76	55	156
	TCCTCACATTCTTTGCCAGACA	22	59.89	45.45	
TAGLN	AACGGCGTGATTCTGAGCAA	20	60.23	47.2	158
	CCACCTGCTCCATTTGCTTG	21	59.78	50	
ALPI	ACACACCTCATGGGCCTCTT	20	61.14	55	199
	TCAGTGCCAGATAAGCCCTG	20	59.46	55	
CNN1	TGGCATCATTCTTTGCGAGTTC	22	59.84	45.45	153
	TCGAAAATGTCGTGGGGCTT	20	60.25	50	

Table 1 Primers used in the qRT-PCR in the present study *(Continued)*

Gene	Sequence (5'-3')	Primer length (mer)	Tm (°C)	GC %	Product length (bp)
LYPD2	TGAGATGCTACACCTGTCACG	21	59.80	52.38	123
	AGAAGGGGTACACTATCTCCAAG	23	58.71	47.83	
pCREB	CCACAACCATCCGTCCTTCT	20	62.26	55	137
	TGTGTGTGTGTGTGTCGGTATGT	23	62.26	47.83	
MMP	GACGACGATGAGCTGTGGA	19	61.02	57.89	115
	TGGTGTATTCCTTGCCGTTG	20	61.85	50	
FABP1	CTGATGAAGGTGCCAAGAACAA	22	62.46	45.45	132
	GCATTTCCTCACTATTTCCCACTC	24	62.3	45.83	

Abbreviation: Tm, melting temperature

number of genes at each time point after infection are shown (Fig. 7). Catalytic activity and metabolic process were the most significantly enriched GO terms in molecular function category and biological process category, respectively. This finding was consistently observed in all of the six groups (6, 12, 18, 24, 72, and 96 hpi) compared to the uninfected control group, suggesting that these processes play fundamental roles in feline response to infection with this parasite.

Functional analysis of the transcriptional response of cat intestine to *T. gondii* infection

Compared to controls, 145 genes were assigned to 62 pathways at 6 hpi, 386 genes were involved in 141 pathways at 12 hpi, 674 genes were involved in 201 pathways at 18 hpi, 890 genes were involved in 206 pathways at 24 hpi, 673 genes were involved in 189 pathways at 72 hpi, and 1321 genes were involved in 238 pathways at 96 hpi. The top 20 most overrepresented pathways in each group are shown in Fig. 8. Interestingly, pathways related to metabolism were enriched in samples from all time points except at 6 hpi. These results agree with the results of GO analysis of DEGs and show that fewer host pathways were identified within 6 h of infection to be uniquely affected by *T. gondii* infection. As shown in Table 3, 36 KEGG pathways were differentially expressed in cat intestine following *T. gondii* infection.

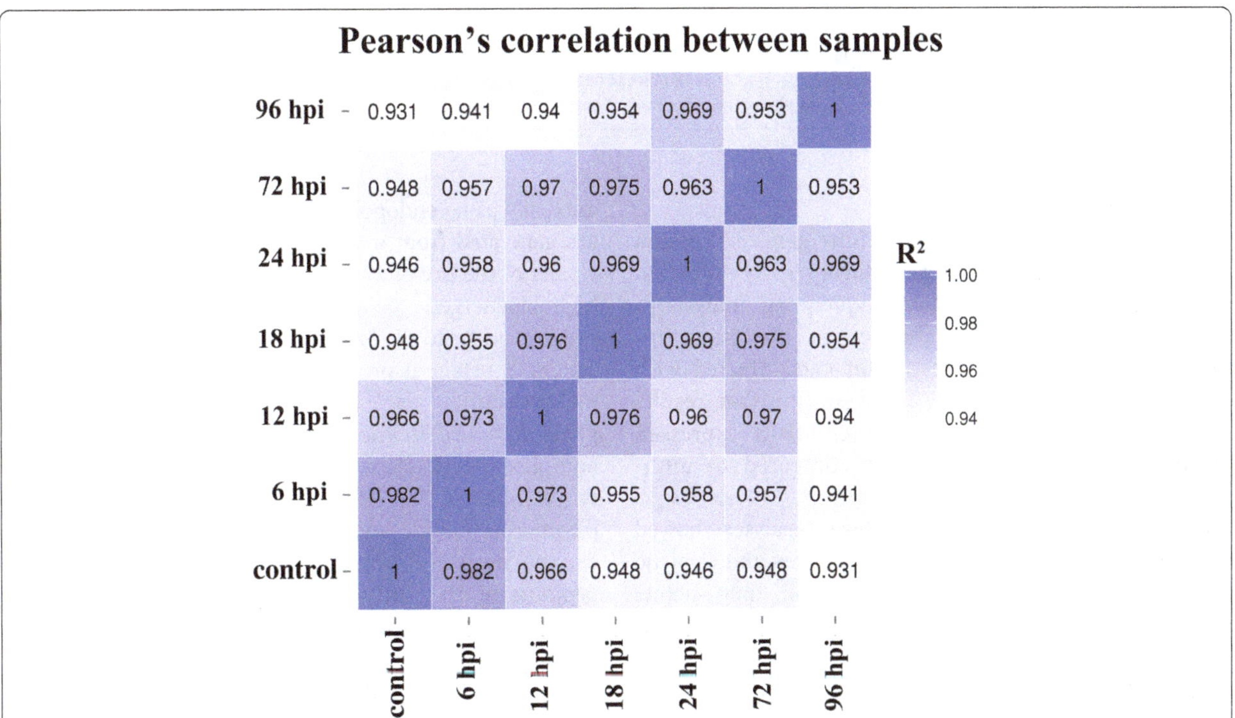

Fig. 1 A heatmap showing the magnitude of the Pearson's correlation coefficient matrix among different groups. The map shows that all correlations in this matrix are positive and of moderate to large value. Variables: 0 (control), 6, 12, 18, 24, 72 and 96 hours post-infection

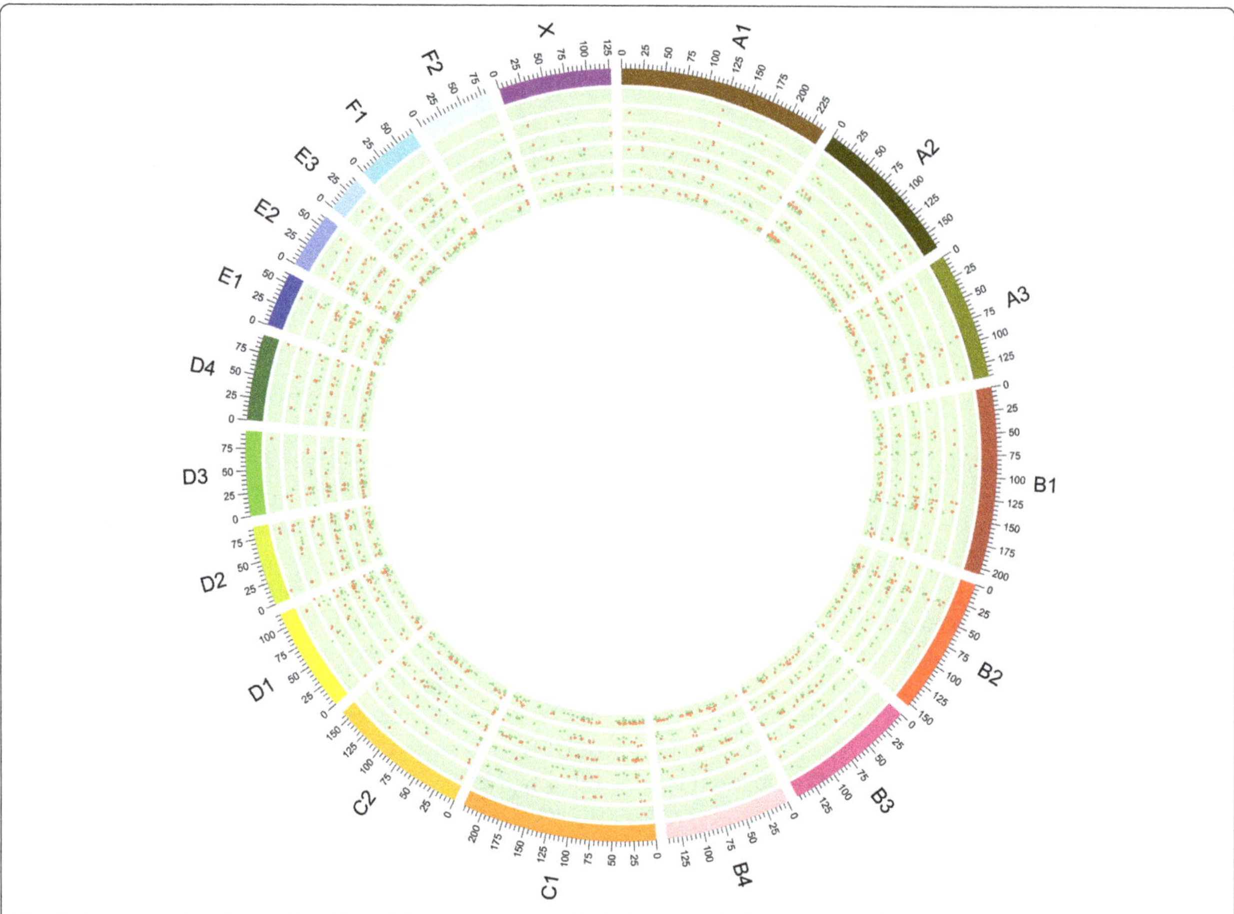

Fig. 2 Chromosomal position of the differentially expressed genes (DEGs) implicated in *T. gondii* interaction with cat intestine. Circos plot shows the relative expression levels of DEGs in the cat chromosomes. Up- and downregulated genes were found on all cat chromosomes; however, the DEGs encoded by chromosome X were mainly downregulated. Chromosome number and bands are identified in the outermost ring. Other tracks from outer to inner compares the cat intestinal transcriptional response to *T. gondii* infection at 6, 12, 18, 24, 72, and 96 hours post-infection. Red and green color represents the upregulated and downregulated genes, respectively

Discussion

This study aimed to investigate how gene expression in the cat intestine is altered during early infection with *T. gondii*. We used RNA sequencing analysis to determine any temporal changes in the transcriptional response of the intestine of cats infected with *T. gondii* at 6, 12, 18, 24, 72 and 96 hpi. Our results showed that 2363 genes were differentially expressed in the intestine of infected cats compared to uninfected control cats.

GO enrichment and KEGG pathway analyses showed that DEGs involved in the metabolic process and catalytic activity were the most enriched at all time points post-infection. A previous study has reported the upregulation of cell growth/maintenance (Translation and Transcription GO categories) and metabolism (Glycolysis and TCA Cycle GO categories)-related genes in the *T. gondii* merozoite stage during intestinal infection of mice [26]. This intraepithelial intestinal stage of *T. gondii* proliferates asexually using endopolygeny, whereby multiple daughters are generated from a single parental organism [27]. The results of the present and previous studies underscore the high bioenergetic demands of the growing parasite, in order to adapt to the low oxygen tension in the cat's intestine, and sustain its proliferation [28].

Our results also showed the downregulation of genes involved in the class I major histocompatibility complex (MHC I) pathway, at 6 and 12 hpi. MHC I is composed of the polymorphic heavy chain, β2-microglobulin, and antigenic peptides. The latter can be derived from endogenous proteins and from proteins of this intracellular parasite. These proteins are degraded by the proteolytic proteasome complex, then transported into the endoplasmic reticulum (ER) where they associate with the class I molecule to form MHC I. One of the physiological functions of MHC I is recognition by the peptide-specific T-cell receptors of cytolytic T lymphocytes (CTLs). These

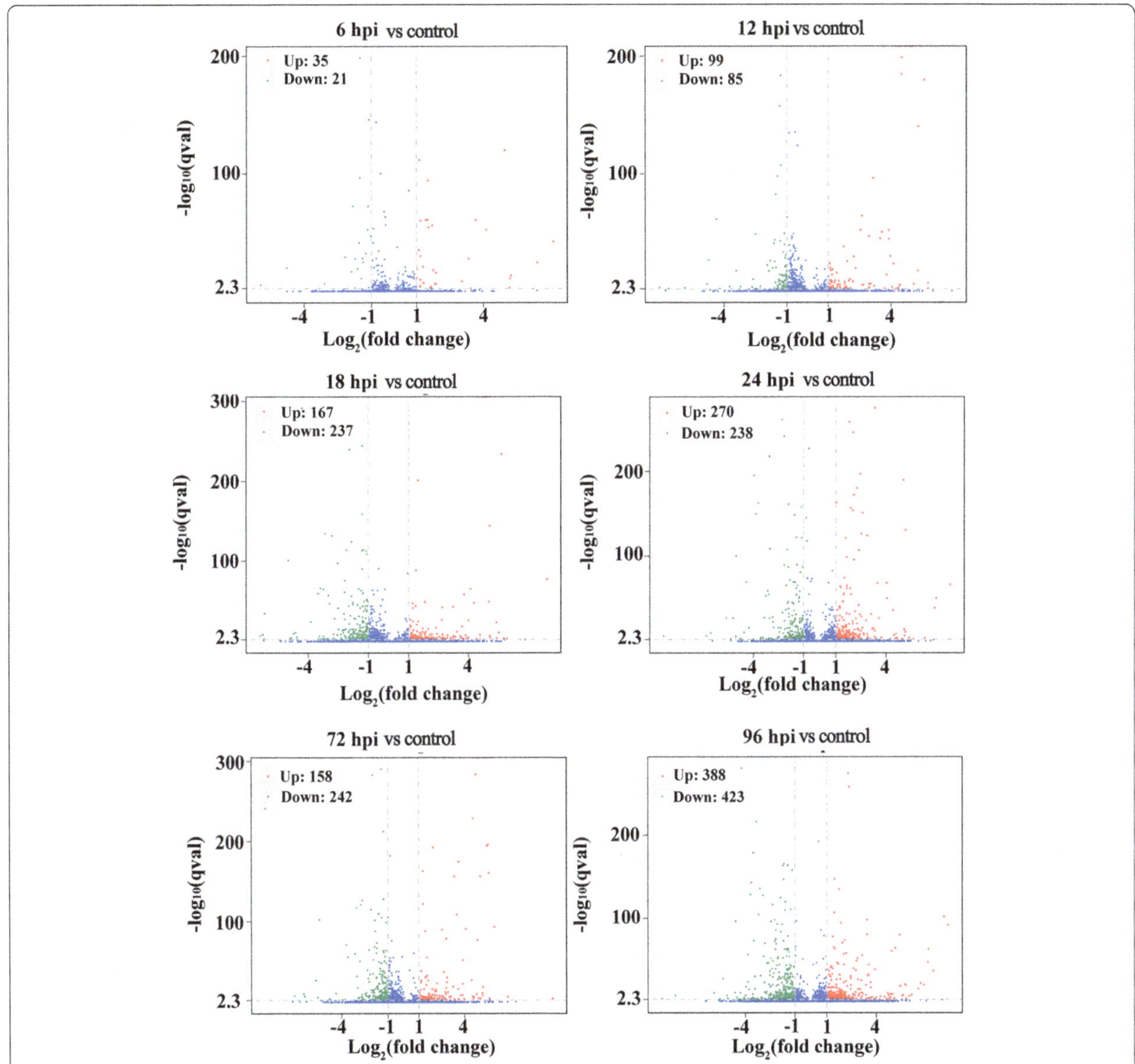

Fig. 3 Volcano plots showing the transcriptional response of cat intestine to infection with *T. gondii* PRU strain at each of the indicated time points after infection compared to those of the uninfected controls. Differentially expressed genes (DEGs) are shown as red (upregulated) or green (downregulated) dots. Non-significant difference between the expressions of genes is indicated by blue dots. The X-axis represents the value of $\log_2$(fold change) and the Y-axis shows the value of $-\log_{10}$(qval)

cells are known to play critical roles in controlling *T. gondii* infection, by limiting the reactivation of latent infection and parasite proliferation during acute infection [29–31]. CTLs eliminate infected cells by recognition of foreign antigens that are processed in a proteasome-dependent pathway and presented by MHC I [32]. Therefore, the downregulation of MHC I genes during the first 12 hours after infection can reduce the antigen-specific CTL cell-mediated killing of *T. gondii*-infected cells [33]. Interferon gamma (IFN-γ) plays a critical role in innate immunity during acute *T. gondii* infection [34]. PA28, a proteasome activator induced by IFN-γ, has been implicated in MHC I antigen processing. The upregulation of the *PA28* gene, observed at 24 hpi, indicates that levels of this IFN-γ-inducible activator protein, PA28, had increased to enhance the cat's defense response. PA28 promotes antigen processing and presentation, through recruiting more immunoproteasomes to proteasomes, and processing more parasite antigens during acute infection [35, 36]. Antigenic peptides resulting from proteasomal degradation are translocated

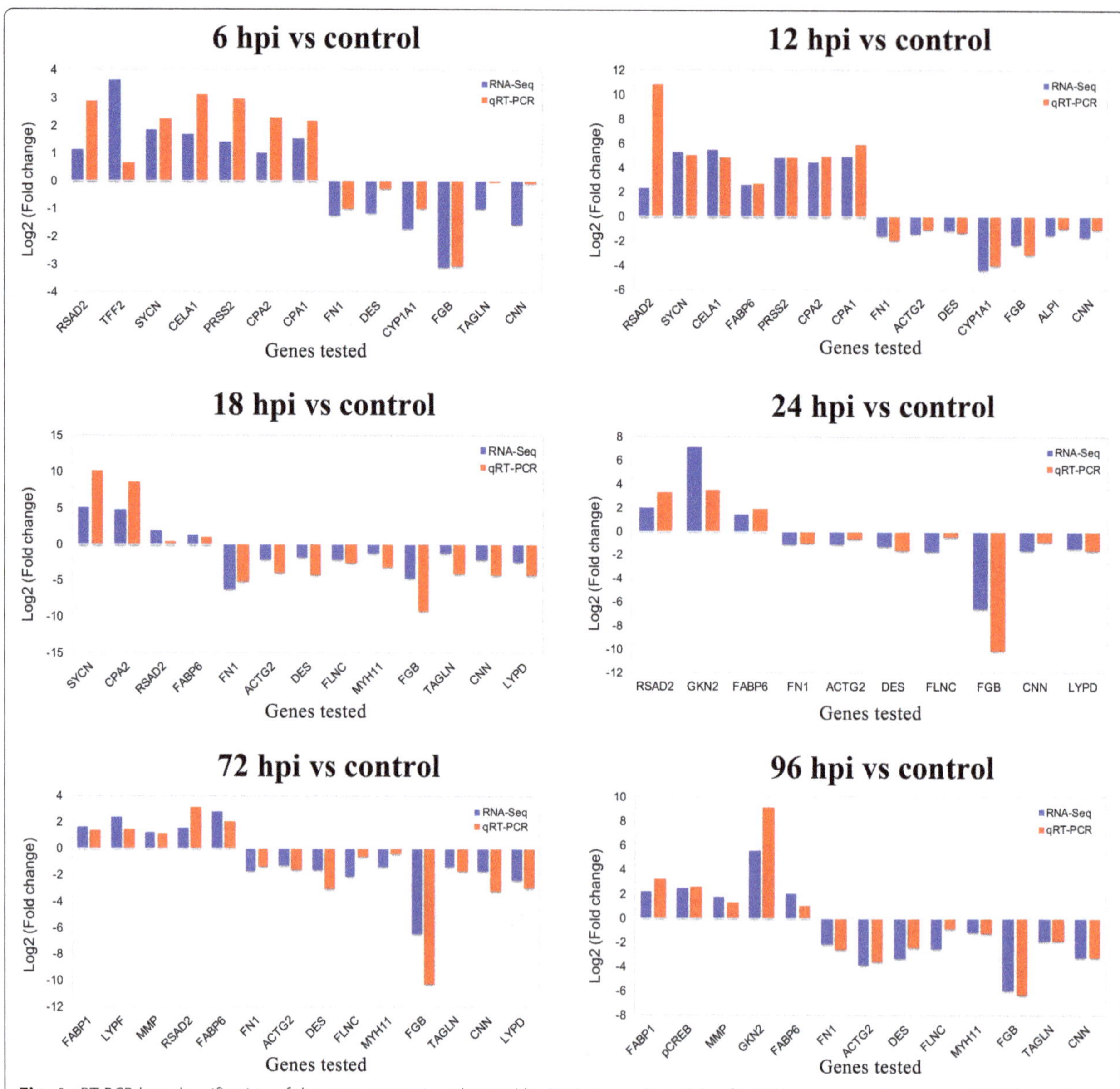

Fig. 4 qRT-PCR-based verification of the gene expression obtained by RNA sequencing. Data of RNA-Seq were confirmed by qRT-PCR at 6, 12, 18, 24, 72 and 96 hours post-infection. The X-axis shows the name of genes tested and the Y-axis represents the relative expression for the genes examined

into the ER lumen *via* transporters associated with antigen processing (*TAP1/2*) [37]. Therefore, the upregulation of the *TAP1/2* gene, observed at 24 hpi, may have also enhanced the cats' intestinal immune response to *T. gondii* infection.

The molecular chaperones heat-shock proteins (HSPs) can stimulate cells of the innate immune response by serving as 'danger'-signaling molecules [38]. After HSP70 binds to the surface of antigen presenting cells, MHC I presentation of the HSP-bound cytosolic antigen occurs, mediated by a transporter associated with antigen processing (TAP) [39]. We did not find any significant changes in the regulation of MHC I gene expression at 18 and 24 hpi; however, *hsp70* and *hsp90* genes were upregulated at both time points, in addition to *PA28* and *TAP1/2* genes at 24 hpi. HSP70 and HSP90 are peptide-binding proteins, and are associated with antigenic epitopes [40]. The upregulation of the HSP70/HSP90 complex may support the immune response, through enhancing antigen processing and presentation *via* proteasome and enhancing cell viability. *hsp70* is expressed in response to a variety of pathological stimuli, and allows the cell to survive lethal insults [41]. The interplay between HSP70 and HSP90 is of crucial

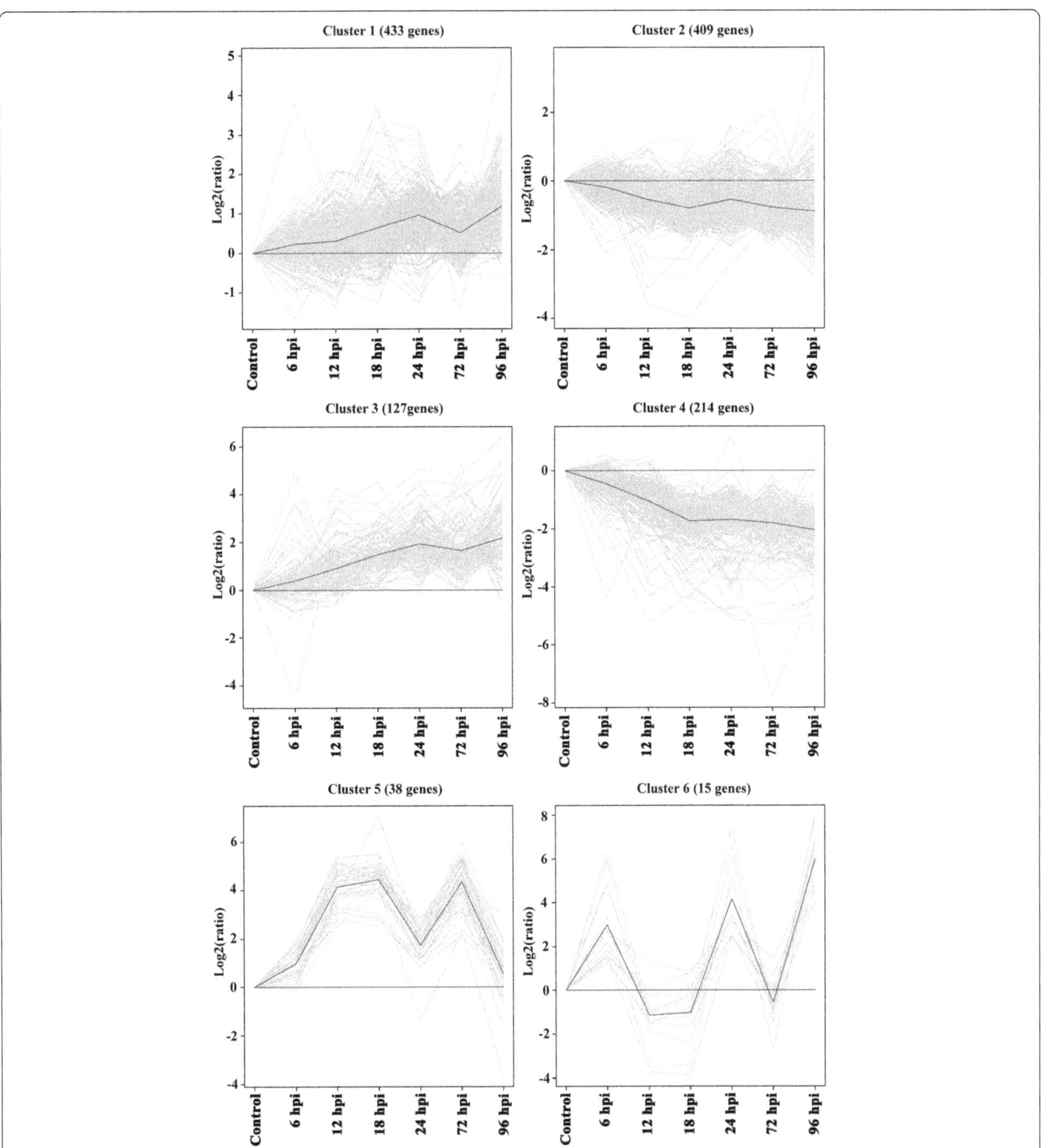

Fig. 5 Expression pattern clustering from RNA-Seq analysis of 2363 DEGs in the intestine of cats infected with *T. gondii*. Differentially expressed, co-regulated genes from adjacent stage pairwise comparisons were analyzed using k-means clustering. The identified DEGs were grouped into 6 clusters based on the similarity of their expression. The six clusters are shown in a graphical format based on the pattern of expression at different time points after infection. The X-axis represents time points after infection and the Y-axis indicates the relative gene expression

importance for cell viability [42]. *Toxoplasma gondii* may benefit from the upregulation of *hsp70*, by maintaining the integrity of surrogate host cells, in order to complete its own growth, and to evade immunological detection. A connection between the upregulation of *HSP* genes and the division of schizont nucleoli has been suggested as nuclear division was not detected after 24 hpi in cat intestine [43].

These results support the hypothesis that *T. gondii*, through the downregulation of MHCI- related genes

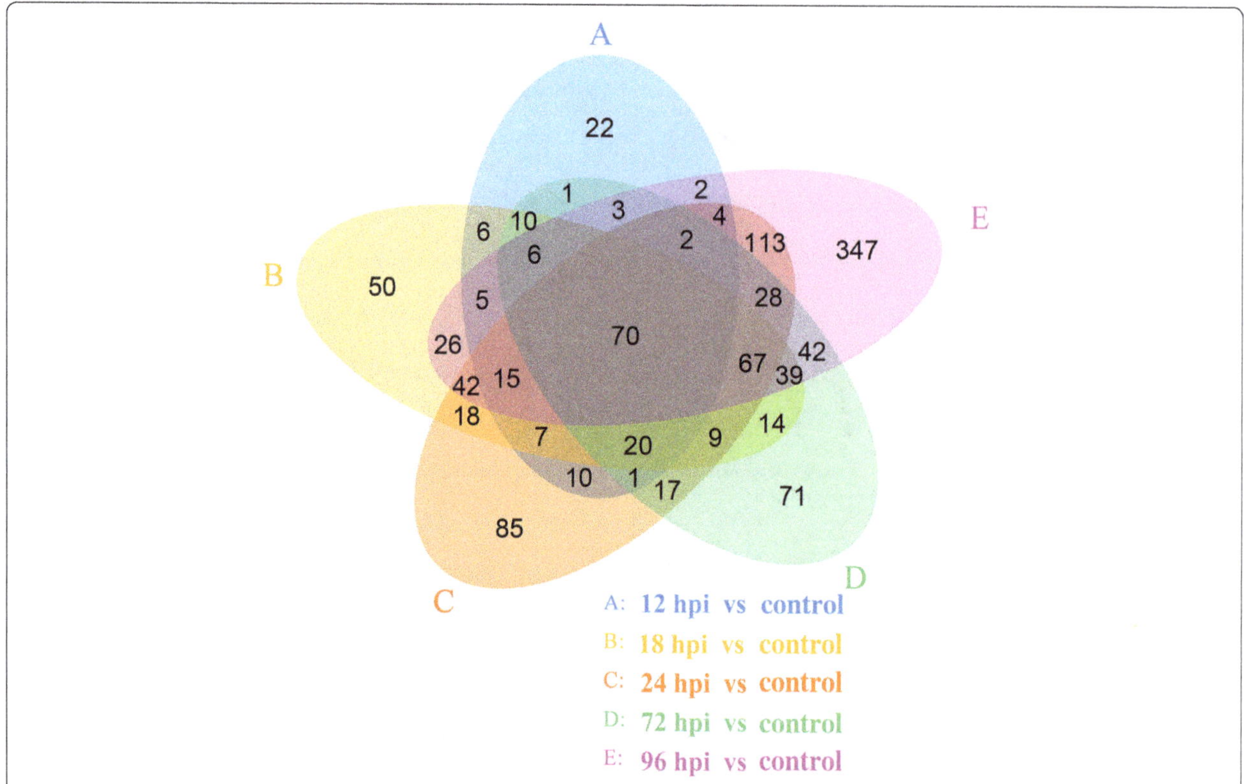

Fig. 6 Venn diagram depicting the respective unique and shared differentially expressed genes among five *Toxoplasma gondii*-infected groups at 12, 18, 24, 72 and 96 hours post-infection. The result of 6 hpi was not shown because this two-dimensional diagram could not display more than five comparisons

evades the immune response in order to facilitate its own growth in the intestine of cats during the first 12 hpi. Host cells, *via* increasing the expression of *HSP70/90*, *PA28*, *TAP*, and *TAP1/2* genes, deploy chaperones, immunoproteasomes and transporters to limit infection, through promoting antigen processing and presentation. In the present study, as infection progressed, the expression of MHC I genes was elevated at 72 and 96 hpi, indicating that the cats may have mounted a CTL response, mediated by MHC I, to limit replication of the parasite. Infecting cultured rat-intestinal epithelial cells with mature sporozoites, induced an elevated expression of genes associated with tumor necrosis factor alpha (TNFα) signaling, *via* NF-κB [44]. This transcriptomic change was not observed in our study, suggesting that anti-*T. gondii* intestinal immunity can vary between different hosts and different parasite stages, and based on whether the infection was established under *in vitro* or *in vivo* conditions.

Fatty acid binding proteins (FABPs) are released from the cytoplasm following the loss of enterocyte membrane integrity. *Toxoplasma gondii* can damage cell integrity, leading to the release of FABPs into the circulatory system. Ileal FABP (Il-FABP), which is located at the distal part of the small intestine, can mediate the uptake of fatty-acids. Peroxisome proliferator-activated receptors (PPARs) are activated by fatty acids and their derivatives. Il-FABP was upregulated in the intestine of cats from 12 to 96 hpi, but was downregulated at 6 hpi. This suggests a correlation between infection-induced alterations in the expression of FABP, and its potential lipid-metabolizing capacity [45] on the activation of PPARs, and the subsequent influence on key biological processes, such as the regulation of glucose, lipid homeostasis, cell survival, inflammation, proliferation and differentiation.

Through metabolic activation caused by phase I enzymes in conjugation with phase II enzymes, xenobiotic compounds such as drugs and chemical pollutants can be eliminated in the urine or bile by phase III transporters [46]. Phase I enzymes include the cytochrome P450 (CYP) superfamily, whereas phase II conjugating enzymes include some enzyme superfamilies; for example sulfotransferase, glutathione S-transferase (GST) and uridine diphosphate-glucuronosyltransferase (UGT). Some CYPs, for example CYP1A1, CYP1A2, CYP1B1 and CYP2A6, are procarcinogen-bioactivating enzymes. By metabolizing xenobiotics into reactive

Table 2 The top 30 differentially expressed GO terms between *T. gondii*-infected and uninfected cats

GO category	GO name	Gene number						FDR corrected *P*-value
		Cluster 1	Cluster 2	Cluster 3	Cluster 4	Cluster 5	Cluster 6	
Biological process	Carbohydrate_metabolic_process	22	28	4	27	1	0	2.03E-04
	Cellular amino acid metabolic process	20	8	8	6	0	0	0.014098
	tRNA metabolic process	20	5	5	3	0	0	0.04415
Cellular component	Extracellular region	30	27	38	6	11	2	3.84E-04
	Extracellular matrix	7	7	14	0	3	0	0.018194
	Extracellular matrix component	1	4	10	0	1	0	0.014935
	Myosin complex	6	2	8	0	1	0	0.021049
	Extracellular region part	13	11	19	0	5	0	0.022411
Molecular function	Catalytic activity	194	93	182	19	40	5	4.44E-16
	Hydrolase activity	95	52	93	15	13	3	3.02E-10
	Ion binding	137	49	117	6	23	1	0.044804
	Nucleotide binding	94	16	48	2	11	0	0.008417
	Small molecule binding	99	19	55	3	12	0	0.001499
	Anion binding	92	18	49	1	10	1	0.020323
	Carbohydrate derivative binding	83	16	42	3	10	0	0.026838
	Pyrophosphatase activity	52	6	24	0	4	0	0.030815
	Nucleoside-triphosphatase activity	51	6	23	0	4	0	0.043152
	Oxidoreductase activity	47	14	41	3	10	1	2.03E-04
	Cofactor binding	23	9	23	2	8	0	0.001491
	Cargo receptor activity	4	3	4	0	0	0	0.001611
	Chemokine receptor binding	5	0	1	0	4	0	0.002826
	Coenzyme binding	15	4	12	1	3	0	0.008153
	G-protein coupled receptor binding	5	0	1	0	4	0	0.012537
	Motor activity	12	2	9	0	1	0	0.012498
	Metalloexopeptidase activity	0	2	2	3	0	0	0.013723
	Metallocarboxypeptidase activity	0	2	1	3	0	0	0.036387
	Tetrapyrrole binding	4	4	7	1	4	0	0.029038
	Cytokine activity	5	0	1	0	4	0	0.033712
	Peroxiredoxin activity	4	0	1	0	0	0	0.037208
	Adenylylsulfate kinase activity	2	1	2	0	0	0	0.044538

oxygenated intermediates (ROMs), which can cause genotoxicity and mutation by covalently binding to nucleic acids and proteins, CYPs can trigger tumor development [46]. In this study, the expression of the *CYP1A1* gene was downregulated from 6 to 96 hpi, except at 72 hpi, and the *GSTA2* gene was upregulated from 18 to 96 hpi. While downregulated *CYP1A1* can reduce the production of ROMs, thus minimizing DNA and protein damage, the upregulation of *GSTA2* may allow cytotoxic xenobiotics to accumulate, possibly triggering tumor development. This may be a mechanism *via* which *T. gondii* contributes to the development of some forms of cancer [47].

The expression of *UGT1A* was decreased from 12 to 96 hpi; however, no significant change in the gene expression was observed at 6 hpi. The UGT1A1 enzyme can detoxify many endogenous and exogenous compounds [48]. For example, irinotecan is widely used for the treatment of metastatic colorectal cancer and is metabolized by esterase to form a SN-38, which is further conjugated to UGT1A1. Patients with the UGT1A1 variant have poor metabolism of SN-38 and are thus prone to irinotecan toxicity because of the difficulty of SN-38 excretion from body in the non-toxic SN-38G form [49]. It is possible to hypothesize that cancer patients concurrently infected with *T. gondii*, if administered irinotecan,

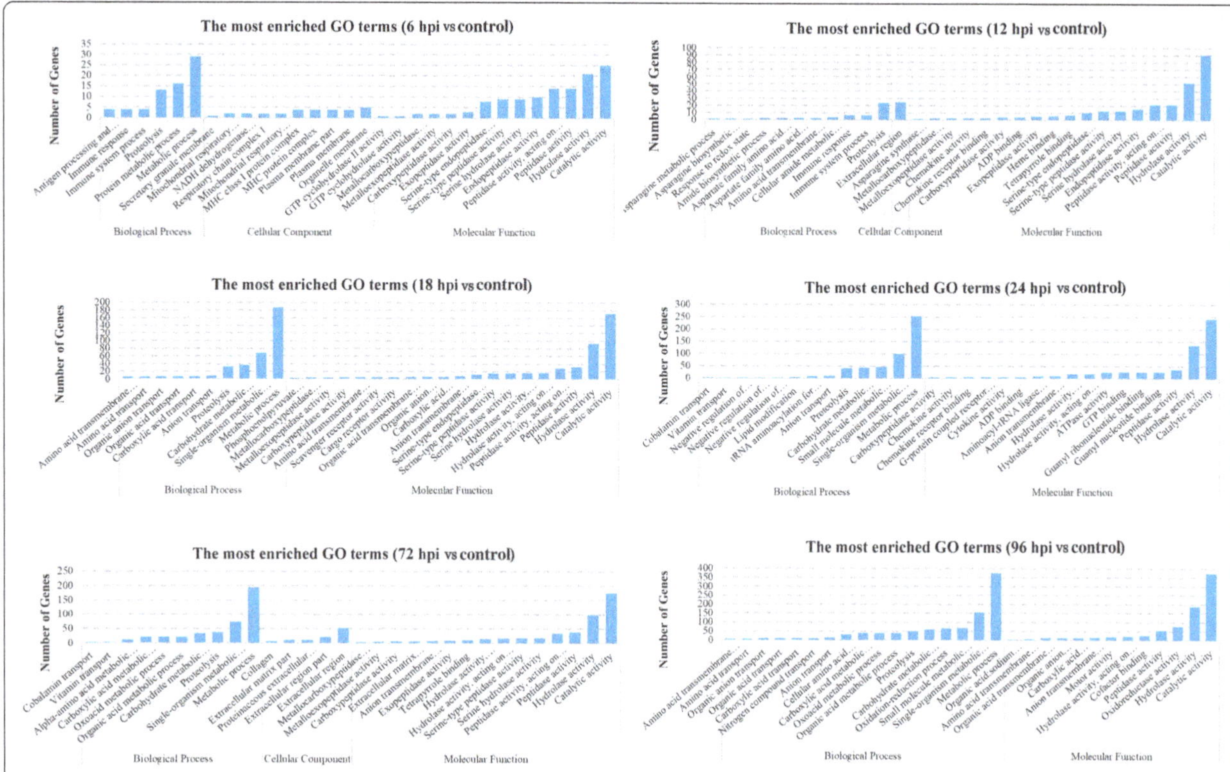

Fig. 7 The gene ontology (GO) analysis of the DEGs. The 30 most significantly enriched GO terms for each time point after infected *versus* control are shown. The GO distributions are summarized in three main categories: biological process, cellular component and molecular function. The X-axis shows different GO terms and the Y-axis indicates the corresponding number of genes in each GO term

may experience serious toxicity due to limited detoxification and increased accumulation of SN-38 caused by reduced expression of *UGT1A*. The expression of *UGT1A* during the *T. gondii*-host interaction raises a new question about the potential impact of parasite infection on irinotecan-treated cancer patients.

A link between *T. gondii* infection and Alzheimer's disease (AD) has also been previously suggested [50–52]. We were intrigued by the observation that the neutral endopeptidase (*NEP*), amyloid-β precursor protein (*APP*) and *APOE* genes were significantly downregulated at 24, 72 and 96 hpi, respectively. The altered expression of the *NEP*, *APP* and *APOE* genes may impact the metabolism of endogenous amyloid-β, putatively a main contributor to AD [53–55]. Here, the downregulation of *NEP*, *APP* and *APOE* genes at 24, 72 and 96 hpi suggests diverse means by which early *T. gondii* may contribute to the development of AD. In this study, we have not quantified the extent of *T. gondii* infection in each cat, nor considered the impact of parasite burden on the hosts' response. Therefore, the differences in host transcript abundance, observed over the course of infection, might have been influenced by changes in parasite burden or changes in parasite life stage development. Quantification of parasite burden, either through qPCR or analyzing parasite reads in RNA-Seq data, should be used to address this issue in future investigations. In addition, looking at differences in host transcript abundance during parasite life stage transitions throughout the course of infection, may provide critical insights in to how the feline host supports sexual reproduction.

Conclusions

Whole-transcriptome profiling, using RNA-Seq technology, of the cat's intestine following infection with *T. gondii* improved our understanding of the signaling pathways that mediate the response of cat intestine to early infection. Comparing the infection groups to the PBS-treated control group, 56, 184, 404, 508, 400 and 811 significantly DEGs were identified at 6, 12, 18, 24, 72 and 96 hpi, respectively. Our data suggest that *T. gondii* can modulate immune response and metabolic pathway to facilitate its development and survival in cat intestine. At 6 and 12 hpi, downregulation of MHC I genes may contribute to the establishment of infection in cat intestine during this early stage of host-parasite interaction. To counter the infection, the cat leverages chaperones, immunoproteasomes and transporters, through the upregulation of *HSP70/90*, *PA28*, *TAP*, and

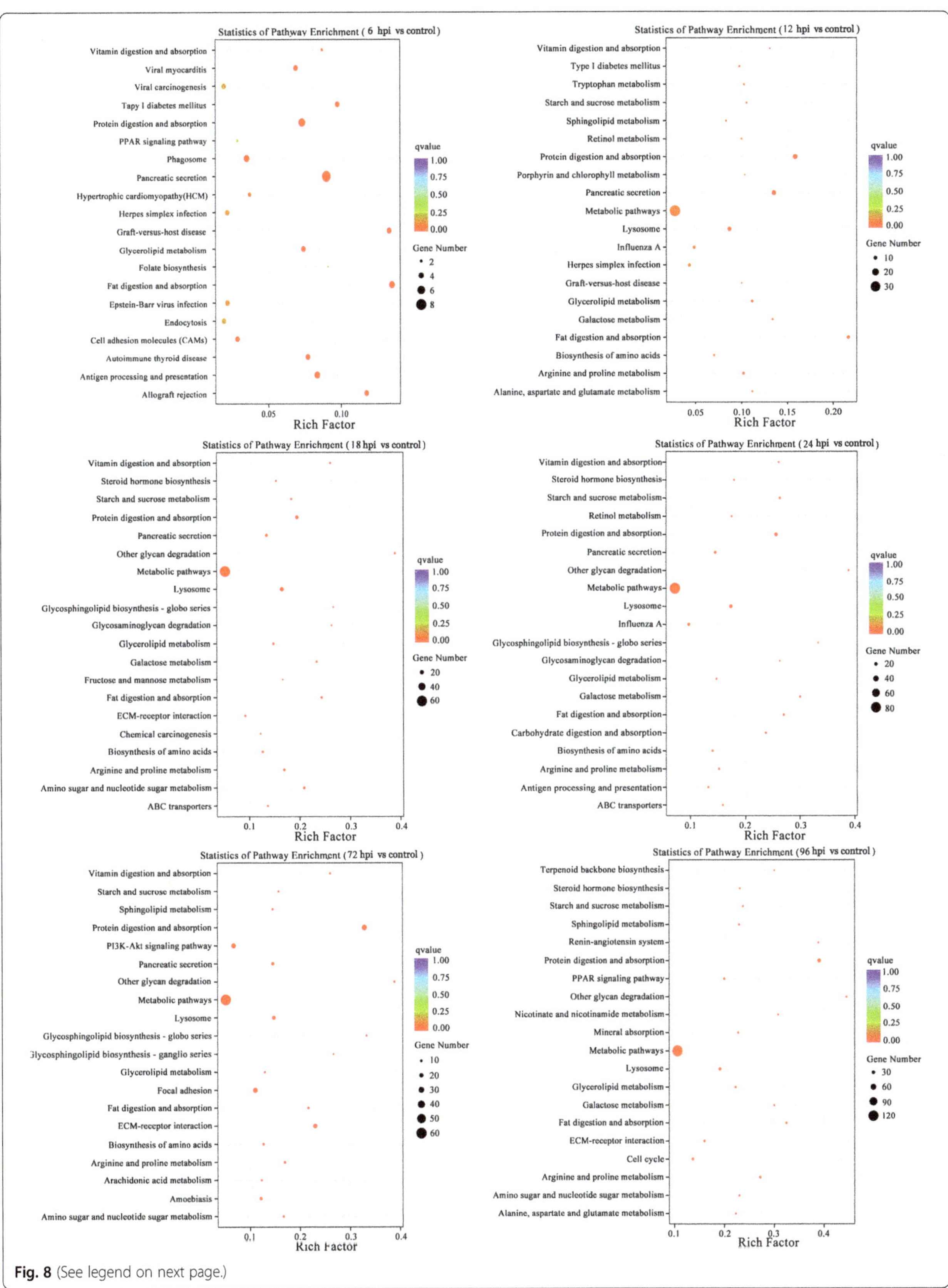

Fig. 8 (See legend on next page.)

(See figure on previous page.)
Fig. 8 Scatter plots of the enriched KEGG pathways statistics. The *q*-value is the corrected *P*-value (range from 0 to 1). The colour and size of the dots represent the range of the *q*-value (level of significance) and the number of DEGs mapped to the indicated pathways, respectively. The X-axis shows the enrichment factor; the Y-axis corresponds to the KEGG Pathway. The top 20 enriched KEGG pathways of the indicated groups are shown. Rich factor is the ratio of the DEG number to the total gene number in a certain pathway

Table 3 Total differentially expressed KEGG pathways overrepresented/enriched by the differentially expressed genes in cat intestine in response to infection with *T. gondii*

KEGG pathway	Gene number						FDR corrected *P*-value
	Cluster 1	Cluster 2	Cluster 3	Cluster 4	Cluster 5	Cluster 6	
Protein digestion and absorption	1	16	1	10	7	1	2.66E-15
Lysosome	3	9	1	13	0	1	4.44E-06
Mineral absorption	0	10	1	3	0	0	5.75E-05
ECM-receptor interaction	0	13	1	5	0	0	0.000222
Pancreatic secretion	4	6	0	0	9	0	0.000232
Galactose metabolism	2	2	1	6	0	0	0.000677
Other glycan degradation	0	3	0	5	0	0	0.001051
Amino sugar and nucleotide sugar metabolism	2	4	1	6	0	0	0.001526
Arginine biosynthesis	1	2	1	4	0	0	0.002527
Bile secretion	1	8	2	3	0	0	0.00304
Alanine, aspartate and glutamate metabolism	1	4	2	3	0	0	0.003204
Retinol metabolism	2	4	0	4	0	0	0.005355
Focal adhesion	4	14	1	7	0	0	0.010981
Starch and sucrose metabolism	0	2	1	5	1	0	0.011597
Sphingolipid metabolism	0	4	1	5	0	0	0.013042
Cell cycle	17	0	1	0	0	0	0.014158
Carbohydrate digestion and absorption	0	2	1	5	1	0	0.014633
Proximal tubule bicarbonate reclamation	1	5	1	0	0	0	0.014947
Arginine and proline metabolism	1	5	0	4	0	0	0.01764
Glycosaminoglycan degradation	1	1	0	4	0	0	0.01764
ABC transporters	2	5	0	2	0	0	0.021963
Glycosphingolipid biosynthesis - globo series	0	1	0	4	0	0	0.023611
Steroid hormone biosynthesis	1	2	1	3	0	1	0.024807
Fructose and mannose metabolism	1	4	1	2	0	0	0.024807
Glycolysis / Gluconeogenesis	2	5	1	3	0	0	0.024807
Chemical carcinogenesis	1	6	0	2	0	0	0.024807
Glutathione metabolism	3	5	1	0	0	0	0.024807
Steroid biosynthesis	6	0	0	0	0	0	0.025842
Drug metabolism - cytochrome P450	1	6	0	1	0	0	0.025842
Complement and coagulation cascades	6	2	3	1	0	0	0.026353
p53 signaling pathway	6	2	3	0	0	0	0.026976
Glycine, serine and threonine metabolism	4	1	2	1	0	0	0.027354
Renin-angiotensin system	1	3	0	2	0	0	0.027354
Pyrimidine metabolism	10	1	2	0	0	0	0.03345
Amoebiasis	3	7	0	4	0	0	0.034505
Nitrogen metabolism	3	0	1	1	0	0	0.034505

TAP1/2 genes, in order to promote potent antigen-specific immunity. Interestingly, *T. gondii* altered the expression of genes which may have relevance to other processes, such as xenobiotic metabolism and the pathogenesis of AD. Elucidation of the roles of these pathways in the protective immunity against *T. gondii* infection may reveal new targets for vaccine design and therapeutic interventions to break the parasite transmission cycle in the definitive host.

Abbreviations
AD: Alzheimer's disease; AIDS: Acquired immune deficiency syndrome; APOE: Apolipoprotein E; APP: Amyloid precursor protein; CYPs: Cytochrome P450s; DC: Dendritic cells; DEGs: Differentially expressed genes; ER: Endoplasmic reticulum; FABPs: Fatty acid binding proteins; FDR: False discovery rate; GO: Gene ontology; GSTs: Glutathione S-transferases; hpi: Hours post-infection; HSP70: 70 kilodalton heat-shock proteins; HSP90: 90 kilodalton heat-shock proteins; IEL: Intraepithelial T lymphocytes; IFN-γ: Gamma interferon; IL 4/5/13/17: Interleukin 4/5/13/17; ILC: Innate lymphoid cells; KEGG: Kyoto Encyclopedia of Genes and Genomes; LP: Lamina propria; M cells: Microfold cells; MAT: Modified agglutination test; MHC I: Major histocompatibility complex I; NEP: Neutral endopeptidase; NK: Natural killer cells; PBS: Phosphate buffered saline; PPARs: Peroxisome proliferator-activated receptors; PSEN1: Presenilin-1 gene; PSEN2: Presenilin-2 gene; qRT-PCR: Quantitative reverse-transcribed polymerase chain reaction; RNA-Seq: RNA sequencing; ROMs: Reactive oxygenated intermediates; TAP: A transporter associated with antigen processing; TCR: T cell receptor; UGT1A1: Uridine diphosphate glucuronosyltransferase A1

Acknowledgements
The authors would like to thank Novogene Bioinformatics Technology Co., Ltd (Beijing, China) for performing the sequencing and preliminary computational analysis.

Funding
Project support was provided by the International Science and Technology Cooperation Project of Gansu Provincial Key Research and Development Program (grant no. 17JR7WA031), the National Natural Science Foundation of China (grant no. 31230073), the Elite Program of Chinese Academy of Agricultural Sciences, and the Agricultural Science and Technology Innovation Program (ASTIP) (grant no. CAAS-ASTIP-2016-LVRI-03).

Authors' contributions
XQZ, JXL, JJH and HME conceived and designed the study, and critically revised the manuscript. MW and FKZ performed the experiment, analyzed the transcriptomic data and drafted the manuscript. HME, NZZ and JJH helped in data analysis and manuscript revision. All authors read and approved the final manuscript.

Competing interests
The authors declare that they have no competing interests.

Author details
[1]State Key Laboratory of Veterinary Etiological Biology, Key Laboratory of Veterinary Parasitology of Gansu Province, Lanzhou Veterinary Research Institute, Chinese Academy of Agricultural Sciences, Lanzhou, Gansu Province 730046, People's Republic of China. [2]Faculty of Medicine and Health Sciences, School of Veterinary Medicine and Science, University of Nottingham, Sutton Bonington Campus, Loughborough LE12 5RD, UK. [3]Jiangsu Co-innovation Center for the Prevention and Control of Important Animal Infectious Diseases and Zoonoses, Yangzhou University College of Veterinary Medicine, Yangzhou, Jiangsu Province 225009, People's Republic of China.

References
1. Dubey JP. Toxoplasmosis of Animals and Humans. Boca Raton: CRC Press; 2010.
2. Dubey JP, Miller NL, Frenkel JK. The *Toxoplasma gondii* oocyst from cat feces. J Exp Med. 1970;132:636–62.
3. Dubey JP. History of the discovery of the life cycle of *Toxoplasma gondii*. Int J Parasitol. 2009;39:877–82.
4. Dubey JP. *Toxoplasma gondii* oocyst survival under defined temperatures. J Parasitol. 1998;84:862–5.
5. Lindsay DS, Dubey JP. Long-term survival of *Toxoplasma gondii* sporulated oocysts in seawater. J Parasitol. 2009;95:1019–20.
6. Jones JL, Dubey JP. Waterborne toxoplasmosis - recent developments. Exp Parasitol. 2010;124:10–25.
7. Jones JL, Dubey JP. Foodborne toxoplasmosis. Clin Infect Dis. 2012;55:845–51.
8. Dubey JP, Prowell M. *Ante-mortem* diagnosis, diarrhea, oocyst shedding, treatment, isolation, and genetic typing of *Toxoplasma gondii* associated with clinical toxoplasmosis in a naturally infected cat. J Parasitol. 2013;99:158–60.
9. Montoya JG, Liesenfeld O. Toxoplasmosis. Lancet. 2004;363:1965–76.
10. Torrey EF, Yolken RH. *Toxoplasma* oocysts as a public health problem. Trends Parasitol. 2013;29:380–4.
11. Shao L, Serrano D, Mayer L. The role of epithelial cells in immune regulation in the gut. Semin Immunol. 2001;13:163–76.
12. Haber AL, Biton M, Rogel N, Herbst RH, Shekhar K, Smillie C, et al. A single-cell survey of the small intestinal epithelium. Nature. 2017;551:333–9.
13. Liesenfeld O. Immune responses to *Toxoplasma gondii* in the gut. Immunobiology. 1999;201:229–39.
14. McLeod R, Estes RG, Mack DG, Cohen H. Immune response of mice to ingested *Toxoplasma gondii*: a model of toxoplasma infection acquired by ingestion. J Infect Dis. 1984;149:234–44.
15. McLeod R, Eisenhauer P, Mack D, Brown C, Filice G, Spitalny G. Immune responses associated with early survival after peroral infection with *Toxoplasma gondii*. J Immunol. 1989;142:3247–55.
16. Herrmann DC, Pantchev N, Vrhovec MG, Barutzki D, Wilking H, Frohlich A, et al. Atypical *Toxoplasma gondii* genotypes identified in oocysts shed by cats in Germany. Int J Parasitol. 2010;40:285–92.
17. Maksimov P, Zerweck J, Dubey JP, Pantchev N, Frey CF, Maksimov A, et al. Serotyping of *Toxoplasma gondii* in cats (*Felis domesticus*) reveals predominance of type II infections in Germany. PLoS One. 2013;8:e80213.
18. Brennan A, Donahoe SL, Beatty JA, Belov K, Lindsay S, Briscoe KA, et al. Comparison of genotypes of *Toxoplasma gondii* in domestic cats from Australia with latent infection or clinical toxoplasmosis. Vet Parasitol. 2016; 228:13–6.
19. Cong W, Zhang XX, He JJ, Li FC, Elsheikha HM, Zhu XQ. Global miRNA expression profiling of domestic cat livers following acute *Toxoplasma gondii* infection. Oncotarget. 2017;8:25599–611.
20. Yan HK, Yuan ZG, Song HQ, Petersen E, Zhou Y, Ren D, et al. Vaccination with a DNA vaccine coding for perforin-like protein 1 and MIC6 induces significant protective immunity against *Toxoplasma gondii*. Clin Vaccine Immunol. 2012;19:684–9.
21. Trapnell C, Pachter L, Salzberg SL. TopHat: discovering splice junctions with RNA-Seq. Bioinformatics. 2009;25:1105–11.
22. Anders S, Huber W. Differential expression analysis for sequence count data. Genome Biol. 2010;11:R106.
23. Young MD, Wakefield MJ, Smyth GK, Oshlack A. Gene ontology analysis for RNA-seq: accounting for selection bias. Genome Biol. 2010;11:R14.

24. Kanehisa M, Araki M, Goto S, Hattori M, Hirakawa M, Itoh M, et al. KEGG for linking genomes to life and the environment. Nucleic Acids Res. 2008;36: D480–4.
25. Mao X, Cai T, Olyarchuk JG, Wei L. Automated genome annotation and pathway identification using the KEGG Orthology (KO) as a controlled vocabulary. Bioinformatics. 2005;21:3787–93.
26. Behnke MS, Zhang TP, Dubey JP, Sibley LD. *Toxoplasma gondii* merozoite gene expression analysis with comparison to the life cycle discloses a unique expression state during enteric development. BMC Genomics. 2014; 15:350.
27. Piekarski G, Pelster B, Witte HM. Endopolygeny in *Toxoplasma gondii*. Z Parasitenkd. 1971;36:122–30 (In German).
28. Hehl AB, Basso WU, Lippuner C, Ramakrishnan C, Okoniewski M, Walker RA, et al. Asexual expansion of *Toxoplasma gondii* merozoites is distinct from tachyzoites and entails expression of non-overlapping gene families to attach, invade, and replicate within feline enterocytes. BMC Genomics. 2015;16:66.
29. Blanchard N, Gonzalez F, Schaeffer M, Joncker NT, Cheng T, Shastri AJ, et al. Immunodominant, protective response to the parasite *Toxoplasma gondii* requires antigen processing in the endoplasmic reticulum. Nat Immunol. 2008;9:937–44.
30. Buaillon C, Guerrero NA, Cebrian I, Blanie S, Lopez J, Bassot E, et al. MHC I presentation of *Toxoplasma gondii* immunodominant antigen does not require Sec22b and is regulated by antigen orientation at the vacuole membrane. Eur J Immunol. 2017;47:1160–70.
31. Khan IA, Ely KH, Kasper LH. Antigen-specific CD8+ T cell clone protects against acute *Toxoplasma gondii* infection in mice. J Immunol. 1994;152: 1856–60.
32. Preckel T, Fung-Leung WP, Cai Z, Vitiello A, Salter-Cid L, Winqvist O, et al. Impaired immunoproteasome assembly and immune responses in PA28-/- mice. Science. 1999;286:2162–5.
33. Combe CL, Curiel TJ, Moretto MM, Khan IA. NK cells help to induce CD8(+)-T-cell immunity against *Toxoplasma gondii* in the absence of CD4(+) T cells. Infect Immun. 2005;73:4913–21.
34. MacMicking JD. Interferon-inducible effector mechanisms in cell-autonomous immunity. Nat Rev Immunol. 2012;12:367–82.
35. Kloetzel PM. Antigen processing by the proteasome. Nat Rev Mol Cell Bio. 2001;2:179–87.
36. Rock KL, Goldberg AL. Degradation of cell proteins and the generation of MHC class I-presented peptides. Annu Rev Immunol. 1999;17:739–79.
37. Bougneres L, Helft J, Tiwari S, Vargas P, Chang BH, Chan L, et al. A role for lipid bodies in the cross-presentation of phagocytosed antigens by MHC class I in dendritic cells. Immunity. 2009;31:232–44.
38. Milani V, Noessner E, Ghose S, Kuppner M, Ahrens B, Scharner A, et al. Heat shock protein 70: role in antigen presentation and immune stimulation. Int J Hyperthermia. 2002;18:563–75.
39. Castellino F, Boucher PE, Eichelberg K, Mayhew M, Rothman JE, Houghton AN, et al. Receptor-mediated uptake of antigen/heat shock protein complexes results in major histocompatibility complex class I antigen presentation *via* two distinct processing pathways. J Exp Med. 2000;191: 1957–64.
40. Srivastava P. Interaction of heat shock proteins with peptides and antigen presenting cells: chaperoning of the innate and adaptive immune responses. Annu Rev Immunol. 2002;20:395–425.
41. Garrido C, Brunet M, Didelot C, Zermati Y, Schmitt E, Kroemer G. Heat shock proteins 27 and 70: anti-apoptotic proteins with tumorigenic properties. Cell Cycle. 2006;5:2592–601.
42. Wegele H, Muller L, Buchner J. Hsp70 and Hsp90 - a relay team for protein folding. Rev Physiol Biochem Pharmacol. 2004;151:1–44.
43. Speer CA, Dubey JP. Ultrastructural differentiation of *Toxoplasma gondii* schizonts (types B to E) and gamonts in the intestines of cats fed bradyzoites. Int J Parasitol. 2005;35:193–206.
44. Guiton PS, Sagawa JM, Fritz HM, Boothroyd JC. An *in vitro* model of intestinal infection reveals a developmentally regulated transcriptome of *Toxoplasma* sporozoites and a NF-kappaB-like signature in infected host cells. PLoS One. 2017;12:e0173018.
45. Furuhashi M, Hotamisligil GS. Fatty acid-binding proteins: role in metabolic diseases and potential as drug targets. Nat Rev Drug Discov. 2008;7:489–503.
46. Nebert DW, Dalton TP. The role of cytochrome P450 enzymes in endogenous signalling pathways and environmental carcinogenesis. Nat Rev Cancer. 2006;6:947–60.
47. Cong W, Liu GH, Meng QF, Dong W, Qin SY, Zhang FK, et al. *Toxoplasma gondii* infection in cancer patients: prevalence, risk factors, genotypes and association with clinical diagnosis. Cancer Lett. 2015;359:307–13.
48. Tukey RH, Strassburg CP. Human UDP-glucuronosyltransferases: metabolism, expression, and disease. Annu Rev Pharmacol. 2000;40:581–616.
49. O'Dwyer PJ, Catalano RB. Uridine diphosphate glucuronosyltransferase(UGT)1A1 and irinotecan: practical pharmacogenomics arrives in cancer therapy. J Clin Oncol. 2006;24:4534–8.
50. Kusbeci OY, Miman O, Yaman M, Aktepe OC, Yazar S. Could *Toxoplasma gondii* have any role in Alzheimer disease? Alzheimer Dis Assoc Disord. 2011;25:1–3.
51. Mahami-Oskouei M, Hamidi F, Talebi M, Farhoudi M, Taheraghdam AA, Kazemi T, et al. Toxoplasmosis and Alzheimer: can *Toxoplasma gondii* really be introduced as a risk factor in etiology of Alzheimer? Parasitol Res. 2016; 115:3169–74.
52. Perry CE, Gale SD, Erickson L, Wilson E, Nielsen B, Kauwe J, et al. Seroprevalence and serointensity of latent *Toxoplasma gondii* in a sample of elderly adults with and without Alzheimer disease. Alzheimer Dis Assoc Disord. 2016;30:123–6.
53. Iwata N, Tsubuki S, Takaki Y, Watanabe K, Sekiguchi M, Hosoki E, et al. Identification of the major Abeta1-42-degrading catabolic pathway in brain parenchyma: suppression leads to biochemical and pathological deposition. Nat Med. 2000;6:143–50.
54. Zhang YW, Thompson R, Zhang H, Xu H. APP processing in Alzheimer's disease. Mol Brain. 2011;4:3.
55. Canter RG, Penney J, Tsai LH. The road to restoring neural circuits for the treatment of Alzheimer's disease. Nature. 2016;539:187–96.

Permissions

All chapters in this book were first published in P&V, by BioMed Central; hereby published with permission under the Creative Commons Attribution License or equivalent. Every chapter published in this book has been scrutinized by our experts. Their significance has been extensively debated. The topics covered herein carry significant findings which will fuel the growth of the discipline. They may even be implemented as practical applications or may be referred to as a beginning point for another development.

The contributors of this book come from diverse backgrounds, making this book a truly international effort. This book will bring forth new frontiers with its revolutionizing research information and detailed analysis of the nascent developments around the world.

We would like to thank all the contributing authors for lending their expertise to make the book truly unique. They have played a crucial role in the development of this book. Without their invaluable contributions this book wouldn't have been possible. They have made vital efforts to compile up to date information on the varied aspects of this subject to make this book a valuable addition to the collection of many professionals and students.

This book was conceptualized with the vision of imparting up-to-date information and advanced data in this field. To ensure the same, a matchless editorial board was set up. Every individual on the board went through rigorous rounds of assessment to prove their worth. After which they invested a large part of their time researching and compiling the most relevant data for our readers.

The editorial board has been involved in producing this book since its inception. They have spent rigorous hours researching and exploring the diverse topics which have resulted in the successful publishing of this book. They have passed on their knowledge of decades through this book. To expedite this challenging task, the publisher supported the team at every step. A small team of assistant editors was also appointed to further simplify the editing procedure and attain best results for the readers.

Apart from the editorial board, the designing team has also invested a significant amount of their time in understanding the subject and creating the most relevant covers. They scrutinized every image to scout for the most suitable representation of the subject and create an appropriate cover for the book.

The publishing team has been an ardent support to the editorial, designing and production team. Their endless efforts to recruit the best for this project, has resulted in the accomplishment of this book. They are a veteran in the field of academics and their pool of knowledge is as vast as their experience in printing. Their expertise and guidance has proved useful at every step. Their uncompromising quality standards have made this book an exceptional effort. Their encouragement from time to time has been an inspiration for everyone.

The publisher and the editorial board hope that this book will prove to be a valuable piece of knowledge for researchers, students, practitioners and scholars across the globe.

List of Contributors

Anubis Vega-Rúa, Lyza Hery and Daniella Goindin
Laboratory of Vector Control Research, Environment and Health Unit, Institut Pasteur de la Guadeloupe, 97183 Les Abymes, Guadeloupe, France

Nonito Pagès
CIRAD, UMR ASTRE, F-97170 Petit Bourg, Guadeloupe, France
ASTRE, CIRAD, INRA, University of Montpellier, Montpellier, France

Albin Fontaine and Lionel Almeras
Unité de Parasitologie et Entomologie, Département des Maladies Infectieuses, Institut de Recherche Biomédicale des Armées, Marseille, France
Aix Marseille Université, IRD, AP-HM, SSA, UMR Vecteurs - Infections Tropicales et Méditerranéennes (VITROME), IHU - Méditerranée Infection, 19–21 bd Jean Moulin, 13385 Marseille, cedex 5, France

Christopher Nuccio
Aix Marseille Université, INSERM, SSA, IRBA, MCT, 13005 Marseille, France

Joel Gustave
Vector Control Service of Guadeloupe, Regional Health Agency, Airport Zone South Raizet, 97139 Les Abymes, Guadeloupe, France

Sanjay A. Desai
The Laboratory of Malaria and Vector Research, National Institute of Allergy and Infectious Diseases, National Institutes of Health, Rockville, MD 20852, USA

Praveen Balabaskaran-Nina
The Laboratory of Malaria and Vector Research, National Institute of Allergy and Infectious Diseases, National Institutes of Health, Rockville, MD 20852, USA

Department of Epidemiology and Public Health, Central University of Tamil Nadu, Thiruvarur, India

Sofía Ocaña-Mayorga and Anita G. Villacís
Centro de Investigación para la Salud en América Latina (CISeAL), Escuela de Ciencias Biológicas, Facultad de Ciencias Exactas y Naturales, Pontificia Universidad Católica del Ecuador, Calle San Pedro y Pamba Hacienda, 170530 Nayón, Ecuador

Simón E. Lobos
Centro de Investigación para la Salud en América Latina (CISeAL), Escuela de Ciencias Biológicas, Facultad de Ciencias Exactas y Naturales, Pontificia Universidad Católica del Ecuador, Calle San Pedro y Pamba Hacienda, 170530 Nayón, Ecuador
Museo de Zoología, Escuela de Ciencias Biológicas, Facultad de Ciencias Exactas y Naturales, Pontificia Universidad Católica del Ecuador, Av. 12 de octubre 1076 y Roca, 170525 Quito, Ecuador

C. Miguel Pinto
Centro de Investigación para la Salud en América Latina (CISeAL), Escuela de Ciencias Biológicas, Facultad de Ciencias Exactas y Naturales, Pontificia Universidad Católica del Ecuador, Calle San Pedro y Pamba Hacienda, 170530 Nayón, Ecuador
Instituto de Ciencias Biológicas, Escuela Politécnica Nacional, Ladrón de Guevara E11-254, 170517 Quito, Ecuador

Mario J. Grijalva
Centro de Investigación para la Salud en América Latina (CISeAL), Escuela de Ciencias Biológicas, Facultad de Ciencias Exactas y Naturales, Pontificia Universidad Católica del Ecuador, Calle San Pedro y Pamba Hacienda, 170530 Nayón, Ecuador
Infectious and Tropical Disease Institute, Department of Biomedical Sciences, Heritage College of Osteopathic Medicine, Ohio University, Athens, OH 45701, USA

Verónica Crespo-Pérez
Laboratorio de Entomología, Escuela de Ciencias Biológicas, Facultad de Ciencias Exactas y Naturales, Pontificia Universidad Católica del Ecuador, Av. 12 de octubre 1076 y Roca, 170525 Quito, Ecuador

Wen X. Li, Hong Zou, Shan G. Wu, Ming Li and Gui T. Wang
Key Laboratory of Aquaculture Disease Control, Ministry of Agriculture, and State Key Laboratory of Freshwater Ecology and Biotechnology, Institute of Hydrobiology, Chinese Academy of Sciences, Wuhan 430072, People's Republic of China

Dong Zhang
Key Laboratory of Aquaculture Disease Control, Ministry of Agriculture, and State Key Laboratory of Freshwater Ecology and Biotechnology, Institute of Hydrobiology, Chinese Academy of Sciences, Wuhan 430072, People's Republic of China
University of Chinese Academy of Sciences, Beijing, People's Republic of China

Ivan Jakovlić, Jin Zhang and Rong Chen
Bio-Transduction Lab, Biolake, Wuhan 430075, People's Republic of China

Carolina Romeiro Fernandes Chagas, Dovilė Bukauskaitė, Mikas Ilgūnas, Tatjana Iezhova and Gediminas Valkiūnas
Institute of Ecology, Nature Research Centre, Akademijos 2, 21, LT-09412 Vilnius, Lithuania

Veronique Dermauw
Department of Biomedical Sciences, Institute of Tropical Medicine, Antwerp, Belgium

Pierre Dorny
Department of Biomedical Sciences, Institute of Tropical Medicine, Antwerp, Belgium
Department of Virology, Parasitology and Immunology, Faculty of Veterinary Medicine, Ghent University, Merelbeke, Belgium

Uffe Christian Braae
One Health Center for Zoonoses and Tropical Veterinary Medicine, Ross University School of Veterinary Medicine, Basseterre, Saint Kitts, Trinidad and Tobago

Brecht Devleesschauwer
Department of Epidemiology and Public Health, Sciensano, Brussels, Belgium
Department of Veterinary Public Health and Food Safety, Faculty of Veterinary Medicine, Ghent University, Merelbeke, Belgium

Lucy J. Robertson
Parasitology, Department of Food Safety and Infection Biology, Faculty of Veterinary Medicine, Norwegian University of Life Sciences, Adamstuen Campus, Oslo, Norway

Anastasios Saratsis
Laboratory of Parasitology, Veterinary Research Institute, Hellenic Agricultural Organization Demeter, Thermi, 57001 Thessaloniki, Greece

Lian F. Thomas
International Livestock Research Institute (ILRI), Nairobi, Kenya
Institute for Infection and Global Health, University of Liverpool, Neston, UK

Deepa Gopinath
MSD Animal Health, 26 Talavera Rd, Macquarie Park, NSW 2113, Australia

Leon Meyer and Jehane Smith
Clinvet International, Uitzich Road, Bainsvlei, Bloemfontein 9338, South Africa

Rob Armstrong
Merck Animal Health, 2 Giralda Farms, Madison, NJ 07940, USA

Miguel A. Mercado-Uriostegui, Juan Mosqueda and Mario Hidalgo-Ruiz
Immunology and Vaccines Laboratory, C. A. Facultad de Ciencias Naturales, Universidad Autónoma de Querétaro, Carretera a Chichimequillas, Ejido Bolaños, 76140 Queretaro, Queretaro, Mexico

Carlos E. Suarez
Animal Disease Research Unit,USDA-ARS, 3003 ADBF, WSU, Pullman, WA 99164-6630, USA

Ruben Hernandez-Ortiz and Juan Alberto Ramos
CENID-Parasitologia Veterinaria / INIFAP, Carretera federal Cuernavaca-Cuautla #8534, Col. Progreso, 62550 Jiutepec, Morelos, Mexico

Edelmira Galindo-Velasco
Facultad de Medicina Veterinaria y Zootecnia, Universidad de Colima, Km.40 carretera Colima-Manzanillo, 28100 Tecoman, Colima, Mexico

Gloria León-Ávila
Departamento de Zoología, Escuela Nacional de Ciencias Biológicas,Instituto Politécnico Nacional, Carpio y Plan de Ayala, Col. Casco de Santo Tomás, 11340 Mexico City, Mexico

José Manuel Hernández
Departamento de Biología Celular, Centro de Investigación y Estudios Avanzados del Instituto Politécnico Nacional, Av. IPN 2508, Col. San Pedro Zacatenco, 07360 Mexico City, Mexico

Benjamin Abuaku, Collins Ahorlu, Sedzro Mensah, William Sackey and Kwadwo A Koram
Epidemiology Department, Noguchi Memorial Institute for Medical Research, College of Health Sciences, University of Ghana, Legon, Legon, Ghana

Paul Psychas
University of Florida, 410 NE Waldo Rd, Gainesville, FL 32641, USA

Philip Ricks
President's Malaria Initiative/Malaria Branch, Centers for Disease Control and Prevention, Atlanta, GA, USA

Samuel Oppong
National Malaria Control Programme, Public Health Division, Ghana Health Service, Accra, Ghana

Soledad Santillán-Guayasamín and Anita G. Villacís
Center for Research on Health in Latin America (CISeAL), School of Biological Sciences, Pontifical Catholic University of Ecuador, Calle Pambahacienda s/n y San Pedro del Valle, Campus Nayón, Quito, Ecuador

Mario J. Grijalva
Center for Research on Health in Latin America (CISeAL), School of Biological Sciences, Pontifical Catholic University of Ecuador, Calle Pambahacienda s/n y San Pedro del Valle, Campus Nayón, Quito, Ecuador
Infectious and Tropical Disease Institute, Department of Biomedical Sciences, Heritage College of Osteopathic Medicine, Ohio University, Athens, OH 45701, USA

Jean-Pierre Dujardin
Center for Research on Health in Latin America (CISeAL), School of Biological Sciences, Pontifical Catholic University of Ecuador, Calle Pambahacienda s/n y San Pedro del Valle, Campus Nayón, Quito, Ecuador
IRD, UMR 177 IRD-CIRAD INTERTRYP, Campus international de Baillarguet, Montpellier, France

Djamel Khelef
École Nationale Supérieure Vétérinaire, Rue Issaad Abbes, El Alia, Alger, Algérie

Djamel Baroudi
École Nationale Supérieure Vétérinaire, Rue Issaad Abbes, El Alia, Alger, Algérie
Division of Foodborne, Waterborne and Environmental Diseases, Centers for Disease Control and Prevention, 1600 Clifton Road, Atlanta, GA 30329, USA

Dawn Roellig
Division of Foodborne, Waterborne and Environmental Diseases, Centers for Disease Control and Prevention, 1600 Clifton Road, Atlanta, GA 30329, USA

Ahcene Hakem
Laboratoire exploration et valorisation des ecosystems steppique, Université Ziane Achor, 17000 Djelfa, Algérie

Haileeyesus Adamu
Department of Biology, Addis Ababa University, Addis Ababa, Ethiopia

Said Amer
Department of Zoology, Faculty of Science, Kafr El Sheikh University, Kafr El Sheikh 33516, Egypt

Karim Adjou
UMR-BIPAR, ANSES-Ecole Nationale Vétérinaire d'Alfort, Maisons-Alfort, Paris, France

Hichem Dahmani
Université Saad Dahleb Blida, Blida, Algérie

Xiaohua Chen
Beijing Tropical Medicine Research Institute, Beijing Friendship Hospital, Beijing 100050, China

Yaoyu Feng and Lihua Xiao
Key Laboratory of Zoonosis of Ministry of Agriculture, College of Veterinary Medicine, South China Agricultural University, Guangzhou 510642, China

Rebecca Cole and Mark Viney
School of Biological Sciences, University of Bristol, Bristol BS8 1TQ, UK

Ana L Lanfranchi, Paola E Braicovich, Delfina M P Cantatore, Manuel M Irigoitia, Verónica Taglioretti and Juan T Timi
Laboratorio de Ictioparasitología, Instituto de Investigaciones Marinas y Costeras (IIMyC), Facultad de Ciencias Exactas y Naturales, Universidad Nacional de Mar del Plata - Consejo Nacional de Investigaciones Científicas y Técnicas (CONICET), (7600) Mar del Plata, 3350 Funes, Argentina

Marisa D Farber
Instituto de Biotecnología, Instituto Nacional de Tecnología Agropecuaria (INTA), Hurlingham, Buenos Aires, Argentina

Hilda M. Hernández and Jorge Sánchez
Centro de Investigaciones, Diagnóstico y Referencia, Instituto de Medicina Tropical "Pedro Kourí", La Habana, Cuba

Annia Alba
Centro de Investigaciones, Diagnóstico y Referencia, Instituto de Medicina Tropical "Pedro Kourí", La Habana, Cuba
University of Perpignan Via Domitia, Interactions Hosts Pathogens Environments UMR 5244, CNRS, IFREMER, Univ. Montpellier, F-66860 Perpignan, France

Antonio A. Vázquez
Centro de Investigaciones, Diagnóstico y Referencia, Instituto de Medicina Tropical "Pedro Kourí", La Habana, Cuba
MIVEGEC, IRD, CNRS, Univ. Montpellier, Montpellier, France

David Duval and Benjamin Gourbal
University of Perpignan Via Domitia, Interactions Hosts Pathogens Environments UMR 5244, CNRS, IFREMER, Univ. Montpellier, F-66860 Perpignan, France

Marion Vittecoq
Centre de recherché de la Tour du Valat, Arles, France

Emeline Sabourin
Centre de recherché de la Tour du Valat, Arles, France
MIVEGEC, IRD, CNRS, Univ. Montpellier, Montpellier, France

Sylvie Hurtrez-Boussés
MIVEGEC, IRD, CNRS, Univ. Montpellier, Montpellier, France

Rita Velez and Montserrat Gállego
ISGlobal, Hospital Clínic - Universitat de Barcelona, Barcelona, Spain
Secció de Parasitologia, Departament de Biologia, Sanitat i Medi Ambient, Facultat de Farmàcia i Ciències de l'Alimentació, Universitat de Barcelona, Barcelona, Spain

Tatiana Spitzova, Laura Willen and Petr Volf
Department of Parasitology, Faculty of Science, Charles University, Prague, Czech Republic.

Ester Domenech and Jordi Cairó
Hospital Veterinari Canis, Girona, Spain

Ruilin Chu, Xinxin Zhang, Limei Chen, Yuhong Li, Yinghua Xuan and Yang Cheng
Laboratory of Pathogen Infection and Immunity, Department of Public Health and Preventive Medicine, Wuxi School of Medicine, Jiangnan University, Wuxi, Jiangsu, People's Republic of China

Jun Cao
Laboratory of Pathogen Infection and Immunity, Department of Public Health and Preventive Medicine, Wuxi School of Medicine, Jiangnan University, Wuxi, Jiangsu, People's Republic of China
Key Laboratory of National Health and Family Planning Commission on Parasitic Disease Control and Prevention, Jiangsu Provincial Key Laboratory on Parasite and Vector Control Technology, Jiangsu Institute of Parasite Diseases, Wuxi 214064, Jiangsu, People's Republic of China

Sui Xu, Jianxia Tang, Jing Chen and Guoding Zhu
Key Laboratory of National Health and Family Planning Commission on Parasitic Disease Control and Prevention, Jiangsu Provincial Key Laboratory on Parasite and Vector Control Technology, Jiangsu Institute of Parasite Diseases, Wuxi 214064, Jiangsu, People's Republic of China

Nengxing Shen, Haojie Zhang, Ran He, Jing Xu, Chunyan Li, Weimin Lai, Xiaobin Gu, Yue Xie and Guangyou Yang
Department of Parasitology, College of Veterinary Medicine, Sichuan Agricultural University, Chengdu 611130, China

Yongjun Ren
Animal Breeding and Genetics Key Laboratory of Sichuan Province, Chengdu 610066, China

Xuerong Peng
Department of Chemistry, College of Life and Basic Science, Sichuan Agricultural University, Chengdu 611130, China

Nadja Rohdich, Eva Zschiesche and Rainer K. A. Roepke
MSD Animal Health Innovation GmbH, Zur Propstei, 55270 Schwabenheim, Germany

Oliver Wolf and Wolfgang Loehlein
Loehlein & Wolf Vet Research, Maistrasse 69, 80337 Munich, Germany

Thierry Pobel and Maria José Gil
TPC Biomed, C/Los Betetas 12-4°D, 42002 Soria, Spain

Sylwia Grzelak, Bożena Moskwa and Justyna Bień
Witold Stefański Institute of Parasitology, Polish Academy of Sciences, Twarda 51/55, 00-818 Warsaw, Poland

Meng Wang, Fu-Kai Zhang, Nian-Zhang Zhang, Jun-Jun He and Jian-Xun Luo
State Key Laboratory of Veterinary Etiological Biology, Key Laboratory of Veterinary Parasitology of Gansu Province, Lanzhou Veterinary Research Institute, Chinese Academy of Agricultural Sciences, Lanzhou, Gansu Province 730046, People's Republic of China

Xing-Quan Zhu
State Key Laboratory of Veterinary Etiological Biology, Key Laboratory of Veterinary Parasitology of Gansu Province, Lanzhou Veterinary Research Institute, Chinese Academy of Agricultural Sciences, Lanzhou, Gansu Province 730046, People's Republic of China
Jiangsu Co-innovation Center for the Prevention and Control of Important Animal Infectious Diseases and Zoonoses, Yangzhou University College of Veterinary Medicine, Yangzhou, Jiangsu Province 225009, People's Republic of China

Hany M. Elsheikha
Faculty of Medicine and Health Sciences, School of Veterinary Medicine and Science, University of Nottingham, Sutton Bonington Campus, Loughborough LE12 5RD, UK

Index

www.ingramcontent.com/pod-product-compliance
Lightning Source LLC
Chambersburg PA
CBHW061301190326
41458CB00011B/3737
9781632428554